Spondylolisthesis

Adam L. Wollowick • Vishal Sarwahi
Editors

Spondylolisthesis

Diagnosis, Non-Surgical Management, and Surgical Techniques

Springer

Editors
Adam L. Wollowick, MD
Assistant Professor of Orthopedic Surgery
Albert Einstein College of Medicine
New York, NY, USA

Vishal Sarwahi, MD
Associate Professor of Orthopedic Surgery
Albert Einstein College of Medicine
Department of Orthopedic Surgery
Montefiore Medical Center
Bronx, NY, USA

ISBN 978-1-4899-7973-5 ISBN 978-1-4899-7575-1 (eBook)
DOI 10.1007/978-1-4899-7575-1

Springer New York Heidelberg Dordrecht London

Softcover reprint of the hardcover 1st edition 2015

Printed on acid-free paper

Springer Science+Business Media LLC New York is part of Springer Science+Business Media (www.springer.com)

This word book would not have been possible without the support of my mentors, friends, and family. I'm grateful to my parents for their love and affection, my dear wife and loving children for their understanding and support, and my teachers for their guidance. This is a labor of love and it is for all of you to enjoy.

-Vishal Sarwahi

This book is dedicated to the memory of my father, Burton Saadia Wollowick, M.D., who was a wonderful physician, mentor, role model, and friend. Without his guidance, I would not be the person that I am today. This book would not have been possible without the support of my mother, family, teachers, and friends. Finally, I am grateful for the gifts of laughter and love that my daughter provides each and every day. Penelope, you are truly my guiding light.

-Adam Laurance Wollowick

Preface

Spondylolisthesis: Diagnosis, Non-Surgical Management, and Surgical Techniques is intended to fill a void in every spine care professional's library. As teachers of medical students, residents, and fellows, we frequently found ourselves being asked for references about spondylolisthesis. We realized that a definitive source covering all aspects of the diagnosis and treatment of this common, yet intricate condition did not exist. As a result, we felt compelled to design and publish a text to meet that need.

The management of the various types of spondylolisthesis requires a thorough understanding of both fundamental principles and subtle nuances, which are highlighted in this text. The book is intended for spine caregivers at all levels of training and from all disciplines of medicine. We also envisioned the book to be useful and accessible to nonsurgical and surgical practitioners alike. We believe that we have achieved these goals and hope you will agree. We are indebted to the chapter authors, who have done an unbelievable job of presenting the latest thinking on these topics, as well as to our editors for helping us bring our vision from idea to reality. We hope that the readers find this text to be a practical and reliable source of knowledge about spondylolisthesis. We welcome any feedback and hope that this book will become the "go to" source for everything spondy!

New York, NY, USA — Adam Laurance Wollowick
Bronx, NY, USA — Vishal Sarwahi

Contents

Part II Surgical Techniques

Part III Results of Treatment and Complications

Contributors

Khalid Abbed, MD Department of Neurosurgery, Yale School of Medicine, New Haven, CT, USA

Todd J. Albert, MD Hospital for Special Surgery, New York, NY, USA

Louis F. Amorosa, MD Department of Orthopaedic Surgery, Westchester Medical Center, New York Medical College, Hawthorne, NY, USA

Jahangir K. Asghar, MD Department of Orthopaedic Surgery, Miami Children's Hospital, Miami, FL, USA

Kelley Banagan, MD Department of Orthopaedics, University of Maryland Medical System, Baltimore, MD, USA

Sigurd H. Berven, MD Department of Orthopaedic Surgery, UC San Francisco, San Francisco, CA, USA

Laurel C. Blakemore, MD Orthopaedics and Rehabilitation, University of Florida College of Medicine, UF Orthopaedics and Sports Medicine Institute, Gainesville, FL, USA

Oheneba Boachie-Adjei, MD Department of Orthopedic Surgery – Scoliosis Service, Hospital for Special Surgery, New York, NY, USA

David C. Briski, MD Department of Orthopaedic Surgery, Ochsner Medical Center, New Orleans, LA, USA

Jacob M. Buchowski, MD, MS Department of Orthopaedic Surgery, Center for Spinal Tumors, BJC Institute of Health, Washington University in St. Louis, St. Louis, MO, USA

Eugene J. Carragee, MD Department of Orthopedic Surgery, Stanford University Hospital and Clinics, Redwood City, CA, USA

Kshitij Chaudhary, MS, DNB (Ortho) Spine Surgery, Sir H.N. Reliance Foundation Hospital, Mumbai, Maharashtra, India

Andrew J. Cordiale, DO, MS Norton Leatherman Spine Center, Louisville, KY, USA

Matthew E. Cunningham, MD, PhD Spine and Scoliosis Service, Hospital for Special Surgery, New York, NY, USA

John R. Dimar II, MD Department of Orthopaedic Surgery, University of Louisville School of Medicine, KY, USA

Norton Leatherman Spine Center, Louisville, KY, USA

Melissa Esparza, BA Department of Orthopaedic Surgery, UC San Francisco, San Francisco, CA, USA

Jeffrey S. Fischgrund, MD Department of Orthopaedics, William Beaumont Hospital, Royal Oak, Michigan Orthopaedic Institute, Royal Oak, MI, USA

John C. France, MD Department of Orthopaedics, West Virginia University, Morgantown, WV, USA

Richard Frisch, MD Southeastern Spine Institute, Mount Pleasant, SC, USA

Gurpreet S. Gandhoke, MD Department of Neurological Surgery, University of Pittsburgh Medical Center, Pittsburgh, PA, USA

Peter C. Gerszten, MD, MPH, FACS Department of Neurological Surgery, University of Pittsburgh Medical Center, Pittsburgh, PA, USA

Christina L. Goldstein, MD, FRCSC Department of Orthopaedic Surgery, University of Missouri, Missouri Orthopaedic Institute, MO, Columbia

Debra J. Green, MD Department of Radiology, Montefiore Medical Center/ Albert Einstein College of Medicine, Bronx, NY, USA

Jeffrey L. Gum, MD Adult and Pediatric Spine Surgeon, Norton Leatherman Spine Center, Louisville, KY, USA

Farah Hameed, MD Department of Rehabilitation and Regenerative Medicine, Columbia University Medical Center, New York, NY, USA

Han Jo Kim, MD Spine and Scoliosis Service, Hospital for Special Surgery, New York, NY, USA

Richard Kim, MD Department of Neurosurgery, Temple University Hospital, Philadelphia, PA, USA

Theodore D. Koreckij, MD Department of Orthopaedic Surgery, University of Missouri-Kansas City School of Medicine, St. Luke's Hospital of Kansas City, Dickson-Diveley Midwest Orthopaedic Clinic, Kansas City Orthopaedic Institute, Leawood, KS, USA

Calvin C. Kuo, MD Norton Leatherman Spine Center, Louisville, KY, USA

Hubert Labelle, MD Department of Surgery, Ste-Justine University Center Hospital/University of Montreal, Montreal, QC, Canada

Leok-Lim Lau, MBChB, FRCS (Orth) University Orthopaedics, Hand and Reconstructive Microsurgery Cluster, National University Health System, Singapore, Singapore

Vu H. Le, MD Newportcare Orthopaedics and Spine Center, CA, USA

Nathan H. Lebwohl, MD Department of Orthopaedics, University of Miami, Miller School of Medicine, Miami, FL, USA

Ronald A. Lehman, MD Department of Orthopaedic Surgery, Walter Reed National Military Medical Center, Bethesda, MD, USA

Stephen J. Lewis, MD, MSc, FRCSC Department of Orthopedics, Toronto Western Hospital, Toronto, ON, Canada

Steven C. Ludwig, MD Department of Orthopaedics, University of Maryland Medical System, Baltimore, MD, USA

Jean-Marc Mac-Thiong, MD, PhD Department of Surgery, Ste-Justine University Center Hospital/University of Montreal, Montreal, QC, Canada

Luis Marchi, MS Department of Minimally Invasive Spine Surgery, Instituto de Patologia da Coluna, São Paulo, SP, Brazil

Ali M. Maziad, MD, MSc Department of Orthopedic Surgery – Scoliosis Service, Hospital for Special Surgery, New York, NY, USA

Venu M. Nemani, MD, PhD Spine and Scoliosis Service, Hospital for Special Surgery, New York, NY, USA

William E. Neway III, DO Department of Orthopaedic Surgery, Spine Service, University of Alabama at Birmingham, Birmingham, AL, USA

Matthew E. Oetgen, MD Department of Orthopaedic Surgery and Sports Medicine, Children's National Medical Center, Washington, DC, USA

Leonardo Oliveira, MS Department of Minimally Invasive Spine Surgery, Instituto de Patologia da Coluna, São Paulo, SP, Brazil

Dana Olszewski, MD, MPH Department of Pediatric Orthopaedics, Texas Scottish Rite Hospital, Dallas, TX, USA

Alpesh A. Patel, MD Department of Orthopaedic Surgery, Northwestern Medical Faculty Foundation, Chicago, IL, USA

Luiz Pimenta, MD, PhD Department of Minimally Invasive Spine Surgery, Instituto de Patologia da Coluna, São Paulo, SP, Brazil

Jeffrey A. Rihn, MD Department of Orthopaedic Surgery, The Rothman Institute, Thomas Jefferson University Hospital, Philadelphia, PA, USA

Benjamin D. Roye, MD, MPH Department of Orthopedic Surgery, Morgan Stanley Children's Hospital of New York, Broadway, New York, NY, USA

Amer F. Samdani, MD Shriners Hospitals for Children – Philadelphia, Philadelphia, PA, USA

Alan H. Schoenfeld, MS Department of Radiology, Montefiore Medical Center/Albert Einstein College of Medicine, Bronx, NY, USA

Gregory D. Schroeder, MD Department of Orthopaedic Surgery, Northwestern Medical Faculty Foundation, Chicago, IL, USA

James D. Schwender, MD Twin Cities Spine Center, Minneapolis, MN, USA

Cara L. Sedney, MD Department of Neurosurgery, West Virginia University, Morgantown, WV, USA

Suken A. Shah, MD Department of Orthopaedics, Nemours/Alfred I. duPont Hospital for Children, Wilmington, DE, USA

Adam C. Shaner, MD Department of Orthopaedic Surgery, Johns Hopkins Hospital, Baltimore, MD, USA

Harry L. Shufflebarger, MD Department of Orthopaedic Surgery, Miami Children's Hospital, Miami, FL, USA

Anuj Singla, MD University of Virginia Health System, Charlottesville, VA, USA

Paul D. Sponseller, MD, MBA Department of Orthopaedic Surgery, John Hopkins Bloomberg Children's Hospital, Baltimore, MD, USA

Michael P. Stauff, MD Department of Orthopedics and Physical Rehabilitation, University of Massachusetts Memorial Medical Center, Worcester, MA, USA

Daniel J. Sucato, MD, MS Department of Orthopaedic Surgery, University of Texas at Southwestern Medical Center, Texas Scottish Rite Hospital, Dallas, TX, USA

Beverly A. Thornhill, MD Department of Radiology, Montefiore Medical Center/Albert Einstein College of Medicine, Bronx, NY, USA

Michael Vitale, MD, MPH Columbia University Medical Center, New York, NY, USA

Scott C. Wagner, MD Department of Orthopaedic Surgery, Walter Reed National Military Medical Center, Bethesda, MD, USA

Joseph M. Zavatsky, MD Spine, Scoliosis and Deformity Institute, Florida Orthopaedic Institute, Tampa, FL, USA

Johnny Zhao, MD, MS Department of Orthopaedic Surgery, Center for Spinal Tumors, BJC Institute of Health, Washington University in St. Louis, St. Louis, MO, USA

Part I

Basic Principles, Diagnosis, and Nonsurgical Management

Spondylolisthesis: A Historical Perspective on Etiology, Diagnosis, and Treatment

1

Vu H. Le and Nathan H. Lebwohl

Introduction

Spondylolisthesis is from the Greek derivatives, "spondylos," meaning vertebra, and "olisthanein," meaning to slip. Essentially, it is defined as the slippage of one vertebra over another. Although it was Kilian who first coined the word "spondylolisthesis" in 1854, it was actually first described by Herbiniaux, a Belgian obstetrician, in 1782 when he reported complete dislocation of the L5 vertebral body over the sacrum, causing narrowing of the birth canal and consequent difficulty with labor and delivery [1, 2]. In fact, many reported cases of spondylolisthesis prior to 1900 were made by obstetricians [3]. In 1888, Neugebauer was one of the first to recognize that the more common form of spondylolisthesis, isthmic, was associated with a separation of the posterior neural arch from the vertebral body [4, 5] (Fig. 1.1). He noted that a bony defect was commonly encountered at the junction of the inferior and superior articulating processes, or pars interarticularis, allowing anterior displacement of the vertebral body while the spinous process and inferior articulating surfaces remained aligned with the posterior sacrum. This bony defect at the pars interarticularis was later termed "spondylolysis." The aim of this chapter is to describe the evolution of the understanding of the etiology, diagnosis, and treatment of spondylolisthesis, particularly, of the isthmic type.

V.H. Le, M.D.
Newportcare Orthopaedics and Spine Center, 3300 West Coast Highway Newport Beach, CA 92663, USA
e-mail: VHL4@yahoo.com

N.H. Lebwohl, M.D. (✉)
Department of Orthopaedics, University of Miami, Miller School of Medicine, 1611 NW 12th Avenue, Miami, FL 33136, USA
e-mail: nlebwohl@miami.edu

Etiology

In the late 1800s and early 1900s, there were multiple studies attempting to identify the cause and incidence of spondylolysis, which was thought to be a major factor in causing spondylolisthesis, especially at the junction of the fifth lumbar vertebra and sacrum. After examining 101 museum specimens in 1888, Neugebauer introduced the anomalous ossification theory as the cause of spondylolysis. He postulated that there were two centers of ossification for each half of the posterior neural arch, and the failure of fusion between these two anomalous centers of ossification was the cause for spondylolysis. However, this conjecture was discredited by numerous studies in the early 1900s showing that there was no evidence of accessory centers in the neural arches.

A.L. Wollowick and V. Sarwahi (eds.), *Spondylolisthesis: Diagnosis, Non-Surgical Management, and Surgical Techniques*, DOI 10.1007/978-1-4899-7575-1_1,

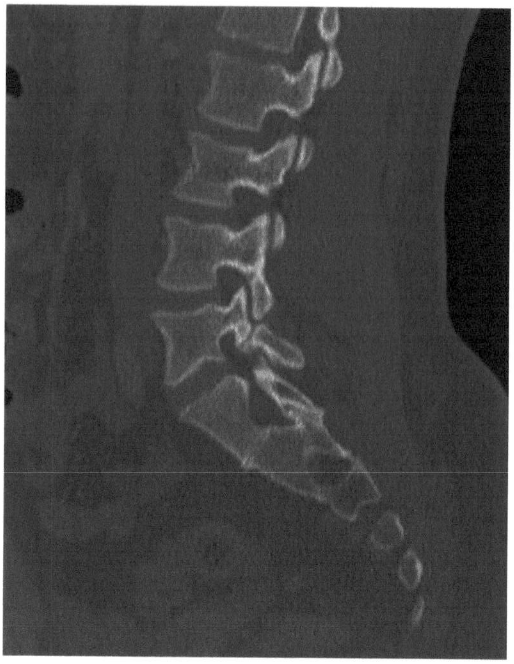

Fig. 1.1 Sagittal view on computed tomography (CT) showing a pars defect of L5

In 1906, Mall inspected 60 embryos less than 100 days old and found no evidence of accessory centers in the neural arches [6]. In 1931, Theodore Willis, from Western Reserve University in Cleveland, Ohio, examined 1,520 human skeletons and found spondylolysis in 79 specimens, or an incidence of 5.2 % of all involved specimens [7]. Like Mall, Willis did not find any evidence of anomalous ossification centers. During the same year, Russell Congdon of Washington State and Henry Meyerding of The Mayo Clinic studied different human populations in an attempt to define the nature of spondylolysis and its association with spondylolisthesis. Congdon evaluated 200 skeletal remains of American aborigines obtained in the Columbia River region and found that bilateral separation of the neural arch was found in ten subjects, or 5 % [8]. In those 5 % with bilateral spondylolysis, nearly 50 % of those subjects displayed spondylolisthesis. Meyerding, in a retrospective case series, looked at 121 patients with spondylolisthesis [3]. Unlike earlier reports, the author found that the condition was more common in males (62 %) than females. Additionally, he introduced the concept of trauma appearing to be a significant factor in the etiology of spondylolysis as approximately 38 % of patients in this series ascribed the cause to trauma. Nevertheless, Meyerding still believed that congenital defects and the apparent instability of the lumbosacral joint may serve as additional factors in creating spondylolysis.

In 1932, Norman Capener tried to explain the pathogenesis of spondylolysis, along with demographics relating to spondylolisthesis, through 34 cases of patients with spondylolisthesis [5]. Like Meyerding, he found that males were more affected than females (53–47 %). Also relating to the trauma concept introduced by Meyerding, Capener described the deleterious effect of the sacrum on the fifth vertebra. He believed that the sacrum acts as a wedge, particularly the posterosuperior apex of the sacrum, which is then driven upwards and splits the fifth lumbar pars interarticularis, creating two portions of the vertebra (Fig. 1.2). Spondylolisthesis, or slipping of the anterior vertebral body with its superior facets, then ensues with continual wedge-like effect of the sacrum as it further displaces the anterior and posterior portions of the fifth vertebral level. He also provided possible reasons that could limit the amount of slippage as he noticed that in the majority of cases, the displaced body comes to a final position of rest after making only a moderate amount of movement. The iliolumbar ligaments can provide checkreins to excessive anterior displacement by the vertebral body, while the bony buttress from the proliferation of bone on the anterior surface of the sacrum can also stop the slippage progression of the L5 vertebra.

From 1939 to 1951, more studies were performed to discern the incidence and etiology of spondylolysis. In 1939, Martin Batts, from the University of Michigan, studied 200 fetal spines and did not find a single instance of double ossification center as mentioned by Neugebauer [9]. Likewise, in 1951, Maurice Roche and George Rowe of Washington University in Saint Louis, Missouri, did not find any consistent association of accessory ossification center with spondylolysis after examining 53 stillborn human fetuses and 20 human embryos [10]. Roche and Rowe also inspected 4,200 human skeletons taken from

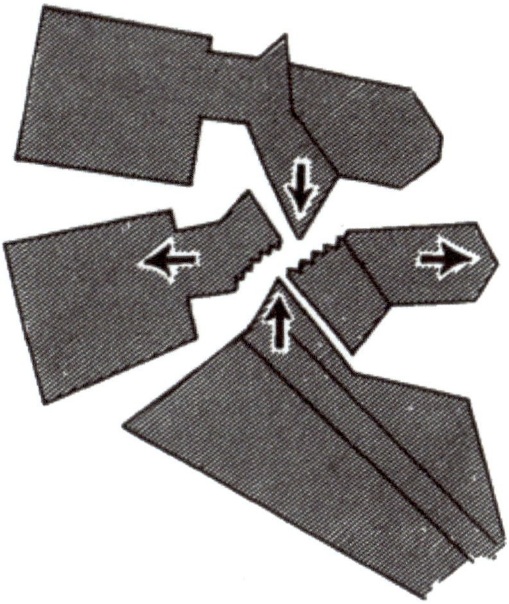

Fig. 1.2 Illustration depicting Capener's theory of the posterosuperior sacrum acting as a wedge to split the pars interarticularis of the fifth lumbar vertebra. [Reprinted from Capener N. Spondylolisthesis. The British J of Surger. 1932; 374-386. With permission from John Wiley & Sons.]

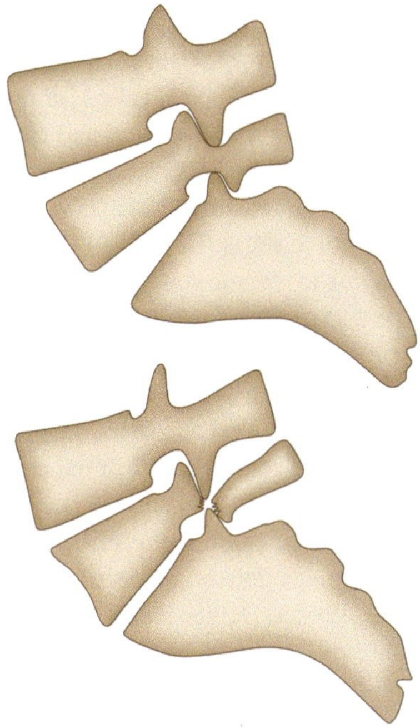

Fig. 1.3 Illustrations depicting Nathan's "pincer effect" theory. The inferior articulating process of the fourth lumbar vertebra and the superior articulating process of the sacrum create a compressive effect on the pars interarticularis of the fifth lumbar vertebra, causing spondylolysis

the Terry Anatomical Collection at Washington University and the Todd Collection at Western Reserve University. They discovered that the incidence of neural arch separation was 4.2 % [11]. Moreover, they further delineated the incidence based on race and sex. Males were more affected than females (6.4–2.3 %), and Caucasians were more likely affected compared to African-Americans. Interestingly, Eskimos have the highest rate, up to 50 %, of developing spondylolysis among different races.

Thus, up to this point, although a congenital factor may still play a large role in creating spondylolysis, the accessory ossification theory had been widely rejected by numerous studies. Consequently, other authors have continued to attempt to explain its etiology. In 1957, Wiltse theorized that the pars lesion may result from congenital weakness [12]. In 1959, Nathan, after inspecting 450 skeletons, ascribed the condition of spondylolysis and its resultant spondylolisthesis to the "pincer effect," and that the presence of preceding bone abnormalities or congenital defects of the pars interarticularis would seem unnecessary for the production of the pars defect [13]. Accordingly, the pars lesion derives from its position between the inferior articulating process of the cephalad vertebral level and the superior articulating process of the caudad level, causing a "pincer grasp" (Fig. 1.3). Continuous compressive effect of these two articular processes on the pars interarticularis can ultimately cause a fracture of the pars. Nathan also explained why spondylolysis commonly occurred at the fifth lumbar and sacrum junction. Due to its inherent hyperlordotic position compared to the upper lumbar spine, the lower lumbar levels transmit more compressive forces to their posterior neural arches, lending to the "pincer effect."

In 1976, Wiltse et al. described one of the more useful classifications of spondylolysis and spondylolisthesis that is commonly used today [14]. The classification distinguishes the multifactorial factors causing these conditions. Type 1 is due to the dysplastic predisposition of the bony architecture of the vertebrae. A congenital deficiency of the superior sacral facet or the posterior neural arch of the fifth lumbar vertebra can allow forward slippage of L5 on S1. Type 2, called isthmic spondylolisthesis, is the most frequent and more commonly involves L5 and S1, is associated with a defect in the pars interarticularis. This defect can be due to chronic stress fracture, an elongated but intact pars due to chronic stress, or acute pars fracture. Type 3 is secondary to the degenerative process and is commonly found at L4 and L5. Unlike its isthmic counterpart, women are more affected than men. Chronic degenerative changes in the discoligamentous complex lead to intersegmental instability of the facet joints and disc space. Types 4 and 5 are less common, but each involves traumatic or pathologic factors, respectively.

In 1979, Wynne-Davies and Scott studied the relationship of inheritance and spondylolisthesis [15]. They followed 147 first-degree relatives of 47 patients with either dysplastic or isthmic spondylolisthesis in Edinburgh. They found that the dysplastic form had a higher proportion of affected relatives (33 %) than the isthmic type (15 %). Due to the higher genetic association in the dysplastic group, they emphasized that affected siblings and children can be identified at an early age.

In 1984, Fredrickson et al. performed a prospective roentgenographic study on 500 first-grade children and made conclusions that align with contemporary beliefs regarding this topic. They reported the incidence of spondylolysis with or without spondylolisthesis to be 4.4 % at the age of six compared with 6 % when reaching adulthood [16]. Although the progression of slip is highest during adolescence, the authors stated that it was unlikely in adulthood. Additionally, they found that spondylolisthesis did not exist at birth.

Diagnosis

In 1782, Herbiniaux described the first case of spondylolisthesis when he discovered difficulty with labor and delivery due to pelvic outlet obstruction associated with the condition. Neugebauer, in the late 1800s, documented a case series of his encounters with spondylolisthesis. In his description of the first clinical case of spondylolisthesis in Freiburg, Germany, Neugebauer portrayed the clinical examination of a female who had undergone an unfortunate delivery and was "attacked with the most violent pains in the right hypogastrium" [17]. His examination of the patient included: "there was a slight lordotic sinking in of the lumbar vertebra, which was more noticeable when the patient laid prone," "the spinal column can be easily felt through the abdominal walls with quite moderate pressure," and "projecting from the anterior surface of the sacrum for about the thickness of a vertebra, immediately behind the vaginal portion, was a hard prominence, which was apparently the last lumbar vertebra."

In 1905, Bradford and Lovett added to the clinical diagnosis of spondylolisthesis [18]. "A disturbance of equilibrium resulting in a faulty carriage, which was shown chiefly by a sharp increase in the lower lumbar curve in even the mildest cases. The spine curved forward sharply from the sacrum, and this gave undue backward prominence to the crest of the ilium and the buttocks. The appearance at first glance was the same as that in cases of double congenital dislocation of the hip."

Capener, in 1932, further described the clinical features of spondylolisthesis [5]. "A shortened trunk in which the lower ribs were depressed, sometimes almost into the pelvis, was associated with a rotation of the pelvis upon a transverse axis so that the sacrum appeared more vertical. There was a small hollow behind the lumbar spinous processes, and at the lower end of this hollow there was a bony projection, which in the commonest type of spondylolisthesis was the tip of the spinous process of the fifth lumbar vertebra. A peculiar waddling gait may be observed. This was due to hyperextension of the hips secondary to the pelvic rotation."

Phalen and Dickson, in 1961, made a significant contribution to the understanding of the muscular imbalance around the hips [19]. They described a case in which a boy "walked on his tarsal pads and thrusted his pelvis violently forward to overcome posterior muscle spasm." The spasm was due to the excessively tight hamstring muscles, which kept the pelvis and the trunk tilted backward and limited the amount of hip flexion. "To pick something from the floor, the child must squat down beside it, since, even with the knees flexed he could not flex his back and hips sufficiently to permit him to bend forward and to reach the floor with his hands."

Before radiographs were introduced in 1895 by Wilhelm Rontgen, Pott's disease was a common differential diagnosis with low back pain. But with radiographic evaluation, especially the lateral view, spondylolisthesis can be easily differentiated from other etiologies of lower back pain. Associated spondylolysis can be viewed on the lateral or oblique radiographs. Computed tomography (CT) later on aided in cases where spondylolysis was difficult to see on plain radiographs.

In order to quantify the severity of the slippage, Meyerding, in 1938, developed a grading system in which the superior endplate of the first sacrum was divided into four quarters [20]. The amount of slippage of the fifth lumbar vertebra on the sacrum corresponded to: grade 1 is slippage of the L5 vertebral body up to 25 % of the sacral endplate's anteroposterior width; grade 2 is up to 50 %; grade 3 is up to 75 %; grade 4 is up to 100 %; and grade 5 is more than 100 % (spondyloptosis). Taillard, in 1954, described a grading system as percentage of displacement of the cephalad vertebral body on the caudad body based on the standing lateral radiograph, which was a modification of the Meyerding classification [21]. In 1983, in addition to quantifying translational displacement, Wiltse standardized terminologies and their methods of measurement related to spondylolisthesis deformity [22]. These included slip angle, sacral inclination, lumbar lordosis, rounding of the first sacral vertebra, sacral slope, lumbosacral joint angle, and lumbosacral angle. The details of these terminologies are beyond the scope of this chapter as they are likely to be mentioned in other chapters.

Treatment

Although the vast majority of patients with spondylolisthesis can be treated conservatively, those who display intractable pain or neurological deficits warrant surgical treatment. In the past, nonoperative treatment consisted of prolonged bedrest and casting, which were not tolerated well [23]. Nonoperative treatment used to involve traction on head and feet in a position of recumbency [4]. The feet were elevated to 35–40° in relation to the torso, with countertraction placed on the head and axillae. Once reduction was accomplished, the patient was placed in a double spica cast extending from the axillae to include both legs for about 6–8 weeks. The cast was reinforced with a steel-back for support.

It was not until the early 1900s that surgery was deemed as a viable option for those who failed conservative treatment. Russell Hibbs and Fred Albee, both of whom were from New York, simultaneously presented the first form of posterior spinal fusion that was later used by many surgeons for spondylolisthesis. Interestingly, both initially devised this surgical technique for deformities caused by Pott's disease. In 1911, both surgeons described methods of fusing the spine, through a posterior midline approach, by partially cutting the local bony elements (spinous processes and laminae) to create a fusion bed and applying the local osteotomized bone over the desired vertebral levels to obtain fusion [24, 25] (Fig. 1.4). In Albee's technique, the spinous process was split and the tibial graft was placed between the halves of the spinous process. Because early posterior spinal fusion did not involve instrumentation to provide stability while the fusion was taking place, Albee and others tended to keep the patients on a fracture bed for 5 weeks, after which a long plaster-of-Paris jacket molded over the buttocks was applied for an additional 2 months [4].

It is unknown when the first posterior fusion operation was performed for spondylolisthesis, but as far as we know, Hibbs and Swift were the first authors to present a case series of 24 patients with spondylolisthesis treated with posterior fusion between 1914 and 1927 [26]. According to this article, the first operation was performed on a 13-year-old patient on 13 October 1914. Of the 24 cases, 16 patients, or 66.9 %, had complete relief of symptoms; 3 patients, or 12.5 %, had some improvement of their symptoms; and 5 patients, or 20.8 %, did not have any improvement in their

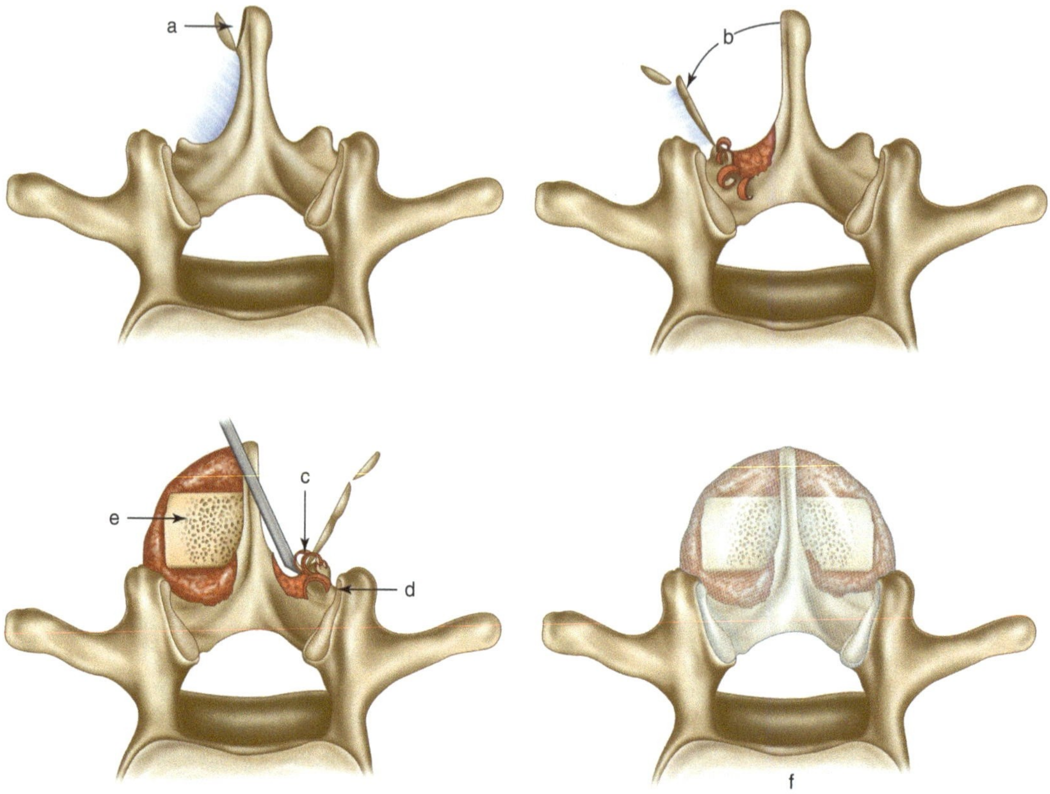

Fig. 1.4 Axial view of posterior spinal fusion technique as described by Meyerding. Partial osteotomies of the spinous process and laminae are created to obtain local bone graft and a fusion bed. Autograft fibula or tibia (e) is then placed into the fusion bed to maximize fusion potential

symptoms. Albee, in his 1915 article, described a posterior fusion procedure for an 18-year-old male with spondylolisthesis [23].

In 1932, Capener theorized a superior technique to stabilize the spine by transfixing the body of the fifth lumbar vertebra to the sacrum through the anterior approach (Fig. 1.5) [5]. Although this might be an excellent way to prevent further slippage, he thought "the technical difficulties of such a procedure, however, preclude their trial."

Capener's theory was later emulated and executed by Burns, Jenkins, Mercer, and Speed. Burns, in 1933, treated a 14-year-old patient with spondylolisthesis by drilling a hole from the anterior aspect of the fifth lumbar vertebral body towards the first sacral body, then filling that bony void with a tibial autograft (Fig. 1.6) [27]. In 1934 and 1938, Jenkins and Speed, respectively, performed similar procedures for patients with spondylolisthesis (Fig. 1.7) [4, 28].

In 1936, Mercer modified the aforementioned anterior spinal fusion [29]. He obtained fusion by removing the intervertebral disc and some adjacent bone and replacing it with bone graft from the ilium (Fig. 1.8). Similar to early posterior spinal fusion, Mercer's procedure required careful postoperative rehabilitation until the bones were fused. Flexion of the back was prohibited to prevent graft displacement and confinement to bed lasted 8 weeks, followed by the use of a steel-back brace until there was evidence of bony fusion.

Since their introduction, both surgical approaches, posterior and anterior, continued to be used and modified. They have also been proven

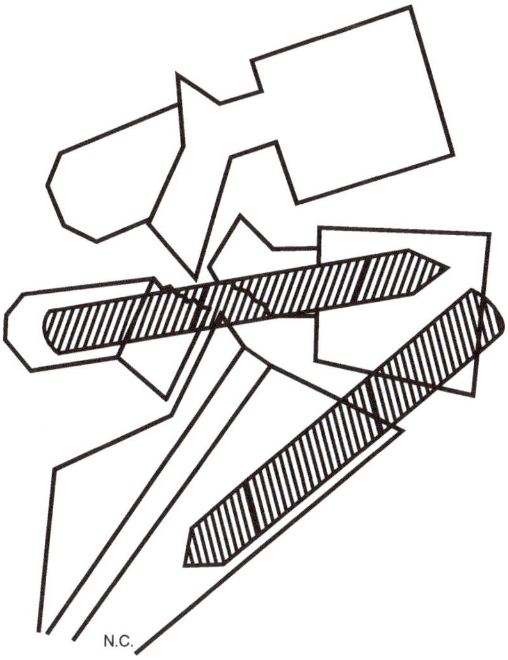

Fig. 1.5 Illustration depicting Capener's vision for anterior fusion of L5 and S1 and direct repair of the spondylolysis. [Reprinted from Capener N. Spondylolisthesis. *The British J of Surger.* 1932; 374-386. With permission from John Wiley & Sons.]

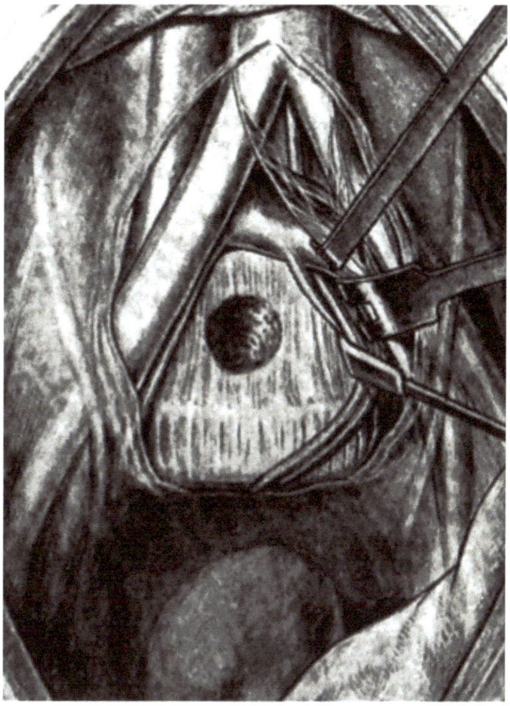

Fig. 1.6 Illustration of the anterior fusion performed by Burns. A drill hole was created starting at the anterior cortex of the fifth lumbar vertebra. [Reprinted from Burns BH. An operation for spondylolisthesis. *The Lancet.* 1933;221(5728):1233. With permission from Elsevier.]

to be relatively effective. In 1943, Meyerding described his experience with a modified version of the Hibbs fusion in 143 patients with spondylolisthesis [30]. In 87.6 % of those cases, patients were able to engage in a gainful occupation after surgery, and in 66.4 % of the cases the patients were able to resume their former occupations. Postoperative complications of infection and phlebitis occurred in 14 patients.

In 1953, Watkins introduced an alternative technique of posterior spinal fusion through a posterolateral fusion technique. Instead of focusing on fusing the spine directly posterior on the spinous process and lamina, bone graft was placed in the inter-transverse interval to obtain fusion across the transverse processes [31]. This was performed through a para-spinal approach instead of the conventional midline approach. The proponents of this technique argued that it was helpful in cases where spinous processes and

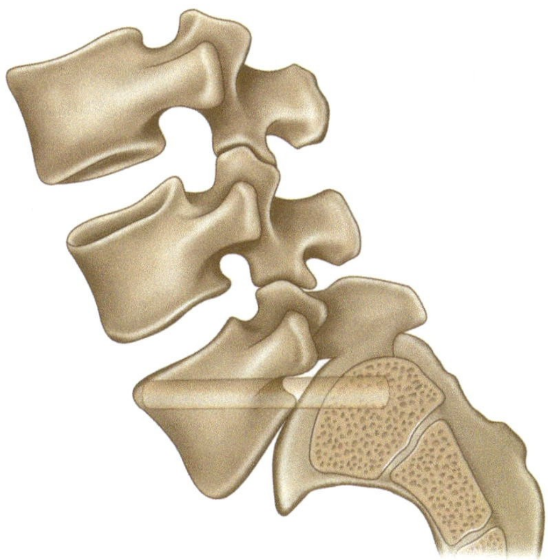

Fig. 1.7 Illustration showing insertion of the strut graft from the anterior aspect of L5 to the body of S1

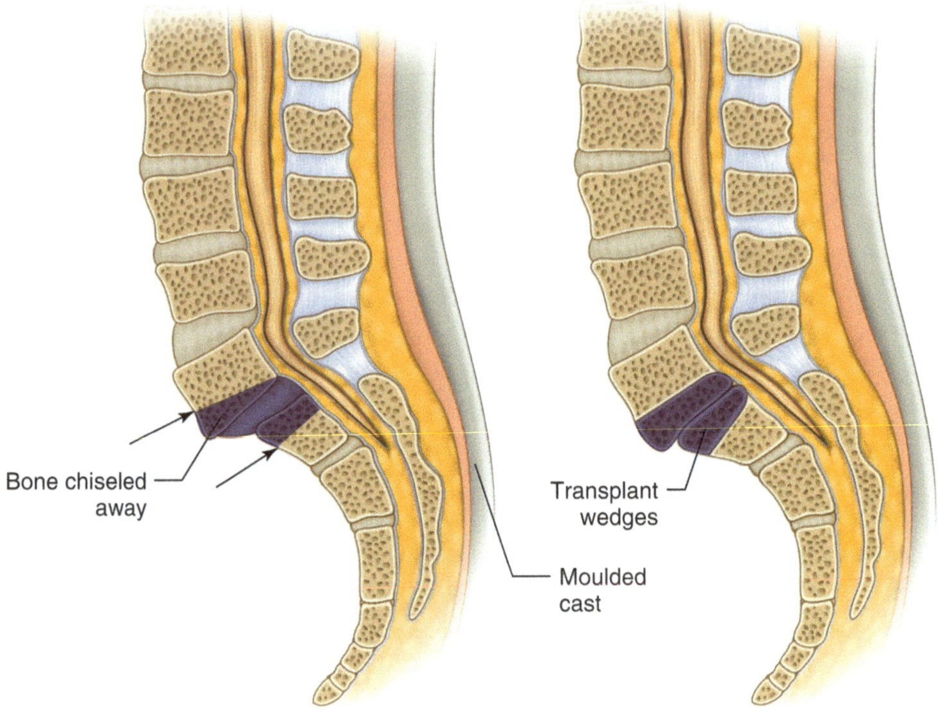

Fig. 1.8 Illustrations portraying Mercer's anterior fusion technique for spondylolisthesis

laminae have to be taken down, such as during decompression; therefore, preventing the creation of a fusion bed needed for the conventional Hibbs fusion. This technique is widely used today, regardless of whether the spinous processes and laminae are taken down or not in order to maximize fusion potential.

For patients with neurological deficits, decompression was generally recommended through the posterior approach. In 1955, Gerald Gill of San Francisco provided another posterior technique for patients who had spondylolisthesis, especially for those with more leg pain than back pain due to nerve impingement [32]. This procedure involved the removal of the lamina and fibrocartilagenous tissue present at the pars defect, which he believed was responsible for the radicular symptoms. For a thorough decompression, complete removal of all offending bone and cartilage from the pars at its junction with the base of the pedicle and transverse process was sometimes necessary. Although this procedure can be performed with or without fusion, Gill recommended this procedure without fusion for elderly patients who have more leg pain than back pain. This was because it was less morbid of a procedure compared with fusion, and he believed the chances of further slippage after decompression alone were not significant in this population.

In 1968, the evolution of the posterior fusion approach continued to progress. Wiltse et al. introduced the modified posterolateral approach [33]. Instead of going lateral to the sacrospinalis muscle to obtain posterolateral fusion, the authors recommended going through the muscle for various reasons. First, it obviated the release of important stabilizing structures such as the supraspinous and interspinous ligaments that was commonly performed through a midline approach. This theoretically prevented further slippage of the spondylolisthesis, especially after decompression. Second, this approach provided the appropriate window to decompress the L5 nerve root and to perform posterolateral fusion as described by Watkins.

As demonstrated, the majority of surgical advancement had been related to the posterior approach aside from Capener's introduction of the anterior approach. This was likely due to the unfamiliarity and the technical challenges of this technique compared to the conventional posterior procedure. Due to these reasons, some authors initially had reservations regarding the ability to attain fusion with anterior surgery. In 1971, Freebody, through a case series of 167 patients with spondylolisthesis who underwent an anterior lumbar fusion similar to that of Mercer's, found that 81 % obtained fusion, 91 % reported excellent or good results, and complications were minimal [34]. However, it was noted that this procedure was done mainly for backache due to the deformity, but not for radicular symptoms as the nerve root could not be adequately decompressed anteriorly. Therefore, it was not unusual to see an anterior interbody fusion combined with posterior decompression with fusion, especially for those with neurological symptoms.

Around this time, instrumentation was introduced to provide reduction of the deformity, especially the lumbosacral kyphosis, and stability after reduction. In 1971, Harrington and Tullos described posterior distractive instrumentation in nine patients with spondylolisthesis through the usage of metal bars connected to sublaminar hooks at L1 cranially and attached to sacral bars caudally [35]. Distraction force was then applied between the sacrum and L1 to reduce L5 on S1. This was done in conjunction with posterior decompression and posterolateral fusion. The authors later added an interbody fusion between L5 and S1 to facilitate fusion and preservation of deformity correction. With instrumentation, the patient was allowed to mobilize within days after the procedure as opposed to prior fusion techniques requiring postoperative casting. Although it was an attractive surgical option, this procedure's complication rates were high as one patient

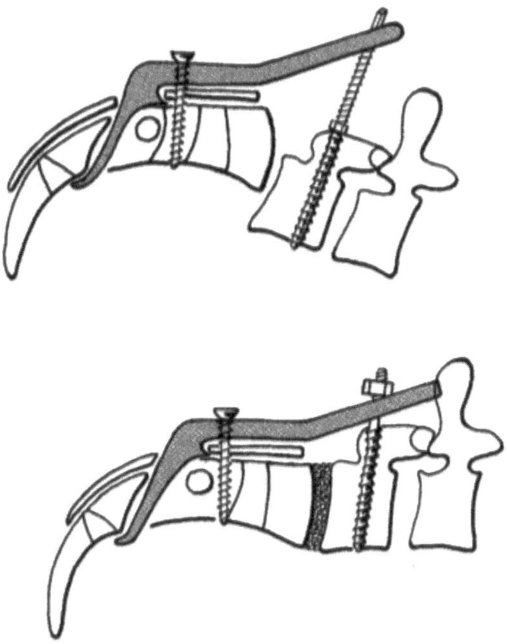

Fig. 1.9 Illustrations of the Schollner technique, involving reduction of L5 towards the plate via double threaded screws. Notice the interbody fusion at L5/S1 using autograft. [Reprinted from Schollner D. One stage reduction and fusion for spondylolisthesis. Int Orthop. 1990;14(2):145-150. With permission from Springer Verlag.]

developed cauda equina syndrome from the sacral bars, one sustained an infection, and four lost some reduction with long-term follow-up. In addition, the biomechanical property of this maneuver did not work favorably as distraction at the posterior apex of the lumbosacral kyphosis worsened the verticality of the sacrum and decreased lordosis in the lumbar region.

In 1973, Schollner described a new method of instrumentation through a one-stage posterior approach [36]. First, it involved decompression of L5 and removal of the L5/S1 disc. Then hooked plates were applied posteriorly through the second sacral foramina and secured to the sacrum with screws. Double threaded screws were then inserted through the pedicles of L5. In order to obtain reduction of L5 onto S1, nuts were then applied on the double threaded screws to bring the L5 vertebra towards the fixed hooked plates (Fig. 1.9). This was also augmented with posterolateral and interbody fusion via the posterior approach. L5 nerve root injury was an important complication. Of the reported 51 cases, one patient developed persistent foot drop, ten patients had temporary foot drop, and infections occurred in three patients.

In 1976, Laurent and Osterman presented their results after treating 91 patients at the Orthopaedic Hospital of the Invalid Foundation in Helsinki with various techniques discussed up to this point in time including posterior fusion, posterior fusion with Knodt's rods, laminectomy and posterior fusion, posterolateral fusion, laminectomy and posterolateral fusion, anterior fusion, and laminectomy alone [37]. They found that the rate of pseudarthrosis after primary operations was 19.5 %. Moreover, there was progression of displacement despite posterior fusion in 14 patients (18 %). The clinical outcomes after surgery were: good in 60 % of patients, satisfactory in 24 %, and unsatisfactory in 16 %.

Between 1978 and 1984, Bradford and Boachie-Adjei treated 22 patients with severe spondylolisthesis by introducing a two-stage approach at Twin Cities Spine Center in Minneapolis, USA [38]. The first stage involved posterior decompression and posterolateral arthrodesis. This was followed by halo-skeletal traction to obtain reduction. Then the second stage was performed by obtaining anterior lumbosacral interbody fusion. Because instrumentation was not involved, casting was implemented for 4 months after the second stage. Four patients developed pseudarthrosis and three sustained neurologic deficits from deformity reductions, which again emphasized the complications of reduction maneuvers.

In the same era, L5 vertebrectomy was introduced for spondyloptosis by Gaines. He later reported his experience with 30 patients who underwent L5 vertebrectomy over 25 years [39]. All had improvements in back and leg pain following surgery. Of the 23 patients who had temporary neurological deficit in the L5 root for 6 weeks to 3 years following their surgeries, all but two recovered fully.

In 1982, Bohlman and Cook combined multiple concepts into a one-stage approach involving decompression and posterolateral and interbody fusion for high-grade spondylolisthesis through a posterior approach which they described in two patients (Fig. 1.10) [40]. The technique consisted of decompression of the posterior elements of L5 and S1. Then the posterosuperior aspect of the S1 body was osteotomized to decompress the dura, preventing cauda equina syndrome. Two guide wires were then introduced between the fifth lumbar and first sacral nerve roots, just lateral to the midline under fluoroscopy, aiming from posterior to anterior towards the anterior cortex of the fifth lumbar vertebra. A cannulated drill was used to drill over the guide wires, but not breaching the anterior cortex of L5 body. Autograft fibular struts were then harvested and placed into these two drill holes, connecting L5 to S1 bodies. Posterolateral fusion was also performed to enhance fusion. Despite the technical difficulty, both patients had relief of their symptoms and achieved solid fusion. This landmark technique provided the blueprints to obviate the need for a separate anterior transabdominal procedure to attain transfixing interbody fusion as proposed by Capener in 1932.

Similar to the technique of sacral osteotomy by Bohlman and Cook, Schoennecker et al. recommended decompression of the cauda equina during arthrodesis in patients who have at least grade 3 or 4 spondylolisthesis due to the fact that the cauda equina can be tethered by the posterosuperior aspect of the sacrum intraoperatively, even during an in situ fusion [41]. In 1990, they reported 12 cases of cauda equina syndrome after in-situ arthrodesis for severe spondylolisthesis. This brought into light that not only was the L5 nerve root susceptible to impingement in isthmic spondylolisthesis, but also the cauda equina, especially in severe forms of the condition. Decompression of the cauda equina can be performed through the osteotomy of the posterosuperior aspect of the S1 body, as described in Bohlman's case reports.

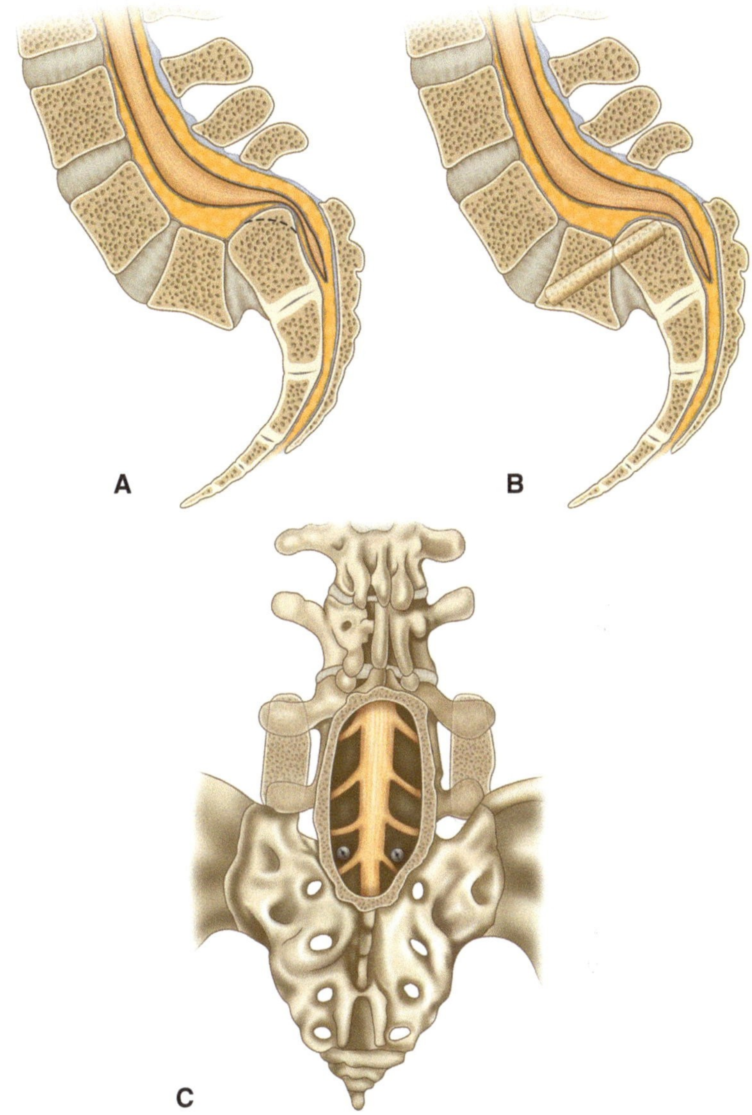

Fig. 1.10 Illustrations of the one-stage posterior interbody and posterolateral fusion with decompression introduced by Bohlman. Notice the osteotomy of the posterosuperior portion of S1 to decompress the cauda equina

In 1988, Steffee and Sitkowski introduced reduction and stabilization by using plates and transpedicular screws, augmented with lumbosacral interbody fusion (Fig. 1.11) [42]. In their case series of 14 patients with severe spondylolisthesis, all had improvements in leg pain symptoms and achieved fusion after undergoing this technique. However, they recommended close somatosensory evoked potential monitoring during the reduction maneuver to prevent neurological complications.

Despite more recent advances in instrumentation, the principles of reduction and stabilization through various fusion techniques for spondylolisthesis can be found in the innovations introduced by the surgeons whose historic work has been reviewed in this chapter.

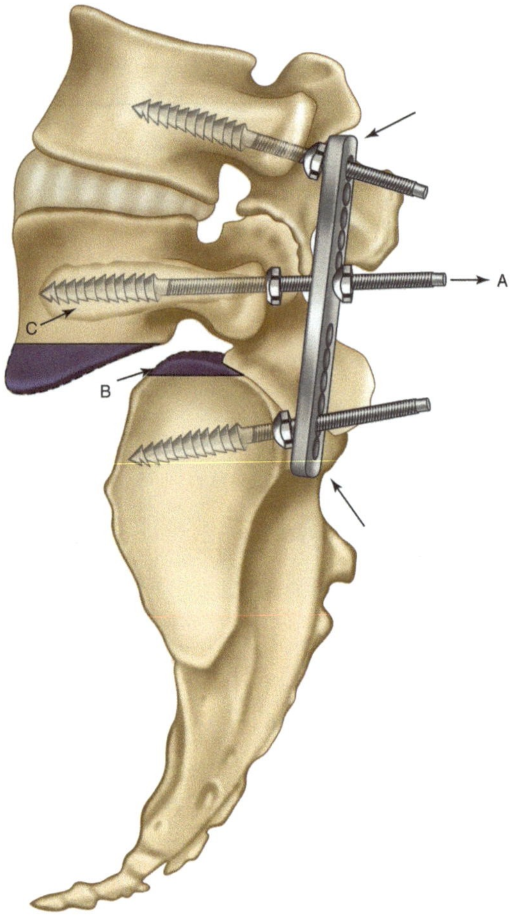

Fig. 1.11 Illustration depicting reduction of L5 through transpedicular screws and plate by pulling the slipped vertebra back to the plate and sacrum

References

1. Herbiniaux G. Traite sur divers accouchemens laborleux et sur les polypes de la matrice. Bruxelles: J. L. DeBoubers; 1782.
2. Kilian HF. Schilderungen neuer eckenformen und ihres verhaltens in Leven. Mannheim: Verlag von Bassermann & Mathy; 1854.
3. Meyerding HW. Spondylolisthesis. J Bone Joint Surg. 1931;13:39–48.
4. Speed K. Spondylolisthesis. Arch Surg. 1938; 37(2):175–89.
5. Capener N. Spondylolisthesis. Br J Surg. 1932; 19:374–86.
6. Mall FP. On ossification centers in human embryos less than one hundred days old. Am J Anat. 1906;5:433–58.
7. Willis TA. An analysis of vertebral anomalies. Am J Surg. 1929;6:163–8.
8. Congdon RT. Spondylolisthesis and vertebral anomalies in skeletons of American aborigines. With clinical notes on spondylolisthesis. J Bone Joint Surg Am. 1932;14(3):511–24.
9. Batts M. The etiology of spondylolisthesis. J Bone Joint Surg Am. 1939;21(4):879–84.
10. Roche MB, Rowe GG. Anomalous centers of ossification for inferior articular processes of the lumbar vertebrae. Anat Rec. 1951;109:253–9.
11. Roche MB, Rowe GG. The incidence of separate neural arch and coincident bone variations. J Bone Joint Surg Am. 1952;34(2):491–3.
12. Wiltse L. Etiology of spondylolisthesis. Clin Orthop. 1957;10:48–59.
13. Nathan H. Spondylolysis its anatomy and mechanism of development. J Bone Joint Surg Am. 1959;41(2): 303–20.
14. Wiltse LL, Newman PH, Macnab I. Classification of spondylolysis and spondylolisthesis. Clin Orthop. 1976;117:23–9.
15. Wynne-Davies R, Scott J. Inheritance and spondylolisthesis. J Bone Joint Surg. 1979;61:301–5.
16. Fredrickson BE, Baker D, McHolick WJ, Yuan HA, Lubicky JP. The natural history of spondylolysis and spondylolisthesis. J Bone Joint Surg. 1984;66: 699–707.
17. Neugebauer FL. The classic: a new contribution to the history and etiology of spondylolisthesis. Clin Orthop Relat Res. 1976;117:4–22.
18. Bradford EH, Lovett RW. Spondylolisthesis. Treatise Orthop Surg. 1905;3:385–8.
19. Phalen G, Dickson J. Spondylolisthesis and tight hamstrings. J Bone Joint Surg. 1961;43:505–12.
20. Meyerding H. Spondylolisthesis as an etiologic factor in backache. JAMA. 1938;111:1971–6.
21. Taillard W. Le spondylolisthesis chez l'enfant et l'adolescent. Acta Orthop. 1954;24:115–44.
22. Wiltse LL, Winter RB. Terminology and measurement of spondylolisthesis. J Bone Joint Surg. 1983;65:768–72.
23. Albee F. Spondylolisthesis. Bone Graft Surg. 1915;134–40.
24. Bick EM. An essay on the history of spine fusion operations. Clin Orthop Relat Res. 1964;35:9–15.
25. Hibbs R. An operation for progressive spinal deformities. N Y Med J. 1911;93:1013.
26. Hibbs R, Swift W. Developmental abnormalities at the lumbosacral juncture causing pain and disability. Surg Gynecol Obstet. 1929;48:604–12.
27. Burns BH. An operation for spondylolisthesis. Lancet. 1933;221:1233.
28. Jenkins J. Spondylolisthesis. Br J Surg. 1934; 24:80–5.
29. Mercer W. Spondylolisthesis. Edinburg Med J. 1936;43:545–72.
30. Meyerding H. Spondylolisthesis: surgical treatment and results. J Bone Joint Surg. 1943;25:65–77.

31. Watkins M. Posterolateral fusion of lumbar and lumbosacral spine. J Bone Joint Surg. 1953;35:1014–8.
32. Gill G, Manning J, White H. Surgical treatment of spondylolisthesis without spinal fusion. J Bone Joint Surg. 1955;37:493.
33. Wiltse L, Bateman G, Hutchinson R, Nelson W. The paraspinal sacrospinalis-splitting approach to the lumbar spine. J Bone Joint Surg. 1968;50:919–26.
34. Freebody D, Bendall R, Taylor RD. Anterior transperitoneal lumbar fusion. J Bone Joint Surg Br. 1971;53:617–27.
35. Harrington P, Tullos H. Spondylolisthesis in children. Clin Orthop Relat Res. 1971;79:75.
36. Schollner D. One stage reduction and fusion for spondylolisthesis. Int Orthop. 1990;14:145–50.
37. Laurent L, Osterman K. Operative treatment of spondylolisthesis in young patients. Clin Orthop Relat Res. 1976;117:85.
38. Bradford D, Boachie-Adjei O. Treatment of severe spondylolisthesis by anterior and posterior reduction and stabilization. J Bone Joint Surg. 1990;72:1060–6.
39. Gaines R. L5 vertebrectomy for the surgical treatment of spondyloptosis. Spine. 2005;30:S66–70.
40. Bohlman H, Cook S. One-stage decompression and posterolateral and interbody fusion for lumbosacral spondyloptosis through a posterior approach. Report of two cases. J Bone Joint Surg Am. 1982;64:415–8.
41. Schoenecker PL, Cole H, Herring J, Capelli A, Bradford D. Cauda equina syndrome after in situ arthrodesis for severe spondylolisthesis at the lumbosacral junction. J Bone Joint Surg. 1990;72:369–77.
42. Steffee A, Sitkowski D. Reduction and stabilization of grade 4 spondylolisthesis. Clin Orthop Relat Res. 1988;227:82–9.

Anatomy and Biomechanics Relevant to Spondylolisthesis

2

Venu M. Nemani, Han Jo Kim, and Matthew E. Cunningham

Introduction

Spondylolisthesis can occur anywhere along the spinal column from the cervical spine down to the lumbosacral junction (LSJ). It occurs most frequently, however, in the middle lumbar spine and the LSJ, less often in the cervical spine, and rarely in the thoracic spine. The exact cause of spondylolisthesis is not entirely understood but likely reflects a combination of familial and acquired factors, which combine to create a specific anatomic and mechanical environment that cause a slip to occur. In this section we will discuss the anatomic and mechanical factors that are thought to be important in the development and progression of spondylolisthesis.

The spine has a complex anatomy, which in the absence of pathology, optimally accomplishes its basic functions which are to transmit load from the head and trunk to the pelvis, allow for truncal motion, and to protect the spinal cord and associated neural elements. While a complete description of spinal anatomy and biomechanics is beyond the scope of this chapter, spinal balance, sacropelvic and spinopelvic alignment, lumbosacral dysplasia, and how they influence the biomechanical properties of the spine are critical to understanding the factors that predispose to spondylolisthesis.

Biomechanics

In addition to hereditary and racial factors, biomechanical factors play an important role in the development and progression of spondylolisthesis. Athletes in sports that involve repetitive hyperextension of the lumbar spine, such as gymnasts, American football offensive linemen, divers, and swimmers who perform the butterfly stroke are all at elevated risk of isthmic spondylolysis, which in some patients can progress to spondylolisthesis.

Biomechanical studies have shown that under normal loading conditions of the lumbar spine, the anterior spinal column, consisting of the vertebral bodies and the discs, supports 80–90 % of the axial load whereas the posterior elements support 10–20 % of the load. The load imparted on a lumbar disc is a combination of an axial force and a shear force due to the oblique orientation of the lumbar vertebral endplates. Further, the lumbar-anchored musculature adds to the shear stress imparted on the lumbar discs. In this loading situation, the posterior elements of the lumbar spine act as a tension band resisting the tendency for anterolisthesis of one vertebral body on another.

V.M. Nemani, M.D., Ph.D. (✉) • H.J. Kim, M.D.
M.E. Cunningham, M.D., Ph.D.
Spine and Scoliosis Service,
Hospital for Special Surgery, 535 E 70th Street,
New York, NY 10021, USA
e-mail: vnemani@gmail.com; hanjokimmd@gmail.com; cunninghamm@hss.edu

A.L. Wollowick and V. Sarwahi (eds.), *Spondylolisthesis: Diagnosis, Non-Surgical Management, and Surgical Techniques*, DOI 10.1007/978-1-4899-7575-1_2,

The annulus fibrosis of the disc as well as the posterior longitudinal ligament additionally provide some resistance against spondylolisthesis [1]. In some cases where bilateral spondylolysis is present, shear forces can result in anterior displacement of the superior vertebral body and its attached anterosuperior pars fragment, which is exacerbated during flexion or in patients with high pelvic incidence, which will be discussed in more detail later. There are specific anatomic factors related to the LSJ and to overall spinal morphology that are critical in understanding the pathogenesis and progression of spondylolisthesis, which will be discussed in greater detail.

Spinal Balance

It has become very clear in recent years that global sagittal plane alignment is a critical factor to consider in both adult and pediatric patients with spondylolisthesis. The spine rather than being completely straight has natural curvatures in the sagittal plane, with cervical and lumbar lordosis and thoracic and sacral kyphosis. These curves are normally balanced resulting in positioning of the head directly over the pelvis, allowing the muscles of gait and posture to work most efficiently. Thus, in the coronal plane, a plumb line dropped from the dens falls through the center of the sacrum and in the sagittal plane, a plumb line falls posterior to the cervical spine, through the C7 vertebral body, anterior to the thoracic spine, posterior to the lumbar spine, and through the body of S1 (Fig. 2.1). When the C7 plumb line falls anterior to the sacrum, the center of rotation of angulation (CORA) at the LSJ is also anterior to the L5–S1 disc further increasing the already significant shear and axial forces present at this level, increasing the susceptibility for spondylolisthesis. In patients with adult spinal deformity, the maintenance of sagittal balance has been closely linked with clinical outcomes [2, 3], underscoring its importance for overall health and function. There is a wide range of normal values for thoracic kyphosis and lumbar lordosis that are generally complementary; however, alterations in spinopelvic morphology can change the amount of lumbar lordosis that is needed to compensate for thoracic kyphosis. In fact, because the relationship of the sacrum to the pelvis is fixed in the absence of sacroiliac motion, the remainder of the pelvis, hips, and spine must adapt to any spondylolisthesis to balance the trunk in the upright posture. Optimal spinopelvic balance in the sagittal plane occurs when a C7 plumb line falls at or behind the femoral heads (center of gravity) ensuring that a minimum amount of energy is necessary to maintain upright posture.

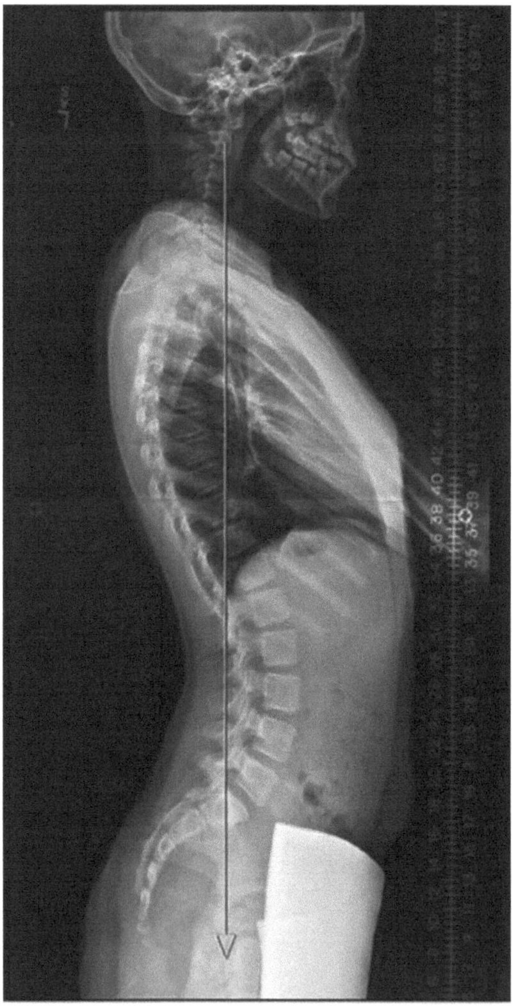

Fig. 2.1 Sagittal spine radiograph showing a plumb line dropped from the dens that intersects the sacrum and falls posterior to the bi-femoral axis showing neutral sagittal balance

With lumbosacral spondylolisthesis and resultant sacral dysplasia, it may be difficult for the body to obtain proper sagittal spinopelvic balance [4–6]. Mac-Thiong and colleagues found that a normal posture was maintained in patients with low-grade spondylolisthesis, but that spinopelvic balance was disturbed in patients with high-grade spondylolisthesis, and particularly so in those with an unbalanced pelvis (pelvic retroversion). These studies emphasize the important role that the local anatomy at the LSJ plays in determining overall spinopelvic balance and alignment.

Sacropelvic Alignment

The LSJ is an area of transition from the relatively mobile lumbar spine with its normal lordotic curve, to the rigid kyphotic sacrococcygeal spine. Because the sacroiliac joints are relatively fixed with little motion, the pelvis and the hip joints play an important role in the overall orientation of the lumbosacral spine and its contribution to overall spinal balance in the sagittal plane. Several authors have described radiographic parameters that can be used to quantify sacropelvic and spinopelvic alignment [7–11]. Further, pelvic and sacral morphology has been cited as an important factor contributing to the development of spondylolisthesis. Some of the important anatomic factors that can be quantified on radiographs include pelvic tilt (PT), sacral slope (SS), pelvic incidence (PI), and lumbar lordosis (LL).

Pelvic tilt describes the orientation of the pelvis with respect to a vertical reference line. Anterior pelvic tilt is also referred to as pelvic flexion, anteversion, and inclination while posterior pelvic tilt is also referred to as pelvic retroversion, extension, or reclination [12]. Pelvic tilt is the angle subtended by a vertical line and a line connecting the center of the superior S1 endplate to a point that bisects the center of rotation of the hip joints (Fig. 2.2a). Pelvic tilt is not only a critical parameter in the evaluation of patients with spondylolisthesis, but also plays an important role in patients undergoing total hip replacement, re-orienting acetabular osteotomies, or treatment for femoro-acetabular impingement. Sacral slope describes the orientation of the superior endplate of the sacrum with respect to a horizontal reference line (Fig. 2.2b). Importantly, both PT and SS are measures of sacropelvic orientation as they are dependent on the position of the individual in space.

Unlike PT and SS, pelvic incidence is a measure of sacropelvic morphology as it is a measurement that is unique and fixed amongst individuals and does not change with positioning (assuming insignificant motion at the sacroiliac joints). Pelvic incidence was first introduced by Duval-Beaupère and colleagues in the early 1990s, and is measured by the angle subtended by a line perpendicular to the endplate of the superior endplate of S1, and a line connecting the middle of the superior endplate of S1 and the hip axis [13] (Fig. 2.2c). Conveniently, PI is the arithmetic sum of PT and SS. Because of this, the morphology of the sacropelvis (as defined by the PI) is closely correlated with the orientation of the pelvis in space. For example, if a patient has a very high PI, then the PT, SS, or both must also be high. Other measurements that have been described to quantify sacropelvic morphology are the pelvic radius angle [14] and pelvic-sacral angle [15]; however, these lack the geometric correlation with SS and PT. Pelvic incidence plays an extremely important role in overall sagittal balance, with higher PI requiring increased lumbar lordosis to maintain an upright balanced posture [9].

There have been several studies examining these measurements in both adult [16] and pediatric [17] populations defining their normal values (Table 2.1). The inter-observer and intra-observer reliability for measurement of PI is excellent [18]. PI has been shown to increase slightly and constantly over the course of childhood before stabilizing in adulthood [19]. Compared to normal patients, several investigators have shown that PI is significantly higher in those patients with spondylolisthesis [20–23]. Interestingly, there is a linear correlation of higher PI with worsening spondylolisthesis (Table 2.1), which makes sense biomechanically. A low PI means low values for pelvic tilt and

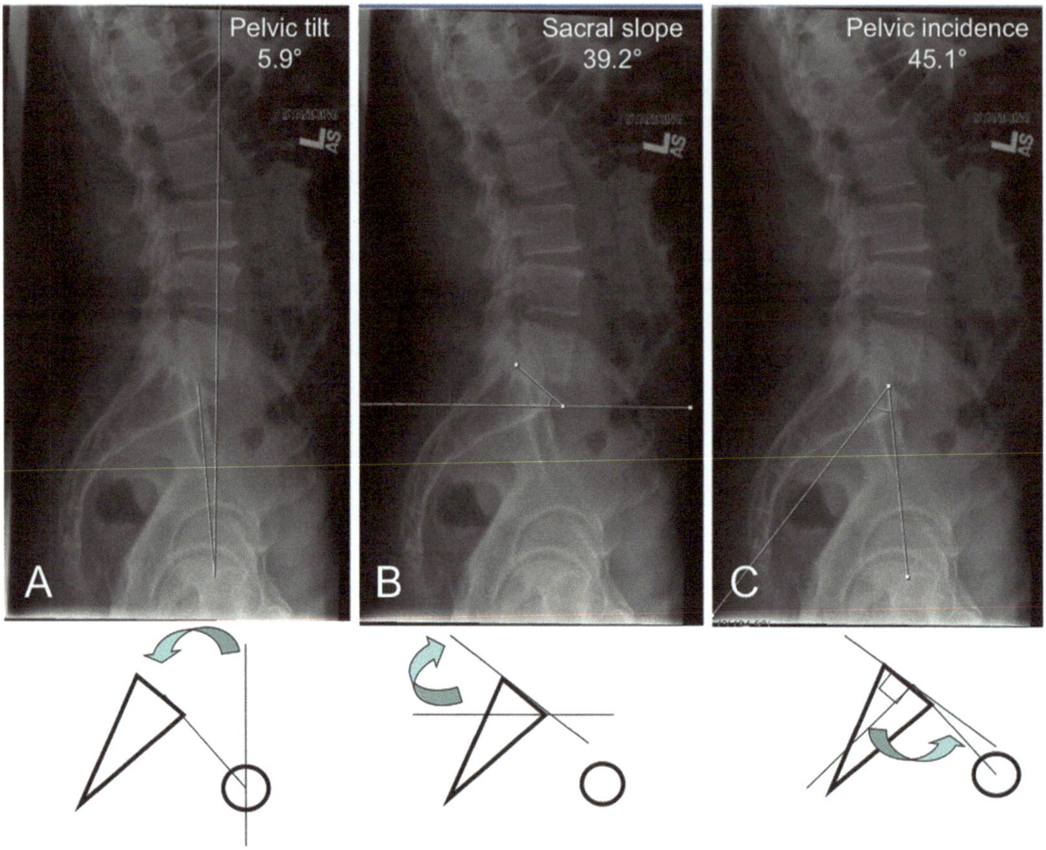

Fig. 2.2 (**a**) Pelvic tilt is the angle of a line connecting the center of the superior endplate of S1 to a point that bisects the center of rotation of the hip joints compared to a vertical reference line. (**b**) Sacral slope is the angle of a line tangential to the superior endplate of S1 compared to a horizontal reference line. (**c**) Pelvic incidence is the angle subtended by a line perpendicular to the superior endplate of S1, and a line connecting the center of the superior endplate of S1 to the center of the bi-femoral axis. It also is the arithmetic sum of pelvic tilt and sacral slope

Table 2.1 Average sagittal sacropelvic measurements in a normal population and patients with spondylolisthesis

	Normal children and adolescents	Normal adults	Developmental spondylolisthesis				
			Grade 1	Grade 2	Grade 3	Grade 4	Grade 5
Pelvic incidence	49.1 (11.0)	51.8 (5.3)	57.7 (6.3)	66.0 (6.9)	78.8 (5.6)	82.3 (7.2)	79.4 (10.2)
Sacral slope	41.4 (8.2)	39.7 (4.1)	43.9 (4.8)	49.8 (4.2)	51.2 (5.7)	48.5 (7.6)	45.9 (13.5)
Pelvic tilt	7.7 (8.0)	12.1 (3.2)	13.8 (3.9)	16.2 (5.4)	27.6 (5.7)	33.9 (5.2)	33.5 (5.4)

Based on data from [16, 17, 22]

sacral slope, which results in a relatively flat lumbar lordosis and a horizontal sacral endplate creating low shear stresses at the LSJ. Alternatively, a high PI means high values for pelvic tilt and sacral slope, increased lumbar lordosis, and a more vertical sacral endplate resulting in higher shear stress across the LSJ. However, no study has yet been able to demonstrate a causative relationship between sacropelvic alignment and the development of spondylolisthesis.

An important point to make is that two individuals with the same sacropelvic morphology (same PI) can have different sacropelvic orientation (Fig. 2.3). The Spine Deformity Study Group has investigated sacropelvic balance in patients with either high vs. low-grade spondylolisthesis.

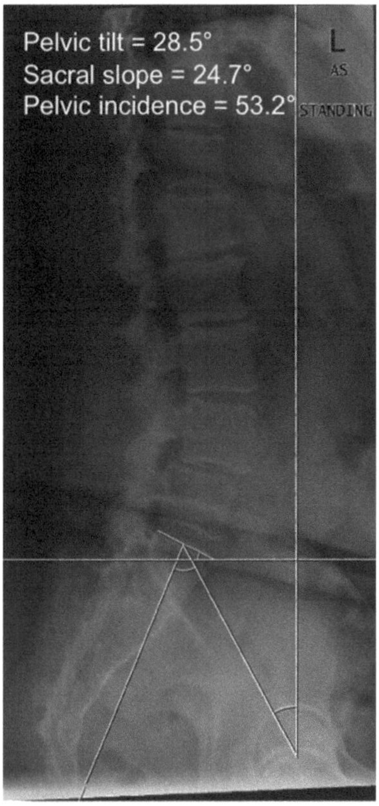

Fig. 2.3 Sagittal radiograph of the lumbar spine showing normal pelvic incidence but markedly different sacropelvic orientation with increased pelvic tilt, decreased sacral slope, and a retroverted pelvis. These differences can be compared to the patient demonstrated in Fig. 2.2, who has a more balanced sacropelvic orientation

Patients with low-grade spondylolisthesis can be subcategorized into two groups: those with low PI (<45°) and those with high PI (>60°). It is thought that patients with high PI suffer tension failure of the pars causing spondylolysis, while patients with low PI undergo pars failure via a "nutcracker" effect, by impingement of the L5 posterior elements between L4 and S1 during extension [24]. Interestingly, patients with high-grade spondylolisthesis almost invariably have high PI, suggesting that low-grade slips with low PI never progress to a high-grade slip. High-grade slips can be subcategorized into those with a balanced pelvis versus those with an unbalanced pelvis. Patients with a balanced pelvis have a low PT and a high SS, with a posture similar to normal individuals with high PI but without spondylolisthesis, whereas those patients with an unbalanced pelvis have a retroverted pelvis with a high PT and low SS.

Lumbosacral Dysplasia

Significant remodeling of the lumbosacral spine can occur in the setting of spondylolisthesis. This remodeling can involve the posterior elements and/or the anterior elements. Dysplasia in the pars interarticularis is causative in dysplastic spondylolisthesis, but can also be secondary from a stress reaction or a malunion after repeated fractures. Dysplasia can also involve the lumbosacral kyphosis (LSK), trapezoidal L5, sacral dysplasia and kyphosis, bifid posterior arch, hypoplastic or aplastic facet joints, dysplasia of the pedicles, lamina or facets, as well as small transverse processes. In fact, Curylo and colleagues showed that 62 % of patients with spondyloptosis had evidence of posterior element dysplasia [20].

Dysplasia at the LSJ contributes to the development and progression of spondylolisthesis by decreasing the mechanical resistance to shear stress in the lumbosacral spine. Only a few studies have attempted to quantify the incidence of posterior element dysplasia and its relationship to spondylolisthesis, and this has mainly been for spina bifida occulta (SBO). While the incidence of SBO in normal individuals at L5 is estimated around 2.2 % [25, 26], the incidence of SBO in Grade 3 or higher spondylolisthesis has been reported to be as high as 42 % [27] and the results of Curylo showing even higher rates of dysplasia in patients with spondyloptosis.

In addition to the translational deformity that can be quantified by the grade of slip as described by Meyerding [28], there is also an angular deformity that is best described as a LSK. Normally, the junction between the lowest lumbar vertebral body and the sacrum is lordotic; however, as the degree of slip progresses to higher grades the relationship becomes kyphotic. There are several described techniques for quantifying LSK, which can be difficult because of the presence of sacral dysplasia involving the S1 endplate.

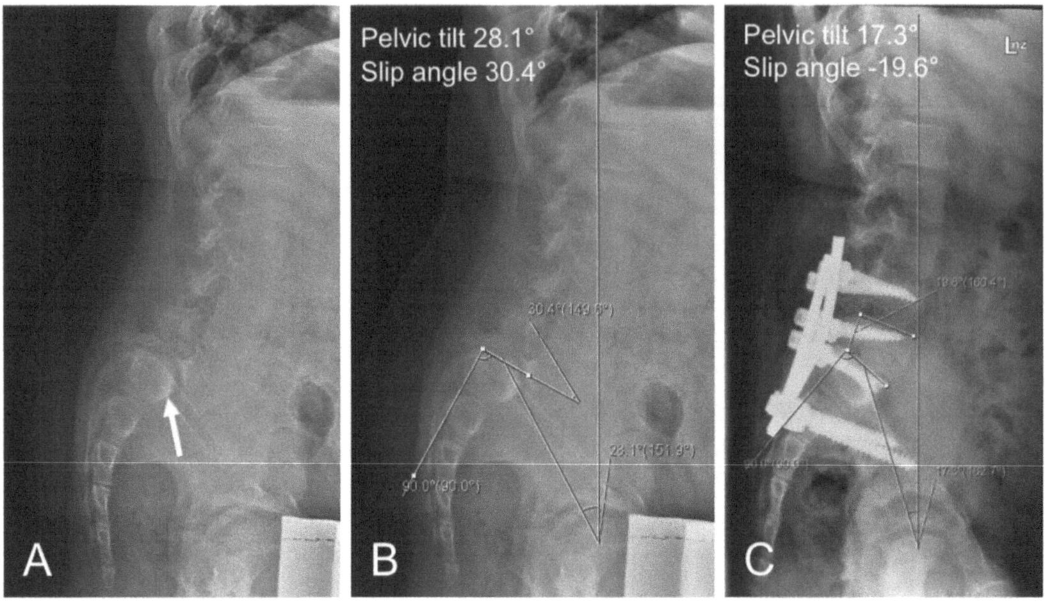

Fig. 2.4 (**a**) Sagittal radiograph of the lumbar spine showing morphologic changes at the S1 endplate (*arrow*) as a result of progressive spondylolisthesis at L5–S1. (**b**) Pre-operative sacropelvic parameters showing increased pelvic tilt and slip angle. (**c**) Post-operative sacropelvic parameters showing reduction of slip and decreased pelvic tilt

One of the most frequently used measures is the slip angle, which was originally described as the angle subtended by a line perpendicular to the posterior cortex of S1, and a line tangential to the inferior endplate of L5 [29], although it is now commonly measured using the superior endplate of L5 because there can be remodeling and distortion of the inferior endplate of L5 secondary to dysplasia (Fig. 2.4). Other measurements that have been described include the Dubousset lumbosacral angle and lumbosacral angle, all of which have excellent reproducibility [30]. Some authors suggest that the amount of LSK is important in determining the risk of progression [29, 31, 32]; however, there is no strong data supporting this idea in the literature. The combination of normal and shear forces at the LSJ leads to altered morphology and remodeling of the sacral endplate, with subsequent appearance of a dome-shaped endplate and progressive anterolisthesis of L5 on S1 (Fig. 2.4). The dome-shape of S1 is specific to spondylolisthesis, and is not seen in its absence. Some investigators believe that the sagittal deformity of the sacrum and LSK seen in spondylolisthesis is secondary, and occurs as a result of abnormal axial stress on the superior S1 endplate causing altered growth according to the Heuter–Volkmann law [23]. However, Wang and colleagues examined 131 children and adolescents with developmental spondylolisthesis and found morphologic changes in the lower sacral segments and in sacral kyphosis, suggesting that a primary abnormality in sacral morphology may play a role in the development or progression of spondylolisthesis [33].

Conclusions

While the precise etiology and risk factors for progression of spondylolysis and spondylolisthesis are not fully understood, it is clear that both local and global anatomic factors play an important role. Sacropelvic morphology and alignment as assessed by pelvic tilt, sacral slope, and pelvic incidence coupled with an understanding of any dysplasia can help classify the spondylolisthesis, and will create a unique biomechanical environment that will guide potential treatment options.

References

1. Steffee AD, Sitkowski DJ. Reduction and stabilization of grade IV spondylolisthesis. Clin Orthop Relat Res. 1988;227:82–9.
2. Glassman SD, et al. The impact of positive sagittal balance in adult spinal deformity. Spine (Phila Pa 1976). 2005;30(18):2024–9.
3. Mac-Thiong JM, et al. Can c7 plumbline and gravity line predict health related quality of life in adult scoliosis? Spine (Phila Pa 1976). 2009;34(15):E519–27.
4. Hresko MT, et al. Classification of high-grade spondylolisthesis based on pelvic version and spine balance: possible rationale for reduction. Spine (Phila Pa 1976). 2007;32(20):2208–13.
5. Labelle H, et al. The importance of spino-pelvic balance in L5-S1 developmental spondylolisthesis: a review of pertinent radiologic measurements. Spine (Phila Pa 1976). 2005;30(6 Suppl):S27–34.
6. Mac-Thiong JM, et al. Postural model of sagittal spino-pelvic alignment and its relevance for lumbosacral developmental spondylolisthesis. Spine (Phila Pa 1976). 2008;33(21):2316–25.
7. Jackson RP, Hales C. Congruent spinopelvic alignment on standing lateral radiographs of adult volunteers. Spine (Phila Pa 1976). 2000;25(21):2808–15.
8. Jackson RP, et al. Compensatory spinopelvic balance over the hip axis and better reliability in measuring lordosis to the pelvic radius on standing lateral radiographs of adult volunteers and patients. Spine (Phila Pa 1976). 1998;23(16):1750–67.
9. Legaye J, et al. Pelvic incidence: a fundamental pelvic parameter for three-dimensional regulation of spinal sagittal curves. Eur Spine J. 1998;7(2):99–103.
10. Vaz G, et al. Sagittal morphology and equilibrium of pelvis and spine. Eur Spine J. 2002;11(1):80–7.
11. Vialle R, et al. Radiographic analysis of the sagittal alignment and balance of the spine in asymptomatic subjects. J Bone Joint Surg Am. 2005;87(2):260–7.
12. Siebenrock KA, Kalbermatten DF, Ganz R. Effect of pelvic tilt on acetabular retroversion: a study of pelves from cadavers. Clin Orthop Relat Res. 2003; 407:241–8.
13. Duval-Beaupere G, Schmidt C, Cosson P. A Barycentremetric study of the sagittal shape of spine and pelvis: the conditions required for an economic standing position. Ann Biomed Eng. 1992;20(4):451–62.
14. Jackson RP, et al. Pelvic lordosis and alignment in spondylolisthesis. Spine (Phila Pa 1976). 2003;28(2): 151–60.
15. During J, et al. Toward standards for posture. Postural characteristics of the lower back system in normal and pathologic conditions. Spine (Phila Pa 1976). 1985; 10(1):83–7.
16. Berthonnaud E, et al. Analysis of the sagittal balance of the spine and pelvis using shape and orientation parameters. J Spinal Disord Tech. 2005;18(1):40–7.
17. Mac-Thiong JM, et al. Sagittal spinopelvic balance in normal children and adolescents. Eur Spine J. 2007;16(2):227–34.
18. Berthonnaud E, et al. A variability study of computerized sagittal spinopelvic radiologic measurements of trunk balance. J Spinal Disord Tech. 2005;18(1): 66–71.
19. Mac-Thiong JM, et al. Sagittal alignment of the spine and pelvis during growth. Spine (Phila Pa 1976). 2004;29(15):1642–7.
20. Curylo LJ, Edwards C, DeWald RW. Radiographic markers in spondyloptosis: implications for spondylolisthesis progression. Spine (Phila Pa 1976). 2002; 27(18):2021–5.
21. Funao H, et al. Comparative study of spinopelvic sagittal alignment between patients with and without degenerative spondylolisthesis. Eur Spine J. 2012;21(11):2181–7.
22. Labelle H, et al. Spondylolisthesis, pelvic incidence, and spinopelvic balance: a correlation study. Spine (Phila Pa 1976). 2004;29(18):2049–54.
23. Whitesides Jr TE, et al. Spondylolytic spondylolisthesis: a study of pelvic and lumbosacral parameters of possible etiologic effect in two genetically and geographically distinct groups with high occurrence. Spine (Phila Pa 1976). 2005;30(6 Suppl):S12–21.
24. Roussouly P, et al. Sagittal alignment of the spine and pelvis in the presence of L5-S1 isthmic lysis and low-grade spondylolisthesis. Spine (Phila Pa 1976). 2006;31(21):2484–90.
25. Fidas A, et al. Prevalence and patterns of spina bifida occulta in 2707 normal adults. Clin Radiol. 1987;38(5):537–42.
26. Saluja PG. The incidence of spina bifida occulta in a historic and a modern London population. J Anat. 1988;158:91–3.
27. Seitsalo S, et al. Progression of spondylolisthesis in children and adolescents. A long-term follow-up of 272 patients. Spine (Phila Pa 1976). 1991;16(4): 417–21.
28. Meyerding HW. Spondylolisthesis. Surg Gynecol Obstet. 1932;54:371–7.
29. Boxall D, et al. Management of severe spondylolisthesis in children and adolescents. J Bone Joint Surg Am. 1979;61(4):479–95.
30. Glavas P, et al. Assessment of lumbosacral kyphosis in spondylolisthesis: a computer-assisted reliability study of six measurement techniques. Eur Spine J. 2009;18(2):212–7.
31. Dubousset J. Treatment of spondylolysis and spondylolisthesis in children and adolescents. Clin Orthop Relat Res. 1997;337:77–85.
32. Speck GR, McCall IW, O'Brien JP. Spondylolisthesis: the angle of kyphosis. Spine (Phila Pa 1976). 1984;9(6):659–60.
33. Wang Z, et al. Influence of sacral morphology in developmental spondylolisthesis. Spine (Phila Pa 1976). 2008;33(20):2185–91.

Pain Generators in Spondylolisthesis

3

Eugene J. Carragee and Michael P. Stauff

Introduction

When treating patients with spinal-area pain, it is fundamental to carefully consider the anatomy and pathophysiology of potential pain generators and the likelihood that one may be a primary source of the apparent pain syndrome. This understanding is of utmost importance in the treatment of patients with spondylolisthesis, or slippage of a vertebra, since this is a common finding in asymptomatic subjects. Patients who have cervical or lumbar spondylolisthesis may have pain coming from one or multiple sources. The confidence with which a provider can identify a true primary pain source has a strong influence on the success of the treatment course, whether it is operative or nonoperative.

In this chapter, we will discuss the pain generators associated with spondylolisthesis of all types. The first part of the chapter will delve into the pain generators in spondylolisthesis that are common with other spinal pathologies. This includes discogenic pain, facetogenic pain, and pain arising from neurologic compression of the spinal cord, nerve roots, and/or cauda equina. In the second half of the chapter, we will focus on pain generators that are unique to spondylolisthesis. This includes pain arising from pathology of the pars interarticularis and axial pain secondary to abnormal sagittal alignment.

Before discussing the multiple pain generators in spondylolisthesis, it should be stressed that many, and perhaps most people with spondylolisthesis are asymptomatic. This is clearly true in patients who have a degenerative spondylolisthesis, but also holds true in patients with isthmic spondylolisthesis. In modern medicine, incidental findings on highly sensitive imaging studies can sometimes lead to missed diagnoses and improper treatment. It is only through careful consideration of a patient's history, physical examination, and clinical data that the spine care provider can effectively treat patients with symptomatic spondylolisthesis.

Discogenic Pain

Axial pain related primarily to disc pathology could manifest in several ways. It may cause deep-seeded posterior midline pain or it may radiate laterally or down the posterior thighs. The

E.J. Carragee, M.D.
Department of Orthopedic Surgery, Stanford University Hospital and Clinics,
450 Broadway Street, Pavilion C, MC 6342,
Redwood City, CA 94063, USA
e-mail: carragee@stanford.edu

M.P. Stauff, M.D. (✉)
Department of Orthopedics and Physical Rehabilitation, University of Massachusetts Memorial Medical Center, Spine Center,
Memorial Campus, 119 Belmont Street,
Worcester, MA 01605, USA
e-mail: michael.stauff@umassmemorial.org

A.L. Wollowick and V. Sarwahi (eds.), *Spondylolisthesis: Diagnosis, Non-Surgical Management, and Surgical Techniques*, DOI 10.1007/978-1-4899-7575-1_3,

variation in its presentation and the overlap with other pain generators make discogenic axial pain a difficult diagnosis in the presence or absence of spondylolisthesis. Afferent nerve fibers are present in intervertebral disc and these can carry pain signals associated with annular stretch or motion, which are both characteristic of spondylolisthesis. In the lumbar spine, the innervation of the lumbar intervertebral has been studied extensively [1]. It has been demonstrated that the nucleus and the inner annulus are devoid of neural tissue, but the outer annulus has innervation that penetrates to a depth of 3 mm [1]. In a review of the lumbar disc innervation, Edgar outlined three sources of innervation of the outer annulus. The sinuvertebral nerves innervate the posterior annulus. There are also direct branches arising from the grey rami communicans or ventral ramus that supplies the posterolateral and lateral aspects of the outer annulus. A number of studies have demonstrated that the anterior annulus has an afferent nerve supply that is carried by branches of the sympathetic trunk. The sensation of pain arises from activation of these nerve fibers by mechanoreceptors in the annulus or inflammatory mediators in the local environment. Some investigators postulate that the multi-faceted innervation of the annulus leads to varying patterns of referred pain. This fact, along with the high prevalence of disc pathology in people over 40 years of age, may be an underlying reason for the diagnostic difficulty in patients with discogenic low back pain. For patients with spondylolisthesis in the lumbar spine, the issue is even more complicated because of the presence of other potential primary axial pain generators.

In the cervical spine, the literature indicates a similar pattern to the lumbar spine, with dual innervation by sensory nerve fibers as well as autonomic nerve fibers. In a recent study by Fujimoto et al. [2], the innervation of the C5–6 intervertebral disc in rats was investigated. The authors demonstrated that the C5–6 disc in rats is innervated in a multisegmental pattern by neurons of the C2–8 dorsal root ganglions, sympathetic ganglions, and parasympathetic ganglions. Overall, they reported that 79.6 % of the innervations arise from sensory afferents, whereas 20.4 % of the innervations arise from autonomic nerves [2]. Because of the complex, multisegmental nature of the intervertebral disc innervation, cervical discogenic pain can manifest in several different patterns, making diagnosis a challenge in a similar way to lumbar discogenic pain. This can make it difficult for a spine care provider to confidently identify the cause or effectively treat the patient with only axial cervical symptoms and cervical spondylolisthesis.

Facet Joints

Axial symptoms can also arise from the facet joints and facet joint arthritis is very common. For this reason, identifying a specific facet joint as a pain source suffers from many of the same diagnostic difficulties as discogenic low back and neck pain. Patients who have facet joint mediated pain classically have paravertebral pain that can radiate cranially or caudally. In the lumbar spine, the pain can radiate into the buttocks or hamstrings, whereas cervical facet joint pain can radiate to the trapezial area or to the occiput. Pain from the facet joint is typically made worse with extension as well as rotation. In some cases, this can be replicated during the physical examination. The physical exam may also be notable for tenderness to palpation over the involved facet joint, but this can be difficult in patients with a large body habitus. Some suggest that inflammation around a facet joint can lead to irritation of exiting nerve roots, mimicking radicular pain [3]. The above factors may lead to the identification of the facet joint as the pain generator, but this can be difficult because of overlap with other pain generators in the cervical and lumbar spine.

The innervation of the facet joint has been studied extensively. The dorsal ramus branches off the nerve root and the first medial branch innervates the facet joint (Fig. 3.1). Pain receptors in the facet capsule and in the facet joint subchondral bone transmit afferent painful stimuli to the central nervous system via the medial branch. The painful stimulus arises from facet capsule stretching and/or abnormal loading of the facet joint subchondral bone. Some clinicians aim to block the

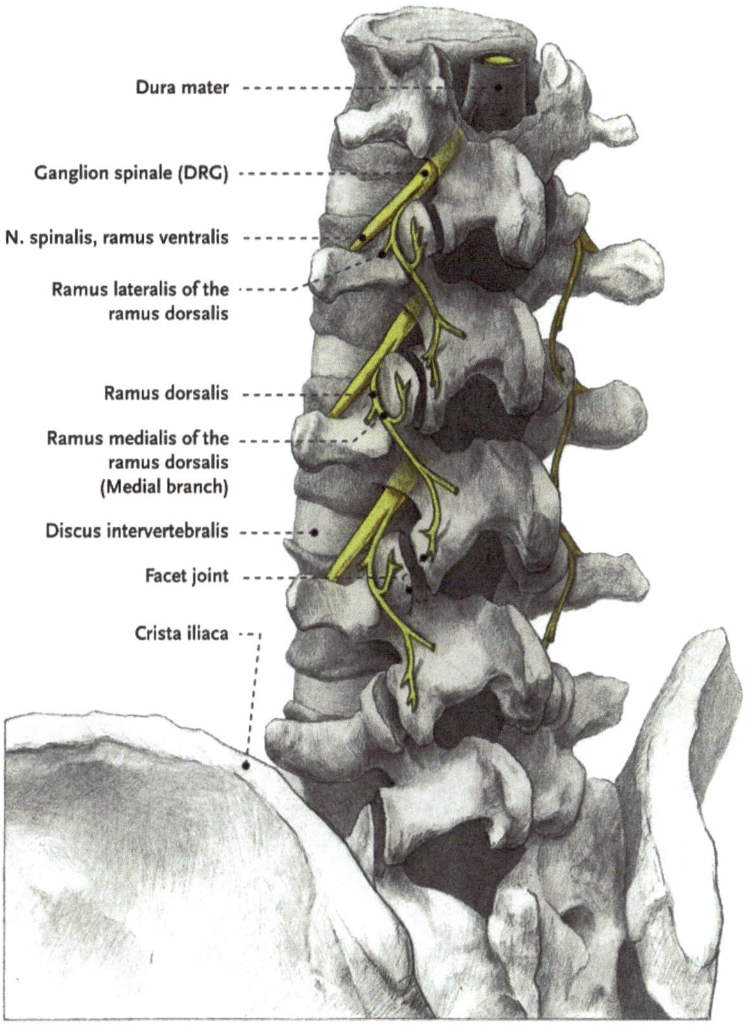

Fig. 3.1 Neuroanatomy of the lumbar spinal nerve roots and branches. [Reprinted from van Kleef M, Vanelderen P, Cohen SP, Lataster A, Van Zundert J, Mekhail N. 12. Pain originating from the lumbar facet joints. Pain practice: the official journal of World Institute of Pain 2010;10:459-69. With permission from John Wiley & Sons, Inc.]

transmission of these painful stimuli using medial branch blocks with local anesthetic as well as radiofrequency ablation in the treatment of primary facetogenic pain. Medial branch blocks are utilized in order to confirm that pain is arising from a particular facet joint, whereas radiofrequency ablation is used in order to effect a more permanent treatment [4, 5]. Facetogenic pain can be a significant contributor to the axial symptoms in patients with spondylolisthesis. This is particularly true in patients who have degenerative spondylolisthesis because these patients very often have degenerated, hypertrophic facet joints that are hypermobile and cause encroachment on the nerve root in the subarticular zone (lumbar spine) or in the foramen (cervical and lumbar spine).

Neurologic Compression

Patients who have spondylolisthesis of any kind are at risk for developing pain related to neurologic encroachment. At the level of the cauda equina, the pain can be categorized as either radiculopathy or neurogenic claudication. Low-grade isthmic spondylolisthesis generally causes a radiculopathy of the exiting nerve root [6, 7], whereas high-grade isthmic spondylolisthesis can also cause central stenosis, leading to a radiculopathy of the traversing nerve or neurogenic claudication. For lumbar degenerative spondylolisthesis, the most commonly affected neurologic structure is the traversing nerve root in the subarticular zone,

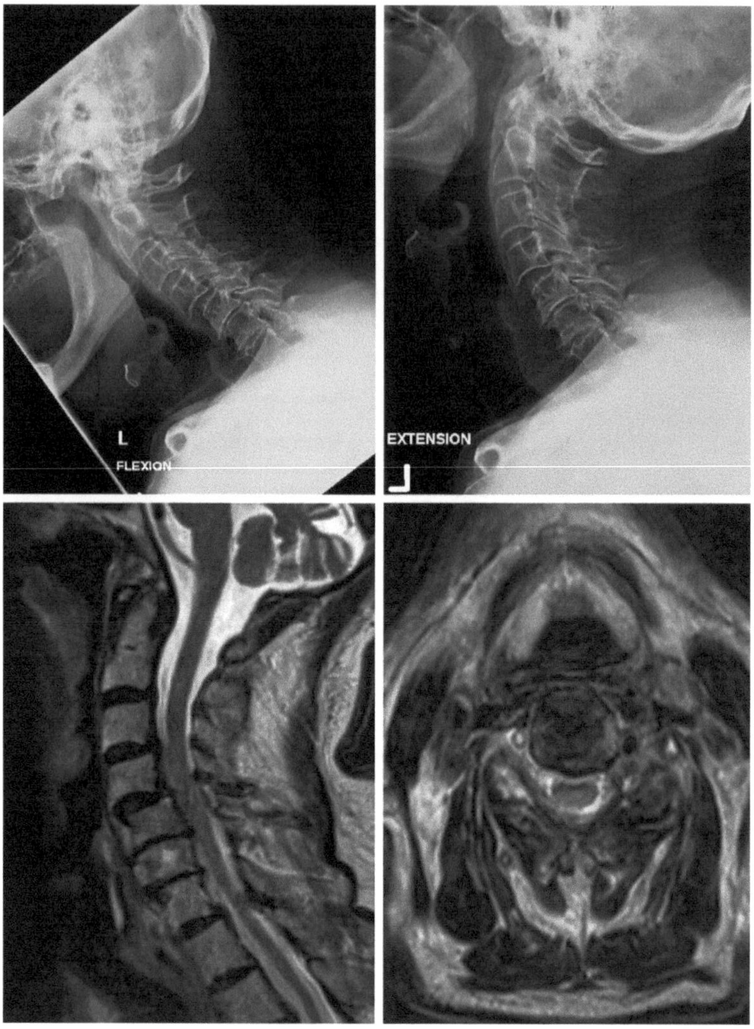

Fig. 3.2 Cervical spondylolisthesis resulting in cervical canal stenosis. The flexion and extension lateral radiographs demonstrate 4 mm of motion at the C4–5 level. The T2 mid-sagittal MRI and an T2 axial MRI slice through the C4–5 segment demonstrates cervical canal stenosis

but these patients may also have central stenosis that leads to neurogenic claudication. Spine care providers must have a thorough knowledge of the specific areas of neurologic impingement in order to effectively guide operative or nonoperative treatment for patients with spondylolisthesis.

Spinal cord level spondylolisthesis is most often found in the cervical spine. These patients can have radicular symptoms but also may have myelopathy from compression of the spinal cord in a static or dynamic fashion (Fig. 3.2). The pain from a radiculopathy in these patients can be very debilitating, whereas the pain arising from compression of the spinal cord and myelopathy may be less severe. Pain from myelopathy can manifest as upper extremity dysesthesia. Although this can be bothersome, this type of pain generated from compression of the spinal cord is not nearly as dangerous as the dysdiadochokinesia, ataxia, and bladder/bowel incontinence that can arise from myelopathy. Figure 3.3 demonstrates how spondylolisthesis in the cervical spine can lead to spinal cord compression and myelopathy. In summary, pain or symptomatology arising from neurologic compression can occur in all types of spondylolisthesis and must be addressed in any treatment algorithm.

Patients with spondylolisthesis in the cervical and lumbar spine can have multiple pain generators. The intervertebral disc, facet joints, or neurologic compression are common pain sources for patients with spondylolisthesis. These pain

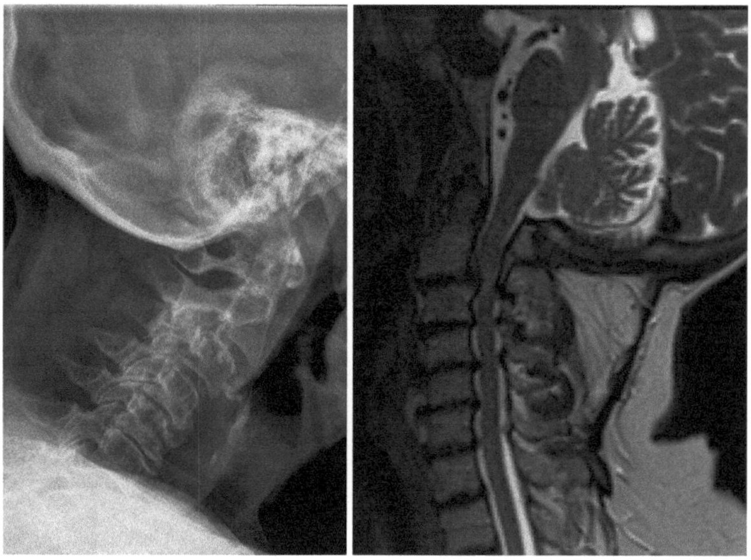

Fig. 3.3 On the left is an upright lateral cervical spine radiograph that demonstrates approximately 7.3 mm anterolisthesis at C2–3 in a 65-year-old female with severe ataxia, bilateral hand dysesthesia, dysdiadochokinesia, and hyper-reflexia. On the right is a mid-sagittal slice of the patient's MRI, which demonstrates significant spinal stenosis at that level with the cord signal change/myelomalacia

sources can also be present in other spinal pathologies. Providers must consider all potential pain generators in patients with spondylolisthesis in order to effectively guide treatment.

Pars Interarticularis

For patients with isthmic spondylolisthesis, pars interarticularis pathology can be a source of pain. It is generally accepted that there are nerve endings at the site of the defect in the pars interarticularis. These nerve endings transmit painful stimuli when there is abnormal motion or stress at the site of the defect. For the patient with an isthmic spondylolisthesis, pain from a pars interarticularis defect (a type of fracture nonunion) may manifest as pain in the paravertebral area and be associated primarily with extension [8]. Because of its proximity to the facet joint, the symptoms from a painful pars interarticularis defect may overlap with the symptoms from a painful facet joint.

The peer-reviewed evidence for the pars interarticularis as a pain generator is sparse. The best evidence in the current literature that supports the pars as a pain generator comes from clinical series in which patients had a positive diagnostic bupivacaine injection and were then treated with a pars repair. Wu et al. [9] reported on a retrospective series on 93 patients who had positive diagnostic injections with bupivacaine. After direct repair of the pars defect, 85 patients had good or excellent results [9]. A more recent, smaller series by Karatas et al. [10] reported on 16 patients who were treated with 2 different pars repair techniques. All patients received diagnostic bupivacaine injections. There were 14/16 patients who achieved good or excellent results following pars repair [10]. Successful outcome following repair of a pars defect after using a positive diagnostic injection as a criteria gives this diagnostic test some credibility. Furthermore, these studies prove that the pars interarticularis can be an isolated pain generator in isthmic spondylolisthesis in those patients without significant anterolisthesis or disc degeneration. While others have purported the use of corticosteroid and bupivacaine injections into the pars interarticularis [8], there is no strong literature to date that supports this treatment modality.

Axial Pain from Sagittal Imbalance

In the last 10 years, a large body of literature has demonstrated the importance of lumbopelvic parameters in the treatment of pediatric and adult

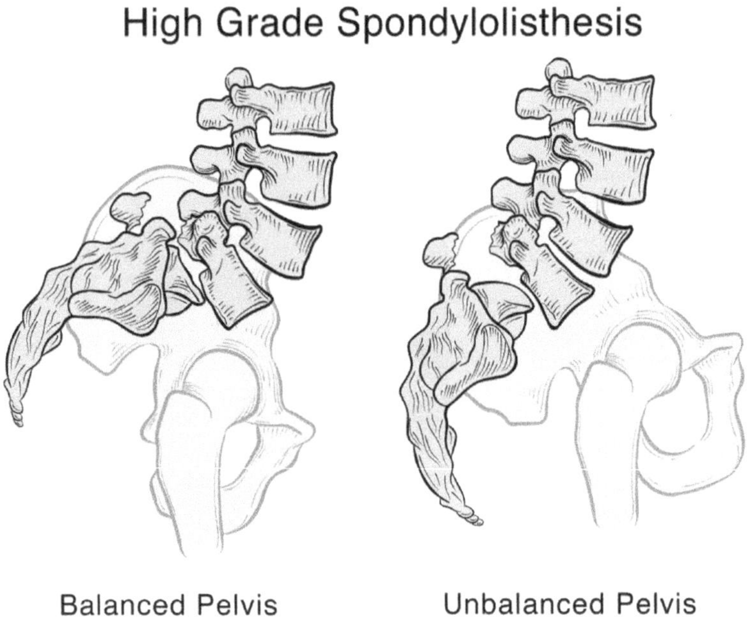

Fig. 3.4 Sagittal view of the pelvis in high-grade spondylolisthesis demonstrating the contrast between a balanced and unbalanced pelvis. Note the relationship between the hip joint and the lumbosacral junction in each picture. The balanced pelvis has a higher sacral slope and lower pelvic tilt, while the unbalanced pelvis has a lower sacral slope with a higher pelvic tilt

scoliosis patients. The concept of lumbopelvic balance has also been applied to patients with spondylolisthesis. In contradistinction to scoliosis, the sagittal malalignment in spondylolisthesis originates from a more focal pathology, typically at one level. Spinopelvic alignment is most relevant to those with isthmic spondylolisthesis, but emerging theory has purported a greater impact in patients with degenerative spondylolisthesis. Indeed, any anterolisthesis can lead to positive sagittal balance. Those patients with dysplastic and spondylolytic spondylolisthesis are more prone to develop a higher-grade slip and hence are more at risk for developing significant sagittal imbalance.

Patients with sagittal imbalance often suffer from axial pain that directly relates to their spinopelvic mismatch. The mismatch forces them to consume more energy in order to maintain an upright posture because of the increased activity of the paraspinal musculature. In the spinal deformity literature, multiple studies have demonstrated a positive correlation between worsening sagittal imbalance and more severe clinical symptoms as well as health related quality of life (HRQOL) [11–13].

The principle of spinopelvic alignment has also been applied to patients with spondylolisthesis. In one of the earliest studies to examine pelvic parameters in spondylolisthesis, Hanson et al. [14] investigated the degree of pelvic incidence in patients with both low and high-grade isthmic spondylolisthesis. They demonstrated that both adult and pediatric patients with isthmic spondylolisthesis had a higher mean pelvic incidence than matched controls. Another more recent study linked the presence of greater sagittal imbalance in isthmic spondylolisthesis with patients' symptoms. Harroud et al. [15] analyzed the sagittal alignment parameters in 149 pediatric and adolescent patients with isthmic spondylolisthesis and correlated them with HRQOL based on SRS-22 scores. They demonstrated worse SRS-22 scores in patients with greater sagittal imbalance. The sagittal imbalance and the HRQOL scores were most significant for the patients with high-grade spondylolisthesis [15].

More recently, some investigators have further characterized lumbopelvic parameters in patients with isthmic spondylolisthesis. The concept of a balanced versus unbalanced pelvis in patients with high-grade isthmic spondylolisthesis was classified by Hresko et al. (Fig. 3.4) [16]. Those patients with an unbalanced pelvis have a higher pelvic tilt and lower sacral slope, while those with a balanced pelvis have a lower pelvic tilt and a higher sacral slope. The concept of pelvic balance is important for the patient because an unbalanced pelvis can theoretically cause more axial low back pain as the patient consumes more energy in order to stay upright. Some authors suggest that reduction of high-grade isthmic spondylolisthesis in patients with an unbalanced pelvis will lead to improved surgical outcomes [17–19]. In theory, normalizing a patient's pelvic parameters in order to address the muscle fatigue pain associated with spinopelvic imbalance is important, but currently there is a dearth of prospective data that directly links improved patient outcomes with successful correction.

More recent literature has applied the concept of spinopelvic mismatch to degenerative spondylolisthesis. Aono et al. [20] and Barrey et al. [21] have demonstrated that patients with degenerative spondylolisthesis have a higher pelvic incidence than controls. Another study [22] compared the spinopelvic parameters of patients with isthmic spondylolisthesis and degenerative spondylolisthesis. Lim and Kim [22] reported significantly higher average pelvic incidence in both experimental cohorts compared with controls. This data is preliminary; however, some investigators suggest that it could lead to a better understanding of the etiology of isthmic and degenerative spondylolisthesis. Also, these alterations in the spinopelvic parameters can predispose to sagittal imbalance, further contributing to the clinical syndrome associated with spondylolisthesis.

The Clinical Scenario

When caring for a patient with spondylolisthesis, it is important to consider all potential pain generators (Fig. 3.5). Individual patients will have different patterns of pathology as well as different patterns of pain. Herein lies the challenge in caring for spondylolisthesis patients, especially when many of the pain generators discussed above contribute to axial pain. The hallmark of spondylolisthesis of any type is the slippage of one vertebrae on another. In this chapter, we have outlined the potential pain generators that may accompany this slippage. The goal of nonoperative and operative treatment of spondylolisthesis, covered in other chapters in this textbook, is to relieve pain. The reader should consider how each treatment affects the above mentioned pain generators.

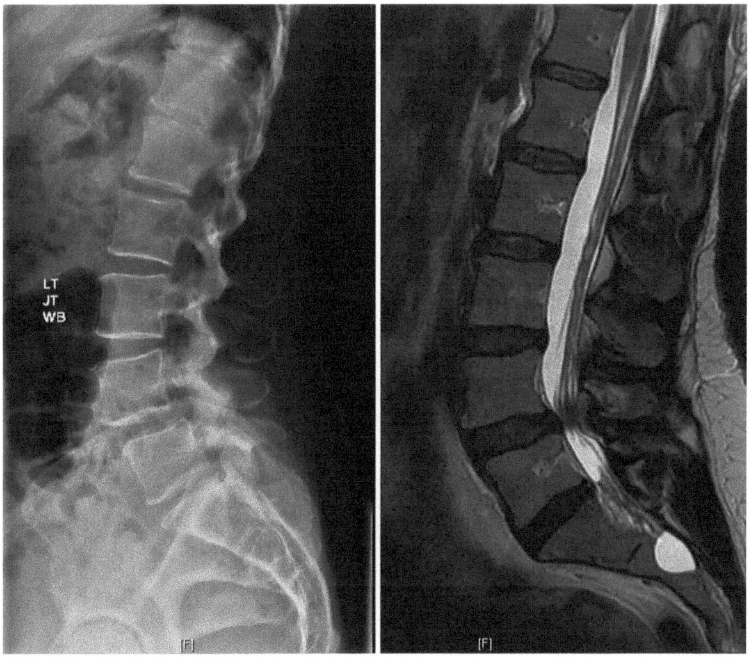

Fig. 3.5 Lumbar degenerative spondylolisthesis. A lateral lumbar radiograph demonstrating L4–5 degenerative spondylolisthesis and a mid-sagittal T2 MRI sequence demonstrating spinal stenosis at the L4–5 segment

References

1. Edgar M. The nerve supply of the lumbar intervertebral disc. J Bone Joint Surg Br. 2007;89:1135–9.
2. Fujimoto K, Miyagi M, Ishikawa T, et al. Sensory and autonomic innervation of the cervical intervertebral disc in rats: the pathomechanics of chronic discogenic neck pain. Spine. 2012;37:1357–62.
3. van Kleef M, Vanelderen P, Cohen SP, Lataster A, Van Zundert J, Mekhail N. 12. Pain originating from the lumbar facet joints. Pain Pract. 2010;10:459–69.
4. Varlotta GP, Lefkowitz TR, Schweitzer M, et al. The lumbar facet joint: a review of current knowledge: Part II: diagnosis and management. Skeletal Radiol. 2011;40:149–57.
5. Smuck M, Crisostomo RA, Trivedi K, Agrawal D. Success of initial and repeated medial branch neurotomy for zygapophysial joint pain: a systematic review. PM R. 2012;4:686–92.
6. Jinkins JR, Rauch A. Magnetic resonance imaging of entrapment of lumbar nerve roots in spondylolytic spondylolisthesis. J Bone Joint Surg Am. 1994;76:1643–8.
7. Wiltse L, Guyer R, Spencer C, Glenn W, Porter I. Alar transverse process impingement of the L5 spinal nerve: the far-out syndrome. Spine. 1984;9:31–41.
8. Petron DJ, Prideaux CC, Likness L. Interventional spine procedures in athletes. Curr Sports Med Rep. 2012;11:335–40.
9. Wu SS, Lee CH, Cheng PQ. Operative repair of symptomatic spondylolysis following a positive response to diagnostic pars injection. J Spinal Disord. 1999;12:10–6.
10. Karatas AF, Dede O, Atanda AA, et al. Comparison of direct pars repair techniques of spondylolysis in pediatric and adolescent patients: pars compression screw versus pedicle screw-rod-hook. J Spinal Disord Tech. 2012 October 16 [Epub ahead of print].
11. Glassman SD, Berven S, Bridwell KH, Horton W, Dimar JR. Correlation of radiographic parameters and clinical symptoms in adult scoliosis. Spine. 2005;30: 682–8.
12. Glassman SD, Bridwell KH, Dimar JR, Horton W, Berven S, Schwab F. The impact of positive sagittal balance in adult spinal deformity. Spine. 2005;30:2024–9.
13. Mac-Thiong JM, Transfeldt EE, Mehbod AA, et al. Can C7 plumbline and gravity line predict health related quality of life in adult scoliosis? Spine. 2009;34:E519–27.
14. Hanson DS, Bridwell KH, Rhee JM, Lenke LG. Correlation of pelvic incidence with low and high grade isthmic spondylolisthesis. Spine. 2002;27: 2026–9.
15. Harroud A, Labelle H, Joncas J, Mac-Thiong JM. Global sagittal alignment and health-related quality of life in lumbosacral spondylolisthesis. Eur Spine J. 2013;22:849–56.
16. Hresko MT, Labelle H, Roussouly P, Berthonnaud E. Classification of high-grade spondylolisthesis based on pelvic version and spine balance – possible rationale for reduction. Spine. 2007;32:2208–13.
17. Labelle H, Roussouly P, Chopin D, Berthonnaud E, Hresko T, O'Brien M. Spino-pelvic alignment after surgical correction for developmental spondylolisthesis. Eur Spine J. 2008;17:1170–6.
18. Labelle H, Mac-Thiong JM, Roussouly P. Spino-pelvic sagittal balance of spondylolisthesis: a review and classification. Eur Spine J. 2011;20 Suppl 5:641–6.
19. Mehta VA, Amin A, Omeis I, Gokaslan ZL, Gottfried ON. Implications of spinopelvic alignment for the spine surgeon. Neurosurgery. 2012;70:707–21.
20. Aono K, Kobayashi T, Jimbo S, Atsuta Y, Matsuno T. Radiographic analysis of newly developed degenerative spondylolisthesis in a mean twelve-year prospective study. Spine. 2010;35:887–91.
21. Barrey C, Jund J, Perrin G, Roussouly P. Spinopelvic alignment of patients with degenerative spondylolisthesis. Neurosurgery. 2007;61:981–6.
22. Lim JK, Kim SM. Difference of sagittal spinopelvic alignments between degenerative spondylolisthesis and isthmic spondylolisthesis. J Korean Neurosurg Soc. 2013;53:96–101.

Clinical Evaluation of Pediatric Patient with Spondylolisthesis

4

Matthew E. Oetgen and Laurel C. Blakemore

Introduction

The clinical presentation of pediatric patients with spondylolysis and spondylolisthesis is highly variable. Available literature on the physical features associated with this condition describes a wide range of symptoms and limited correlation of severity of spondylolisthesis with the physical manifestations [1–4]. As such, much of the information concerning the physical exam in pediatric patients with spondylolisthesis is based on commonly held beliefs and anecdotal experience.

Despite the limited documentation in the literature, the clinical evaluation of pediatric patients presenting with spondylolisthesis should follow general principles of examining pediatric patients with spinal deformities. The exam starts with a thorough history of the presenting symptoms, including onset and location with specific attention paid to complaints of back and leg pain, weakness, numbness, or tingling of the lower extremities. Other signs of subtle neurologic compromise should be inquired about including changes in gait, coordination, or stamina, and issues associated with the cauda equine such as bowel or bladder incontinence, urinary retention, and saddle or perineal anesthesia. The examining physician should inquire about aggravating or relieving postures or activities and times of onset, as well as prior therapies which have or have not been beneficial.

The basic elements of the physical exam of the pediatric spine consist of inspection of the back and trunk for overall coronal and sagittal alignment, rotational deformities, and skin abnormalities, such as creases, dimples, hairy patches, and pigment abnormalities. Palpation of the spine is performed to assess for step-offs, usually at the lumbosacral junction, and tenderness, followed by assessment of the overall range of motion of the spine in flexion and extension and rotation. Evaluation of the patient's gait is important, with particular attention paid to the fluidity of gait, abnormalities in the stride length, presence of a crouch posture or toe-walking. A complete neurologic exam is required to assess the strength and sensation of the lower extremities, the deep tendon and abdominal reflexes, and in some cases the rectal tone. Finally, there are some specific tests which are important in the evaluation of the pediatric patient with spondylolisthesis.

A thorough and complete physical exam in these patients is extremely important to assist the

M.E. Oetgen, M.D. (✉)
Department of Orthopaedic Surgery and Sports Medicine, Children's National Medical Center, 111 Michigan Avenue, Washington, DC 20010, USA
e-mail: moetgen@childrensnational.org

L.C. Blakemore, M.D.
Orthopaedics and Rehabilitation, University of Florida College of Medicine, UF Orthopaedics and Sports Medicine Institute, PO Box 112727, Gainesville, FL 32611-2727, USA
e-mail: blakelc@ortho.ufl.edu

A.L. Wollowick and V. Sarwahi (eds.), *Spondylolisthesis: Diagnosis, Non-Surgical Management, and Surgical Techniques*, DOI 10.1007/978-1-4899-7575-1_4,

clinician in deciding on what type of advanced imaging might be appropriate. Additionally, in cases requiring operative management a baseline exam and documentation of the symptoms may guide surgical treatment and is important due to the possibility of complications or symptoms post operatively. In cases of significant deformity with a significant risk of post-operative complications, an independent pre-operative neurologic evaluation by a pediatric neurologist (who is available to evaluate the patient in the post-operative period) can be helpful to ensure all pre-operative symptoms are properly documented.

History

One of the most common complaints in patients with spondylolisthesis is back pain with or without concomitant radicular pain [1, 2, 5–12]. Pain may be insidious in onset and chronic in nature; however, some patients will have a specific event which they can recall which started the symptoms.

The nature of the pain is often dull and chronic with an area of pain identified in a band like pattern over the entire lumbar spine. Hyperextension activities may exacerbate the pain, which is usually activity related and improved with rest. Pain radiating into the posterior aspect of the legs is not uncommon, and usually limited to the upper posterior thigh and buttock region [6]. This can be unilateral or bilateral in nature. It is sometimes difficult to know if this is true radicular pain or an extension of the lumbar pain described above. True radicular pain which radiates past the knee in a specific nerve root distribution is rare, but can be seen in higher grade spondylolisthesis and requires more urgent evaluation.

The incidence of back pain in children with spondylolisthesis is unknown, as many children are asymptomatic. Due to the commonly held association of back pain in the pediatric population with spondylolisthesis, there have been a number of studies examining this link. The number of children presenting with anatomic findings for their back pain in these studies has decreased over the years, but the incidence of spondylolisthesis has remained relatively stable. Turner in 1989 and Bhatia et al. in 2008 demonstrated a decrease in the number of children with identifiable pathology causing back pain, from 50 % in 1989 to about 22 % in 2008; however, the percentage of subjects diagnosed with spondylolysis or spondylolisthesis remained relatively unchanged at 13 % in 1989 and 12 % in 2008 [13, 14]. This suggests a lowered threshold for orthopedic evaluation of back pain in more recent years, rather than a true change in the pathology of pediatric back pain.

In addition to isolated back pain, radicular type pain is reported by pediatric patients with spondylolysis and spondylolisthesis as well. As described above, this radicular pain is usually isolated to the upper buttock and thigh. The incidence of radicular pain, either isolated or in combination with back pain ranges in the literature from 20 to 80 % with the specific dermatomal patterns of radiating pain is usually difficult to determine on exam [1, 8, 9]. The etiology of this nerve root irritation is unknown, but suggested causes include disc herniation associated with the spondylolisthesis, sacral dome or L5 pedicle impingement, neuroforaminal stenosis, or nerve root compression between the sacral ala and the anterior lumbosacral ligaments [6].

Evaluation

The examination begins with an overall evaluation of the posture of the child. In patients with spondylolysis without any spondylolisthesis, there is typically little deviation in the coronal or sagittal alignment of the spine. As the deformity progresses and the spondylolisthesis worsens, the anatomic abnormalities of the spine will lead to distinct physical findings. Some authors have noted that this postural deformity may be the only finding which leads to the initial orthopedic referral [5]. As the spondylolisthesis progresses, the lower portion of the spine (typically the sacrum in an L5 spondylolisthesis) will rotate and become more vertical [15]; this sacral malalignment together with hamstring tightness which develops causes a distinct postural alignment [2, 16]. Children with this deformity are

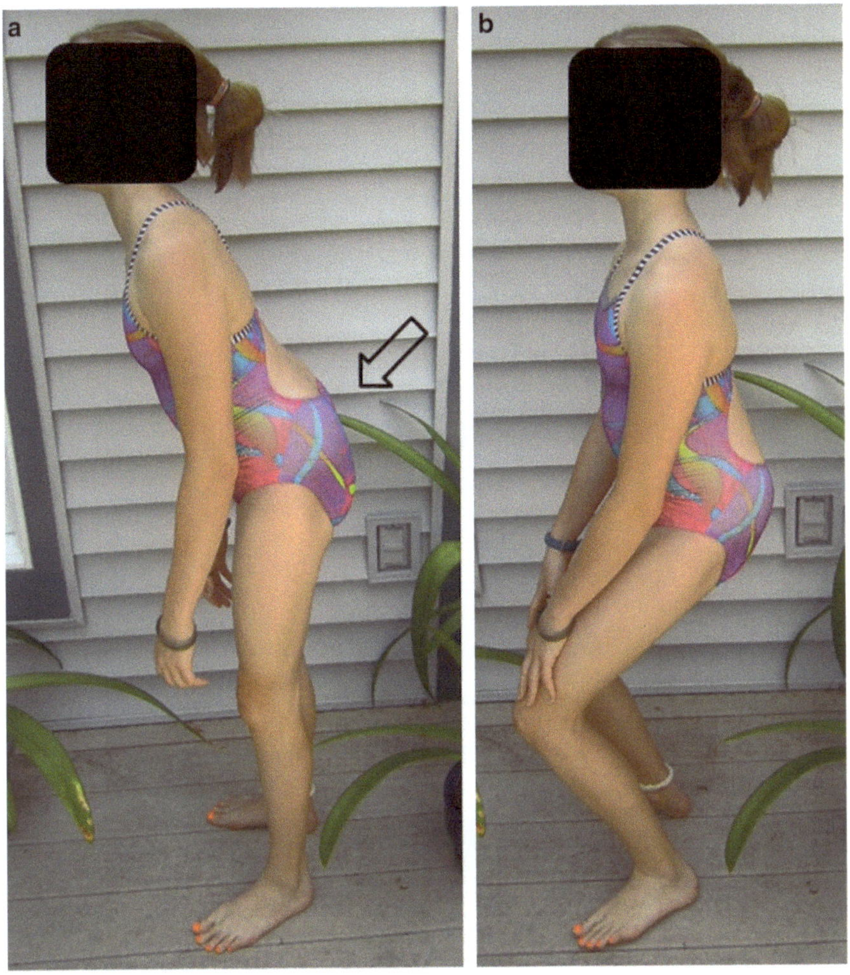

Fig. 4.1 (**a**) Standing sagittal view of a patient with a high grade spondylolisthesis. Notice the flattened buttock (*black arrow*), flattened lumbar lordosis and the positive overall sagittal balance when standing with the knees straight. (**b**) A crouch stance and gait is used to improve the overall sagittal balance due to the spinal imbalance and tight hamstrings

often found to have a prominent and flattened buttock (due to the vertical alignment of the sacrum), flattening of the lumbar lordosis, and a crouched stance with flexion of the hips and knees to keep the overall sagittal alignment in a neutral position (Fig. 4.1a, b). Additionally, as the sacrum becomes more vertical and the lumbar lordosis is flattened, examination of the abdomen may reveal a horizontal abdominal crease above the umbilicus which is caused by the translation of the proximal portion of the spine on the vertical sacrum (Fig. 4.2).

In some cases, when an Adam's forward bend test is performed, scoliosis will be noted in the upper lumbar and thoracic region of the spine. McPhee and O'Brien have described three categories of scoliosis which are associated with spondylolisthesis [17]. The first is idiopathic scoliosis which is unrelated to the spondylolisthesis. The deformity has the typical appearance of thoracic or thoracolumbar idiopathic scoliosis, and is identified in about 5–10 % of patients with spondylolisthesis [2] (Fig. 4.3). The second type of scoliosis is a rotational deviation of the upper

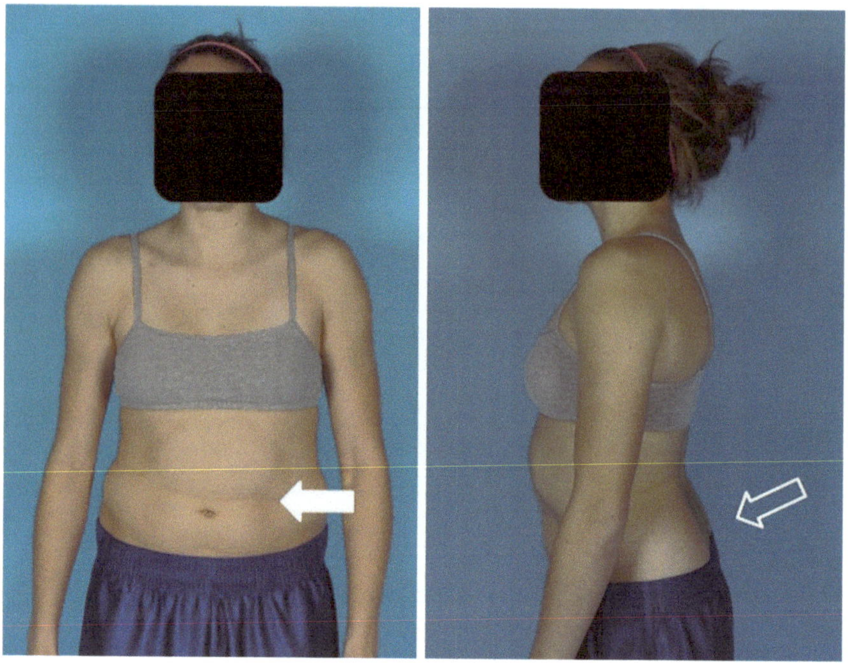

Fig. 4.2 Coronal and sagittal view of an adolescent with a high grade spondylolisthesis. Notice the abdominal crease (*white closed arrow*) and flattening of the lumbar spine and buttock (*white open arrow*)

Fig. 4.3 AP and lateral radiograph showing a grade 1 L5–S1 spondylolisthesis and a 55° idiopathic scoliosis

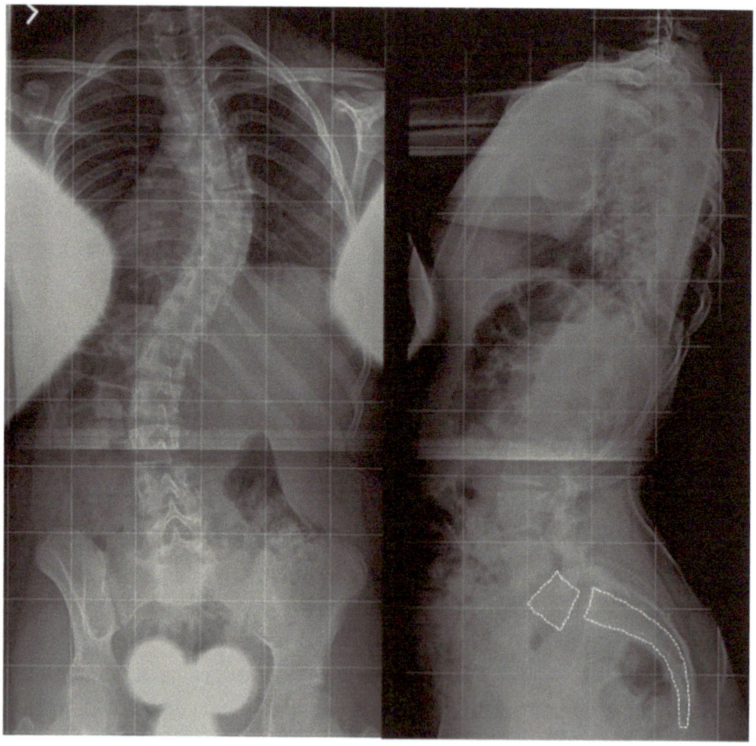

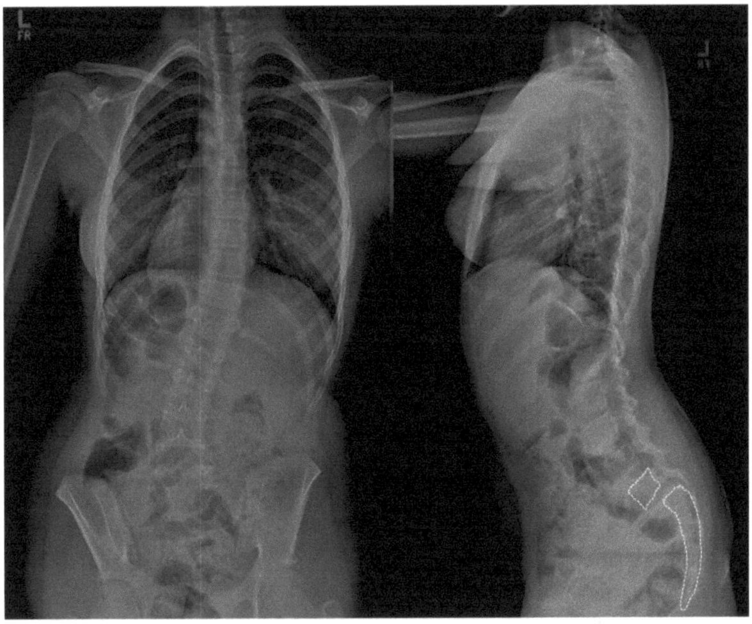

Fig. 4.4 AP and lateral radiograph showing a grade 3 L5–S1 spondylolisthesis and a 25° olisthetic scoliosis

spine due to an asymmetric slippage of the spondylolisthesis, more on one side than the other. In the third category the scoliosis is due to pain or muscle spasm caused by the spondylolisthesis and resultant nerve root irritation. This scoliosis, termed olisthetic scoliosis, has an atypical appearance and is non-structural (Fig. 4.4). Treatment of this third category of scoliosis is often aimed at the spondylolisthesis with subsequent expected resolution of the scoliosis [17].

Palpation

Palpation of the spine in children with spondylolisthesis is typically unremarkable. Pain is usually not exacerbated with palpation of the lumbar spine in these patients, even those reporting back pain. The pain is usually exacerbated with range of motion of the spine, specifically hyperextension. Occasionally in thin patients with high grade spondylolisthesis a step-off is appreciated at the lumbosacral junction, especially when assessed during Adams' forward bend test. This step-off correlates with the prominent posterior elements of the vertebral body immediately caudal to the level of the spondylolisthesis (Fig. 4.5).

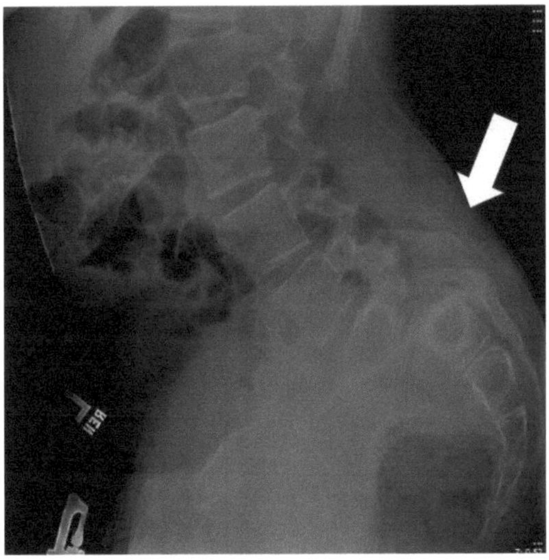

Fig. 4.5 Lateral lumbosacral radiograph demonstrating the prominence of the posterior elements of the sacrum (*white arrow*) caudal to the spondylolisthesis. This area is easily palpated on exam due to prominence

Range of Motion

As is the case with many of the physical findings in a child with spondylolysis or spondylolisthesis, the range of motion of the spine can range from full and unaffected to severely limited.

This motion is somewhat correlated to the degrees of displacement of the spondylolisthesis and the degrees of back pain and nerve root irritation. Flexion of the lumbar spine is typically unencumbered by the anatomic deformity of the spine, but may be limited by associated hamstring tightness. Extension is typically limited by pain in the lumbar spine. The rotation and lateral bending of the spine may also by limited by pain [7].

Tightness of the hamstrings is a classic physical finding associated with pediatric spondylolysis and spondylolisthesis. Originally described by Phalen and Dickson in association with spondylolisthesis, this is found in up to 80 % of symptomatic patients [4]. The etiology of this finding remains unclear. One leading theory is this tightness is due to irritation of the lower lumbar and upper sacral nerve roots which innervate the hamstring muscles and cause muscle spasticity. Some people believe this irritation is from stretching of the nerve roots due to the deformity while others believe it is caused by hypertrophic granulation tissue at the site of the pars defect which impinges on the traversing nerve roots. Others suspect the rotation of the pelvis leads to a mechanical tightness of the hamstrings. No one theory has been shown to be the definitive cause to this point [18, 19].

Gait

Evaluation of the gait of a patient with suspected spondylolisthesis is important. Many of the anatomic abnormalities found can lead to gait alterations. It is most helpful to have the child dressed in shorts, a bathing suit, or a small exam gown so the entire lower extremities and trunk can be evaluated. Shoes and socks are removed and the child is asked to walk back and forth down a long hallway. Often times it is helpful to have the child walk multiple times so different segments of the body can be watched, from the trunk to the pelvis and hip, to the knees and finally the feet. Additionally, in children with spondylolisthesis, it is helpful to evaluate the gait from the front and side of the child to assess both the coronal and sagittal plane.

As discussed above, severe spondylolisthesis typically results in a more vertically oriented sacrum, a forward displacement of the proximal spine and trunk, and tightness of the hamstrings. These deformities will lead to distinct gait abnormalities seen in these patients. In general, patients with significant spondylolisthesis will be found to have a shortened stride length due to the hamstring tightness. In extreme cases, this hamstring tightness and limited stride length can be so severe the child will need to walk sideways to move around effectively. As the spinal deformity, hamstring tightness and sacral malalignment worsen and a crouch alignment becomes more fixed, the child may begin to walk on their tiptoes to compensate for this flexed hip and knee deformity [20].

Neurologic Exam

A detailed neurologic exam is required when evaluating children with spondylolysis and spondylolisthesis. This exam should include documentation of a full lumbar root motor and sensory exam, evaluation of the deep tendon reflexes at the knee and ankle and the abdominal reflexes. Sacral root sensory testing and rectal exam are typically deferred to cases of severe deformity, pre-operative evaluation, and in those patients who complain of bowel or bladder dysfunction.

A complete evaluation of the lower extremity strength and sensation should be completed and documented in a systematic fashion. The typical root levels and exam findings are found in Table 4.1.

Deep tendon reflexes which are noted to be abnormal are often found to be depressed, with complete loss of the ankle jerk reflex in severe cases. This is due to the irritation of the lower motor nerve as it by-passes the deformity near the neural foramina, as opposed to an upper motor nerve irritation, which will more typically cause hyperreflexia. In patients complaining of even subtle bladder dysfunction, formal evaluation with urodynamic studies can identify neurologic issues associated with this finding.

Special Tests

The child being evaluated for spondylolysis or spondylolisthesis often will be found to have significant tightness of the hamstrings. While this is not pathognomonic for this issue, tightness of the hamstrings is often found to some degree in these patients. The most common method to evaluate this issue is to measure the popliteal angle (Fig. 4.6). This is performed with the patient lying supine on the exam table. One leg is gently held down on the table in an extended position by the examiner. The other leg is flexed at the hip and knee. When the hip is held at 90° of flexion, the knee is extended to the maximal amount. The angle subtended by the axis of the thigh and the anterior aspect of the leg is measured and recorded as the popliteal angle. As can be seen with significant tightness of the hamstrings, the leg is unable to be extended very much with the hip held at 90° and the popliteal angle is relatively large. In patients without hamstring tightness, the leg can be fully extended, even with the hip help at 90° of hip flexion.

The Lasegue test, or the straight leg raise test, can also be helpful to distinguish back pain from radicular pain. In this test the child is positioned supine on the examining table (Fig. 4.7). With the contralateral leg gently held in extension on the exam table, the ipsilateral leg is extended at the hip with the knee held in extension. If this maneuver produces pain down the back of the leg to below the knee in a radicular pattern, this is an indication of nerve root irritation. Pain produced in the posterior thigh to the level of the knee is more indicative of irritation of tight hamstrings and does not necessarily due to nerve root irritation.

Finally, the so-called Stork test has been described to assess for pain associated with spondylolysis or spondylolisthesis. This test is performed by having the child balance on one leg, flex at the knee with the opposite leg held off the ground. The patient then hyperextends the lumbar spine (Fig. 4.8). A positive test is one which

Table 4.1 Neurologic examination findings in the lower extremities

Nerve root	Motor distribution	Sensatory distribution	Deep tendon reflex
L1	Iliopsoas (hip flexion)	Anterior hip	None
L2	Hip adductors (hip adduction)	Lateral thigh	None
L3	Quadriceps (knee extension)	Medial thigh and knee	Knee jerk
L4	Tibialis anterior (ankle dorsiflexion)	Medial leg	None
L5	Extension digitorum longus (great toe dorsiflexion)	Lateral leg and great toe	None
S1	Gastroc-soleus complex (ankle plantarflexion)	Lateral foot and toes	Ankle jerk

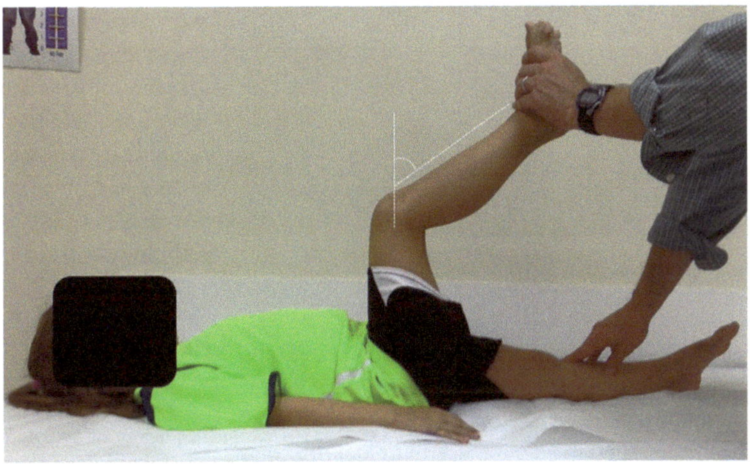

Fig. 4.6 Measurement of the popliteal angle. Angle is measured as shown by the *dotted lines*, 50° in this patient

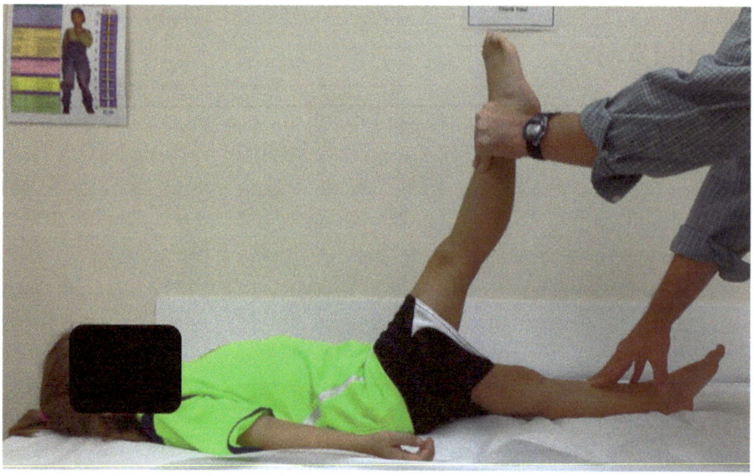

Fig. 4.7 Demonstration of the Lasegue test, or the straight leg raise test

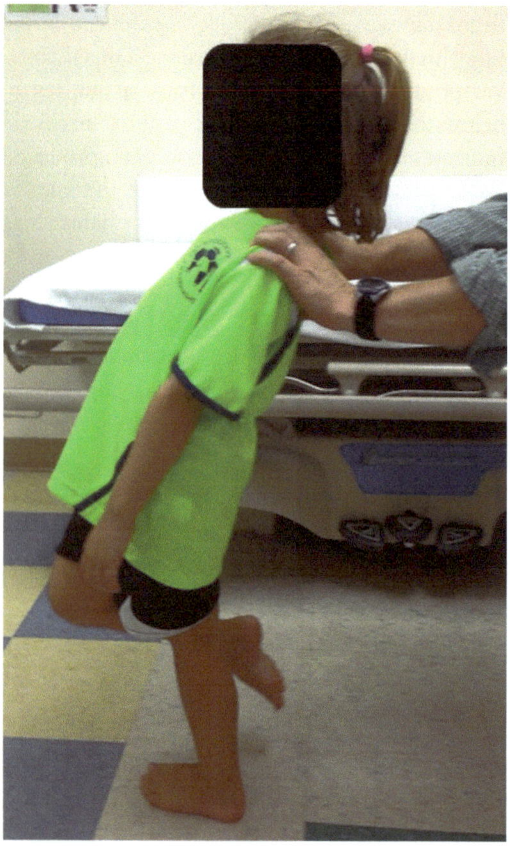

Fig. 4.8 Demonstration of the "Stork" test

exacerbates the back pain. Unilateral symptoms indicate a unilateral pars defect, while bilateral symptoms indicate bilateral defects. This test has been suggested to be quite useful to identify even subtle pars defects [21–23].

Conclusion

Pediatric patients are presenting to the orthopedic surgeons office for evaluation with increasing frequency, and approximately 12 % of those will be diagnosed with spondylolysis or spondylolisthesis. While back pain may be the presenting complaint, occasionally the initial finding is simply spinal deformity or abnormal gait. Reported symptoms may be minimal in the pediatric population with spondylolisthesis, and scoliosis of several types may also be present, so a careful and complete history and physical exam is essential. The exam begins by documenting a thorough history including presenting symptoms, duration, and aggravating or relieving factors. A thorough physical examination including gait assessment and neurologic evaluation is mandatory for the assessment of these children. Complaints or findings of motor weakness, sensory changes, or urologic abnormalities which are identified require further evaluation or imaging. A thorough initial history and physical exam will allow the treating physician to fully assess the impact of the spinal pathology and select appropriate treatment.

References

1. Frennered AK, Danielson BI, Nachemson AL. Natural history of symptomatic isthmic low-grade spondylolisthesis in children and adolescents: a seven-year follow-up study. J Pediatr Orthop. 1991;11:209–13.

2. Hensinger RN. Spondylolysis and spondylolisthesis in children and adolescents. J Bone Joint Surg Am. 1989;71:1098–107.
3. Hu SS, Tribus CB, Diab M, et al. Spondylolisthesis and spondylolysis. J Bone Joint Surg Am. 2008;90: 656–71.
4. Tsirikos AI, Garrido EG. Spondylolysis and spondylolisthesis in children and adolescents. J Bone Joint Surg Br. 2010;92:751–9.
5. Beguiristain JL, Diaz-de-Rada P. Spondylolisthesis in pre-school children. J Pediatr Orthop B. 2004;13 :225–30.
6. Halperin N, Copeliovitch L, Schachner E. Radiating leg pain and positive straight leg raising in spondylolysis in children. J Pediatr Orthop. 1983;3:486–90.
7. Jalanko T, Helenius I, Remes V, et al. Operative treatment of isthmic spondylolisthesis in children: a long-term, retrospective comparative study with matched cohorts. Eur Spine J. 2011;20:766–75.
8. Karampalis C, Grevitt M, Shafafy M, et al. High-grade spondylolisthesis: gradual reduction using Magerl's external fixator followed by circumferential fusion technique and long-term results. Eur Spine J. 2012;21 Suppl 2:S200–6.
9. Muschik M, Zippel H, Perka C. Surgical management of severe spondylolisthesis in children and adolescents. Anterior fusion in situ versus anterior spondylodesis with posterior transpedicular instrumentation and reduction. Spine (Phila Pa 1976). 1997;22:2036–42. discussion 2043.
10. Seitsalo S. Operative and conservative treatment of moderate spondylolisthesis in young patients. J Bone Joint Surg Br. 1990;72:908–13.
11. Seitsalo S, Osterman K, Poussa M, et al. Spondylolisthesis in children under 12 years of age: long-term results of 56 patients treated conservatively or operatively. J Pediatr Orthop. 1988;8:516–21.
12. Sherman FC, Rosenthal RK, Hall JE. Spine fusion for spondylolysis and spondylolisthesis in children. Spine (Phila Pa 1976). 1979;4:59–66.
13. Bhatia NN, Chow G, Timon SJ, et al. Diagnostic modalities for the evaluation of pediatric back pain: a prospective study. J Pediatr Orthop. 2008;28:230–3.
14. Turner PG, Green JH, Galasko CS. Back pain in childhood. Spine (Phila Pa 1976). 1989;14:812–4.
15. Antoniades SB, Hammerberg KW, DeWald RL. Sagittal plane configuration of the sacrum in spondylolisthesis. Spine (Phila Pa 1976). 2000;25:1085–91.
16. Herring JA, Bradford DS. Severe spondylolisthesis. J Pediatr Orthop. 1985;5:737–9.
17. McPhee IB, O'Brien JP. Scoliosis in symptomatic spondylolisthesis. J Bone Joint Surg Br. 1980;62-B: 155–7.
18. Barash HL, Galante JO, Lambert CN, et al. Spondylolisthesis and tight hamstrings. J Bone Joint Surg Am. 1970;52:1319–28.
19. Harnach ZG, Gotfryd O, Baudysova J. Spondylolisthesis with hamstring spasticity. A case report. J Bone Joint Surg Am. 1966;48:878–82.
20. Shelokov A, Haideri N, Roach J. Residual gait abnormalities in surgically treated spondylolisthesis. Spine (Phila Pa 1976). 1993;18:2201–5.
21. Cassidy RC, Shaffer WO, Johnson DL. Spondylolysis and spondylolisthesis in the athlete. Orthopedics. 2005;28:1331–3.
22. Gurd DP. Back pain in the young athlete. Sports Med Arthrosc. 2011;19:7–16.
23. Ralston S, Weir M. Suspecting lumbar spondylolysis in adolescent low back pain. Clin Pediatr (Phila). 1998;37:287–93.

Clinical Evaluation of Adult Patient with Spondylolisthesis

5

Gregory D. Schroeder and Alpesh A. Patel

Introduction

Spondylolisthesis is defined as the translation of one vertebra in relation to the adjacent level and is commonly referenced as an anterolisthesis of the cranial segment on the caudal segment. Wiltse initially classified spondylolisthesis into five different types: dysplastic, isthmic, degenerative, traumatic, and pathologic [1]. Since the initial publication, a sixth type, post-surgical has been added. This chapter will focus on the evaluation of adult patients with either isthmic or degenerative spondylolisthesis.

Isthmic Spondylolisthesis

Introduction

Classically, it has been thought that isthmic spondylolisthesis is caused by repeated impaction of the inferior articular process of the cephalad vertebra onto the pars interarticularis of the caudal vertebra [2, 3]. This repetitive microtrauma can lead to a stress fracture and, eventually, a defect in the pars interarticularis. This mechanism has been supported by the correlation of isthmic spondylolisthesis and hyperextension activities [4, 5]. More recently, however, additional etiologies, such as increased shear stress across the par interarticularis, related to pelvic morphology and lumbar lordosis, have also been postulated [6, 7].

Isthmic spondylolisthesis has been divided into three subtypes: In subtype A, there is a stress fracture leading to a complete pars defect; in subtype B, the pars is intact but elongated due to the healing of micro fractures; and in subtype C, the rarest of all, there is an acute pars fracture [8–10]. Spondylolisthesis is most commonly classified according to the Meyerding grading system, which is based on the amount of translation of the cephalad vertebra relative to the caudal vertebra [11]. Translation less than 25 % is grade one; 26–50 % is grade two; 51–75 % is grade three; 76–100 % is grade four; and more than 100 % (spondyloptosis) is grade five [11] (Fig. 5.1). This classification can be further simplified by grouping grades one and two together as low grade, and grouping grades three, four, and five together as high grade [12].

In a classic study, Frederickson et al. [13] prospectively followed 500 first grade students for 45 years and found that the prevalence of spondylolysis in adults was 5.4 % whereas the prevalence of isthmic spondylolisthesis was 4 %. More recent literature utilizing advanced imaging has reported a significantly higher incidence of

G.D. Schroeder, M.D. • A.A. Patel, M.D. (✉)
Department of Orthopaedic Surgery, Northwestern Medical Faculty Foundation, 676 N. Saint Clair, Suite 1350, Chicago, IL 60611, USA
e-mail: gregdschroeder@gmail.com; alpesh.patel@nmff.org

A.L. Wollowick and V. Sarwahi (eds.), *Spondylolisthesis: Diagnosis, Non-Surgical Management, and Surgical Techniques*, DOI 10.1007/978-1-4899-7575-1_5,

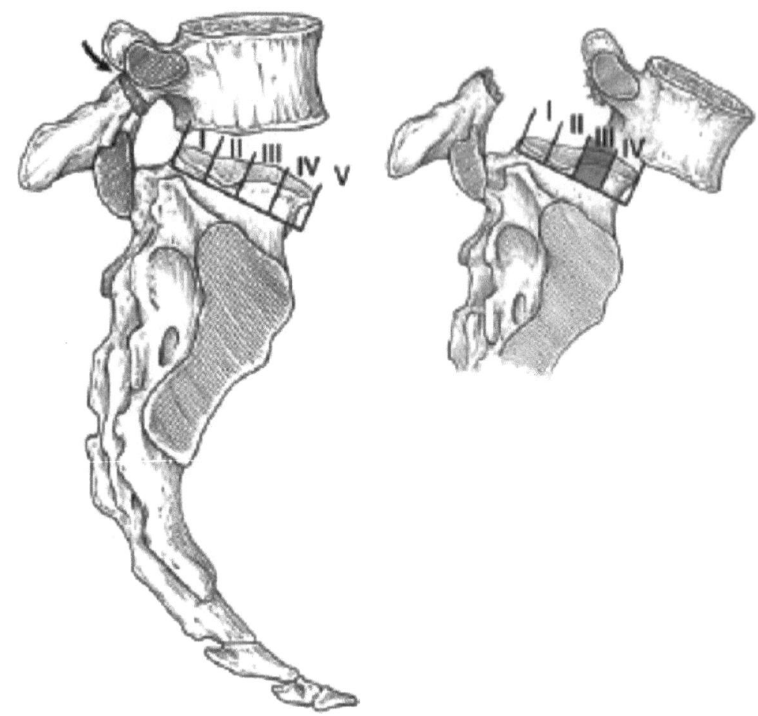

Fig. 5.1 The Meyerding grading scale for the severity of a slip is determined by dividing the superior endplate of the caudal vertebra in quartiles, and measuring the location of the posterior edge of the cephalad vertebra. [© 2009 American Academy of Orthopaedic Surgeons. Adapted from the Journal of the American Academy of Orthopaedic Surgeons, Volume 17(1), pp. 609-617 with permission.]

isthmic spondylolisthesis. In a cross-sectional study of 188 patients in the Framingham Heart Study group, Kalichman et al. [14] reported an 8.2 % prevalence of isthmic spondylolisthesis on a CT scan. While the prevalence varies in the literature, L5/S1 is consistently the most common level in all studies [14, 15].

Both gender and race affect the prevalence of isthmic spondylolisthesis. It is about twice as common in males, however, the slip progression may be higher in females [13]. Additionally, African Americans are less frequently affected (2.8 and 1.1 % in males and females, respectively), whereas the prevalence may be as high as 50 % in the Inuit population [16, 17].

Patient History

The first step to evaluating a patient with a possible isthmic spondylolisthesis is to obtain a complete history of the symptoms. Because isthmic spondylolisthesis often starts during adolescence, it is not uncommon for adults to have prolonged episodic symptoms with intervening pain-free intervals. Additionally, a complete social history dating back to athletic activities during adolescence is relevant, as hyperextension activities such as ballet, gymnastics, baseball, and football are associated with isthmic spondylolisthesis [4, 5].

Low Back Pain

It is critical to differentiate between patients with predominately low back pain and patients with neurogenic leg pain. While patients with isthmic spondylolisthesis may present with low back pain, multiple studies have demonstrated that there is not an increased risk of low back pain in patients with an isthmic spondylolisthesis compared to the general population [13–15]. In a 45-year natural history study of patients with isthmic spondylolisthesis, the diagnosis—regardless of slip progression—did not significantly increase the risk of low back pain [15]. More recently, this has been corroborated by Kalichman et al. [14], who also found no significant increase in the risk of low back pain for patients with isthmic spondylolisthesis.

While the majority of patients with an isthmic spondylolisthesis do not have low back pain, Saraste [18, 19] has reported that patients with an isthmic spondylolisthesis at L4/5 have both an increased frequency and intensity of low back symptoms compared to patients with an L5/S1 slip. He also reported patients with translation greater than 25 % may be at an increased risk for low back pain [18, 19].

Because the majority of individuals with isthmic spondylolisthesis do not have back pain, it is vital to obtain as much information about the pain as possible, including any inciting event, the exact location of the pain, the chronicity of the pain, exacerbating and alleviating factors, and any neurologic symptoms. When patients do have low back pain, it is often worsened with activity and relieved by rest [8]. Other possible etiologies for low back pain in the setting of isthmic spondylolisthesis include chronic muscle strains from lumbar hyperlordosis, sagittal malalignment, and referred pain from degenerative disks or facet joints [15, 19, 20].

Neurologic Symptoms

For patients that present predominantly with leg pain, a thorough investigation of neurologic symptoms is critical. This should include the location, quality and severity of leg pain, as well as any aggravating or alleviating factors. The patient should be asked about numbness, paresthesias, weakness, and bowel and bladder function.

While neurologic symptoms are rare (2 %) at the initial presentation of an isthmic spondylolisthesis in an adolescent, Saraste reported that over the next 29 years, up to 55 % of adults with isthmic spondylolisthesis may develop at least transient radiculopathy, and 16 % of patients will report daily radicular symptoms [19]. These symptoms often occur within the exiting nerve root's distribution due to impingement of the root in the foramen by either a hypertrophic fibrocartilaginous mass (Gill lesion) at the site of the pars interarticularis defect, or vertebral end plate osteophytes. Additionally, symptoms may be caused by nerve root traction from static or dynamic listhesis [21, 22]. Rarely, in patients with a minimum of 20 % translation, unilateral or bilateral compression of the L5 nerve root can occur between an abnormally large transverse process and the sacral ala [23].

Other neurologic presentations are rare, but severe neurologic symptoms such as cauda equina syndrome can occur [10]. These severe neurologic injuries may be more common in patients with a high-grade spondylolisthesis and an elongated, but intact (subtype B), pars interarticularis [20].

Physical Exam

A full spine and neurologic exam should be completed including gait analysis, range of motion, palpation, manual motor testing, sensory testing, reflex testing, and provocative nerve tests. Often the patient will have paraspinal tenderness, and there may be a step-off at the spinous process above the slip [8, 20]. Patients will often have decreased flexion due to paraspinal muscle spasm as well as worsening pain with extension of the spine [8, 20]. In patients with high-grade slips, the patient may present with trunk shortening, tight hamstrings, hyperlordosis, and sagittal imbalance.

The motor strength examination is commonly normal [24]. If the patient is having radicular symptoms, there may be weakness in the distribution of the exiting nerve root. Most commonly this will be weakness in the extensor hallucis longus secondary to L5 compression [24]. Similarly to the motor exam, the sensory exam is often normal, but there may be decreased sensation in the exiting nerve root's dermatome [24]. Even in patients with radicular pain, the straight leg raise test is often negative [24]. Reflexes should be equal bilaterally and may be diminished [24], and the patient should have no upper motor neuron signs (hyper-reflexia, clonus, babinksi). All patients should undergo a full hip examination as well to ensure that the low back and leg pain does not originate from the hip.

Imaging

Diagnosis

All patients who are being evaluated for possible spondylolisthesis should undergo standard upright AP and lateral radiographs of the lumbar spine.

Adult isthmic spondylolisthesis is diagnosed by visualization of a defect or a lengthening of the pars interarticularis as well as the translation of the cephalad vertebra on a lateral radiograph.

Traditionally, oblique radiographs have been utilized to better evaluate the pars interarticularis. What is seen on these radiographs is known as the "Scotty dog" profile—the superior articular process is the ear, the inferior articular process is the front limb, and the pars interarticularis is the neck connecting the superior and inferior process. The defect is often referred to as either the collar or a broken neck [9]. However, a recent high quality study (Level I evidence) by Beck et al. [25] demonstrated that oblique views do not increase the sensitivity or specificity in identifying spondylolysis.

Along with standard upright AP and lateral films, some authors advocate for both upright and supine lateral radiographs or flexion and extension radiographs in an effort to identify instability [9, 26]. Additionally, full-length radiographs are critical to identifying any deformity that may be associated with a high-grade spondylolisthesis. These films should also include the femoral heads, as they are the crucial landmarks for many lumbo-pelvic measurements.

Once the diagnosis of adult isthmic spondylolisthesis has been made, multiple different measurements have been described. Three broad categories of measurements include lumbosacral analysis, spinopelvic analysis, and global sagittal balance.

Lumbosacral Analysis

Level and Degree of Slip

The level of the spondylolisthesis is important, as it will help with the clinical presentation as well as the future progression. Neurologic symptoms, when present, often occur due to compression of the exiting nerve root, and it is important to correlate the symptoms with the imaging. While L5/S1 is the most common location for an isthmic spondylolisthesis, an L4/5 isthmic spondylolisthesis is a significant risk factor for slip progression and symptoms [19, 27]. Additionally the percent of slip at initial diagnosis is one of the most important factors in predicting future progression. In a 14.3-year follow-up of 272 patients, the only predictor of slip progression was the amount of slip at initial diagnosis; patients with an initial slip greater than 20 % have a significantly increased risk of progression [28].

Lumbosacral Angle

The lumbosacral angle, or the slip angle, is a measurement of the sagittal alignment of L5 and S1. There are multiple descriptions of how to calculate this value. It can be calculated by measuring the angle produced by a line parallel to the inferior end plate of L5 and one perpendicular to the posterior aspect of the S1 body; [26] or it can be calculated using the angle produced by lines along the inferior end plate of L5 and the sacral end plate [29]. However, caution is warranted when measuring the inferior L5 end plate, as it can be dysplastic and, therefore, distorted, in spondylolisthesis [30]. Unfortunately, while much of the literature emphasizes the slip angle, it has not been found to be of prognostic value for clinical symptoms or slip progression [15, 28] (Fig. 5.2).

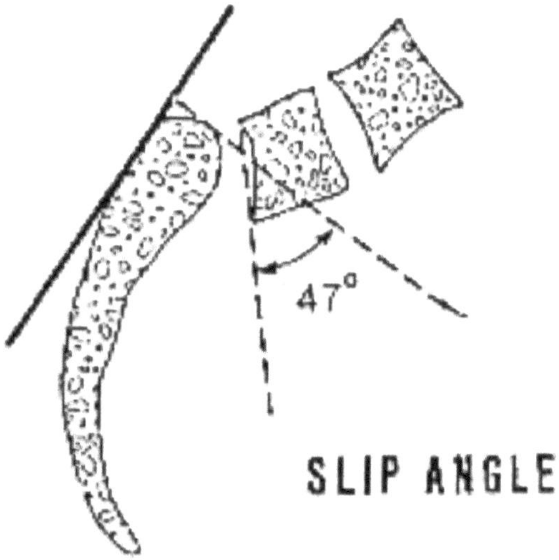

Fig. 5.2 Measurement of the slip angle is calculated by measuring the angle formed by a line parallel to the inferior end plate of L5 and one perpendicular to the posterior aspect of the S1 body. [Reprinted from Beutler WJ, Fredrickson BE, Murtland A, Sweeney CA, Grant WD, Baker D. The natural history of spondylolysis and spondylolisthesis: 45-year follow-up evaluation. Spine (Phila Pa 1976). May 15 2003;28(10):1027-1035; discussion 1035. With permission from Lippincott Williams & Wilkins]

Lumbar Index

The lumbar index is a measurement designed to quantify the change in the shape (i.e., dysplasia) of the L5 vertebral body from a square to a trapezoid in patients with isthmic spondylolisthesis. The lumbar index is calculated by dividing the height of the posterior vertebral body of L5 by the height of the anterior vertebral body of L5 [26, 31]. The average lumbar index in patients with isthmic spondylolisthesis ranges between 0.70 and 0.76; patients without an isthmic spondylolisthesis have a lumbar index around 0.90 [1, 30–32]. In patients in adolescence and early adulthood, the lumbar index has not been found to have any prognostic value for slip progression, but at a 45-year follow-up, Beutler et al. found a lower lumbar index was associated with an increased slip progression [15, 28] (Fig. 5.3).

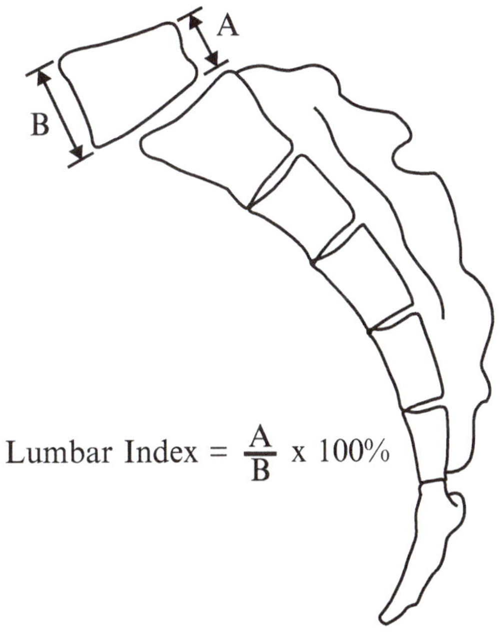

Fig. 5.3 The lumbar index is calculated by dividing the height of the posterior vertebral body of L5 by the height of the anterior vertebral body of L5. [Reprinted from Beutler WJ, Fredrickson BE, Murtland A, Sweeney CA, Grant WD, Baker D. The natural history of spondylolysis and spondylolisthesis: 45-year follow-up evaluation. Spine (Phila Pa 1976). May 15 2003;28(10):1027-1035; discussion 1035. With permission from Lippincott Williams & Wilkins]

Sacral Inclination

Sacral inclination is a measure of the vertical orientation of the sacrum. It is calculated by measuring the angle formed by a line parallel to the posterior S1 vertebral body, and a line perpendicular to the floor [26]. While often reported, there is no evidence that sacral inclination affects slip progression or clinical symptoms. It is, however, related to pelvic incidence and pelvic tilt. With that relationship, sacral inclination (also called sacral slope) may have a role in the development of isthmic spondylolisthesis as well as sagittal balance (Fig. 5.4).

Sacral Rounding

Sacral rounding is a change to the sacral morphology (i.e., dysplasia) leading to a more rounded or dome shape. It is graded zero to three, with zero having no sacral rounding, one having less than 33 % sacral rounding, two having between 33 and 66 %, and three being more than 66 % [26]. While there has been no definitive link to the amount of sacral rounding and slip progression [28], in a case series of 27 patients with spondyloloptosis, all patients had significant sacral rounding [33] (Fig. 5.5).

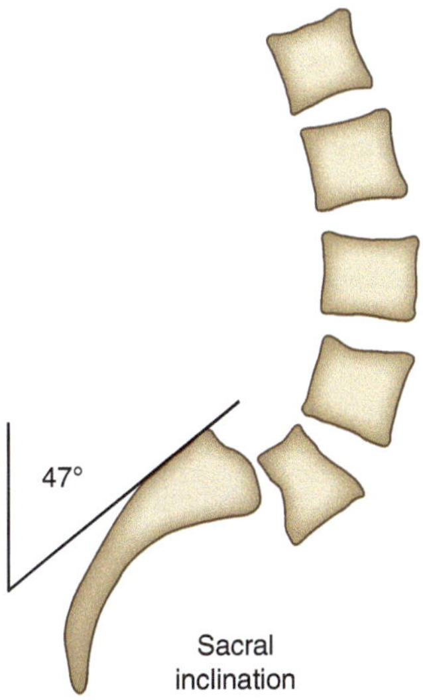

Fig. 5.4 Sacral inclination is a measure of the vertical orientation of the sacrum. It is calculated by measuring the angle formed by a line parallel to the posterior S1 vertebral body, and a line perpendicular to the floor

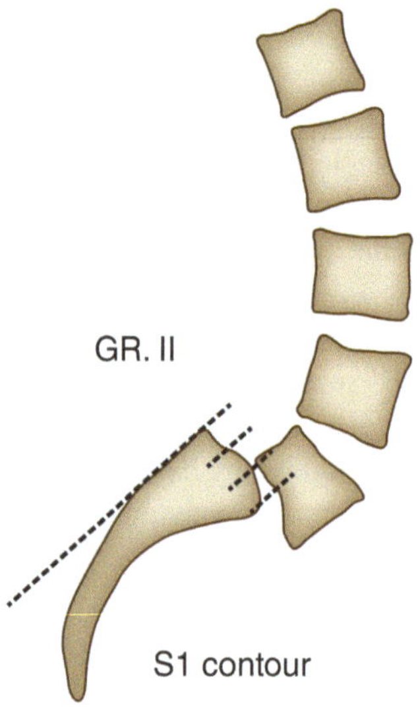

Fig. 5.5 Sacral rounding is a change to the sacral morphology leading to a more rounded shape

Spina Bifida Occulta

Thirty percent of adult patients with isthmic spondylolisthesis have spina bifida occulta [13], and while it is more common in severe slips, it does not increase the risk of slip progression [28].

Spinopelvic Analysis and Sagittal Balance

While traditionally radiographic measurements for isthmic spondylolisthesis have focused almost entirely on the lumbar vertebrae and the sacrum, recent literature has focused on the importance of pelvic morphology and global sagittal alignment, as these measurements are closely related to slip progression and health-related quality of life outcome measures [34–38].

Pelvic Incidence, Sacral Slope and Pelvic Tilt

Duval-Beaupère et al. [39] initially described pelvic incidence in 1992 as an angle formed by a line drawn from the center of the sacral end plate to the center of the femoral head, and a line drawn through the center of the sacral end plate that is perpendicular to the end plate. The average pelvic incidence in adults is 52°, with a normal range for men of 53.2° ± 7.0° and 48.7° ± 7.0° for women [40].

Sacral slope is the angle created by a horizontal line and a line drawn down the sacral end plate [41]. The average sacral slope is 39.4° ± 9.3° [35]. The pelvic tilt is the angle formed by a line that runs from the center of the sacral end plate to the center of the femoral head and a vertical line through the center of the femoral head. The average pelvic tilt is 12.3° ± 5.9° [35], and an increase in pelvic tilt correlates to a retroverted pelvis.

Due to the geometric relationships of these measures, the pelvic incidence is the sum of the sacral slope and the pelvic tilt, and while the overall pelvic incidence remains constant in adulthood, the sacral slope and pelvic tilt change based on the position of the pelvis [41, 42] (Fig. 5.6). The pelvic incidence is therefore a measure of pelvic morphology, while pelvic tilt and sacral slope are measures of pelvic orientation.

Pelvic incidence is correlated strongly to isthmic spondylolisthesis and is significantly higher in patients with both low-grade (68.5°) and high-grade (79.0°) slips compared to controls. Additionally, patients with a high-grade slip have a significantly higher pelvic incidence than those with a low-grade slip [40]. With this relationship being better understood, multiple authors have discussed the possibility of two different mechanisms for isthmic spondylolisthesis depending on the pelvic incidence. Patients with an increased pelvic incidence have more shear stress across the pars interarticularis resulting in the primary mechanism of isthmic spondylolisthesis in this population. Comparatively, patients with a low pelvic incidence may be predisposed to impingement of the posterior elements leading to repeated microtrauma [6, 7]. However there has been no literature to date that can definitively show any causality between pelvic incidence and isthmic spondylolisthesis [7]. Additionally, while there is a correlation between high-grade slips and increased pelvic incidence, there is no evidence that an increased pelvic incidence increases the risk of slip progression after initial diagnosis [43].

Global Sagittal Balance

An abundance of recent literature has established the importance of the global sagittal balance in adult spinal deformity patients. These patients have significantly better health-related quality of life outcomes if normal sagittal balance is maintained [36, 37, 44, 45]. Patients with low-grade

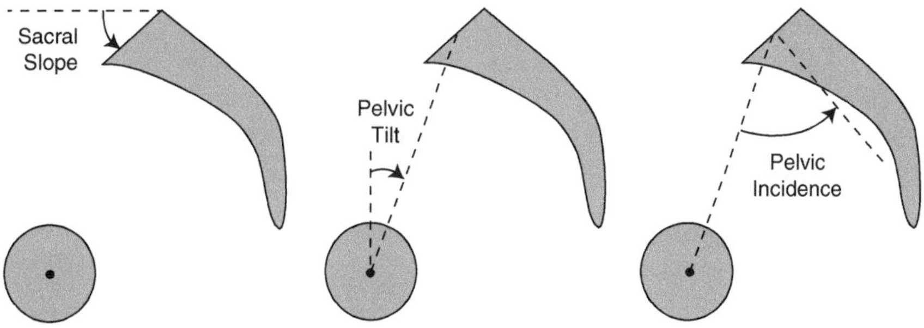

Fig. 5.6 The pelvic incidence is the sum of the sacral slope and the pelvic tilt. The sacral slope is the angle created by a horizontal line and a line drawn down the sacral end plate. The pelvic tilt is the angle formed by a line from the center of the sacral end plate to the center of the femoral head and a vertical line through the center of the femoral head. The pelvic incidence is the angle formed by a line drawn from the center of the sacral end plate to the center of the femoral head, and a line drawn through the center of the sacral end plate that is perpendicular to the end plate. [Reprinted from Schwab F, Patel A, Ungar B, Farcy JP, Lafage V. Adult spinal deformity-postoperative standing imbalance: how much can you tolerate? An overview of key parameters in assessing alignment and planning corrective surgery. Spine (Phila Pa 1976). Dec 1 2010;35(25):2224-2231. With permission from Lippincott Williams & Wilkins]

isthmic spondylolisthesis are typically not at an increased risk of sagittal malalignment [46, 47], however, patients with a high-grade slip are at an increased risk of global sagittal malalignment [48, 49].

Pelvic incidence correlates the plane of the sacral endplate to the axis of rotation of the femoral head, and since the pelvic incidence is fixed, the pelvis and spine adapt to balance the trunk in the upright position [7]. In patients with a high-grade slip and sagittal imbalance, balance is restored initially through an increase in lumbar lordosis with a corresponding linear increase in sacral slope. Additional balance is achieved through an increase in pelvic tilt leading to a retroverted pelvis [35, 38, 41, 48, 50] (Fig. 5.7). When attempting to evaluate the global sagittal balance, multiple metrics must be used: the sagittal vertical axis (SVA) should be less than 50 mm; the pelvic tilt should be less than 20°; and a patient's lumbar lordosis should be within 9° of the pelvic incidence [36, 38] (Fig. 5.8).

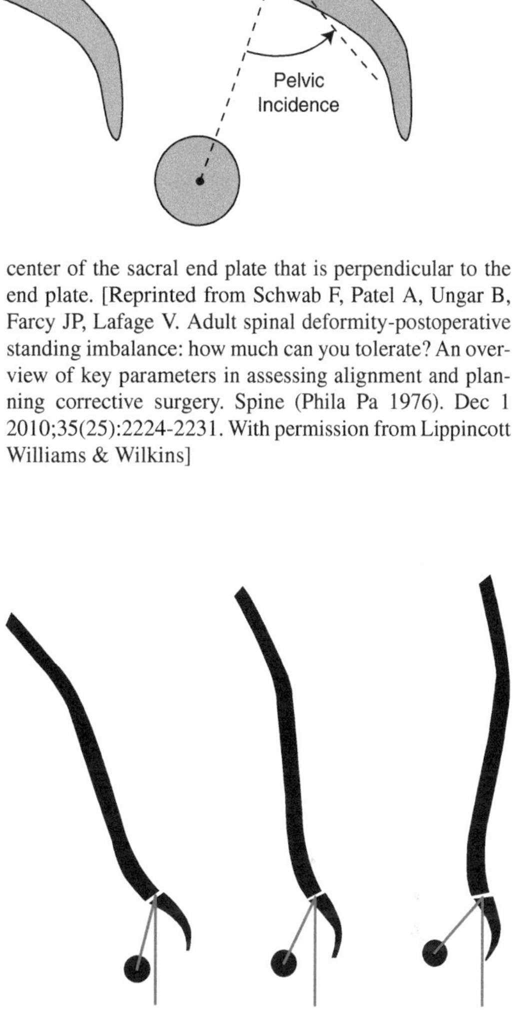

Fig. 5.7 In the drawing on the left, the patient has a positive SVA and no pelvic retroversion. In the drawing in the middle, the patient has decreased the SVA through increasing pelvic retroversion, and the drawing on the right demonstrates how significant pelvic retroversion can normalize the SVA. [Reprinted from Schwab F, Patel A, Ungar B, Farcy JP, Lafage V. Adult spinal deformity-postoperative standing imbalance: how much can you tolerate? An overview of key parameters in assessing alignment and planning corrective surgery. Spine (Phila Pa 1976). Dec 1 2010;35(25):2224-2231. With permission from Lippincott Williams & Wilkins]

It is important not to focus only on one of these values in isolation. While Harroud et al. [45] found a significant decrease in health-related quality of life measurements in patients with a high-grade spondylolisthesis whose SVA fell anterior to the center of the hip, some patients may achieve a balanced SVA by severely retroverting the pelvis. Lafage et al. [36] established that patients with an SVA less than 50 mm and a pelvic tilt less than 25° have better health-related quality of life measurements, compared to patients with either an SVA less than 50 mm or patients with a pelvic tilt less than 25°.

In an effort to incorporate a patient's spinopelvic parameters and global balance into the spondylolisthesis classification system, the Spinal Deformity Study Group has developed a new classification based on the degree of slip, the pelvic incidence, and the sagittal balance [7] (Fig. 5.9).

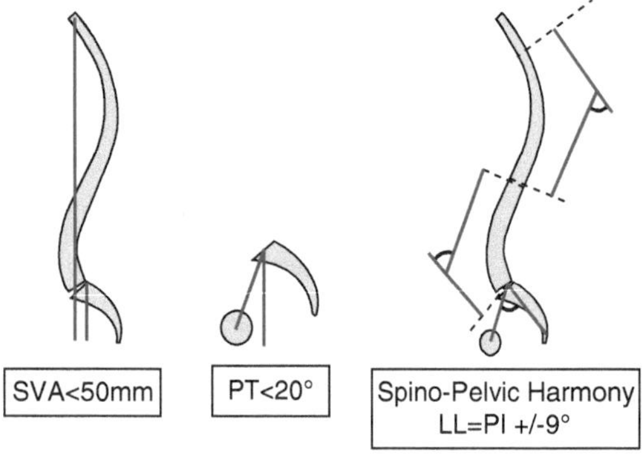

Fig. 5.8 When attempting to evaluate the global sagittal balance, multiple metrics must be used including: the sagittal vertical axis (*SVA*) should be less than 50 mm; the pelvic tilt should be less than 20°, and a patient's lumbar lordosis should be within 9° of the pelvic incidence. [Reprinted from Schwab F, Patel A, Ungar B, Farcy JP, Lafage V. Adult spinal deformity-postoperative standing imbalance: how much can you tolerate? An overview of key parameters in assessing alignment and planning corrective surgery. Spine (Phila Pa 1976). Dec 1 2010;35(25):2224-2231. With permission from Lippincott Williams & Wilkins]

Advanced Imaging

Once the diagnosis has been made, patients with neurologic symptoms can undergo an MRI to evaluate for nerve root compression. If the patient is unable to undergo an MRI, a CT myelogram can help identify possible areas of nerve compression.

Degenerative Spondylolisthesis

Introduction

There are multiple important differences when comparing degenerative spondylolisthesis to isthmic spondylolisthesis. The most obvious is that the posterior arch remains intact in degenerative spondylolisthesis. Another key difference is the natural history of degenerative spondylolisthesis. Kirkaldy-Willis described three phases of degenerative spondylolisthesis. In the dysfunction stage, there is minimal anatomical change. In the instability phase, there is disc height collapse, bulging of the annulus fibrosis, laxity of the facet capsules, and articular cartilage deterioration which leads to increased abnormal motion. Lastly, the third stage is restabilization. In this stage fibrosis in

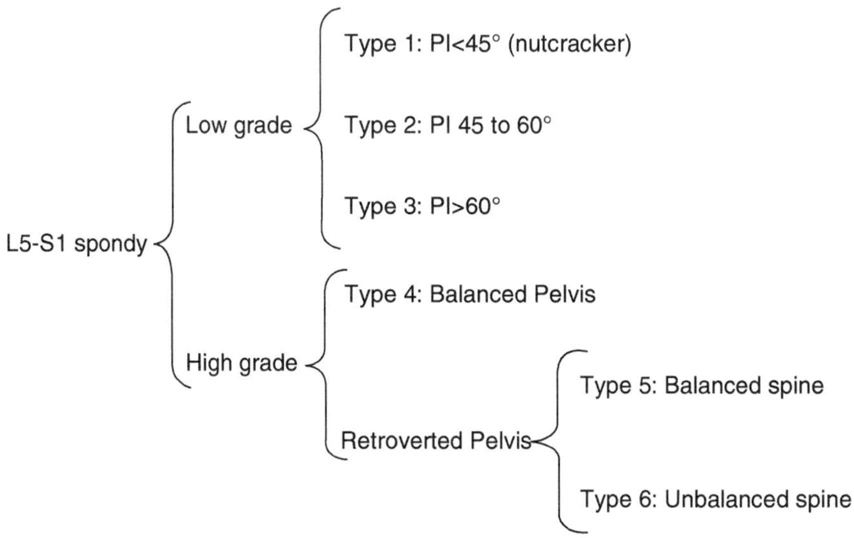

Fig. 5.9 The Spinal Deformity Study Group breaks down isthmic spondylolisthesis into six categories based on the severity of the slip, the total pelvic incidence and the overall sagittal balance. [Reprinted from Labelle H, Mac-Thiong JM, Roussouly P. Spino-pelvic sagittal balance of spondylolisthesis: a review and classification. Eur Spine J. Sep 2011;20 Suppl 5:641-646. With permission from Springer Verlag.]

the posterior joints and osteophyte formation stabilizes the segment [51].

A third key difference is that most common level to develop a degenerative spondylolisthesis is L4/5, and this is thought to be due to the sagittal alignment of the L4/5 facets and the more coronal alignment of the L5/S1 facets [14, 52]. Additionally, as one would expect in a degenerative condition, the onset begins later in life, with most patients being diagnosed above the age of 50 years [14, 53, 54].

The epidemiology of degenerative spondylolisthesis also is quite different when compared to isthmic spondylolisthesis. In a cross-sectional epidemiological survey of more than 4,000 patients, Jacobsen et al. [54] found the prevalence in men is 2.7 % and the prevalence in women is 8.4 %. The increased prevalence in women may be due to an elevated expression of estrogen receptors in the facet joints cartilage [55]; alternatively, other authors have postulated that the increased prevalence in females may be due to an increased ligamentous laxity [56]. Race also affects the prevalence, however unlike in isthmic spondylolisthesis, it is more common in patients of African decent than patients of European decent [53].

Patient History

When evaluating a patient for a degenerative lumbar condition, it is important to obtain a complete medical and social history along with a complete history of the current problem. While there has been no significant link established between heavy lifting or smoking and the development of degenerative spondylolisthesis, an increased BMI has been associated with degenerative spondylolisthesis [54]. Additionally, while comorbidities such as smoking and diabetes have not demonstrated involvement in the pathogenesis of degenerative spondylolisthesis, these will place the patient at an increased risk of vascular claudication: a source of pain similar to neurogenic claudication.

Low Back Pain

Classically, low back pain has been attributed to degenerative spondylolisthesis [57, 58], and it has been described as mechanical in origin. Often it can be exacerbated by hyperextension as well as rising from a seated position [59], as opposed to discogenic low back pain, which may be worsened by forward bending [57, 58]. However, recent literature has questioned the association of low back pain with degenerative spondylolisthesis. Twenty-three patients with a degenerative spondylolisthesis were identified in a cross-sectional study of 188 patients, and the patients with a degenerative slip did not report a significant increase in low back pain [14]. Additionally, when low back pain from degenerative spondylolisthesis does occur, it is likely transient in nature as osteoarthritic changes stabilize the slip. Matsunaga et al. reported 10-year follow-up data on 145 patients who presented with a symptomatic degenerative spondylolisthesis and underwent non-operative treatment. He found that 77 % of the patients with isolated low back pain without neurologic symptoms reported improvement with conservative care. The average length of an acute low back pain exacerbation was 3.2 months, and the frequency decreased over time. The decrease in symptoms was directly related to a decrease in intervertebral disc height [60].

Neurogenic Claudication and Radiculopathy

It is crucial to identify patients who have neurologic symptoms, as the presence or absence of neurologic symptoms greatly affects the natural history as well as proposed treatment. In the aforementioned study, Matsunaga et al. demonstrated good results for conservative care for patients with isolated low back pain. However, 83 % of patients who presented with neurologic symptoms, such as neurogenic claudication, had progressive worsening of their symptoms [60].

Neurogenic claudication is leg pain associated with walking, and is one of the classic findings of patients with lumbar spinal stenosis [61]. In patients with a degenerative spondylolisthesis, the stenosis may be due to the vertebral slippage, as well as hypertrophy of the ligamentum flavum and hypertrophic facets [58]. Patients often complain of pain in buttocks as well as the proximal thigh that can be accompanied by numbness, tingling, and weakness in the legs [58]. Pain is the most sensitive symptom with 94 % of patients with spinal stenosis reporting pain. While numbness (63 %) and weakness (43 %) are common, the absence of these symptoms does not preclude the diagnosis of spinal stenosis [62].

Importantly neurogenic claudication must be differentiated from vascular claudication. Pain from vascular claudication is brought on by walking, but not by prolonged standing; in contrast, prolonged standing can incite pain due to neurogenic claudication. Additionally, pain from vascular claudication is not affected by the position of the lumbar spine, but neurogenic claudication can often be relieved by lumbar flexion (i.e., the shopping cart sign). Because of the position of the lumbar spine, riding a bicycle often does not elicit pain due to neurogenic claudication, but it does cause pain from vascular claudication [58]. This clinical finding has been validated by Inufusa et al. [63] who demonstrated that nerve root compression is significantly worse in lumbar extension compared to flexion in a cadaveric model. Finally, patients with prolonged symptoms may also present with hip flexion contractures, due to prolonged periods in the forward flexed position [57].

An isolated radicular presentation is less common in patients with lumbar stenosis. While 88 % of patients with spinal stenosis have pain distal to the buttocks, only about 56 % have pain distal to the knee [62]. When it does occur, it is most commonly due to compression of the L5 nerve root in the lateral recess [57]. Compression of the L5 nerve root often causes pain and sometimes numbness in the posterolateral thigh continuing to the lateral calf and possibly into the dorsum of the foot [59]. An L5 radiculopathy can also lead to weakness in the extensor hallucis longus. While less common, a degenerative spondylolisthesis can lead to L4 foraminal stenosis causing pain and numbness along the anterior thigh and continuing past the knee to the anterior shin [59], as well as weakness with ankle dorsiflexion.

Physical Exam

A full spine and neurologic exam should be completed including gait analysis, range of motion, palpation, manual motor testing, sensory testing, reflex testing and provocative nerve tests. Often the patient will have paraspinal tenderness, and palpation may or may not demonstrate and obvious palpable step-off [57]. Compared to patients with isthmic spondylolisthesis, patients with degenerative spondylolisthesis often maintain their lumbar range of motion, and in some cases patients may be hypermobile [57, 58]. Patients may also present with a loss of lumbar lordosis [58], as opposed to the hyperlordosis that can be present with isthmic spondylolisthesis.

Patients will often walk with a wide-based gait and a forward flexed posture [62]. The motor exam is often normal, with only 47 % of patients presenting with weakness on exam [62]. However, patients with lateral recess stenosis can often present with increased weakness compared to patients with central stenosis [64].

Similar to the motor exam, the sensory exam is often normal with only about 50 % of patients with lumbar stenosis presenting with a focal area of numbness [62, 64]. Reflexes are often diminished, most commonly the Achilles reflex [64], and the patient should have no upper motor neuron signs.

Along with a neurologic exam, all patients should undergo a vascular exam evaluating the dorsalis pedis and the posterior tibial pulse. Additionally, other signs of vascular disease such as a distal extremity alopecia and decreased capillary refill should be assessed. All patients should undergo a hip examination as well, ensuring that low back and buttock pain does not originate from the hip.

Radiographic Exam

Radiographic Diagnosis

Patients can undergo standard upright static and dynamic radiographs of the lumbar spine. Similar to isthmic spondylolisthesis, the location and the amount of translation is important and is graded using the Meyerding classification system. However, in degenerative spondylolisthesis, progression beyond 30 % is rare [60].

Degenerative spondylolisthesis can be a dynamic process, so it is critical the initial lateral radiographs are upright [65], as up to 22 % of patients with a degenerative spondylolisthesis on upright films are completely reduced on a supine MRI [66]. Flexion and extension films can also be obtained to better evaluate a degenerative spondylolisthesis and to attempt to identify patients with instability.

While identifying a small slip on radiographs is relatively straightforward, determining what constitutes instability is much more challenging. Most asymptomatic patients have less than 3 mm of translation on flexion and extension radiographs, however up to 20 % of asymptomatic patients may have 4 mm of translation at the L4/5 segment [67, 68].

Another important factor to evaluate is the disc space height. While slip progression is rare, it almost exclusively happens in patients whose disc height is maintained [60]. Additionally, as disc space height decreases, there is a decrease in lumbar back pain [60].

Advanced Imaging

Once the diagnosis has been made, patients with neurologic symptoms should undergo an MRI to evaluate for the presence and location of nerve root compression. Compression can be located centrally, in the lateral recess or in the foramen, with lateral recess stenosis being the most common. If the patient is unable to undergo an MRI, a CT myelogram can help identify possible areas of nerve compression.

Along with evaluating neurologic compression, there has been a significant amount of recent literature attempting to correlate MRI findings to the stability of a degenerative spondylolisthesis. One area of interest has been the presence of T2 signal and gaping within the facet joint, often described as a facet effusion (Fig. 5.10). While at times, the dynamic properties of a degenerative spondylolisthesis can make the slip unidentifiable on a supine MRI [66, 69], multiple studies have demonstrated that the presence of a facet signal or gaping is indicative of instability and a reduced spondylolisthesis [66, 69, 70]. Specifically, a signal of greater than 1.5 mm is highly suggestive of a degenerative spondylolisthesis, even in the absence of a visible slip on a supine MRI [66]. Since this is a sign of slip instability, as the degenerative spondylolisthesis progresses to the stabilized phase, the joint signal often decreases or completely resolves [66, 71].

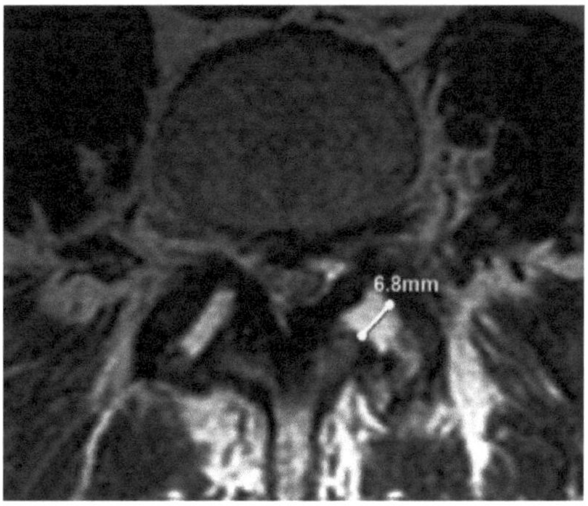

Fig. 5.10 An axial MRI image demonstrating a large 6.8 mm facet effusion. [Reprinted from Chaput C, Padon D, Rush J, Lenehan E, Rahm M. The significance of increased fluid signal on magnetic resonance imaging in lumbar facets in relationship to degenerative spondylolisthesis. Spine (Phila Pa 1976). Aug 1 2007;32(17):1883-1887. With permission from Lippincott Williams & Wilkins.]

Due to the potential limitations of supine MRI, there have also been multiple studies evaluating the benefits of an upright or axial loaded MRI (Fig. 5.11). Upright MRIs increase the sensitivity of identifying a dynamic degenerative spondylolisthesis that may be reduced in a supine MRI [72, 73]. Ferreiro Perez et al. reported on 45 patients who underwent both a supine and an upright MRI, and they found 36 % of anterior spondylolisthesis were missed on supine imaging. Additionally, the slip increased in the upright position in 64 % of the cases [72]. In another study by Hiwatashi

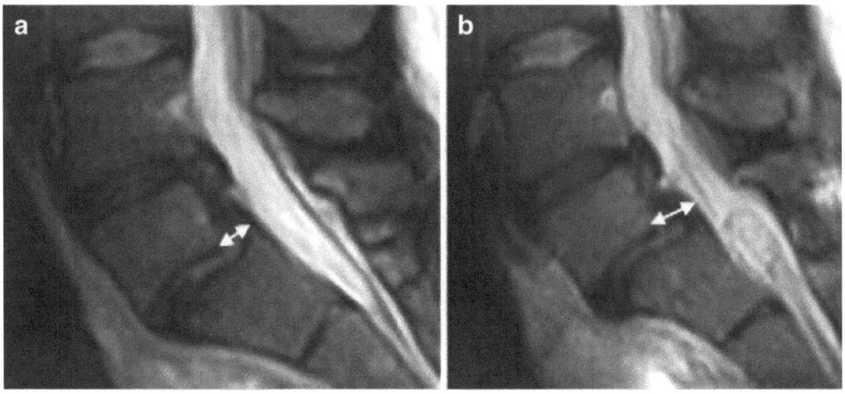

Fig. 5.11 There is increased slip on the upright sagittal MRI image on the right (**a**) compared to the supine sagittal MRI image on the left (**b**). [Reprinted from Tarantino U, Fanucci E, Iundusi R, et al. Lumbar spine MRI in upright position for diagnosing acute and chronic low back pain: statistical analysis of morphological changes. J Orthop Traumatol. Mar 2013;14(1):15-22. With permission from Springer Verlag.] [75]

et al. [74], it was found that not only does an upright MRI increase the sensitivity of detecting spondylolisthesis, it also significantly changes the amount of stenosis and may potentially alter a surgeon's treatment algorithm. However, there is insufficient evidence to support the routine use of upright or dynamic MRI.

Clinical Correlation

When evaluating a patient with either isthmic or degenerative spondylolisthesis, correlating a patient's history and physical exam to the patient's imaging is crucial. The first step is identifying if the patient has primarily low back pain or neurologic symptoms, as the treatment algorithm will vary significantly. If the patient does have neurologic symptoms, a physical exam can often help localize the dermatomal or myotomal area of pathology. Upright AP and lateral radiographs will allow the physician to make the diagnosis of either isthmic or degenerative spondylolisthesis, and a combination of full-length radiographs and advanced imaging will help shape the treatment algorithm. Finally correlating advanced imaging to patient-specific symptoms is important. Many patients may have degenerative changes identified on MRI that are not related to their symptom pattern (dermatome, myotome, or left/ride sidedness). A critical analysis of both the patient's symptoms and direct visualization of the MRI (not just the radiologist's interpretations) is critical to making a correct diagnosis and initiating the appropriate care for the patient.

References

1. Wiltse LL, Newman PH, Macnab I. Classification of spondylolisis and spondylolisthesis. Clin Orthop Relat Res. 1976;117:23–9.
2. Farfan HF, Osteria V, Lamy C. The mechanical etiology of spondylolysis and spondylolisthesis. Clin Orthop Relat Res. 1976;117:40–55.
3. Wiltse LL, Widell Jr EH, Jackson DW. Fatigue fracture: the basic lesion is inthmic spondylolisthesis. J Bone Joint Surg Am. 1975;57(1):17–22.
4. Ferguson RJ, McMaster JH, Stanitski CL. Low back pain in college football linemen. J Sports Med. 1974; 2(2):63–9.
5. Jackson DW, Wiltse LL, Cirincoine RJ. Spondylolysis in the female gymnast. Clin Orthop Relat Res. 1976;117:68–73.
6. Roussouly P, Gollogly S, Berthonnaud E, Labelle H, Weidenbaum M. Sagittal alignment of the spine and pelvis in the presence of L5-s1 isthmic lysis and low-grade spondylolisthesis. Spine (Phila Pa 1976). 2006;31(21):2484–90.
7. Labelle H, Mac-Thiong JM, Roussouly P. Spino-pelvic sagittal balance of spondylolisthesis: a review and classification. Eur Spine J. 2011;20 Suppl 5:641–6.
8. McGuire Jr R. Adult isthmic spondylolisthesis. In: Harry N, Herkowitz SRG, Eismont FJ, Bell GR, Balderston R, editors. Rothman-Simeone the spine, vol. 2. Philadelphia: Elsevier Saunders; 2011. p. 1254–62.

9. Hu SS, Tribus CB, Diab M, Ghanayem AJ. Spondylolisthesis and spondylolysis. J Bone Joint Surg Am. 2008;90(3):656–71.
10. Ganju A. Isthmic spondylolisthesis. Neurosurg Focus. 2002;13(1):E1.
11. Meyerding H. Spondylolisthesis. Surg Gynecol Obstet. 1932;54:371–7.
12. Marchetti P, Bartolozzi P. Classification of spondylolisthesis as a guideline for treatment. In: Bridwell K, DeWald R, Hammerberg K, et al., editors. The textbook of spinal surgery. 2nd ed. Philadelphia: Lippincott-Raven; 1997. p. 1211–54.
13. Fredrickson BE, Baker D, McHolick WJ, Yuan HA, Lubicky JP. The natural history of spondylolysis and spondylolisthesis. J Bone Joint Surg Am. 1984;66(5): 699–707.
14. Kalichman L, Kim DH, Li L, Guermazi A, Berkin V, Hunter DJ. Spondylolysis and spondylolisthesis: prevalence and association with low back pain in the adult community-based population. Spine (Phila Pa 1976). 2009;34(2):199–205.
15. Beutler WJ, Fredrickson BE, Murtland A, Sweeney CA, Grant WD, Baker D. The natural history of spondylolysis and spondylolisthesis: 45-year follow-up evaluation. Spine (Phila Pa 1976). 2003;28(10): 1027–35. discussion 1035.
16. Roche MB, Rowe GG. The incidence of separate neural arch and coincident bone variations; a summary. J Bone Joint Surg Am. 1952;34-A(2):491–4.
17. Stewart TD. The age incidence of neural-arch defects in Alaskan natives, considered from the standpoint of etiology. J Bone Joint Surg Am. 1953; 35-A(4):937–50.
18. Saraste H. Symptoms in relation to the level of spondylolysis. Int Orthop. 1986;10(3):183–5.
19. Saraste H. Long-term clinical and radiological follow-up of spondylolysis and spondylolisthesis. J Pediatr Orthop. 1987;7(6):631–8.
20. Jones TR, Rao RD. Adult isthmic spondylolisthesis. J Am Acad Orthop Surg. 2009;17(10):609–17.
21. Edelson JG, Nathan H. Nerve root compression in spondylolysis and spondylolisthesis. J Bone Joint Surg Br. 1986;68(4):596–9.
22. Jinkins JR, Rauch A. Magnetic resonance imaging of entrapment of lumbar nerve roots in spondylolytic spondylolisthesis. J Bone Joint Surg Am. 1994;76(11): 1643–8.
23. Wiltse LL, Guyer RD, Spencer CW, Glenn WV, Porter IS. Alar transverse process impingement of the L5 spinal nerve: the far-out syndrome. Spine (Phila Pa 1976). 1984;9(1):31–41.
24. Moller H, Sundin A, Hedlund R. Symptoms, signs, and functional disability in adult spondylolisthesis. Spine (Phila Pa 1976). 2000;25(6):683–9. discussion 690.
25. Beck NA, Miller R, Baldwin K, et al. Do oblique views add value in the diagnosis of spondylolysis in adolescents? J Bone Joint Surg Am. 2013;95(10): e651–7.
26. Boxall D, Bradford DS, Winter RB, Moe JH. Management of severe spondylolisthesis in children and adolescents. J Bone Joint Surg Am. 1979; 61(4):479–95.
27. Grobler LJ, Novotny JE, Wilder DG, Frymoyer JW, Pope MH. L4-5 isthmic spondylolisthesis. A biomechanical analysis comparing stability in L4-5 and L5-S1 isthmic spondylolisthesis. Spine (Phila Pa 1976). 1994;19(2):222–7.
28. Seitsalo S, Osterman K, Hyvarinen H, Tallroth K, Schlenzka D, Poussa M. Progression of spondylolisthesis in children and adolescents. A long-term follow-up of 272 patients. Spine (Phila Pa 1976). 1991; 16(4):417–21.
29. Wiltse LL, Winter RB. Terminology and measurement of spondylolisthesis. J Bone Joint Surg Am. 1983;65(6):768–72.
30. Antoniades SB, Hammerberg KW, DeWald RL. Sagittal plane configuration of the sacrum in spondylolisthesis. Spine (Phila Pa 1976). 2000;25(9): 1085–91.
31. Laurent LE, Einola S. Spondylolisthesis in children and adolescents. Acta Orthop Scand. 1961;31:45–64.
32. Slim GP. Vertebral contour in spondylolisthesis. Br J Radiol. 1973;46(544):250–4.
33. Yue WM, Brodner W, Gaines RW. Abnormal spinal anatomy in 27 cases of surgically corrected spondyloptosis: proximal sacral endplate damage as a possible cause of spondyloptosis. Spine (Phila Pa 1976). 2005;30(6 Suppl):S22–6.
34. Vialle R, Levassor N, Rillardon L, Templier A, Skalli W, Guigui P. Radiographic analysis of the sagittal alignment and balance of the spine in asymptomatic subjects. J Bone Joint Surg Am. 2005;87(2):260–7.
35. Vaz G, Roussouly P, Berthonnaud E, Dimnet J. Sagittal morphology and equilibrium of pelvis and spine. Eur Spine J. 2002;11(1):80–7.
36. Lafage V, Schwab F, Patel A, Hawkinson N, Farcy JP. Pelvic tilt and truncal inclination: two key radiographic parameters in the setting of adults with spinal deformity. Spine (Phila Pa 1976). 2009;34(17): E599–606.
37. Glassman SD, Bridwell K, Dimar JR, Horton W, Berven S, Schwab F. The impact of positive sagittal balance in adult spinal deformity. Spine (Phila Pa 1976). 2005;30(18):2024–9.
38. Schwab F, Patel A, Ungar B, Farcy JP, Lafage V. Adult spinal deformity-postoperative standing imbalance: how much can you tolerate? An overview of key parameters in assessing alignment and planning corrective surgery. Spine (Phila Pa 1976). 2010;35(25): 2224–31.
39. Duval-Beaupere G, Schmidt C, Cosson P. A Barycentremetric study of the sagittal shape of spine and pelvis: the conditions required for an economic standing position. Ann Biomed Eng. 1992;20(4):451–62.
40. Hanson DS, Bridwell KH, Rhee JM, Lenke LG. Correlation of pelvic incidence with low- and

high-grade isthmic spondylolisthesis. Spine (Phila Pa 1976). 2002;27(18):2026–9.
41. Li Y, Hresko MT. Radiographic analysis of spondylolisthesis and sagittal spinopelvic deformity. J Am Acad Orthop Surg. 2012;20(4):194–205.
42. Mac-Thiong JM, Berthonnaud E, Dimar 2nd JR, Betz RR, Labelle H. Sagittal alignment of the spine and pelvis during growth. Spine (Phila Pa 1976). 2004;29(15):1642–7.
43. Huang RP, Bohlman HH, Thompson GH, Poe-Kochert C. Predictive value of pelvic incidence in progression of spondylolisthesis. Spine (Phila Pa 1976). 2003;28(20):2381–5. discussion 2385.
44. Mac-Thiong JM, Transfeldt EE, Mehbod AA, et al. Can C7 plumbline and gravity line predict health related quality of life in adult scoliosis? Spine (Phila Pa 1976). 2009;34(15):E519–27.
45. Harroud A, Labelle H, Joncas J, Mac-Thiong JM. Global sagittal alignment and health-related quality of life in lumbosacral spondylolisthesis. Eur Spine J. 2013;22(4):849–56.
46. Jackson RP, Phipps T, Hales C, Surber J. Pelvic lordosis and alignment in spondylolisthesis. Spine (Phila Pa 1976). 2003;28(2):151–60.
47. Mac-Thiong JM, Wang Z, de Guise JA, Labelle H. Postural model of sagittal spino-pelvic alignment and its relevance for lumbosacral developmental spondylolisthesis. Spine (Phila Pa 1976). 2008;33(21): 2316–25.
48. Labelle H, Roussouly P, Berthonnaud E, Dimnet J, O'Brien M. The importance of spino-pelvic balance in L5-s1 developmental spondylolisthesis: a review of pertinent radiologic measurements. Spine (Phila Pa 1976). 2005;30(6 Suppl):S27–34.
49. Hresko MT, Labelle H, Roussouly P, Berthonnaud E. Classification of high-grade spondylolistheses based on pelvic version and spine balance: possible rationale for reduction. Spine (Phila Pa 1976). 2007; 32(20):2208–13.
50. Stagnara P, De Mauroy JC, Dran G, et al. Reciprocal angulation of vertebral bodies in a sagittal plane: approach to references for the evaluation of kyphosis and lordosis. Spine (Phila Pa 1976). 1982;7(4): 335–42.
51. Kirkaldy-Willis W. Presidential symposium on instability of the lumbar spine. Spine (Phila Pa 1976). 1985;10:254.
52. Grobler LJ, Robertson PA, Novotny JE, Pope MH. Etiology of spondylolisthesis. Assessment of the role played by lumbar facet joint morphology. Spine (Phila Pa 1976). 1993;18(1):80–91.
53. Rosenberg NJ. Degenerative spondylolisthesis. Predisposing factors. J Bone Joint Surg Am. 1975; 57(4):467–74.
54. Jacobsen S, Sonne-Holm S, Rovsing H, Monrad H, Gebuhr P. Degenerative lumbar spondylolisthesis: an epidemiological perspective: the Copenhagen Osteoarthritis Study. Spine (Phila Pa 1976). 2007; 32(1):120–5.
55. Ha KY, Chang CH, Kim KW, Kim YS, Na KH, Lee JS. Expression of estrogen receptor of the facet joints in degenerative spondylolisthesis. Spine (Phila Pa 1976). 2005;30(5):562–6.
56. Bird HA, Eastmond CJ, Hudson A, Wright V. Is generalized joint laxity a factor in spondylolisthesis? Scand J Rheumatol. 1980;9(4):203–5.
57. Vibert BT, Sliva CD, Herkowitz HN. Treatment of instability and spondylolisthesis: surgical versus nonsurgical treatment. Clin Orthop Relat Res. 2006;443: 222–7.
58. Majid K, Fischgrund JS. Degenerative lumbar spondylolisthesis: trends in management. J Am Acad Orthop Surg. 2008;16(4):208–15.
59. Bell GR. Degenerative spondylolisthesis. In: Harry N, Herkowitz SRG, Eismont FJ, Bell GR, Balderston R, editors. Rothman-Simeone the spine, vol. 2. Philadelphia: Elsevier Saunders; 2011. p. 1101–17.
60. Matsunaga S, Ijiri K, Hayashi K. Nonsurgically managed patients with degenerative spondylolisthesis: a 10- to 18-year follow-up study. J Neurosurg. 2000; 93(2 Suppl):194–8.
61. Verbiest H. A radicular syndrome from developmental narrowing of the lumbar vertebral canal. J Bone Joint Surg Br. 1954;36-B(2):230–7.
62. Katz JN, Dalgas M, Stucki G, et al. Degenerative lumbar spinal stenosis. Diagnostic value of the history and physical examination. Arthritis Rheum. 1995; 38(9):1236–41.
63. Inufusa A, An HS, Lim TH, Hasegawa T, Haughton VM, Nowicki BH. Anatomic changes of the spinal canal and intervertebral foramen associated with flexion-extension movement. Spine (Phila Pa 1976). 1996;21(21):2412–20.
64. Jonsson B, Stromqvist B. Symptoms and signs in degeneration of the lumbar spine. A prospective, consecutive study of 300 operated patients. J Bone Joint Surg Br. 1993;75(3):381–5.
65. Bendo JA, Ong B. Importance of correlating static and dynamic imaging studies in diagnosing degenerative lumbar spondylolisthesis. Am J Orthop (Belle Mead NJ). 2001;30(3):247–50.
66. Chaput C, Padon D, Rush J, Lenehan E, Rahm M. The significance of increased fluid signal on magnetic resonance imaging in lumbar facets in relationship to degenerative spondylolisthesis. Spine (Phila Pa 1976). 2007;32(17):1883–7.
67. Boden SD, Wiesel SW. Lumbosacral segmental motion in normal individuals. Have we been measuring instability properly? Spine (Phila Pa 1976). 1990;15(6):571–6.
68. Hayes MA, Howard TC, Gruel CR, Kopta JA. Roentgenographic evaluation of lumbar spine flexion-extension in asymptomatic individuals. Spine (Phila Pa 1976). 1989;14(3):327–31.
69. Lattig F, Fekete TF, Grob D, Kleinstuck FS, Jeszenszky D, Mannion AF. Lumbar facet joint effusion in MRI: a sign of instability in degenerative spondylolisthesis? Eur Spine J. 2012;21(2):276–81.

70. Ben-Galim P, Reitman CA. The distended facet sign: an indicator of position-dependent spinal stenosis and degenerative spondylolisthesis. Spine J. 2007;7(2):245–8.
71. Oishi Y, Murase M, Hayashi Y, Ogawa T, Hamawaki J. Smaller facet effusion in association with restabilization at the time of operation in Japanese patients with lumbar degenerative spondylolisthesis. J Neurosurg Spine. 2010;12(1):88–95.
72. Ferreiro Perez A, Garcia Isidro M, Ayerbe E, Castedo J, Jinkins JR. Evaluation of intervertebral disc herniation and hypermobile intersegmental instability in symptomatic adult patients undergoing recumbent and upright MRI of the cervical or lumbosacral spines. Eur J Radiol. 2007;62(3):444–8.
73. Jayakumar P, Nnadi C, Saifuddin A, Macsweeney E, Casey A. Dynamic degenerative lumbar spondylolisthesis: diagnosis with axial loaded magnetic resonance imaging. Spine (Phila Pa 1976). 2006;31(10):E298–301.
74. Hiwatashi A, Danielson B, Moritani T, et al. Axial loading during MR imaging can influence treatment decision for symptomatic spinal stenosis. AJNR Am J Neuroradiol. 2004;25(2):170–4.
75. Tarantino U, Fanucci E, Iundusi R, et al. Lumbar spine MRI in upright position for diagnosing acute and chronic low back pain: statistical analysis of morphological changes. J Orthop Traumatol. 2013;14(1):15–22.

Imaging Techniques for the Diagnosis of Spondylolisthesis

6

Beverly A. Thornhill, Debra J. Green, and Alan H. Schoenfeld

Abbreviations

AP	Anteroposterior
CAT	Computed axial tomography
CBCT	Cone beam computed tomography
CT	Computed tomography
EM	Electromagnetic
H_E	Effective dose
ICRP	International Commission on Radiological Protection
kVp	Peak kilovoltage
LSA	Lumbosacral angle
mA	Milliampere
mAs	Milliamperes × seconds
MRI	Magnetic resonance imaging
mSv	Millisievert
PA	Posteroanterior
PD	Proton-density
PET	Positron-emission tomography
PI	Pelvic index
SI	Sacral inclination
SPECT	Single-photon emission computed tomography
STIR	Short-tau inversion recovery
T1W	T1-weighted
T2W	T2-weighted
UV	Ultraviolet

B.A. Thornhill, M.D. (✉) • D.J. Green, M.D.
A.H. Schoenfeld, M.S.
Department of Radiology, Montefiore Medical Center/Albert Einstein College of Medicine, 111 E. 210th Street, Bronx, NY 10467, USA
e-mail: bthornhi@montefiore.org; degreen@montefiore.org; aschoenf@montefiore.org

Introduction

Since the initial use of the term spondylolisthesis by Killian in 1853, the advances in imaging have provided increased facility in the diagnosis and analysis of the disease process. The major modalities, including radiography, computed tomography (CT), and magnetic resonance imaging (MRI), are readily available for widespread use. Nuclear medicine studies can add valuable information. An understanding of the strengths and limitations of these modalities is important for accurate and efficient diagnosis.

Imaging studies are useful for the classification of spondylolisthesis, determination of the severity of disease, assessment of progression of disease, and pre-operative planning. In most cases, radiography is the initial examination performed. The decision to proceed with further imaging studies will depend upon the specific information needed. The choice should be made with full knowledge of the likely yield, radiation burden, and feasibility of obtaining an adequate study [1].

Correlation between imaging findings and the clinical scenario is essential. Modern imaging provides a high sensitivity for the detection of spondylolisthesis and its associated findings.

A.L. Wollowick and V. Sarwahi (eds.), *Spondylolisthesis: Diagnosis, Non-Surgical Management, and Surgical Techniques*, DOI 10.1007/978-1-4899-7575-1_6,

However, these abnormalities are often seen in patients who are asymptomatic or in whom the spondylolisthesis is not the cause of the presenting complaints.

Radiography

Radiography requires the use of X-rays, energy waves on the spectrum of electromagnetic (EM) radiation; EM radiation is energy in the form of waves that travel and spread. The other types of EM radiation that make up the spectrum, in order of increasing energy, are radio waves, microwaves, infrared light, visible light, ultraviolet light, and gamma rays. X-rays fall between ultraviolet (UV) light and gamma rays on the spectrum. The higher energy UV light waves, along with X-rays and gamma rays, carry sufficient energy to ionize tissues and are therefore types of ionizing radiation that have the potential to damage tissues. The lower energy forms of radiation on the EM spectrum are non-ionizing.

In medical radiography, X-rays enter a patient and undergo variable attenuation and absorption as they travel through on the way to a detector (radiographic film or digital detector). Dense tissues such as bones allow fewer X-rays to pass through and so appear whiter, or more opaque, on conventional radiographs in comparison with thinner tissues such as the lungs.

The advantages of radiography include availability, ease of performance, and low cost. While one should remain vigilant about minimizing patient exposure to ionizing radiation, the radiation doses involved in radiography are relatively low.

Radiographic Examinations

A radiographic examination of the spine includes a minimum of a frontal view and a neutral lateral view. Optional views include coned-down lateral views, oblique views (also termed lateral obliques), and lateral views in flexion and extension. The patient may be examined on the radiographic table in supine, prone, and decubitus positions using vertical or cross-table lateral radiographic beam orientation. Radiographs can also be obtained with patients sitting or standing. Positioning and the number of views obtained reflect preferences among institutions, radiologists, and referring clinicians.

Frontal Radiographs

Frontal views may be performed in the anteroposterior (AP) or posteroanterior (PA) projection. AP radiographs are obtained with the patient's back against the detector and the radiographic beam enters the patient anteriorly; the reverse is true for PA radiographs. AP radiographs are preferable because the spine is closer to the detector and therefore the bony details are sharper and less magnified. However, AP radiographs result in higher radiation exposure to the breasts, of particular concern in adolescents, when the thoracic region is included. Standing frontal views can be obtained using AP or PA beam direction, while tabletop frontal views are almost always obtained with the patient supine and are therefore AP images.

Lateral Radiographs

Upright lateral views can be performed with either the left or right side of the patient against the detector. The tabletop lateral is usually performed with the patient in the lateral decubitus position (lying on the right or left side); a cross-table lateral view is an option if the patient is unable to assume the lateral decubitus position.

Oblique Radiographs

Oblique views and coned-down lateral views may afford better visualization of spondylolysis (a defect in the posterior neural arch commonly associated with spondylolisthesis) than the full-size lateral view. Lateral flexion and extension views are useful for evaluation of spinal stability.

Radiographic Anatomy

Frontal Radiographs

On frontal radiographs, vertebral body heights and alignment are evaluated; scoliosis and lateral spondylolisthesis are demonstrated if present (Fig. 6.1). Anatomic landmarks seen on frontal radiographs include the intervertebral disc spaces, transverse processes, articular facets, and laminae. The pedicles and spinous processes are seen *en face* (Fig. 6.2).

Lateral Radiographs

Vertebral body alignment and height are best assessed on well-positioned lateral radiographs (Fig. 6.1). Optimal positioning yields a single line denoting the posterior cortex of each vertebral body; a line along these posterior cortices will form a smooth, uninterrupted curve when the

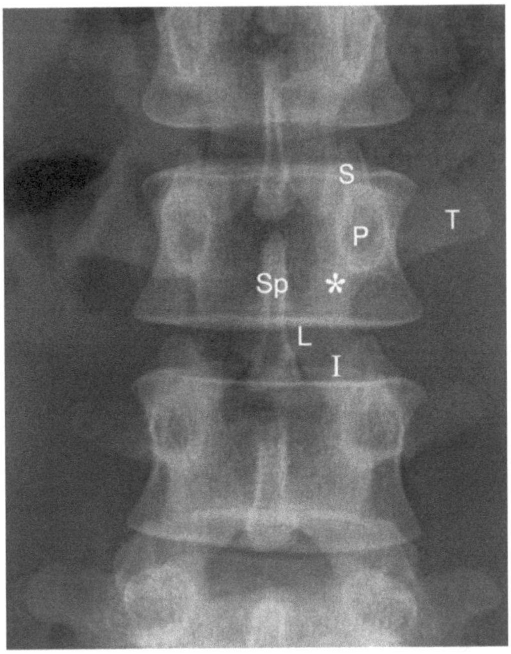

Fig. 6.2 Normal anatomy in the AP projection demonstrated at L3: Superior articular facet (*S*), inferior articular facet (*I*), pedicle (*P*), pars interarticularis (*), transverse process (*T*), lamina (*L*), and spinous process (*Sp*)

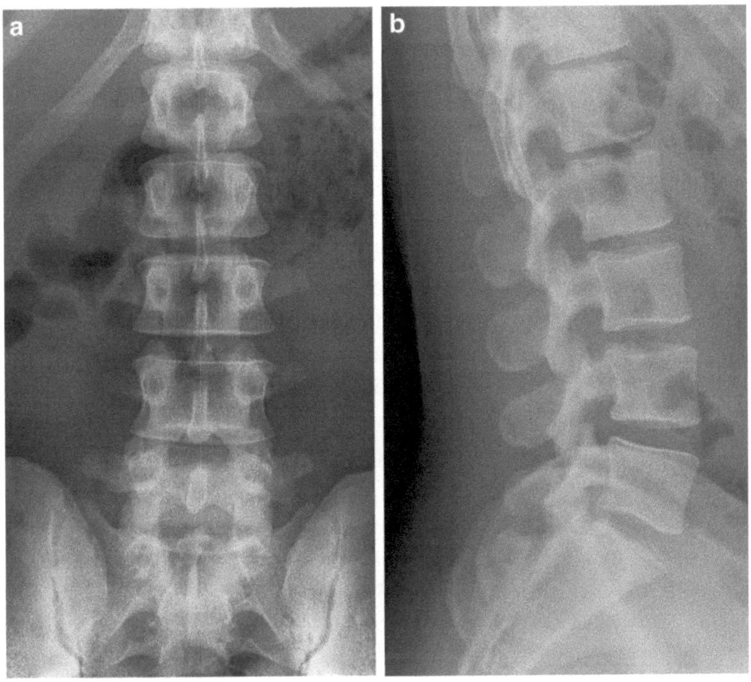

Fig. 6.1 Normal frontal (**a**) and lateral (**b**) lumbosacral spine radiographs

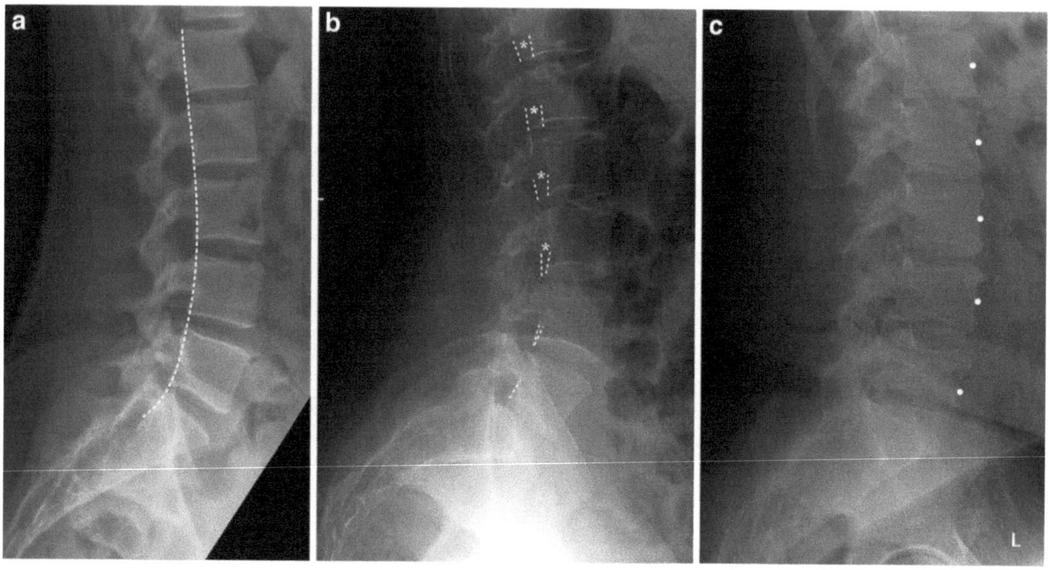

Fig. 6.3 Assessment of vertebral body alignment on lateral radiographs with and without patient rotation. There is normal alignment in the examples shown. (**a**) Lateral lumbosacral spine radiograph with optimal positioning. A smooth, uninterrupted line is drawn along the posterior vertebral body margins of L1–S1 (*dashed line*). (**b**) Lateral view with patient rotation. The posterior vertebral margin of L5 is demarcated with a *single dashed line*. At L4 and above, two posterior margins are evident (*dashed lines*), with gradual divergence superiorly. Normal alignment is confirmed by visualizing a smooth line connecting the midpoints (*) between the *dashed lines*. (**c**) Another lateral view with patient rotation. Alignment in this case is assessed by visualizing a smooth line connecting the midpoints of the anterior borders of the vertebral bodies (*dots*)

vertebral alignment is normal. However, lateral views are often compromised by patient rotation. With rotation, two posterior vertebral body cortices may be evident at the rotated levels; a line connecting the midpoints of the spaces between these cortices can be visualized and should again form a smooth curve when the alignment is normal. Alternatively the midpoints of the anterior aspects of the vertebral bodies should be smoothly aligned (Fig. 6.3). Vertebral anatomic landmarks demonstrated on lateral radiographs include the pedicles, superior and inferior articular facets, facet joints, neural foramina, intervertebral disc spaces, and spinous processes. The portion of the neural arch between the superior and inferior articular facets, the pars interarticularis (plural, pars interarticulari; Latin plural partes interarticulares) can be seen, of particular interest in spondylolisthesis (Fig. 6.4). Most of the radiographic measurements related to spondylolisthesis are performed on lateral views.

Oblique Radiographs

Oblique views are performed in the AP projection with the patient rotated 45° to his or her left (left posterior oblique) and right (right posterior oblique). In these views, the shape of the vertebral posterior elements is reminiscent of a Scottish terrier; hence, the term "Scottie dog" is used. The parts of the Scottie dog that can be identified include the eye (pedicle), snout or nose (transverse process), ear (superior articular facet), foot (inferior articular facet), and neck (pars interarticularis) (Fig. 6.5).

Radiographic Diagnosis and Grading of Spondylolisthesis

The diagnosis of spondylolisthesis is most commonly made on lateral lumbar spine radiographs where anterior slippage (anterolisthesis)

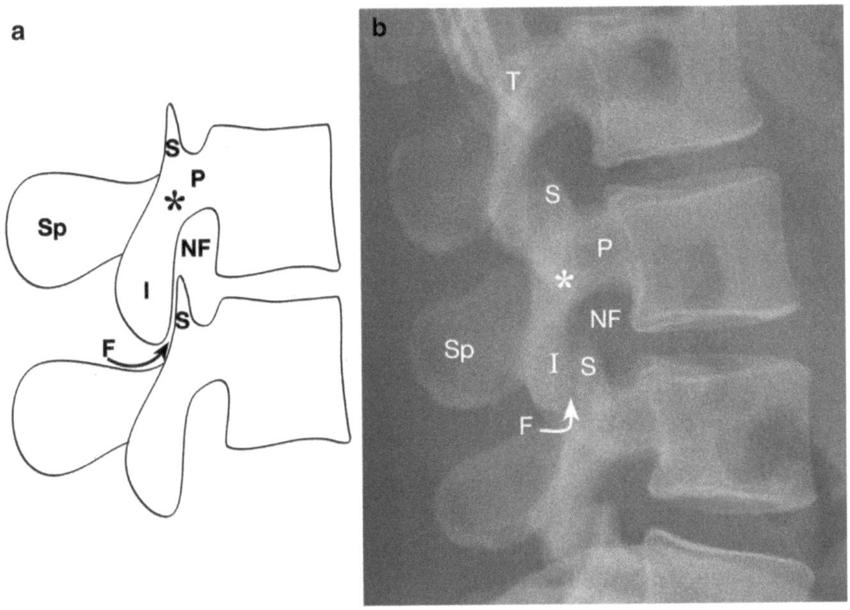

Fig. 6.4 Normal anatomy in the lateral projection on diagram (**a**) and lateral radiograph centered at L3 (**b**). Superior articular facet (*S*), inferior articular facet (*I*), facet joint (*F*), pedicle (*P*), pars interarticularis (*), neural foramen (*NF*), and spinous process (*Sp*). The transverse process of L2 (*T*) is seen *en face* in (**b**)

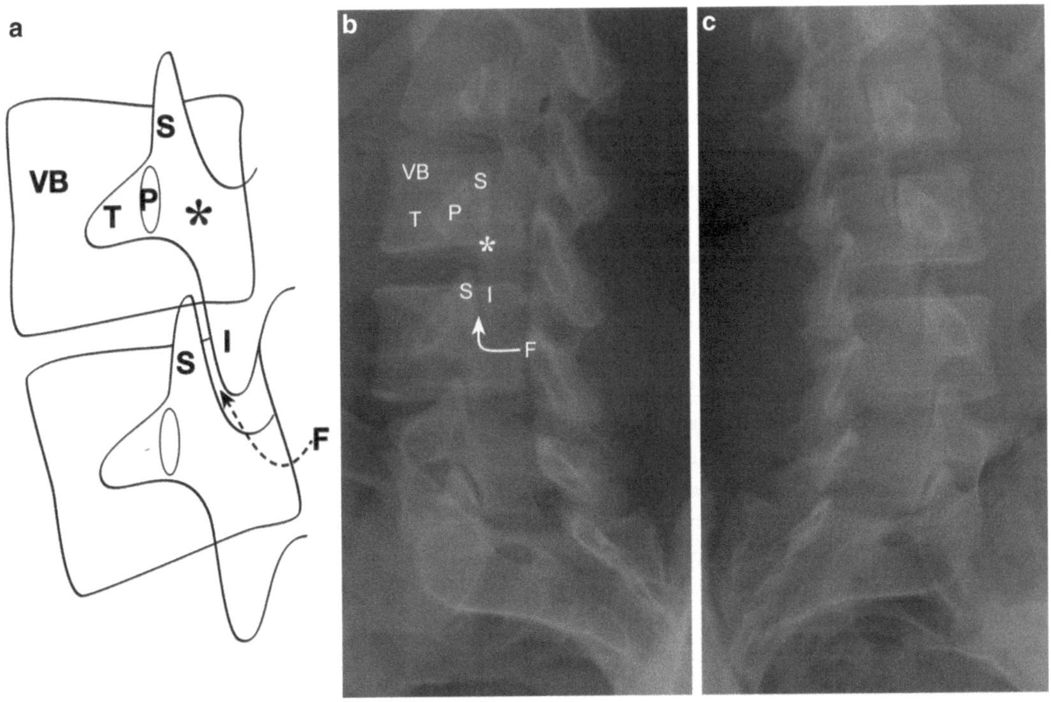

Fig. 6.5 Normal "Scottie dog" anatomy in the oblique projection on diagram (**a**) and right posterior oblique radiograph (**b**). Superior articular facet (*S*)=dog's ear, inferior articular facet (*I*)=foot, pedicle (*P*)=eye, pars interarticularis (*)=neck, transverse process (*T*)=snout. Also noted are the facet joint (*F*) and vertebral body (*VB*). (**c**) Unlabelled normal left posterior oblique projection

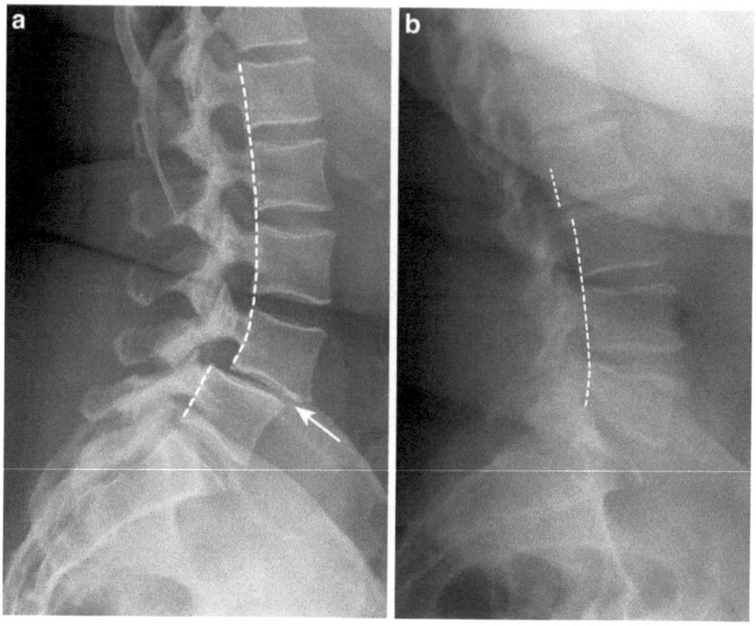

Fig. 6.6 (**a**) Anterolisthesis at L4–5. (**b**) Retrolisthesis at L2–3. *Dashed lines* on each image denote step-offs in alignment. Intervertebral disc space narrowing is noted at L4–5 in (**a**) (*arrow*)

or posterior slippage (retrolisthesis) of a vertebral body is noted in relation to the vertebral body directly below (Fig. 6.6). Spondylolisthesis, either anterior or posterior, is usually found at a single level but may be seen at multiple levels (Fig. 6.7) [2]. Again, the radiographic finding of spondylolisthesis, especially when mild, may not correlate with symptomatology.

In the radiographic grading of spondylolisthesis, the most commonly used tools are the classification systems of Meyerding [3] and Taillard [4] both of which have been shown to yield results with high intra- and inter-observer agreement [5].

Meyerding's system is based on division of the superior endplate of the vertebra below the slipped vertebra into four equal parts. Alignment of the listhesed or slipped vertebra in relation to the divisions in the endplate below determines the grade. Slippages between 0 and 25 % of the endplate below are grade I, between 25 and 50 % are grade II, between 50 and 75 % are grade III, and between 75 and 100 % are grade IV. Anteriorly slipped vertebrae that descend anterior and inferior to the endplate below are classified as grade V, also called spondyloptosis (Fig. 6.8).

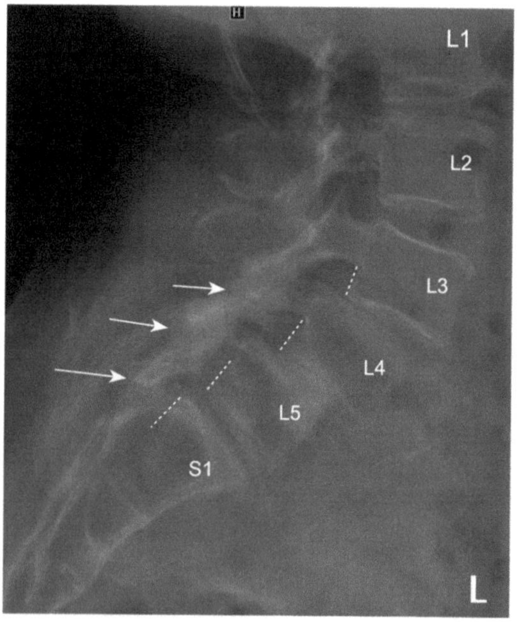

Fig. 6.7 Multilevel degenerative spondylolisthesis. There are anterolistheses at L3–4, L4–5, and L5–S1 (*dashed lines*). Degenerative narrowing with sclerosis is seen along the facet joints indicating arthropathy (*arrows*). Intervertebral disc space narrowing is noted at these levels, most severe at L4–5

Taillard's assessment method is also referred to as the "percentage slip" measurement. The distance between the posterior margins of the slipped vertebra and the vertebra below is divided by the anteroposterior dimension of the inferior vertebral endplate and expressed as a percentage (Fig. 6.9).

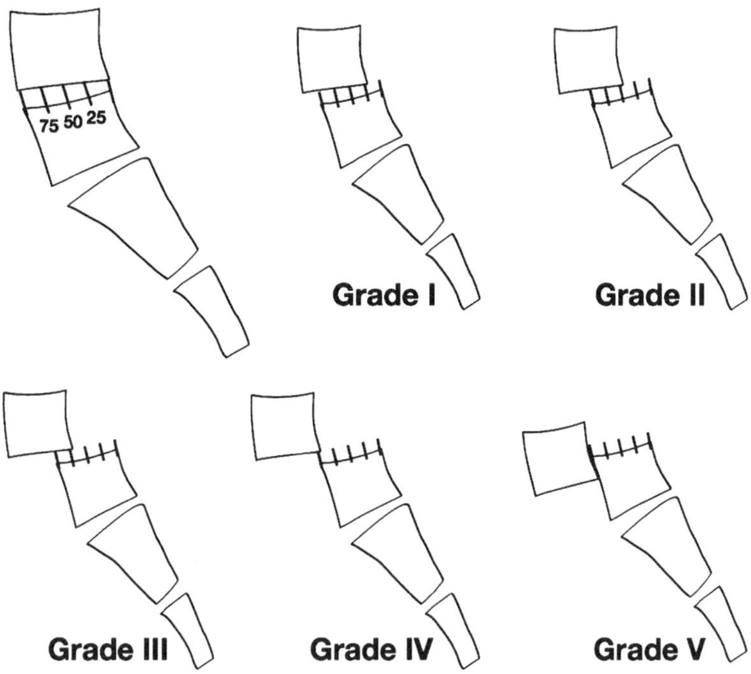

Fig. 6.8 Meyerding grading system of spondylolisthesis. This method is based on division of the superior endplate of the lower vertebra at the level of spondylolisthesis into four equal parts from 0 to 100 %. In anterolisthesis, the posterior aspect of the lower endplate is 0 % and the anterior aspect of the endplate is 100 %. The 25, 50, and 75 % marks are shown on the *upper left drawing*. In retrolisthesis, the frame of reference would be the inferior endplate of the upper vertebral body. Grade I = slippage up to 25 %. Grade II = 25–50 %. Grade III = 50–75 %. Grade IV = 75–100 %. Grade V = anterior and inferior displacement of superior vertebral body (spondyloptosis)

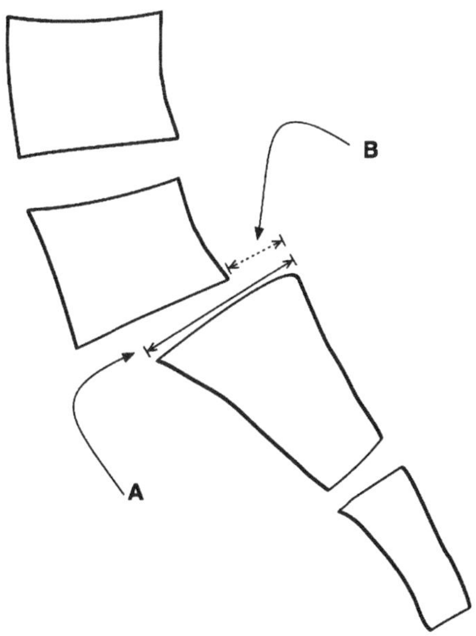

Fig. 6.9 Taillard method of measuring spondylolisthesis ("percentage slip"). A = AP dimension of the superior endplate of the lower vertebra at the level of spondylolisthesis. B = measurement of anterior or posterior displacement of the superior vertebra. The % slippage = $(B \div A) \times 100$

In the cervical spine and thoracic spine, spondylolisthesis is commonly measured in millimeters rather than grades or percentage slip.

Progression of spondylolisthesis can be assessed radiographically, provided that follow-up examinations are similar to prior studies in technique and positioning (Fig. 6.10).

Additional Radiographic Observations in Spondylolisthesis

Spondylolysis

Spondylolysis, a defect in the pars interarticularis, is a common radiographic finding in spondylolisthesis. The abnormality, discussed in detail in the section on isthmic spondylolisthesis, can be detected on lateral or coned-down lateral views (Fig. 6.11). On oblique views, a lucency in the pars interarticularis (representing a break in or collar on the Scottie dog's neck) indicates spondylolysis

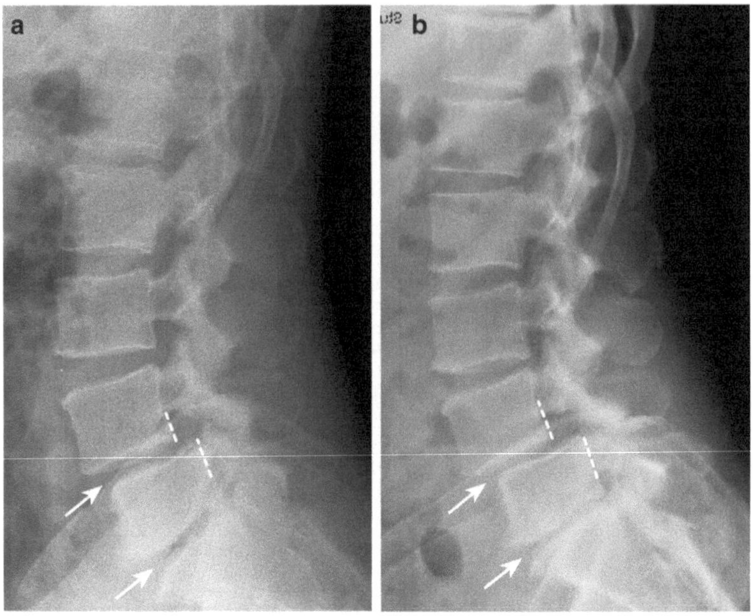

Fig. 6.10 Progression of spondylolisthesis. (**a**) Lateral lumbosacral spine radiograph shows a grade I anterolisthesis at L4–5 (*dashed lines*) with intervertebral disc space narrowing at L4–5 and L5–S1 (*arrows*). (**b**) Two years later, the spondylolisthesis has progressed to grade II (*dashed lines*) and there is further narrowing of the disc spaces at L4–5 and L5–S1 (*arrows*)

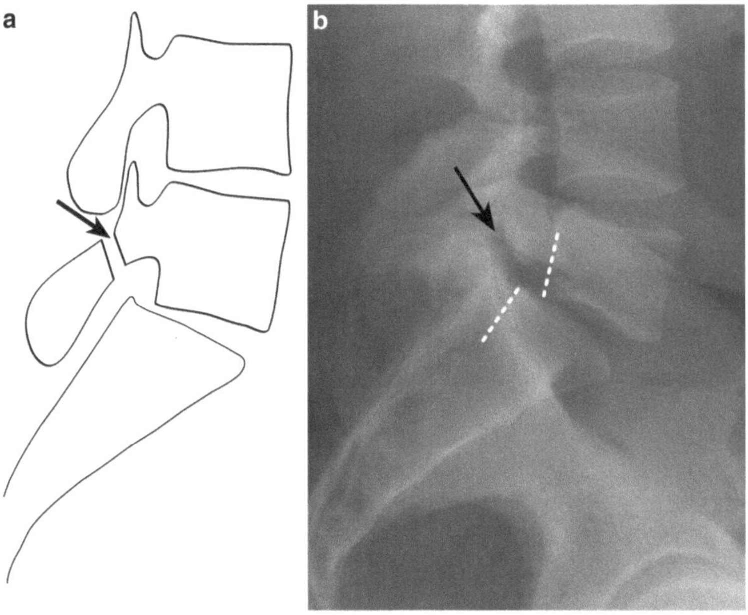

Fig. 6.11 Spondylolysis and spondylolisthesis in the lateral projection. *Arrows* on diagram (**a**) and lateral radiograph (**b**) demonstrate the pars interarticularis defect. Spondylolisthesis is denoted by *dashed lines* in (**b**)

(Fig. 6.12). In the presence of spondylolysis, a vertebral body can move forward (anterolisthesis) without its spinous process, resulting in a step-off between this spinous process and the spinous processes above (Figs. 6.13 and 6.14).

Dysplastic or Dystrophic Changes

Dysplastic or dystrophic changes may be detected on radiographs in patients with spondylolisthesis. Dysplastic changes reflect abnormal development

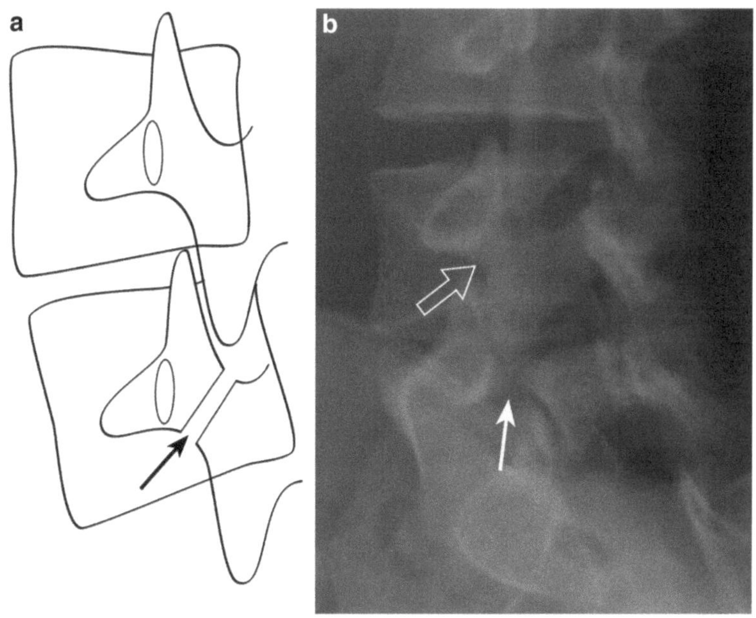

Fig. 6.12 Spondylolysis in the oblique projection. *Arrows* on diagram (**a**) and right posterior oblique radiograph (**b**) demonstrate the broken Scottie dog neck (pars interarticularis). Note the normal Scottie dog neck at the level above (*open arrow* in **b**)

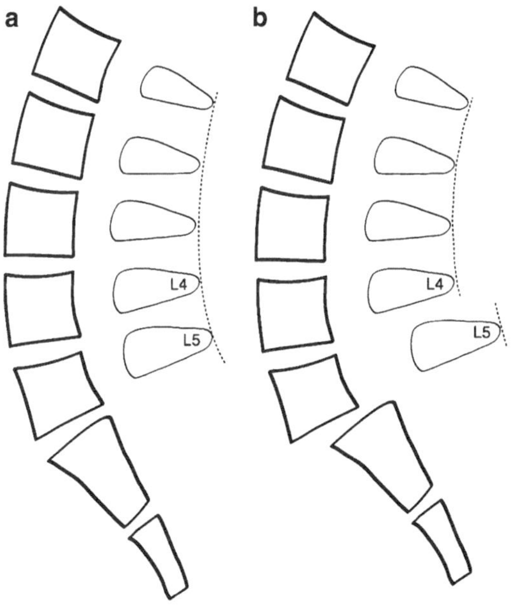

Fig. 6.13 Spinous process step-off in spondylolisthesis (illustrated here at L5–S1) with spondylolysis. A *dotted line* runs along the posterior aspects of the spinous processes. (**a**) Normal alignment. The *dotted line* forms a smooth arc from L1 to L5. (**b**) Anterolisthesis at L5–S1 with spondylolysis. As the L5 vertebra and the vertebrae above move forward, the posterior elements of L1–4 also move forward. The spinous process of L5 remains in its original position (or in some cases slips posteriorly), resulting in disruption of the *dotted line* with a step-off between L4 and L5

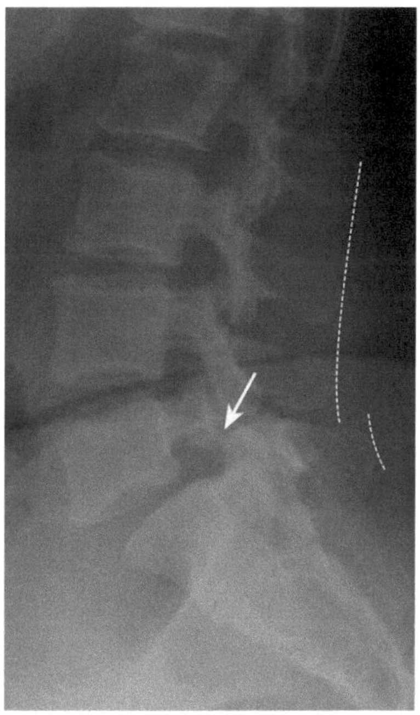

Fig. 6.14 Radiographic demonstration of spinous process step-off in spondylolisthesis with spondylolysis. A grade I anterolisthesis at L5–S1 is noted with defects in the pars interarticulari (*arrow*). The L5 vertebral body remains aligned with L2–4. In contrast, the spinous process of L5 is now situated posterior to the spinous processes above (*dotted lines*)

of the spinal elements, while dystrophic changes reflect sequelae of spondylolisthesis which occur in areas that had originally developed normally. In some cases, particularly in the pars interarticularis, dystrophic changes may not be distinguishable from dysplastic changes; evaluation of the remaining vertebral body elements is often helpful in these instances. Dysplastic changes related to spondylolisthesis include abnormalities of the pars interarticulari (defects or elongation), spina bifida, posterior element hypoplasia, rounding of the superior endplate of S1 and posterior wedging of L5. Dystrophic changes described by Vialle et al. [6] include bony condensation and sclerosis of the anterior portion of the S1 superior endplate and posterior portion of the L5 inferior endplate, a bony protuberance at the posterior part of the S1 endplate, and convexity of the S1 superior endplate. At a pars interarticularis defect, dystrophic sclerosis and attenuation may be seen.

Degenerative Intervertebral Disc Disease and Facet Arthropathy

Degenerative disc disease and facet arthropathy can be demonstrated on radiography. While these findings are most commonly associated with degenerative spondylolisthesis, they can be found in any of the other types of spondylolisthesis, especially in cases of instability. The radiographic hallmarks of degenerative disc disease are disc space narrowing, endplate sclerosis, and osteophyte formation. The frequently associated disc protrusions and bulges cannot be assessed on radiography. The vacuum phenomenon of disc degeneration may be present (Fig. 6.15).

Sclerosis and bony overgrowth at the facet joints indicate arthropathy (Fig. 6.7). Facet arthropathy may be overestimated on lateral views in the lower lumbosacral spine due to the overlying density of the pelvic bones, and should be confirmed on frontal or oblique views. Review of previous imaging,

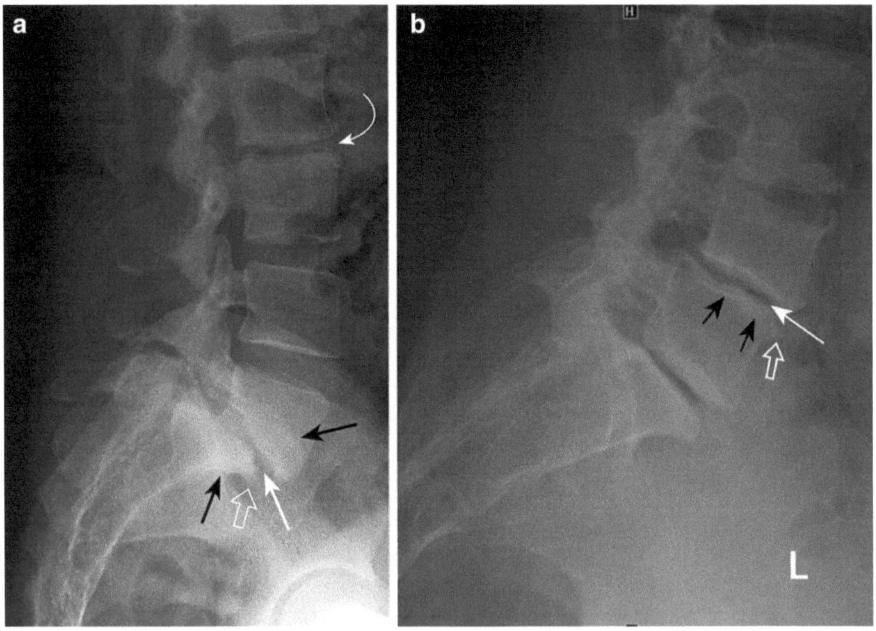

Fig. 6.15 Spondylolisthesis with degenerative disc disease in two patients. (**a**) Lateral radiograph of the lower lumbosacral spine demonstrates anterolisthesis at L5–S1. The hallmarks of degenerative disc disease are seen at this level including disc space narrowing (*straight white arrow*), osteophyte formation (*open white arrow*), and endplate sclerosis (*black arrows*). Similar but less severe changes are seen at L2–3 (*curved white arrow*). (**b**) In this patient with anterolisthesis at L4–5, the vacuum phenomenon of disc degeneration is present (*white arrow*) along with endplate sclerosis (*black arrows*) and an anterior osteophyte (*open white arrow*). Similar changes are present at the level below without spondylolisthesis

such as abdominal CT scans done for medical indications, often yields the desired information about the presence or absence of facet arthropathy. Generally, intervertebral disc degeneration is believed to precede facet joint degeneration and to be a primary cause of anterolisthesis [7, 8].

Spondylolisthesis in Patients with Scoliosis

Spondylolisthesis may be initially encountered in the workup of scoliosis (Fig. 6.16). The incidence of spondylolysis and spondylolisthesis in patients

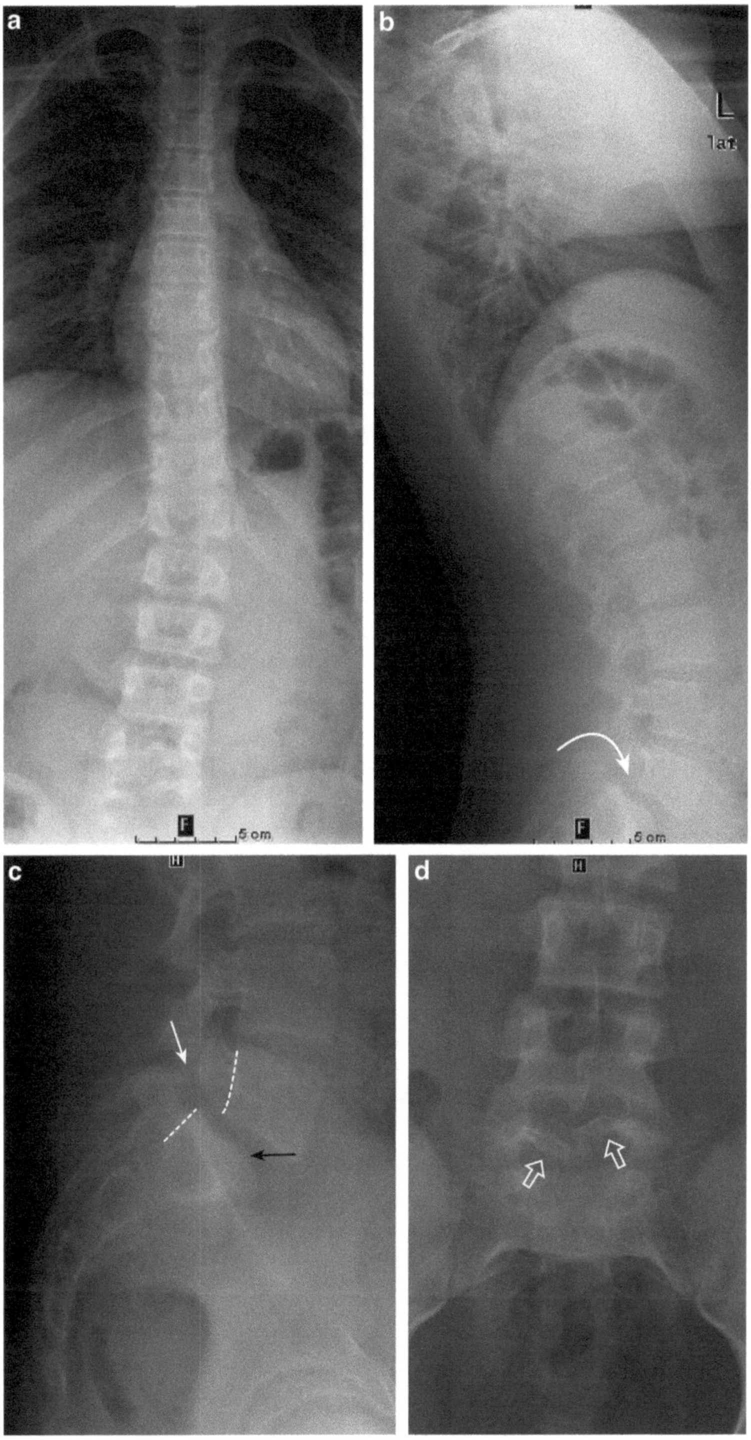

Fig. 6.16 Scoliosis and dysplastic spondylolisthesis. (**a**) AP thoracolumbar radiograph demonstrates mild S-shaped scoliosis in a teenager. (**b**) Lateral thoracolumbar radiograph demonstrates spondylolisthesis at the lower edge of the image (*curved arrow*). (**c**) Dedicated lateral lumbosacral spine radiograph was later performed, clearly showing spondylolisthesis (*dashed lines*) at L5–S1 with spondylolysis of L5 (*white arrow*) and convexity of the superior endplate of S1 (*black arrow*). (**d**) Dedicated AP view at the same time as (**c**) demonstrates dysplastic changes in the posterior elements of L5 (*open arrows*)

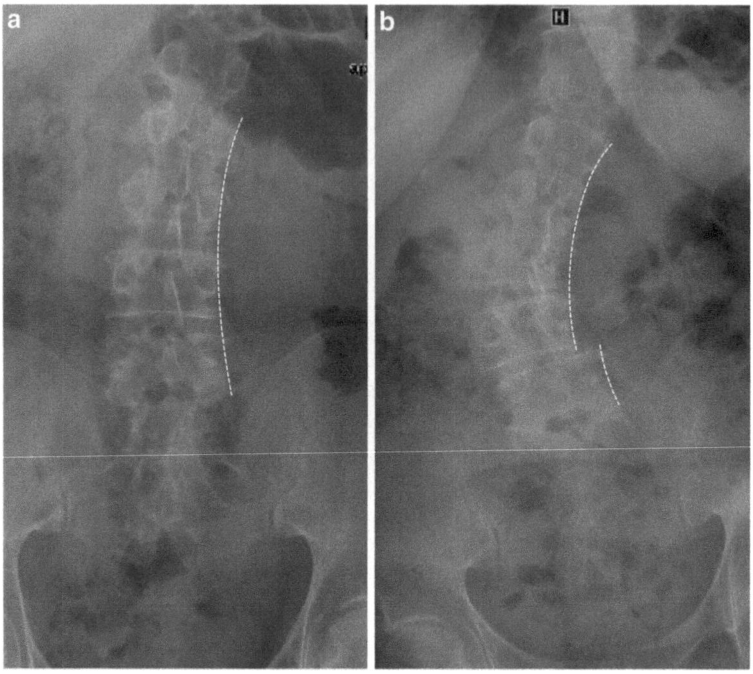

Fig. 6.17 Lateral spondylolisthesis in a patient with progression of scoliosis. (**a**) Dextroscoliosis measures 17° and there is no step-off in the coronal plane (*dashed lines*). (**b**) Four years later, the dextroscoliosis has progressed to 35° and there is right lateral translation of L4 with respect to L5 (*dashed lines*)

with idiopathic scoliosis has been shown to be equal to or only slightly higher than the general population. The two processes are generally, though not always, thought to be unrelated [9].

In the adult population with scoliosis, lateral spondylolisthesis can be seen on frontal radiographs, either initially or with progression of disease (Fig. 6.17). Terms that are used synonymously with lateral spondylolisthesis include translatory shift, lateral subluxation, rotatory subluxation, and lateral slip. A significant correlation between lateral translation and vertebral rotation has been found, and nerve root compression by the convex superior articular facet of the inferior vertebra has been described [10].

"Inverted Napoleon's Hat" Sign

In cases of high-grade L5 spondylolisthesis, the extreme anterior shift and tilting of L5 results in the superimposition of L5 over the sacrum on frontal radiographs. The rounded anterior margin of L5, now seen *en face*, resembles the dome of an inverted Napoleon's hat, with the transverse processes forming the brim of the hat [11] (Fig. 6.18). The sign is not specific, being present in some cases of extreme lumbar lordosis without spondylolisthesis.

Spinous Process Tilt or Rotation

Tilting and/or lateral rotation of a spinous process on frontal radiographs of the lumbar spine has been described in cases of par interarticularis abnormalities with or without spondylolisthesis [12, 13]. These signs reflect rotational instability in patients with pars interarticularis defects (spondylolysis) or unequally elongated or attenuated pars interarticulari. Ravichandran found lateral rotation of the spinous process to be more pronounced in patients with spondylolysis who had associated spondylolisthesis than in patients with spondylolysis alone [13] (Fig. 6.19).

Radiographic Measurements

In addition to the measurement systems of Meyerding and Taillard, several radiographic measurements have been proposed in evaluating lat-

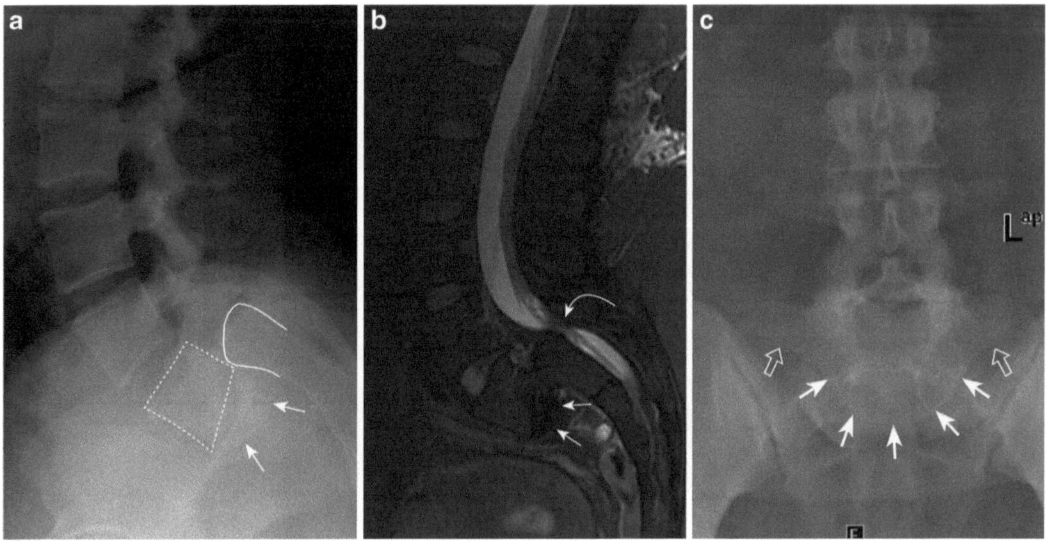

Fig. 6.18 Spondyloptosis with inverted Napoleon's hat sign. (**a**) Lateral radiograph shows displacement of L5 (*dotted lines*) anterior and inferior to superior aspect of S1 (*solid line*). There is curved ossification at the inferior aspect of L5 (*arrows*). (**b**) Sagittal fat-suppressed T2W MRI shows marked central spinal canal stenosis (*curved arrow*). The *dark low signal* area beneath L5 (*arrows*) corresponds to the ossification demonstrated in (**a**) which is seen along the anterior and inferior aspects of the L5–S1 disc that was displaced with L5 (note absence of disc at the superior endplate of S1). (**c**) AP radiograph demonstrates the inverted Napoleon's hat sign related to the marked coronal orientation of the L5 endplate. The crown of the hat is formed by the anterior border of L5 (*straight arrows*) and the brim corresponds to the transverse processes (*open arrows*)

eral lumbosacral spine radiographs in cases of spondylolisthesis but are not as commonly used. Among these measurements are pelvic incidence (PI), lumbosacral angle (LSA), sagittal pelvic tilt index, slip angle, angle of kyphosis, sagittal rotation, sacral inclination (SI), sacral slope, and lumbar index [5, 14, 15]. The various assessments were developed in efforts to better evaluate the overall severity of disease in addition to the amount of displacement, which might improve the ability to predict and measure the progression of disease. Dubousset reported that the increasing kyphosis over time measured by the LSA correlated with worsening of disease which could have surgical implications [15]. Curylo et al. suggested that patients with low-grade spondylolisthesis and higher PI angles could be at greater risk for progression to high-grade spondylolisthesis especially in the context of posterior element dysplasia [16]. In a review of six of the measurements listed above, only the SI measurement was shown to have inter- and intra-observer reliability comparable to those of Meyerding and Taillard [5].

Radiographic Assessment of Instability

Lateral views in flexion and extension (Fig. 6.20) are used to assess stability at the site of spondylolisthesis or to elicit spondylolisthesis. These can be performed on the tabletop with the patient in a lateral decubitus position, or with the patient standing. Proponents of standing views note that weight-bearing views may better approximate normal daily activities. However, patients may achieve a higher degree of flexion and extension in the decubitus tabletop position. In other attempts to elicit the greatest movement at sites of spondylolisthesis, axial compression–traction techniques have been used [17]. Putto proposed that the flexion view be done with the patient seated and their hips flexed, while the extension view be done with the patient standing with hips against the radiography table [18].

Two types of instability are assessed. Parallel instability refers to movement of the upper vertebra

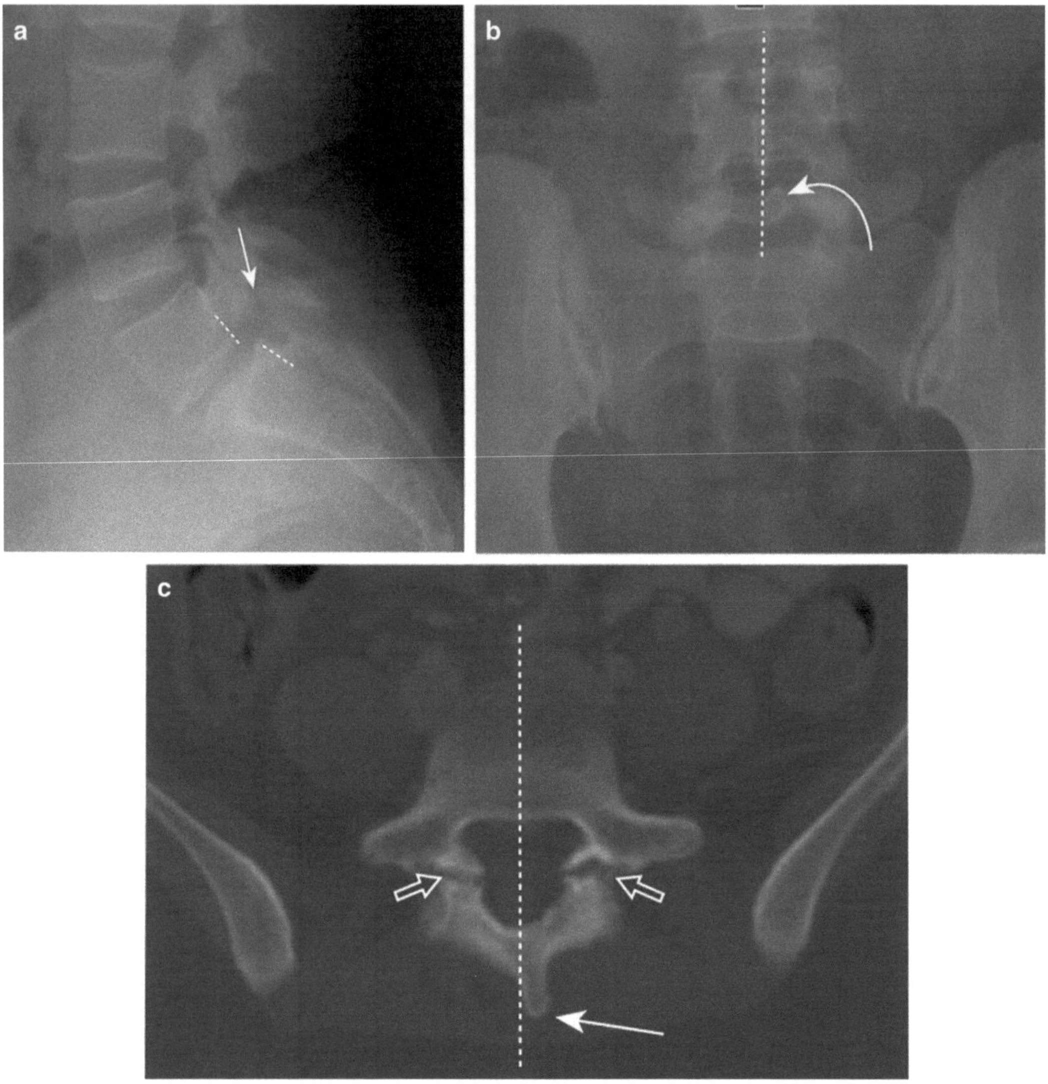

Fig. 6.19 Spinous process rotation and tilt as signs of spondylolysis with spondylolisthesis. (**a**) Lateral radiograph demonstrates anterolisthesis of L5–S1 (*dashed lines*). There is spondylolysis at L5 (*arrow*). (**b**) On the AP radiograph, the spinous process of L5 (*curved arrow*) is rotated to the left of an extension of the *vertical line* drawn through the spinous processes of L3 and L4 (*dashed line*) and appears tilted. (**c**) Axial CT slice through L5 confirms the spondylolyses (*open arrows*) and the rotation of the spinous process (*arrow*) relative to the midline (*dashed line*)

in relation to the lower vertebra anteriorly with flexion or posteriorly with extension. The angle between the two vertebral endplates does not change significantly (Fig. 6.21). Angular instability is defined as an abnormal change in the angle between the endplates of the listhesed vertebra and the vertebra below (Fig. 6.22). Wide variations in vertebral body motion on flexion and extension have been reported. In an extensive review, Leone et al. concluded that between flexion and extension, the upper limit of normal total parallel excursion is 4 mm and the upper limit of normal angular change is 10° [19]. It should be noted that patients with normal alignment in the neutral position may demonstrate spondylolisthesis on flexion or extension (Fig. 6.23).

While flexion and extension radiographs are the most common method of assessing stability,

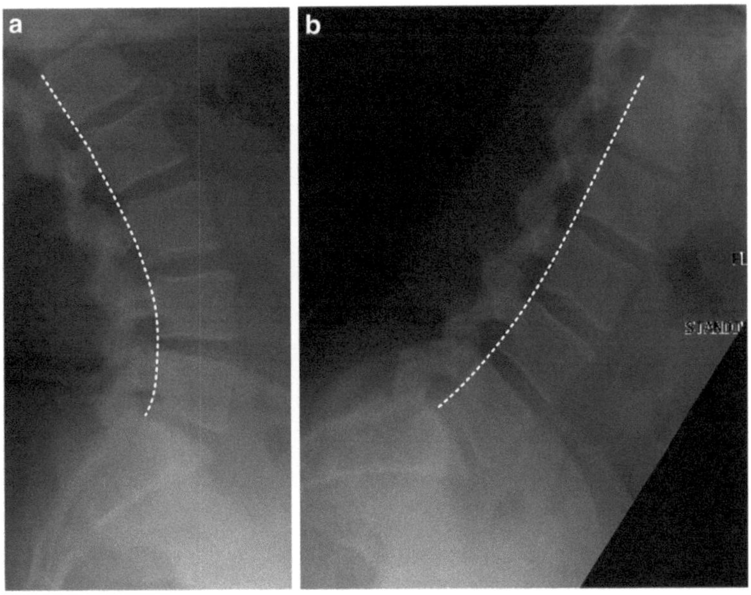

Fig. 6.20 Normal flexion (**a**) and extension (**b**) lateral radiographs. The vertebral bodies remain smoothly aligned in both views

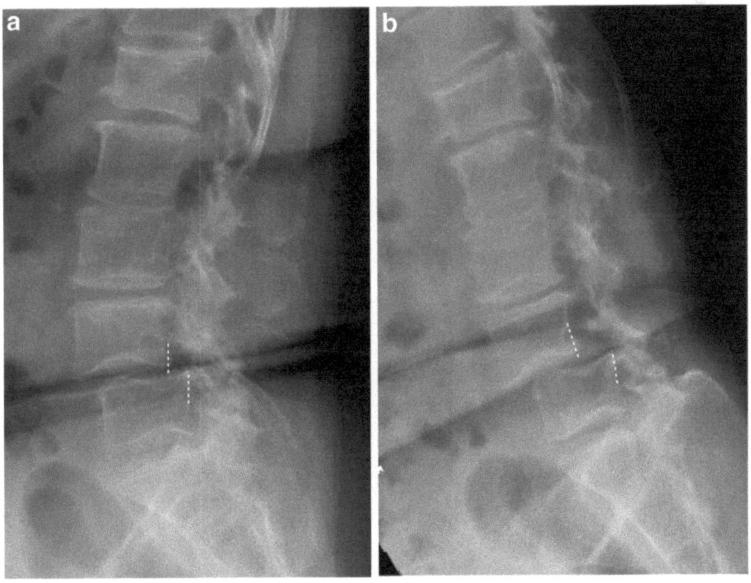

Fig. 6.21 Parallel instability. (**a**) Anterolisthesis at L4–5 is seen (*dashed lines*). (**b**) The percentage slip at L4–5 increases from grade I to grade II with flexion (*dashed lines*), without significant change in angulation between the inferior endplate of L4 and superior endplate of L5

comparison between modalities may provide similar information. For instance, if the severity of spondylolisthesis changes between a neutral radiograph and a supine MRI study, instability has been effectively demonstrated (Fig. 6.24).

Progression of instability in spondylolisthesis can be assessed on serial studies. However, reproducibility of flexion and extension views is difficult and slight variations in patient positioning or angulation of the radiographic beam can result in discrepancies in the range of vertebral displacement.

Magnetic Resonance Imaging

MRI is a powerful cross-sectional imaging modality that detects the behavior of the nuclei of hydrogen atoms, the most abundant atoms in the human

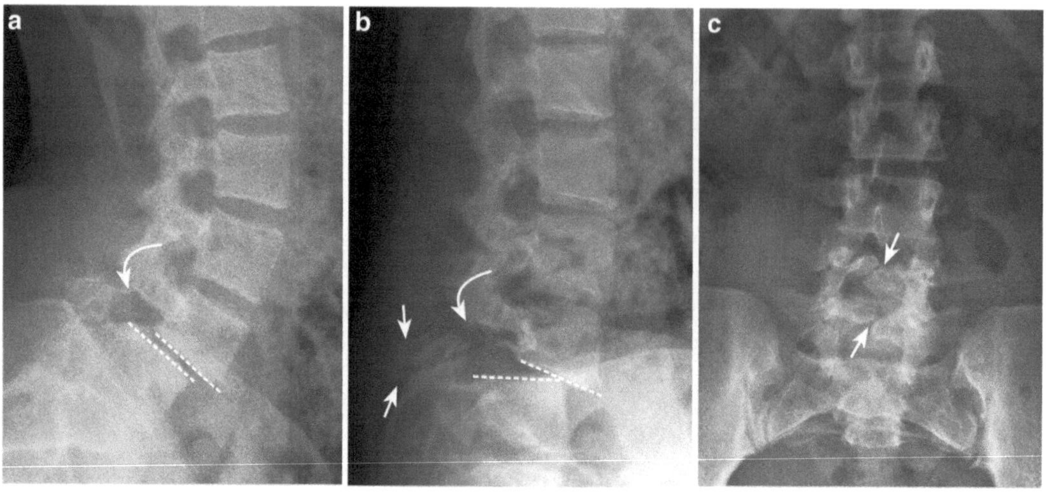

Fig. 6.22 Angular instability in spondylolisthesis. (**a**) Lateral radiograph in the neutral position demonstrates anterolisthesis at L4–5. A defect is seen in the L4 pars interarticularis (*curved arrow*). The inferior endplate of L4 is approximately parallel to the superior endplate of L5 (*dashed lines*). (**b**) Lateral radiograph in flexion demonstrates a change in the angle between the involved endplates (*dashed lines*) with L4 appearing to be perched on L5. The L4 spondylolysis defect (*curved arrow*) has widened compared to the neutral position. Spinous process dysplastic changes are seen at L4 (*arrows*). (**c**) On the AP radiograph, *arrows* denote dysplastic posterior elements of L4 and L5

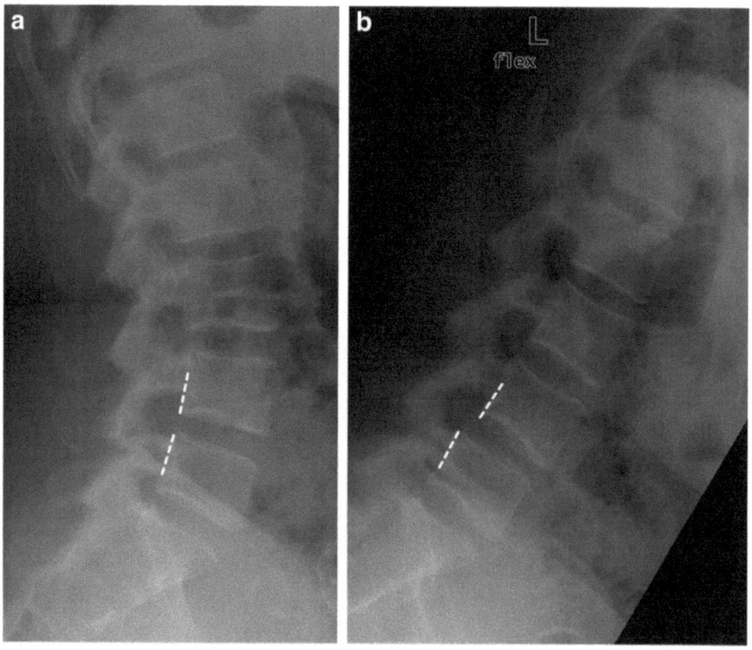

Fig. 6.23 Spondylolisthesis on flexion in a patient with normal neutral alignment. (**a**) Neutral lateral radiograph demonstrates normal alignment at L4–5 (*dashed lines*). (**b**) Lateral radiograph in flexion demonstrates grade I anterolisthesis at L4–5 (*dashed lines*)

body, in the context of a strong magnetic field. The physics concepts related to MRI are complex and are beyond the scope of this text. Very simply put, patients undergoing MRI are placed within the strong magnetic field of the machine; this magnetic field is always "on." Current is applied to a coil over the body part to be imaged and the coil produces energy in the form of a rapidly changing

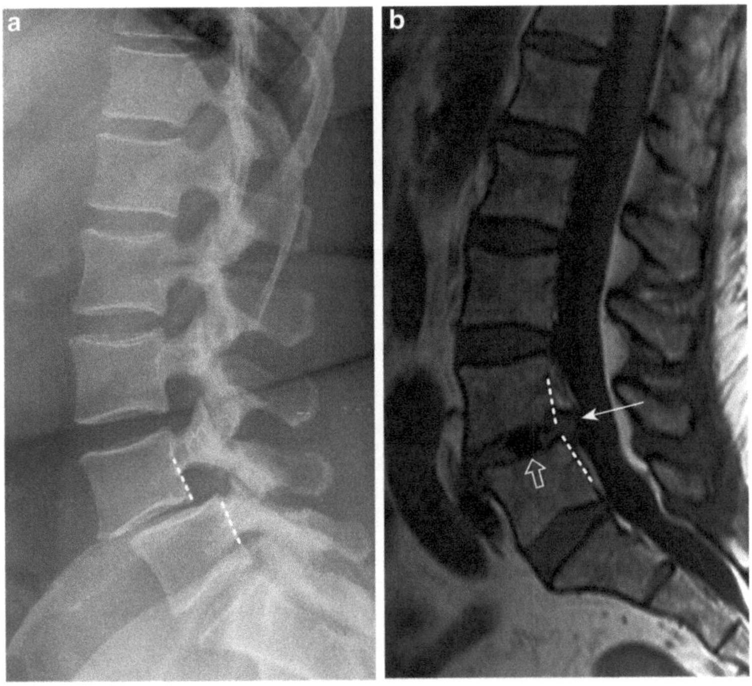

Fig. 6.24 Comparison between modalities illustrates instability. (**a**) Upright lateral lumbosacral spine radiograph demonstrates anterolisthesis at L4–5 (*dashed lines*). (**b**) With the patient supine for MRI, the anterolisthesis reduces (*dashed lines*). A posterior disc protrusion (*arrow*) and vacuum phenomenon of disc degeneration (*open arrow*) are noted

magnetic field. This energy falls within the energy frequency range commonly used in radio broadcasts, and is therefore called radiofrequency energy. While radiofrequency energy is on the same EM spectrum as X-rays, it is of a much higher wavelength (lower frequency and therefore lower energy) and cannot ionize tissues. Thus the risks associated with the ionizing radiation of radiography, computed tomography, and nuclear medicine studies do not apply to MRI.

The radiofrequency energy from the coil causes alterations in the spin of the hydrogen nuclei. When the radiofrequency waves are turned off, the hydrogen nuclei "relax" to assume their original orientation. As they relax, they give off energy which is detected by a receiver coil; the information is then processed by computer and an image is generated. An array of coils and MRI scanning parameters are available for use depending on the body part and the type of information sought.

MRI is the cross-sectional imaging modality of choice in the workup of spondylolisthesis as excellent soft tissue differentiation is achieved without exposing the patient to ionizing radiation.

MRI Scanning Sequences and Anatomy

The studies should include sequences using a variety of parameters. T1-weighted (T1W) images are useful for visualizing fracture lines and excluding abnormal marrow infiltration. Proton-density (PD) or T2-weighted (T2W) images provide good spatial resolution. Short-tau inversion recovery (STIR) sequences are excellent for detection of bone marrow edema as are fat-suppressed PD or T2W sequences. Various gradient-echo (GE) sequences are available and are useful in evaluating the intervertebral disc contours particularly in the cervical spine.

Sagittal images demonstrate vertebral body heights and alignment, and are also used to evaluate intervertebral disc heights and disc hydration. The central spinal canal and neural foramina can be assessed on both sagittal and axial images. The axial sequences should include a "stacked" set of slices that are contiguous and parallel to each other, rather than angled for disc evaluation,

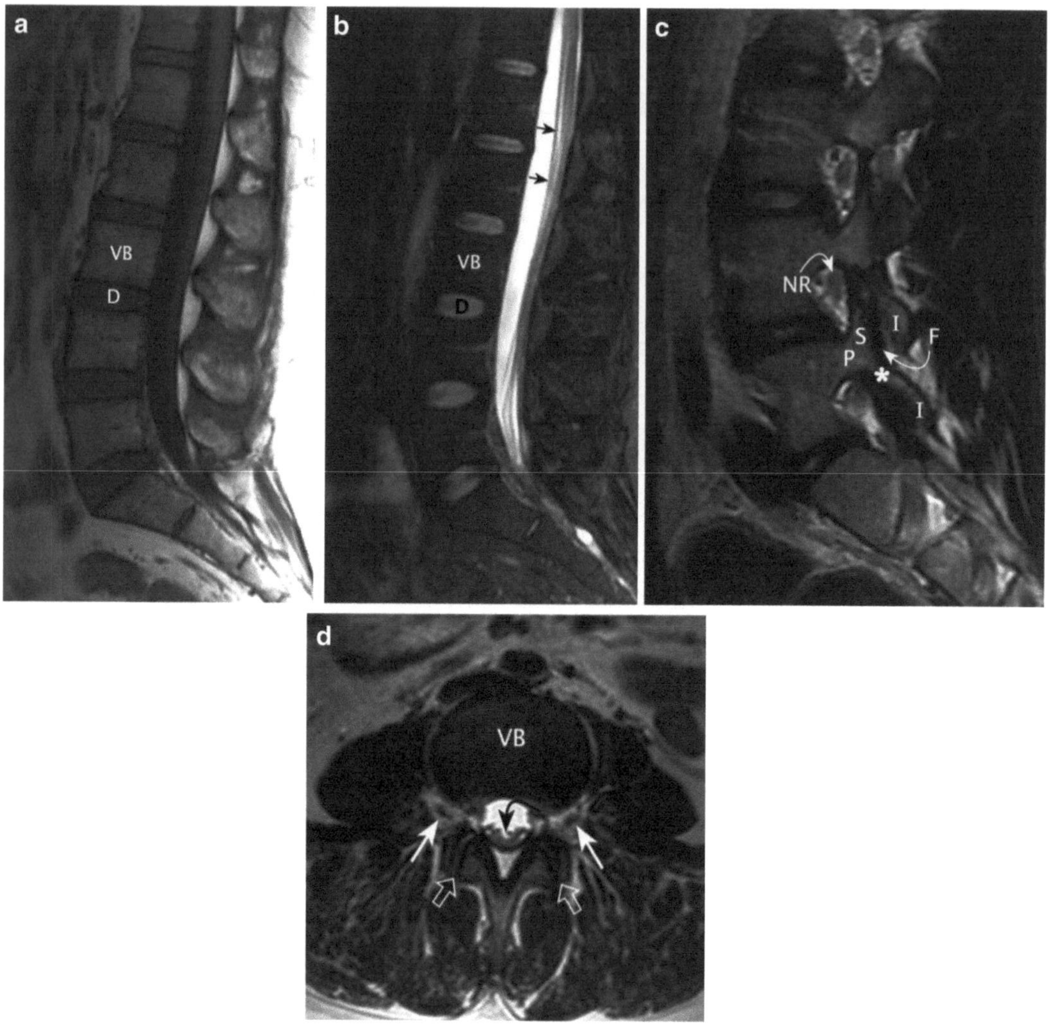

Fig. 6.25 Normal MRI of lumbosacral spine. (**a**) Midline sagittal T1W image demonstrates normal vertebral body alignment. The bone marrow signal in the vertebra (*VB*) is brighter than the signal in the intervertebral disc (*D*). On the sagittal STIR image (**b**), the vertebra (*VB*) is now darker than the disc (*D*). Individual nerve roots can be seen as linear low signal foci (*arrows*) within the bright cerebrospinal fluid. (**c**) Sagittal T2W image through the left neural foramina demonstrates the superior articular facet (*S*), inferior articular facet (*I*), facet joint (*F*), pedicle (*P*), pars interarticularis (*), and nerve root (*NR*). (**d**) Axial T2W slice through the neural foramina demonstrates the vertebral body (*VB*), exiting nerve roots (*white arrows*), facet joints (*open white arrows*), and layering descending nerve roots (*curved black arrow*)

in order to gain optimal visualization of the pars interarticulari. Coronal images are useful for visualization of scoliosis and lateral spondylolisthesis. Figure 6.25 shows normal lumbosacral spine anatomy on MRI.

MRI Findings in Spondylolisthesis

MRI is of great value in the demonstration of central spinal canal and neural foraminal stenosis associated with spondylolisthesis (Figs. 6.26 and 6.27).

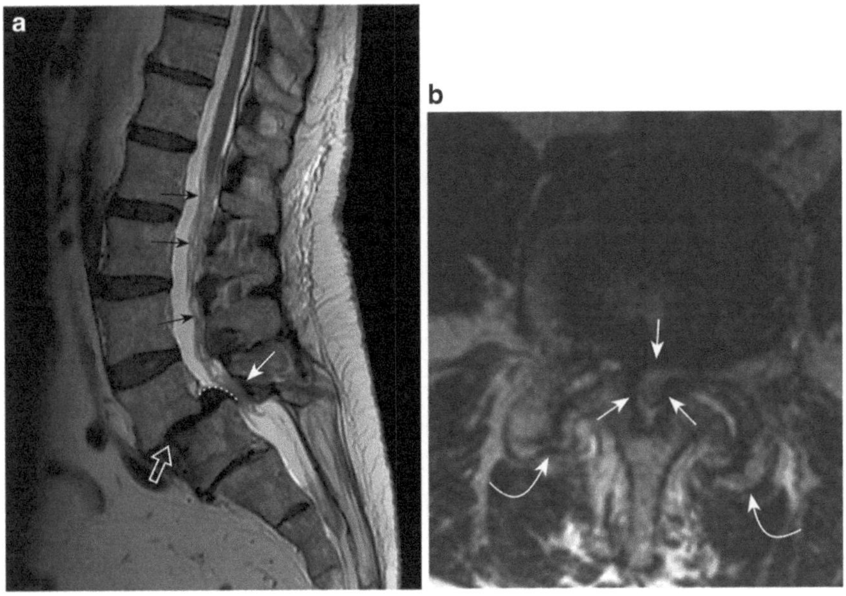

Fig. 6.26 Central spinal canal stenosis in spondylolisthesis. (**a**) A sagittal T2W midline slice shows marked central spinal canal stenosis (*white arrow*) related to a grade II anterolisthesis at L4–5. Redundancy of the descending nerve roots (*black arrows*) is associated with the central spinal canal stenosis. The L4–5 disc remains aligned with the L5 vertebra and is uncovered (*dotted line*), contributing to the canal stenosis. Note significant disc space narrowing at L4–5 (*open white arrow*). (**b**) Axial T2W MRI slice through the L4–5 disc shows severe central spinal canal stenosis (*straight arrows*) and severe facet joint arthropathy (*curved arrows*)

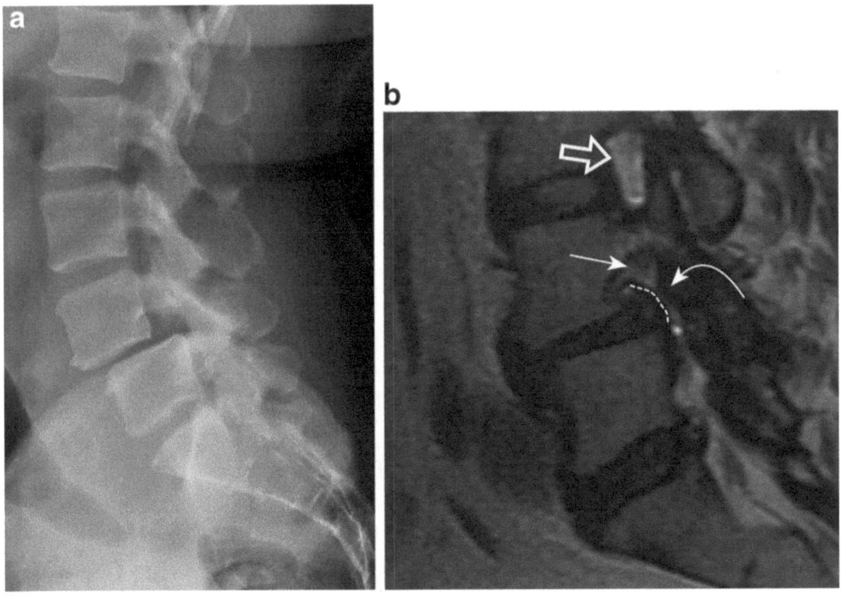

Fig. 6.27 Neural foraminal stenosis in spondylolisthesis. (**a**) The lateral radiograph demonstrates a grade II anterolisthesis at L4–5 with associated intervertebral disc space narrowing. (**b**) On a sagittal T2W MRI slice, the L4–5 intervertebral disc remains aligned with L5 (*dotted line*), and is uncovered due to forward slippage of L4. There is marked stenosis of the neural foramen (*curved arrow*) with entrapment of the exiting L4 nerve root (*straight arrow*). Note the normal appearance of the neural foramen above (*open arrow*)

Nerve root redundancy, a known sequelae of central spinal canal stenosis [20], is readily seen. Facet arthropathy and degenerative disc disease are also well visualized. The appearance of disc uncovering (also termed pseudo-bulge) in spondylolisthesis is related to a disc remaining in alignment with the inferior vertebral body as the superior vertebra slips forward.

Limitations of MRI

Limitations in the use of MRI include the high cost of MRI examinations, claustrophobia, and contraindications such as the presence of a pacemaker or a cochlear implant. The spatial resolution allowing visualization of fine bone details is lower than that of CT. Additionally, MRI scan times are longer than those of CT. In the presence of orthopedic hardware, the MRI images may be significantly degraded due to susceptibility artifacts; metal artifact reduction software should be used for these examinations. On occasion, objects that are not MRI safe are inadvertently allowed to enter the magnetic field and act as missiles that may cause injuries to patients.

Computed Tomography

CT, also known as computed axial tomography (CAT), involves the use of X-rays but differs from conventional radiography in that cross-sectional images (slices) are generated. The slice data is generated using an X-ray source that rotates around the patient; X-ray sensors are positioned on the opposite side of the circle from the X-ray source. As the source rotates continuously, the patient is moved through the gantry and data is recorded. With state-of-the-art multidetector CT scanners, multiple rows of detectors are used to capture multiple cross-sections simultaneously resulting in short scan times.

CT is superior to other imaging modalities for visualization of fine bony detail, important for the detection of subtle spondylolyses. However, as CT involves ionizing radiation, it is not commonly used as the first cross-sectional examination in spondylolisthesis. Rather, CT is generally reserved for cases in which questions remain following MRI or for patients who cannot undergo MRI. The raw data obtained on multidetector CT scans can be used for 2-dimensional reformatting in any plane desired, as well as 3-D reformatting. Bone marrow edema cannot be detected by single energy CT which is the most commonly available and widely used type of CT. However, promising data is emerging regarding detection of bone marrow edema using dual-energy CT [21].

CT Anatomy and Findings in Spondylolisthesis

Similar to MRI, CT demonstrates spinal anatomy including the central spinal canal and neural foramina (Fig. 6.28). Abnormalities of the pars interarticulari (spondylolyses, attenuation, or sclerosis), central spinal canal stenosis, neural foraminal stenosis, degenerative disc disease, and facet arthropathy can all be demonstrated (new Figs. 6.29 and 6.30). The exceptional bony detail afforded by CT can be instrumental in the detection of spondylolyses that may not be discerned on radiographs or MRI. In some instances, CT can detect nondisplaced or incomplete defects in the pars interarticulari that would not result in vertebral slippage at this stage; early recognition and proper management of these cases may minimize progression of disease and therefore potentially prevent the development of spondylolisthesis (Fig. 6.31).

CT Myelography

CT myelography can afford improved anatomic visualization over conventional CT, such as delineation of nerve roots, but is generally reserved for post-operative cases or other complicated cases (Fig. 6.32). The examination requires the administration of intrathecal iodinated contrast. While complications are rare, theoretical risks include hemorrhage, cerebrospinal fluid leak, infection, and arachnoiditis.

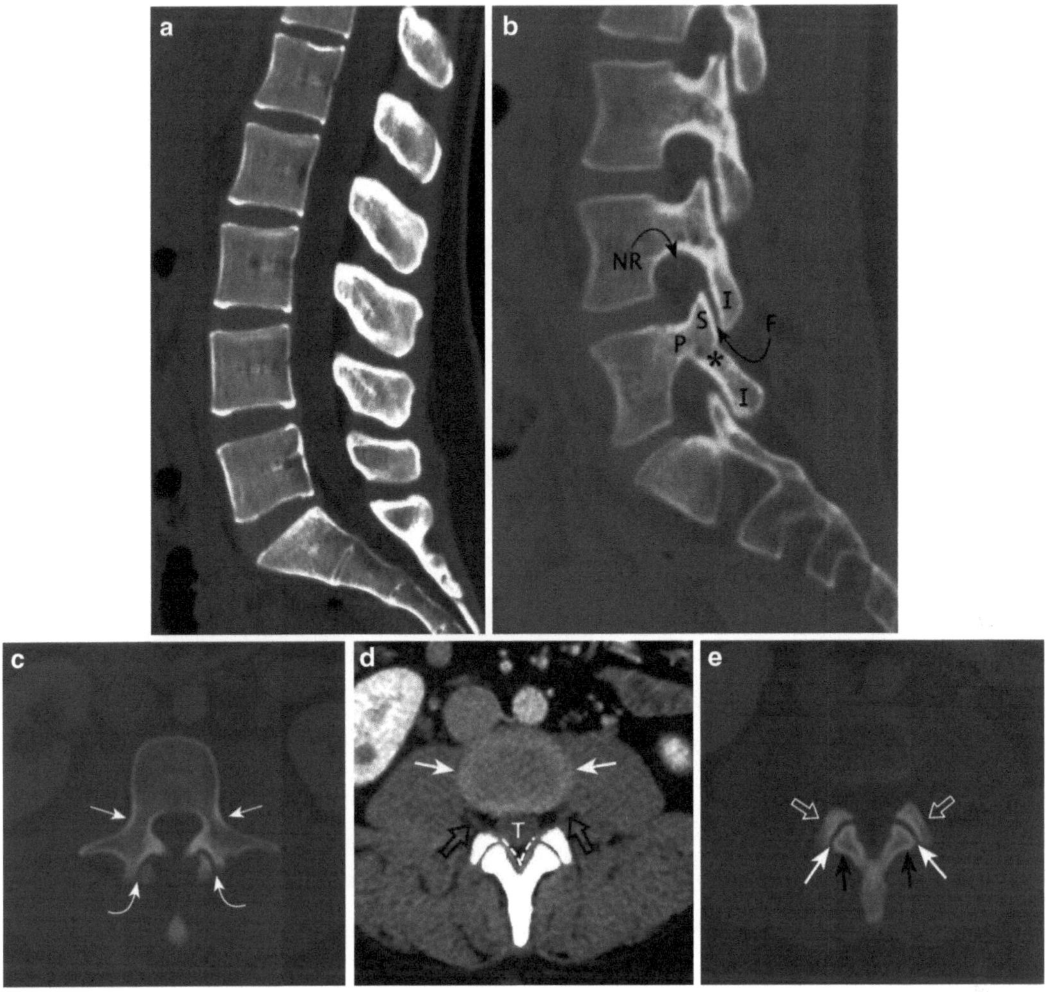

Fig. 6.28 Normal CT of lumbosacral spine. (**a**) Midline sagittal reformatted CT demonstrates normal alignment of the vertebral bodies and spinous processes. (**b**) Sagittal reformatted slice through left neural foramina (lateral to midline) demonstrates the superior articular facet (*S*), inferior articular facet (*I*), facet joint (*F*), pedicle (*P*), pars interarticularis (*), and nerve root (*NR*). (**c**) Axial slice through L2 demonstrates the pedicles (*straight arrows*) and inferior aspects of the L1–2 facet joints (*curved arrows*). (**d** and **e**) Axial slice below (**c**) through the L2–3 intervertebral disc is viewed in soft tissue (**d**) and bone (**e**) windows. In (**d**), the disc (*solid arrows*), thecal sac (*T*), exiting L2 nerve roots (*open arrows*), and ligamentum flavum (*dashed lines*) are shown. (**e**) Shows the osseous details of the L2–3 facet joints (*solid white arrows*). The inferior articular facets of L2 (*solid black arrows*) are posterior to the superior articular facets of L3 (*open white arrows*)

Nuclear Medicine Studies

The basic principle of nuclear scintigraphy is the detection of gamma rays, emitted from the decay of a radionuclide, by a gamma camera. Radionuclides, also known as radiopharmaceuticals, radioisotopes, or radiotracers, are injected intravenously, consumed, inhaled, or otherwise instilled into the body. The gamma rays emitted during decay of these agents are a form of electromagnetic radiation, along the same spectrum as X-rays used in radiography and radiofrequency waves produced during MRI examinations. Gamma rays are of slightly higher energy than X-rays and therefore, similar to X-rays, gamma rays

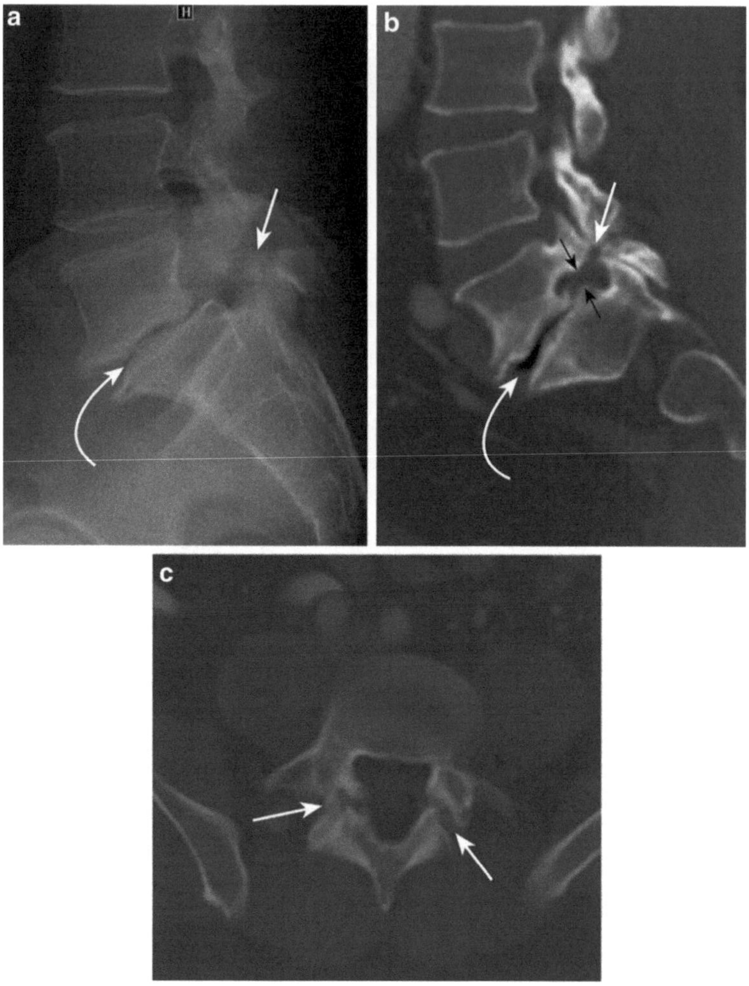

Fig. 6.29 Spondylolisthesis with degenerative disc disease, spondylolysis and neural foraminal narrowing. (**a**) Coned-down lateral radiograph of the lower lumbosacral spine demonstrates disc space narrowing at L5–S1 with a faint vacuum phenomenon (*curved arrow*). Endplate sclerosis and osteophytes are also seen at that level. Poor bony definition in the region of the pars interarticularis suggests spondylolysis (*straight arrow*). (**b**) Sagittal CT reformatted image through the left neural foramina better demonstrates the vacuum phenomenon at L5–1 (*curved white arrow*). The neural foramen is markedly narrowed in its cephalocaudad dimension (*black arrows*). Spondylolysis is confirmed at the left L5 pars interarticularis (*straight white arrow*). (**c**) Axial CT slice through the L5 pars interarticulari demonstrates bilateral spondylolysis

cause tissue ionization. The type of radionuclide and the amount used depends on several factors including the body part being imaged.

Bone Scintigraphy with Single-Photon Emission Computed Tomography

Conventional planar bone scintigraphy is performed after the intravenous injection of Technetium-99m methylene diphosphonate (MDP), a bone-seeking agent radionuclide. Images are obtained using a stationary gamma camera. Single-photon emission computed tomography (SPECT) can be added to a planar bone scan, yielding increased sensitivity for abnormal radioisotope activity and improved localization of abnormalities. An additional radionuclide injection is not required. SPECT images are obtained as the gamma camera is rotated around the patient; images are acquired at defined points during the rotation, typically 3–6° apart, followed by computer processing.

The addition of SPECT to planar bone scintigraphy has proven to be of value in the detection of spondylolysis as the radiotracer uptake is better localized to the area of the pars interarticularis (Fig. 6.33), however SPECT does not provide specific anatomic detail [22]. A follow-up CT or MRI examination may be necessary to confirm the presence of a pars interarticularis defect and/or exclude other causes of abnormal uptake in the region of the pars interarticularis.

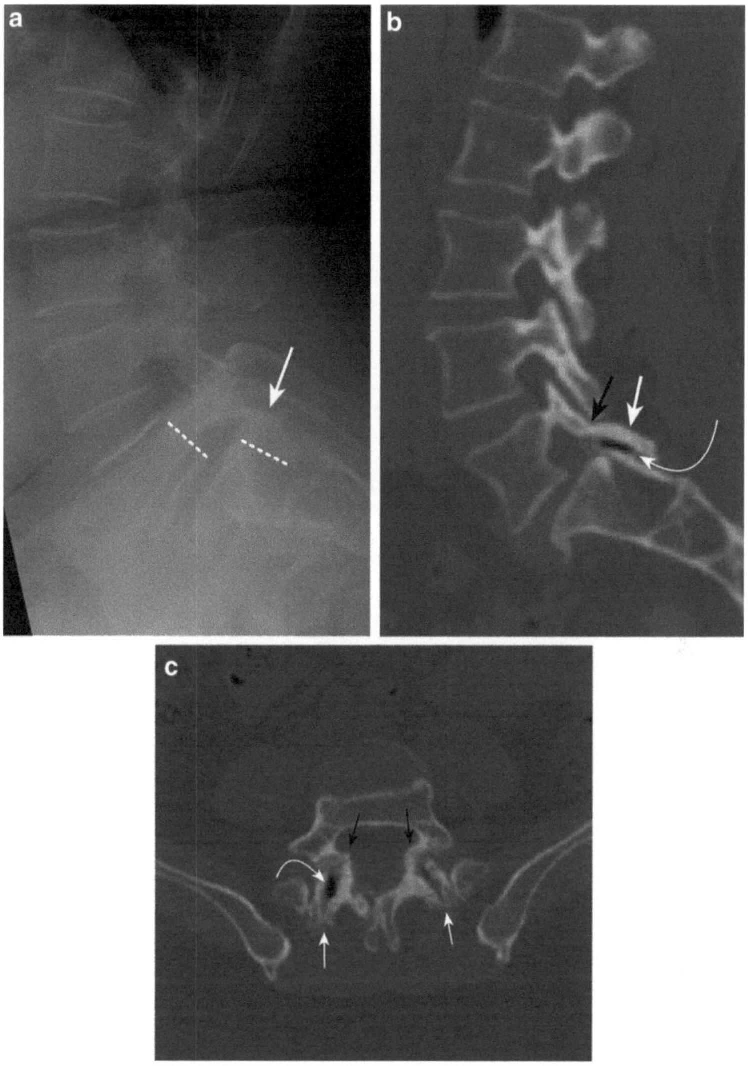

Fig. 6.30 Spondylolisthesis with pars interarticulari attenuation and facet arthropathy. (**a**) Lateral radiograph of the lumbosacral spine demonstrates spondylolisthesis at L5–S1 (*dashed lines*). There is a suggestion of sclerosis in the region of the L5–S1 facet joints (*arrow*). (**b**) Sagittal CT reformatted image shows thinning of the right pars interarticularis (*black arrow*) and facet arthropathy at L5–S1 on the right with sclerosis (*straight white arrow*) and a vacuum phenomenon (*curved white arrow*). (**c**) Axial CT slice through the L5–S1 posterior elements confirms the thinning of the pars interarticulari (*black arrows*). Facet arthropathy (*straight white arrows*) is seen with vacuum phenomena, more prominent on the right (*curved arrow*)

Similarly, SPECT cannot provide information about the presence or absence of spondylolisthesis. With proper equipment, SPECT can be combined with conventional CT in one examination (SPECT/CT).

Positron-Emission Tomography Bone Scintigraphy

Positron-emission tomography (PET) is similar to SPECT in that the examination provides improved localization of radiotracer activity over planar scintigraphy. However, the radiotracers used in PET are different from SPECT as they do not directly emit gamma rays, but rather they emit protons that interact with the surrounding tissues to produce gamma rays indirectly.

Although not commonly used, PET bone scans following administration of the bone-specific radiotracer fluorine-18 sodium fluoride (^{18}F NaF) may be superior to SPECT bone scans in the assessment of spondylolysis [23].

Similar to SPECT, PET does not provide specific anatomic detail unless combined with CT (PET/CT). The cost of PET is higher than SPECT but some of the relative expense may be offset by improved patient flow through the imaging facility as scan times for PET are shorter than those for SPECT.

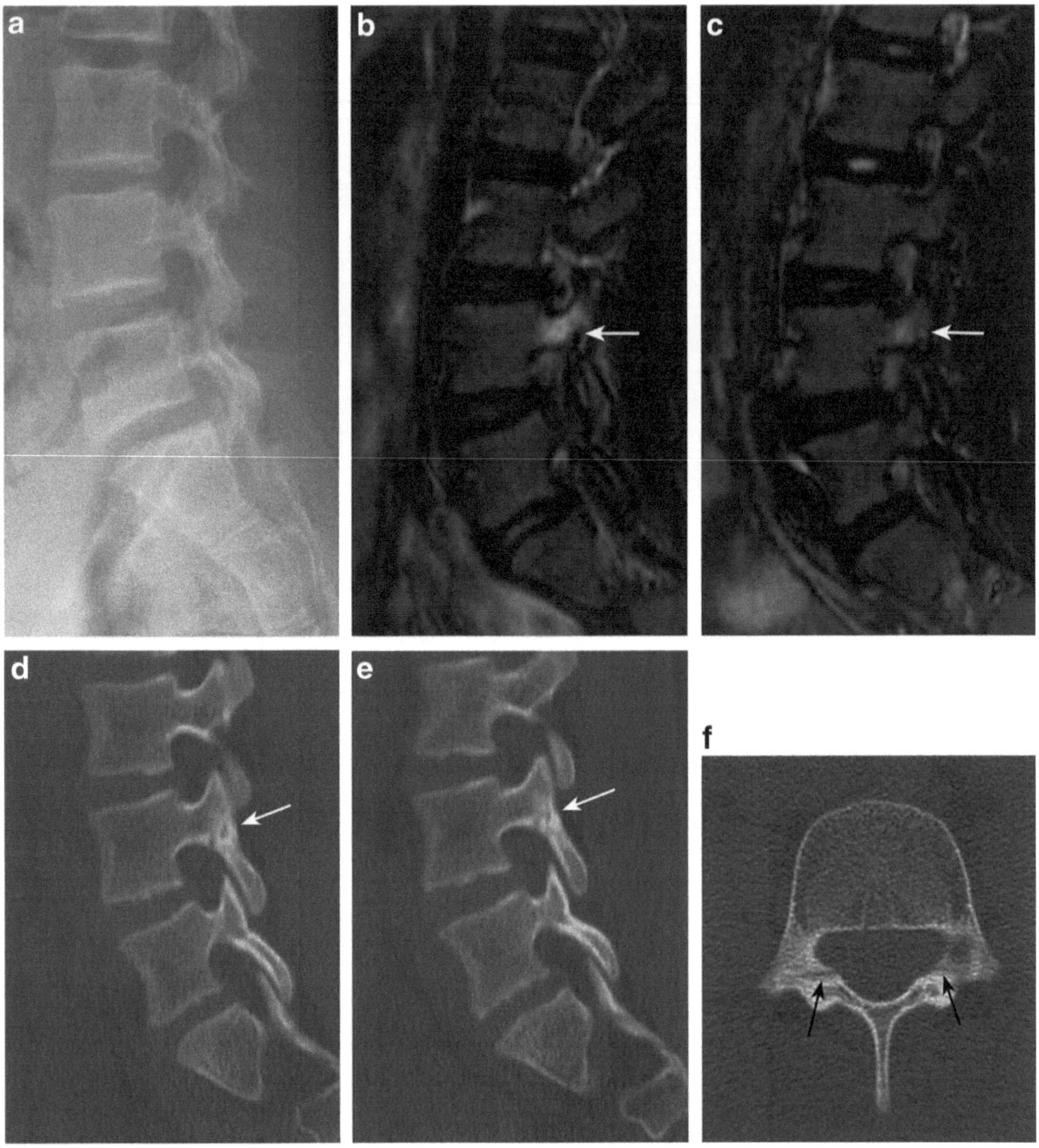

Fig. 6.31 Incomplete bilateral spondylolysis at L4. (**a**) Lateral lumbosacral spine radiograph appears normal. Sagittal MRI STIR images demonstrate edema in the pedicles of L4, greater on the right (**b**) than on the left (**c**). Sagittal reformatted CT images demonstrate lucencies with surrounding sclerosis in the pars interarticulari, greater on the right (**d**) than on the left (**e**). (**f**) Axial CT slice through the L4 pars interarticulari confirms the incomplete spondylolyses, more pronounced on the right than the left

Imaging Findings in Spondylolisthesis According to Etiology

The classification of spondylolisthesis proposed by Wiltse et al. [24] is based on the etiology of the spondylolisthesis and remains in general use today. The original classification includes five categories: dysplastic, isthmic, degenerative, traumatic, and pathological spondylolisthesis. Post-operative spondylolisthesis has been added as a sixth group. There are imaging similarities and differences among the groups. The choice of imaging beyond radiographs may be influenced by the type of spondylolisthesis.

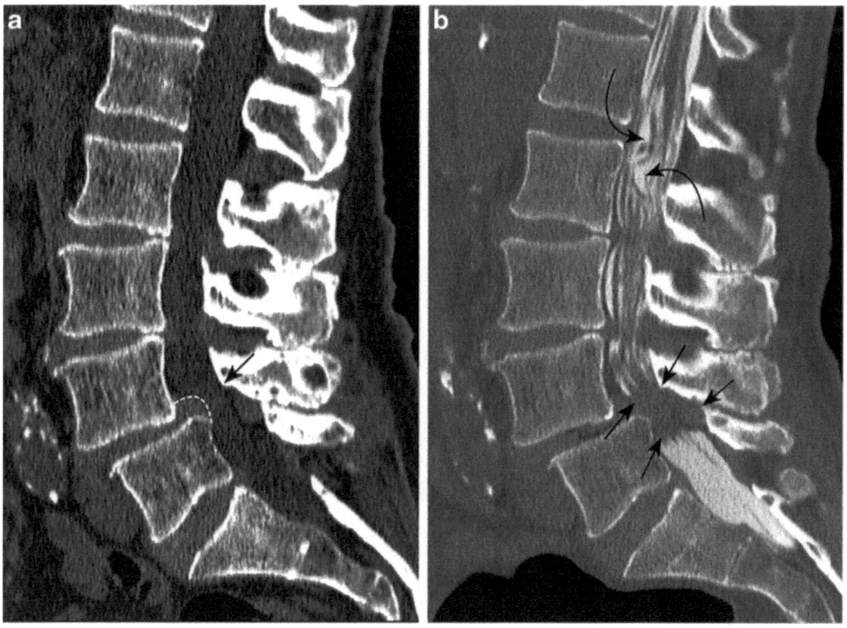

Fig. 6.32 Myelography in spondylolisthesis. (**a**) Reformatted sagittal CT image demonstrates anterolisthesis at L4–5. The L4–5 intervertebral disc is uncovered as it remains aligned with L5 (*dotted line*). Central spinal canal stenosis is evident (*arrow*). (**b**) Image from a CT myelogram demonstrates a filling defect in the spinal canal at the level of the stenosis, indicating a high-grade block to cerebrospinal fluid flow (*straight arrows*). There is redundancy of the descending nerve roots related to the spinal canal stenosis (*curved arrows*)

Dysplastic Spondylolisthesis

Dysplastic spondylolisthesis includes cases of congenital dysplasia of the upper sacrum or the posterior elements of L5, such as spina bifida (Figs. 6.16 and 6.34). The pars interarticulari may remain normal, allowing only a grade I slip. More frequently, the pars interarticulari are elongated or separated [24]. When the pars interarticularis is elongated or separated in dysplastic spondylolisthesis, the process may be difficult to distinguish from isthmic spondylolisthesis; attention to the caudal end of the sacrum and the remainder of the neural arch of L5 is essential for diagnosis.

Isthmic Spondylolisthesis

In isthmic spondylolisthesis, the most common type of spondylolisthesis in patients below age 50, the primary abnormality is in the pars interarticularis, the segment of bone between the superior and inferior articular facets of the neural arch. Spondylolyses can be demonstrated on radiography (Figs. 6.11, 6.12, and 6.19), CT (Figs. 6.19 and 6.29) or MRI (Fig. 6.33). The abnormality occurs most commonly at L5 [24, 25]. In the majority of patients with spondylolysis, the finding is bilateral [24]. Intervertebral disc degeneration and facet arthropathy are characteristically absent in adolescents with isthmic spondylolisthesis especially in milder slips [26].

In subtype A of isthmic spondylolisthesis, there is a discrete defect and the consensus at present is that the defect is a fatigue fracture. Thus, evaluation of spine radiographs in adolescents with spondylolisthesis should include a meticulous search for spondylolysis, particularly in athletes participating in sports such as diving, weightlifting, and wrestling [27]. The edges of the pars interarticulari defects are usually somewhat smoothed and may show sclerosis. In unilateral spondylolysis, sclerosis may also been seen in the opposite side of the neural arch related to stress changes, indicating the possibility of a developing spondylolysis. Subset B includes patients with elongation of the pars

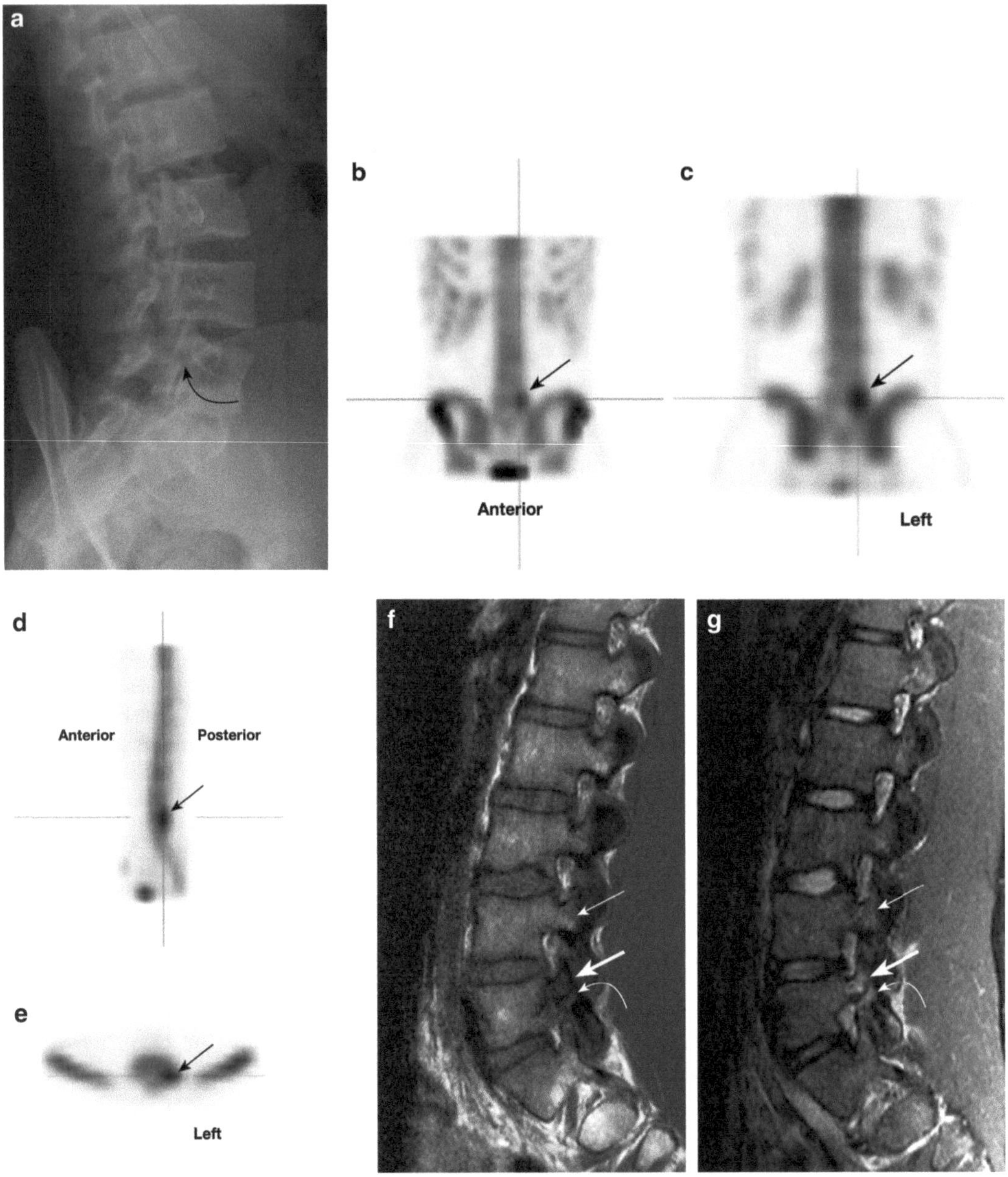

Fig. 6.33 SPECT bone scan and MRI in spondylolisthesis. (**a**) Left posterior oblique radiograph demonstrates a questionable lucency in the left L5 pars interarticularis (*curved arrow*). (**b**) Standard Tc-99m MDP bone scan shows a focus of increased radioisotope activity at L5 on the left (*arrow*). (**c–e**) SPECT bone scan images in coronal (**c**), sagittal (**d**), and axial (**e**) planes further localize the site of radioisotope activity to the left posterior elements of L5 (*arrows*). (**f**) Sagittal T1W MRI slice to the left of midline delineates a defect in the left pars interarticularis (*curved arrow*) with decreased signal in the adjacent pedicle (*thick straight arrow*) indicating marrow edema. Note the normal signal in the pedicle above (*thin white arrow*). (**g**) Increased signal intensity in the pedicle on the STIR MRI sequence confirms the presence of marrow edema (*thick white arrow*) with normal marrow signal in the pedicle above (*thin white arrow*). Increased signal intensity is seen at the pars interarticularis defect (*curved arrow*)

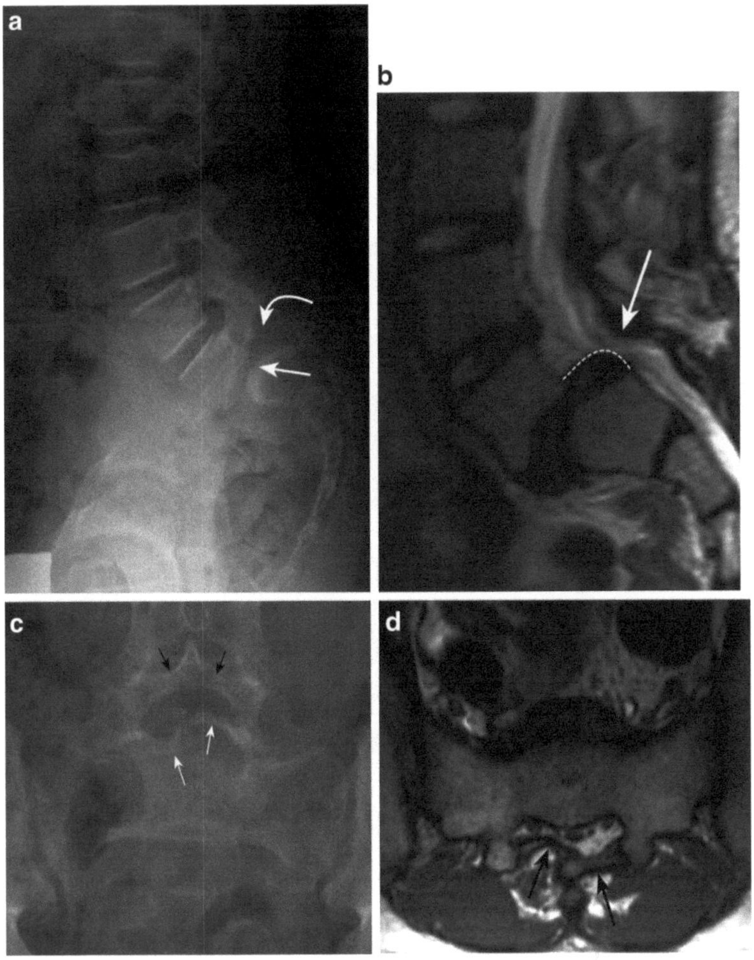

Fig. 6.34 Dysplastic spondylolisthesis. (**a**) Lateral radiograph demonstrates anterolisthesis at L5–S1 with a gaping defect in the pars interarticularis of L5 (*curved arrow*). There is convexity of the superior endplate of S1 with sclerosis (*straight arrow*). (**b**) Sagittal T2W MRI slice demonstrates uncovering of the L5–S1 disc (*dashed line*) with central spinal canal stenosis (*arrow*). (**c**) Frontal radiograph demonstrates dysplastic changes of the posterior elements of S1 (*white arrows*) with a normal appearance of the laminae and spinous process of L5 (*black arrows*). (**d**) Axial T1W MRI confirms the dysplastic changes of S1 (*black arrows*) with central canal stenosis more pronounced on the right

interarticularis without separation. The finding is thought to be related to serial microfractures with subsequent deformity (Fig. 6.35). Subset C of isthmic spondylolisthesis refers to rare acute fractures of the pars interarticulari secondary to severe trauma. A sharp fracture line in the pars interarticularis may indicate an acute finding in the proper clinical setting.

Regarding the sensitivity of radiographs in spondylolysis, a 1,500-patient study of six-view examinations reported an incidence of spondylolysis of 3.7 % [28], just slightly lower than a 4,200-cadaver study where the incidence was 4.2 % [25]. In the former study, the six views included AP, lateral, angled-up AP, collimated lateral, and obliques. The single most sensitive view was the collimated lateral view which detected 84 % of the lyses; 10 % of lyses were seen only on the oblique views. Libson et al. reported that almost 19 % of spondylolyses in their series were seen only on the oblique views [29]. Oblique radiographs carry a higher degree of difficulty for the technologist than lateral views with regard to optimal positioning and technique. Even in the best of hands, lyses at L5, the most common level, may be difficult to demonstrate on the obliques. In view of concerns about radiation exposure, a prudent approach would include evaluation of the routine lateral view before proceeding to a collimated lateral view and/or lateral obliques. If the radiographs are equivocal or negative in the setting of strong

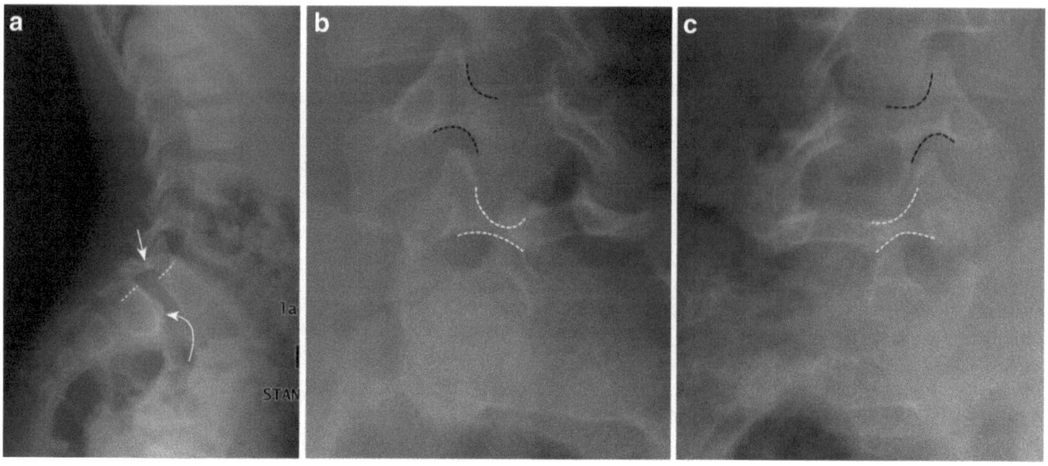

Fig. 6.35 Isthmic spondylolisthesis, subset B. (**a**) Lateral lumbosacral spine radiograph in a 7-year-old demonstrates a grade I anterolisthesis at L5–S1 (*dashed lines*), dystrophic convexity and sclerosis of the superior endplate of the sacrum (*curved arrow*), and thinning of the pars interarticularis (*straight arrow*). (**b** and **c**) Oblique views demonstrate elongation and thinning of the *right* (**b**) and *left* (**c**) L5 pars interarticulari (*white dotted lines*). Note the normal L4 Scottie dog necks (pars interarticulari) outlined by *black dotted lines*

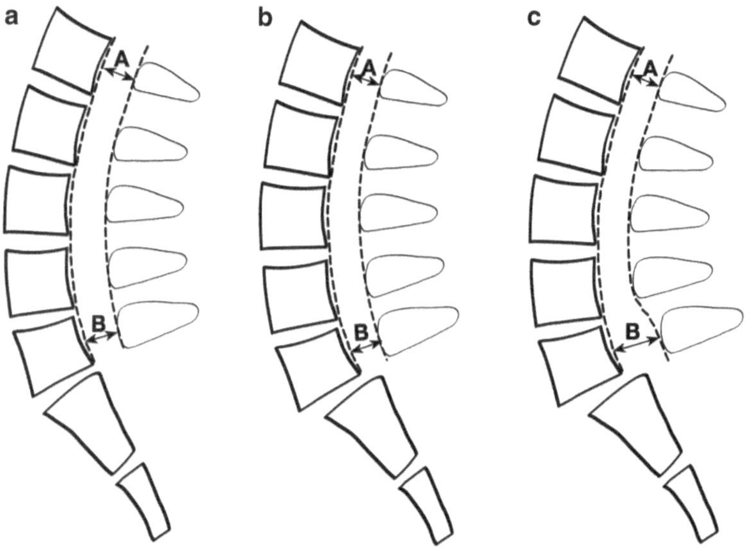

Fig. 6.36 Spinal canal caliber in spondylolisthesis (illustrated here at L5–S1) with and without spondylolysis. The spinal canal is delineated anteriorly by a *dashed line* that runs along the posterior vertebral body margins. Posteriorly, the canal is defined by a *dashed line* running along the anterior aspects of the spinous processes. A = spinal canal width posterior to L1. B = canal width posterior to L5. (**a**) Normal alignment. B is $<1.25 \times A$. (**b**) Anterolisthesis at L5–S1 without spondylolysis. L5 and the vertebrae above move forward with their posterior elements. B is $<1.25 \times A$. (**c**) Anterolisthesis at L5–S1 with spondylolysis resulting in "wide canal" sign. As L5 and the vertebrae above move forward, the spinous process of L5 remains in its original position (or in some cases slips posteriorly). B is $\geq 1.25 \times A$

clinical suspicion for spondylolysis, the next step in the workup would be cross-sectional imaging.

In patients with isthmic spondylolisthesis, MRI and CT may reveal a widened appearance to the spinal canal at the level of slippage. The finding of a wide canal reflects anterior displacement of the involved vertebral body without its spinous process (Figs. 6.36 and 6.37) [30].

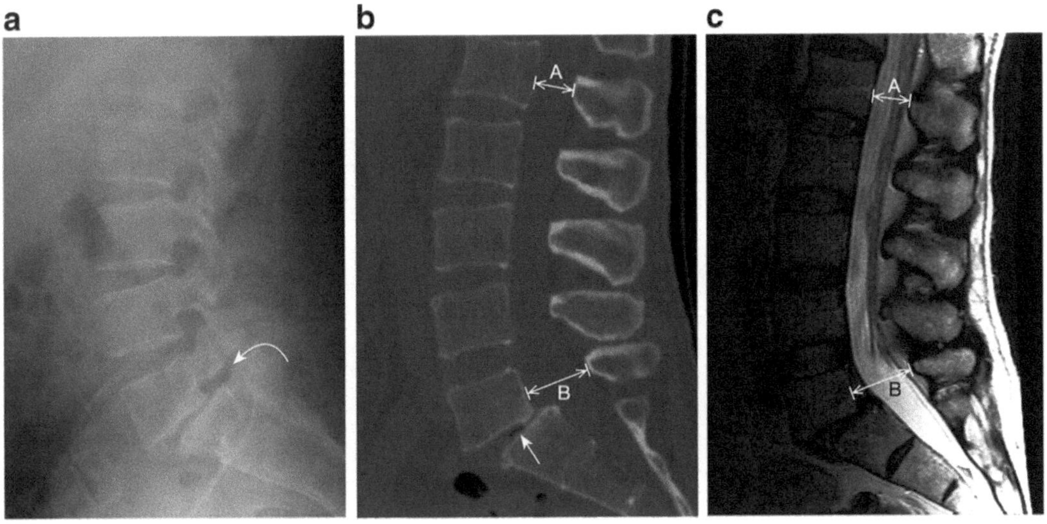

Fig. 6.37 "Wide canal" sign of spondylolisthesis with spondylolysis. (**a**) Lateral radiograph demonstrates anterolisthesis of L5 over S1 with spondylolysis (*curved arrow*). (**b**) Midline sagittal CT reformatted image shows discrepancy between the AP diameters of the spinal canal at L1 (*A*) versus L5 (*B*), with increased AP diameter of the canal at L5 as a result of anterior displacement of the L5 vertebral body without its spinous process. Also noted is L5–S1 disc space narrowing with the vacuum phenomenon of disc degeneration (*arrow*). (**c**) Discrepancy in AP canal diameter is shown on sagittal T2W MRI in the same patient between L1 (A) and L5 (*B*)

An important advantage of MRI in the evaluation of spondylolysis is that once the diagnosis is established by any imaging modality, the presence or absence of bone marrow edema at the site of the spondylolysis can be assessed on MRI and is thought to correlate with the degree of metabolic activity (Fig. 6.33) [31, 32]. However, one must be aware that for the initial detection of spondylolysis, MRI is not as reliable as CT (Fig. 6.31) [33]. This is related to the fact that the spatial resolution that is necessary to visualize fine bone detail is inherently lower in MRI than CT. In addition, the sagittal plane used in MRI does not parallel the orientation of the pars interarticulari.

Degenerative Spondylolisthesis

Degenerative spondylolisthesis is typically found in the older patient population [34]. Unlike isthmic spondylolisthesis which is most common at L5–S1, degenerative anterolisthesis is most common at L4–5 and degenerative retrolisthesis is most common at L2–3 [33]. The commonly accepted theory is that degenerative spondylolisthesis is related to longstanding intersegmental instability with intervertebral disc degeneration, ligamentous insufficiency, and facet joint degeneration [7, 8].

Much attention has been given to the configuration of the facet joints as visualized on cross-sectional imaging in degenerative spondylolisthesis. Often the hypertrophied and sclerotic lumbar facets in degenerative spondylolisthesis are more sagittally (vertically) oriented on axial CT or MRI images compared to normal joints. This may result in decreased resistance to anterior–posterior stresses compared to normal lumbar facet joints. Most authors believe that progressive facet joint degeneration results in a change in the joint orientation. Others, however, believe that the sagittal facet orientation found in spondylolisthesis is a developmental abnormality that causes facet degeneration [34, 35].

As discussed, cross-sectional imaging is of particular value in assessing sequelae of degenerative spondylolisthesis such as central spinal canal stenosis and neural foraminal stenosis. These stenoses are usually related to a combination of findings including forward slippage of the posterior elements, uncovering of the interverte-

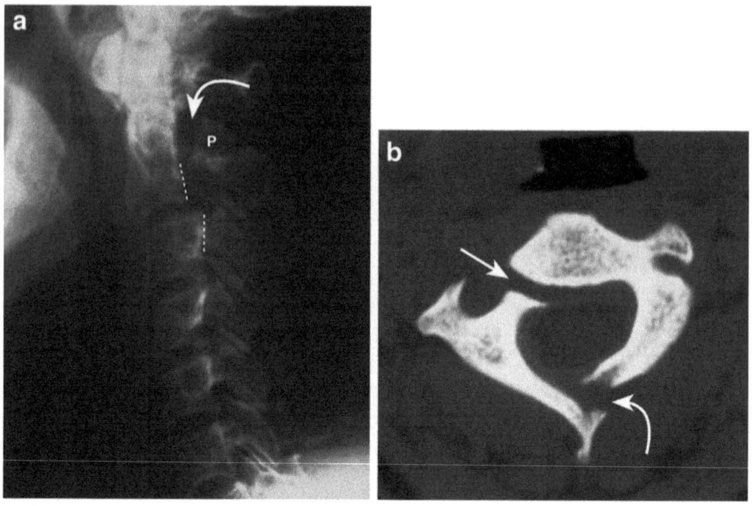

Fig. 6.38 Traumatic spondylolisthesis following a motor vehicle accident. (**a**) Lateral radiograph demonstrates anterolisthesis at C2–3 (*dashed lines*). At C2, there is a fracture (*curved arrow*) at the junction between one of the pedicles (*P*) and the vertebral body, with posterior displacement of the pedicle. (**b**) Axial CT slice confirms the fracture at the junction between the C2 vertebral body and the right pedicle (*arrow*) and a fracture through the left C2 lamina (*curved arrow*)

bral disc, facet joint hypertrophy, and ligamentum flavum hypertrophy (Figs. 6.26, 6.27, and 6.30). Central spinal canal stenosis from any cause may result in redundancy of descending nerve roots or blockage of the flow of cerebrospinal fluid (Figs. 6.26 and 6.32).

Traumatic Spondylolisthesis

Traumatic spondylolisthesis was described by Wiltse as vertebral slippage secondary to a fracture or fractures within the posterior vertebral arch not including the pars interarticularis (Fig. 6.38) [24]. This type of spondylolisthesis must be distinguished from subtype C of isthmic spondylolisthesis where isolated acute fractures of the pars interarticulari are present.

Pathological Spondylolisthesis

Spondylolisthesis in the setting of generalized or localized bone disease is termed pathological spondylolisthesis. Any process resulting in sufficient compromise of the neural arch can be responsible for vertebral slippage (Fig. 6.39). Osteopetrosis, arthrogryposis, infection, Paget's disease, osteoporosis, and tumor are among the many causes.

Post-operative Spondylolisthesis

Spondylolisthesis may develop or progress following posterior spinal decompression procedures. Sienkiewicz and Flatley found that post-operative spondylolisthesis occurred more commonly in women, most often at L4–5 [36]. Radiographic diagnosis involves comparison of pre-operative and post-operative lateral views. Care should be taken to insure that the images are of similar technique and positioning (Fig. 6.40).

Radiation Safety

Patient Radiation Dose

The interest in patient radiation dose has been stimulated by the knowledge that ionizing radiation is a carcinogen coupled with the reported significant increase in computed tomography and nuclear medicine exams in the USA from the

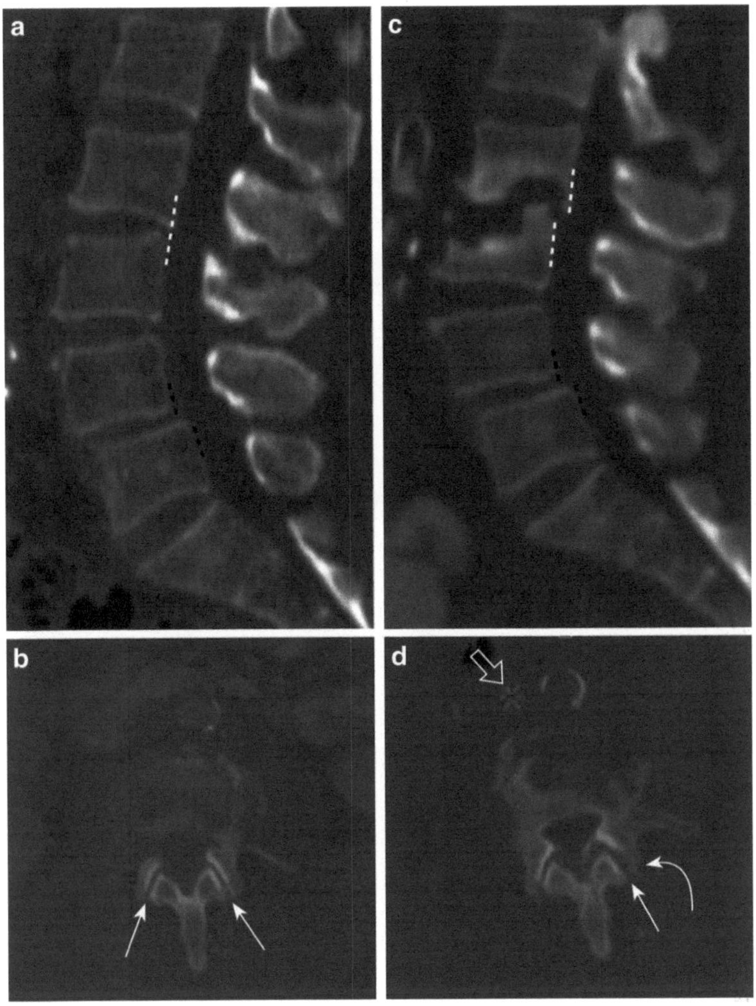

Fig. 6.39 Pathologic spondylolisthesis secondary to discitis and osteomyelitis with spread to the posterior elements. (**a**) Sagittal midline CT reformatted image early in the clinical course of the disease prior to CT evidence of infection demonstrates normal alignment at L2–3 (*white dashed line*). Unrelated disc space narrowing and degenerative anterolisthesis at L4–5 is noted (*black dashed lines*). (**b**) Axial CT slice from same study as (**a**) demonstrates a normal appearance of the L2–3 facet joints (*arrows*). (**c**) Several weeks later, there is marked bone destruction on both sides of the L2–3 disc with new retrolisthesis at L2–3 (*white dashed lines*); there is no change in the unrelated L4–5 anterolisthesis (*black dashed lines*). (**d**) axial CT slice from same scan as (**c**) demonstrates bone destruction at the *left* L2–3 facet joint secondary to infection (*straight arrow*), most pronounced at the posterolateral aspect of the superior articular facet of L3 (*curved arrow*) resulting in instability of the facet joint, the neural arch component of the pathologic spondylolisthesis. Incidentally noted is an inferior vena caval filter (*open arrow*) to the right of the calcified aorta

early 1990s through 2006 [37]. During the period between 1993 and 2006, the number of CT procedures in the USA increased from 18.3 to 62 million, an increase of 240 %, while the population increased by only 16.4 %.

Various reports have been published estimating the risk of cancer induction from computed tomography radiation doses in pediatric and adult patients [38, 39]. While these reports remain controversial with regard to the radiation risk factors used in their calculations, they have stimulated the radiology community to create more awareness of the radiation dose associated with imaging procedures with the Image Gently and Image

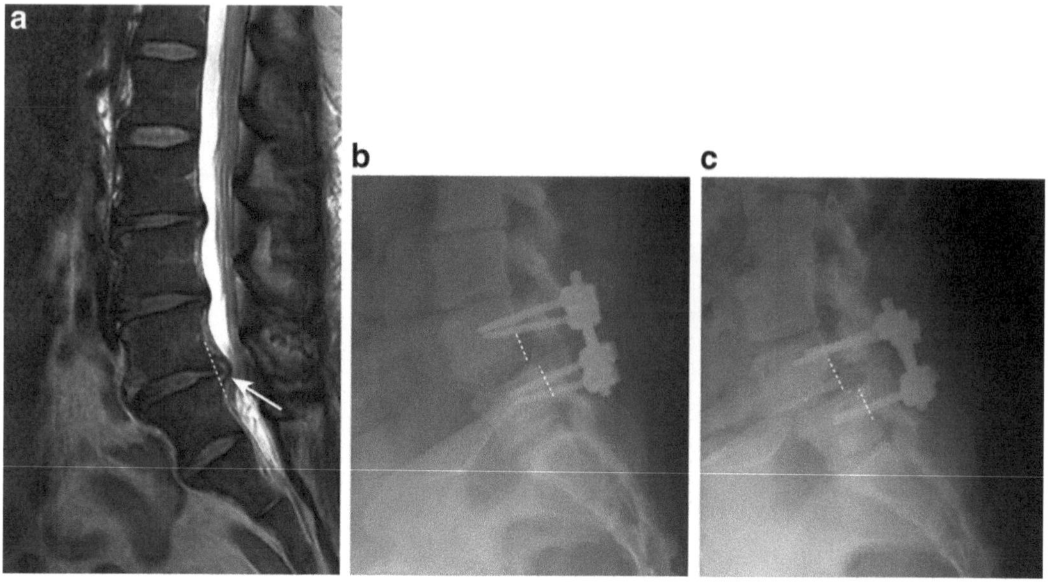

Fig. 6.40 Post-operative spondylolisthesis. (**a**) Pre-operative sagittal T2W MRI demonstrates normal alignment at L4–5 (*dashed line*). There is central spinal canal stenosis related to a disc protrusion (*arrow*). (**b**) Two months after posterior spinal decompression including L4 and L5 laminectomies, there is mild anterolisthesis at L4–5 (*dashed lines*). (**c**) Twenty-six months after surgery, the anterolisthesis has progressed (*dashed lines*)

Wisely campaigns [40, 41]. Efforts have been proposed within these campaigns for imaging facilities to review their CT protocols and radiographic technique factors with the goal of reducing radiation dose as long as the image quality is not significantly compromised.

Effective Dose

The dose metric most widely used to compare different imaging modalities is the effective dose. This dose metric, utilized by the International Commission on Radiological Protection (ICRP), represents the weighted average of the mean absorbed dose to various organs and tissues of the body [42].

The effective dose, H_E, is calculated by summing up the dose equivalent, multiplied by specific weighting factors, for 28 different tissues and organs of the body; these coefficients were most recently revised by the ICRP in 2007 [43].

Since it is not feasible to measure the dose to the tissues during an imaging procedure, Monte Carlo computer codes have been written to estimate the individual tissue doses and calculate the effective dose. The effective dose is widely used to compare the radiation dose for different imaging procedures that utilize ionizing radiation, but it should be noted that the Monte Carlo computer codes usually use an anatomic model of an "average male" or an "average female" mathematical phantom which is not applicable to most patients. The relative uncertainty in the calculation of effective dose for a reference patient has been estimated to be as high as 40 % [44].

Radiography

There are several factors which affect patient effective dose including radiographic technique factors such as peak kilovoltage (kVp), tube current in milliamperes (mA), and exposure time in seconds. The mA×time in seconds equals the mAs. The use of grids, and distance between the X-ray tube, patient, and image receptor also affect the effective dose. In conventional radiography the user has a choice of different speed film/screen systems, and with computed radiography and digital radiography the user can chose different values of a speed class and/or exposure index. As a result of the multiple variables indicated above, there is a range of effective dose values reported in the literature.

Several groups have estimated the effective dose for lumbar spine and scoliosis radiography for film/screen, computed radiography, and digital radiography for adult and pediatric patients. For adult lumbar spine radiography a summary of effective doses included in the United Nations Scientific Committee on the Effects of Atomic Radiation 2008 report indicated a range of 0.309–1.5 millisievert (mSv) for both the AP plus lateral views while other groups reported 3.70 mSv for the same exam [45, 46].

For scoliosis examinations in a patient age range of 13–18 years, Hansen et al. estimated an effective dose for the PA and lateral views of 1.03 mSv for film/screen exams utilizing a grid compared to 0.078 mSv for computed radiography with an air gap technique, a reduction in dose by more than a factor of 10 [47].

Several authors presented data for both AP and PA projections [47, 48]. The effective dose for an AP projection is larger than the PA projection by approximately a factor of 2. The PA projection is preferred to the AP view to minimize the breast dose as well as the effective dose.

Computed Tomography

CT scans deliver a much larger dose of radiation to patients than conventional radiography [49]. For instance, the effective dose for a chest CT is approximately 7 mSv while that for PA and lateral radiographs is only 0.1 mSv [50].

As with radiographic imaging, factors which affect CT radiation dose include kilovoltage, tube current, and rotation time. The radiation dose also depends upon CT parameters such as detector collimation and helical pitch. In most modern CT scanners, the tube current can also be automatically adjusted to accommodate differences in patient thickness as the X-ray tube rotates around the patient and as the table moves through the gantry, allowing for optimization of the tube current and the effective dose [51]. The latest dose reduction strategy utilizes a new CT reconstruction algorithm, adaptive statistical iterative reconstruction, which results in less image noise from the same raw data and has allowed some users to achieve a 50 % dose reduction [52].

Reported values of effective dose for CT examinations of the whole lumbar spine range from 4.5 to 19.15 mSv [47, 53, 54]. However, an effort to reduce the effective dose for scoliosis examinations using 80 kVp and very low mAs resulted in an average effective dose value of 0.37 mSv without any reduction in image quality for the assessment of screw placement, a marked reduction in dose compared to that for trauma CT of the lumbar spine [55].

Nuclear Medicine Imaging

Useful nuclear medicine studies for lumbar spine imaging include SPECT with ^{99m}TcMDP and PET with ^{18}Fl sodium fluoride [56]. The effective doses associated with these imaging studies depend upon the activity (mega Becquerel units) of the isotope injected into the patient and typical values are 4.2–5.3 mSv for SPECT and 4.4–8.9 mSv for PET.

Intraoperative Imaging

There has been an increase in the use of image guided spinal navigation systems which incorporate a C-arm fluoroscope capable of rotational motion around the patient with the subsequent reconstruction of CT format images. This type of unit, often incorporating a flat panel detector, is referred to a cone beam CT (CBCT) scanner. Standard C-arm fluoroscopy is also used during lumbar spine surgery.

The mean effective dose for typical posterior thoracolumbar instrumental spinal procedures using the Medtronic O-Arm in "standard mode" was estimated to be 3.24 mSv for a "small patient" and 8.09 mSv for a "large patient" using a single scan [57]. If the entire procedure contains scans for both navigation and confirmation of instrumentation placement, the total effective dose will be higher. For example, a single-level fusion requiring two scans would double the mean effective dose indicated above, resulting in 6.48 and 16.18 mSv for the "small" and "large" patients, respectively.

For 3-D navigated spinal surgery using a C-arm CBCT, Kraus et al. reported an effective dose of 0.4 mSv for lumbar dorsal spinal fusion (four screws) and 0.51 mSv for sacroiliac single screw insertions [58]. Their 3-D navigational results were markedly lower than the effective doses they measured for conventional fluoroscopy, 5.03 mSv for spinal fusion and 2.5 mSv for sacroiliac screw insertions.

Another group measured the effective dose for lumbar spine fusion for conventional fluoroscopy to be 1.0 mSv [59]. This group also measured an effective dose range for preoperative CT guided surgery of 2.4–4.1 mSv.

It is clear that effective dose levels from CBCT scanners used in image guided surgery can approach and exceed the effective doses delivered by conventional multi-slice CT units for exams of the chest, abdomen, and pelvis [50].

Radiation Risk Factors

The risk factors for radiation-induced cancer have been derived from studies of Japanese survivors of the atomic bomb blasts at the end of World War II. These risk factors have been used in several reports to estimate the cancer risk for individuals exposed to diagnostic imaging dose levels [38, 39, 54]. For example, Richards et al. estimated the cancer risk for a CT scan of the whole lumbar spine with an effective dose of 5.6 mSv to be 1 in 3,200 [54].

Since there are major differences between the instantaneous total body exposure of Japanese survivors and the partial body exposure of patients undergoing imaging procedures, the extrapolation of Japanese survivor data to medical imaging studies has been regarded by some as debatable. However, a recent study of 180,000 pediatric patients who underwent 280,000 CT scans in the United Kingdom between 1985 and 2002 revealed a small but significant risk of brain cancer and leukemia for patients who underwent one head CT in the first decade of life [60]. Although the risk was revealed to be relatively small (one excess brain tumor and one excess case of leukemia per 10,000 patients who underwent head CT before age 10), prudent use of imaging studies that use ionizing radiation is an important goal of the medical community.

Summary

With proper understanding and use of available imaging modalities, the diagnosis and evaluation of spondylolisthesis can be carried out effectively with little or no risk to the patient. Radiography, MRI, CT and nuclear medicine scans are best used with knowledge of their advantages and disadvantages including radiation exposure to the patient. Radiography is usually the first examination to be performed, and in many cases will provide all the information that is needed such as grade, etiology, and presence or absence of spondylolysis. Cross-sectional imaging is particularly useful in assessing the central spinal canal and neural foramina. In evaluation of associated spondylolysis, CT provides added sensitivity over MRI, and provides more specific information than scintigraphy, while MRI and SPECT bone scans can provide information about the activity of disease in pars interarticularis defects.

References

1. American College of Radiology. ACR Appropriateness Criteria®-low back pain radiographs; 2013. http://www.acr.org/~/media/ACR/Documents/AppCriteria/Diagnostic/LowBackPain.pdf. Accessed 23 July 2013.
2. Iguchi T, Wakami T, Kurihara A, Kasahara K, Yoshiya S, Nishida K. Lumbar multilevel degenerative spondylolisthesis: radiological evaluation and factors related to anterolisthesis and retrolisthesis. J Spinal Disord Tech. 2002;5(2):93–9.
3. Meyerding HW. Spondylolisthesis. Surg Gynecol Obstet. 1932;54:371–7.
4. Taillard W. Le spondylolisthesis chez l'enfant et l'adolescent. Acta Orthop Scand. 1954;24(1–40):115–44.

5. Timon SJ, Gardner MJ, Wanich T, Poynton A, Pigeon R, Widmann RF, Rawlins BA, Burke SW. Not all spondylolisthesis grading instruments are reliable. Clin Orthop Relat Res. 2005;434:157–62.
6. Vialle R, Schmit P, Dauzac C, Wicart P, Glorion C, Guigui P. Radiological assessment of lumbosacral dystrophic changes in high-grade spondylolisthesis. Skeletal Radiol. 2005;34(9):528–35.
7. Butler D, Trafimow JH, Andersson GBJ, McNeill TW, Huckman MS. Discs degenerate before facets. Spine. 1990;15(2):111–3.
8. Herkowitz HN. Spine update: degenerative spondylolisthesis. Spine. 1995;20(9):1084–90.
9. Fisk JR, Moe JH, Winter RB. Scoliosis, spondylolysis, and spondylolisthesis. Their relationship as reviewed in 539 patients. Spine (Phila Pa 1976). 1978;3(3): 234–45.
10. Toyone T, Tanaka T, Kato D, Kaneyama R, Otsuka M. Anatomic changes in lateral spondylolisthesis associated with adult lumbar scoliosis. Spine (Phila Pa 1976). 2005;30(22):E671–5.
11. Talangbayan LE. The inverted Napoleon's hat sign. Radiology. 2007;243(2):603–4.
12. Ravichandran G. A radiologic sign in spondylolisthesis. AJR Am J Roentgenol. 1980;134(1): 113–7.
13. Maldague BE, Malghem JJ. Unilateral arch hypertrophy with spinous process tilt: a sign of arch deficiency. Radiology. 1976;121(3 Pt. 1):567–74.
14. Schwab FJ, Farcy JP, Roye Jr DP. The sagittal pelvic tilt index as a criterion in the evaluation of spondylolisthesis. Preliminary observations. Spine (Phila Pa 1976). 1997;22(14):1661–7.
15. Dubousset J. Treatment of spondylolysis and spondylolisthesis in children and adolescents. Clin Orthop Relat Res. 1997;337:77–85.
16. Curylo LJ, Edwards C, DeWald RW. Radiographic markers in spondyloptosis: implications for spondylolisthesis progression. Spine (Phila Pa 1976). 2002; 27(18):2021–5.
17. Kälebo P, Kadziolka R, Swärd L, Zachrisson BE. Stress views in the comparative assessment of spondylolytic spondylolisthesis. Skeletal Radiol. 1989; 17(8):570–5.
18. Putto E, Tallroth K. Extension-flexion radiographs for motion studies of the lumbar spine. A comparison of two methods. Spine (Phila Pa 1976). 1990;15(2): 107–10.
19. Leone A, Guglielmi G, Cassar-Pullicino VN, Bonomo L. Lumbar intervertebral instability: a review. Radiology. 2007;245(1):62–77.
20. Maus T. Imaging of the spine and nerve roots. Phys Med Rehabil Clin N Am. 2002;13:487–544.
21. Nicolaou S, Liang T, Murphy DT, Korzan JR, Ouellette H, Munk P. Dual-energy CT: a promising new technique for assessment of the musculoskeletal system. AJR Am J Roentgenol. 2012;199(5 Suppl): S78–86.
22. Zukotynski K, Curtis C, Grant FD, Micheli L, Treves ST. The value of SPECT in the detection of stress injury to the pars interarticularis in patients with low back pain. J Orthop Surg Res. 2010;5:13.
23. Lim R, Fahey FH, Drubach LA, Connolly LP, Treves ST. Early experience with fluorine-18 sodium fluoride bone PET in young patients with back pain. J Pediatr Orthop. 2007;27(3):277–82. PMID: 17414009.
24. Wiltse LL, Newman PH, Macnab I. Classification of spondylolisis and spondylolisthesis. Clin Orthop Relat Res. 1976;117:23–9.
25. Roche MB, Rowe GG. The incidence of separate neural arch and coincident bone variations; a survey of 4,200 skeletons. Anat Rec. 1951;109(2):233–52.
26. Paajanen H, Tertti M. Association of incipient disc degeneration and instability in spondylolisthesis. A magnetic resonance and flexion-extension radiographic study of 20-year-old low back pain patients. Arch Orthop Trauma Surg. 1991;111(1):16–9.
27. Rossi F, Dragoni S. The prevalence of spondylolysis and spondylolisthesis in symptomatic elite athletes: radiographic findings. Radiography. 2001;7(1):37–42.
28. Amato M, Totty WG, Gilula LA. Spondylolysis of the lumbar spine: demonstration of defects and laminal fragmentation. Radiology. 1984;153(3):627–9.
29. Libson E, Bloom RA, Dinari G. Symptomatic and asymptomatic spondylolysis and spondylolisthesis in young adults. Int Orthop. 1982;6(4):259–61.
30. Ulmer JL, Elster AD, Mathews VP, King JC. Distinction between degenerative and isthmic spondylolisthesis on sagittal MR images: importance of increased anteroposterior diameter of the spinal canal ("wide canal sign"). AJR Am J Roentgenol. 1994;163(2):411–6.
31. Hollenberg GM, Beattie PF, Meyers SP, Weinberg EP, Adams MJ. Stress reactions of the lumbar pars interarticularis: the development of a new MRI classification system. Spine (Phila Pa 1976). 2002;27(2): 181–6.
32. Leone A, Cianfoni A, Cerase A, Magarelli N, Bonomo L. Lumbar spondylolysis: a review. Skeletal Radiol. 2011;40(6):683–700.
33. Yamaguchi Jr KT, Skaggs DL, Acevedo DC, Myung KS, Choi P, Andras L. Spondylolysis is frequently missed by MRI in adolescents with back pain. J Child Orthop. 2012;6(3):237–40.
34. Hession PR, Butt WP. Imaging of spondylolysis and spondylolisthesis. Eur Radiol. 1996;6(3):284–90.
35. Love TW, Fagan AB, Fraser RD. Degenerative spondylolisthesis: developmental or acquired? J Bone Joint Sur Br. 1999;81-B(4):670–4.
36. Sienkiewicz PJ, Flatley TJ. Postoperative spondylolisthesis. Clin Orthop Relat Res. 1987;221:172–80.
37. National Council on Radiation Protection and Measurements. Ionizing radiation exposure of the population of the United States. NCRP Report No. 160. Bethesda, MD: National Council on Radiation Protection and Measurements; 2009.
38. Brenner DJ, Elliston CD, Hall EJ, Berdon WE. Estimated risks of radiation-induced fatal cancer from pediatric CT. AJR Am J Roentgenol. 2001; 176:289–96.

39. Smith-Bindman R, Lipson J, Marcus R, Kim KP, Mahesh M, Gould R, Berrington de Gonza'lez A, Miglioretti DL. Radiation dose associated with common computed tomography examinations and the associated lifetime attributable risk of cancer. Arch Intern Med. 2009;169:2078–86.
40. Image Gently Web site. http://www.imagegently.org/. Accessed 19 Aug 2013.
41. Image Wisely Web site. http://www.imagewisely.org/ Accessed 19 Aug 2013.
42. 1990 Recommendations of the International Commission on Radiological Protection. ICRP publication 60. Ann ICRP. 1991;21(1–3):1–201.
43. The 2007 Recommendations of the International Commission on Radiological Protection. ICRP publication 103. Ann ICRP. 2007;37(2–4):1–332.
44. Martin CJ. Effective dose: how should it be applied to medical exposures? Br J Radiol. 2007;80:639–47.
45. United Nations Scientific Committee on the Effects of Atomic Radiation. Sources and effects of ionizing radiation. UNSCEAR 2008 Report to the General Assembly with Scientific Annexes. New York: United Nations; 2010.
46. Simpson AK, Whang PG, Jonisch A, Haims A, Grauer JN. The radiation exposure associated with cervical and lumbar spine radiographs. J Spinal Disord Tech. 2008;21:409–12.
47. Hansen J, Joric AG, Fiirgaard B, Egund N. Optimisation of scoliosis examination in children. Pediatr Radiol. 2003;33:752–65.
48. Gialousis G, Yiakoumakis EN, Makri TK, Papadoupoulou D, Karlatira M, Karaisakos P, Papaodysseas S, Evlogias N, Dimitriou PA, Georgiou EK. Comparison of dose from radiological examination for scoliosis in children among two pediatric hospitals by Monte Carlo simulation. Health Phys. 2008;94:471–8.
49. Brenner DJ, Hall EJ. Computed tomography – an increasing source of radiation exposure. N Engl J Med. 2007;357:2277–84.
50. Mettler Jr FA, Huda W, Yoshizumi TT, Mahesh M. Effective doses in radiology and diagnostic nuclear medicine: a catalog. Radiology. 2008;248:254–63.
51. Kalra MK, Maher MM, Toth TL, Hamberg LM, Blake MA, Shepard J, Saini S. Strategies for CT radiation dose optimization. Radiology. 2004;230:619–28.
52. Silva AC, Lawder HJ, Hara A, Kujak J, Pavlicek W. Innovations in CT dose reduction strategy: application of the adaptive statistical iterative reconstruction algorithm. AJR Am J Roentgenol. 2010; 194:191–9.
53. Biswas D, Bible JE, Bohan M, Simpson AK, Whang PG, Grauer JN. Radiation exposure from musculoskeletal computerized tomographic exams. J Bone Joint Surg Am. 2009;91:1882–9.
54. Richards PJ, Goerge J, Metelko M, Brown M. Spine computed tomography doses and cancer induction. Spine. 2010;35:430–3.
55. Kasim AK, Overgaard A, Maly P, Ohlin A, Gunnarsson M, Sundgren PC. Low-dose helical computed tomography (CT) in the perioperative workup of adolescent idiopathic scoliosis. Eur Radiol. 2009;19:610–8.
56. ACR-SPR practice guideline for the performance of skeletal scintigraphy (bone scan). American College of Radiology; 2012.
57. Lange J, Karellas A, Street J, Eck JC, Lapinsky A, Connolly PJ, DiPaola CP. Estimating the effective radiation dose imparted to patients by intraoperative cone-beam computed tomography in thoracolumbar spinal surgery. Spine. 2013;38:E306–12.
58. Kraus MD, Krischak G, Keppler P, Gebhard FT, Schuetz UHW. Can computer-assisted surgery reduce the effective dose for spinal fusion and sacroiliac screw insertion? Clin Orthop Relat Res. 2010; 468:2419–29.
59. Slomczykowski M, Roberto M, Schneeberger P, Ozdoba C, Vock P. Radiation dose for pedicle screw insertion. Fluoroscopic method versus computer-assisted surgery. Spine. 1999;24:975–82.
60. Pearce MS, Salotti JA, Little MP, McHugh K, Lee C, Kim KP, Howe NL, Ronckers CM, Rajaraman P, Sir Craft AW, Parker L, Berrington de González A. Radiation exposure from CT scans in childhood and subsequent risk of leukaemia and brain tumours: a retrospective cohort study. Lancet. 2012;380:499–505.

Classification of Spondylolisthesis

7

Richard Kim, Anuj Singla, and Amer F. Samdani

Introduction

Spondylolisthesis is described as the ventral translation of the proximal vertebral body in relation to the distal vertebral body. The pathophysiology involves pars fractures or lengthening which causes the body, pedicles, transverse processes, and superior articular processes to slip forward in varying degrees. The angle of L5 in relation to S1 potentiates this movement, especially in patients with ligamentous and/or bony instability at this level, and accounts for the relatively high incidence at the lumbosacral junction. While most common at this level, spondylolisthesis can occur at any level.

The management of spondylolisthesis is difficult because both surgical intervention and patient selection can be complex. While some patients are asymptomatic from seemingly severe spondylolisthesis, some are extremely symptomatic from a radiographically mild slip. Because of this wide range of patient presentations and radiographic appearances, classification systems are helpful in delineating prognosis and management. The ideal classification system has several key characteristics. First, it should be simple to recall and apply. Systems that are too complex will prohibit the user from being consistent with diagnosis and treatment in addition to deterring its use. Second, inter- and intraobserver variances must be low. This follows from the first requirement and allows consistent management of the pathology across patient populations and across physician populations. Third, the classification system must accurately reflect natural history of the disease so proper counseling can take place. Lastly, the classification system must guide the physician as to the proper treatment of spondylolisthesis; otherwise, it becomes useless in designing a treatment plan for a specific patient.

Classification systems will necessarily evolve over time. Advancements in diagnostic techniques can change how diseases are categorized. The advent of CT and MRI techniques has contributed significantly to the understanding of spondylolisthesis and has influenced how we classify and treat this disease. Evolving surgical techniques may also be the impetus for improving existing systems or developing new systems altogether. Improvements in fusion technologies may allow more aggressive treatment of spondylolisthesis and force surgeons to redefine what is treatable and what is not.

R. Kim, M.D.
Department of Neurosurgery, Temple University Hospital, 3401 North Broad Street, Philadelphia, PA 19140, USA
e-mail: kimrk@temple.edu

A. Singla, M.D.
University of Virginia Health System, 400 Ray C. Hunt Drive, Charlottesville, VA 22903, USA
e-mail: anujrajsingla@gmail.com

A.F. Samdani, M.D. (✉)
Shriners Hospitals for Children – Philadelphia, 3551 North Broad Street, Philadelphia, PA 19140, USA
e-mail: amersamdani@gmail.com

A.L. Wollowick and V. Sarwahi (eds.), *Spondylolisthesis: Diagnosis, Non-Surgical Management, and Surgical Techniques*, DOI 10.1007/978-1-4899-7575-1_7,

Meyerding Classification

In his article from 1932, Meyerding recognizes the rising importance of spondylolisthesis and its role in back pain and disability [1]. While he discussed the role of various factors contributing to spondylolisthesis, he did not incorporate them into the classification system. These factors included constant stress on the pars, congenital defects, and trauma, and he also revealed the value of X-ray in evaluation of this pathology. In addition, he describes his clinical parameters for diagnosis including a depression above the sacrum, sway back, muscle spasm, and prominent sacrum. In fact, he only eludes to the classification system which is described mostly in his figure. He admits that this system is purely for descriptive purposes only. Briefly, his system for grading is based on the percentage of slippage. Grade 1 is 0–25 %, Grade 2 is 25–50 %, Grade 3 is 50–75 %, and Grade 4 is 75–100 % (Table 7.1 and Fig. 7.1). This system holds its value in the fact that it is simple to

Table 7.1 Meyerding classification

Grade	Percentage slip
1	0–25
2	25–50
3	50–75
4	75–100

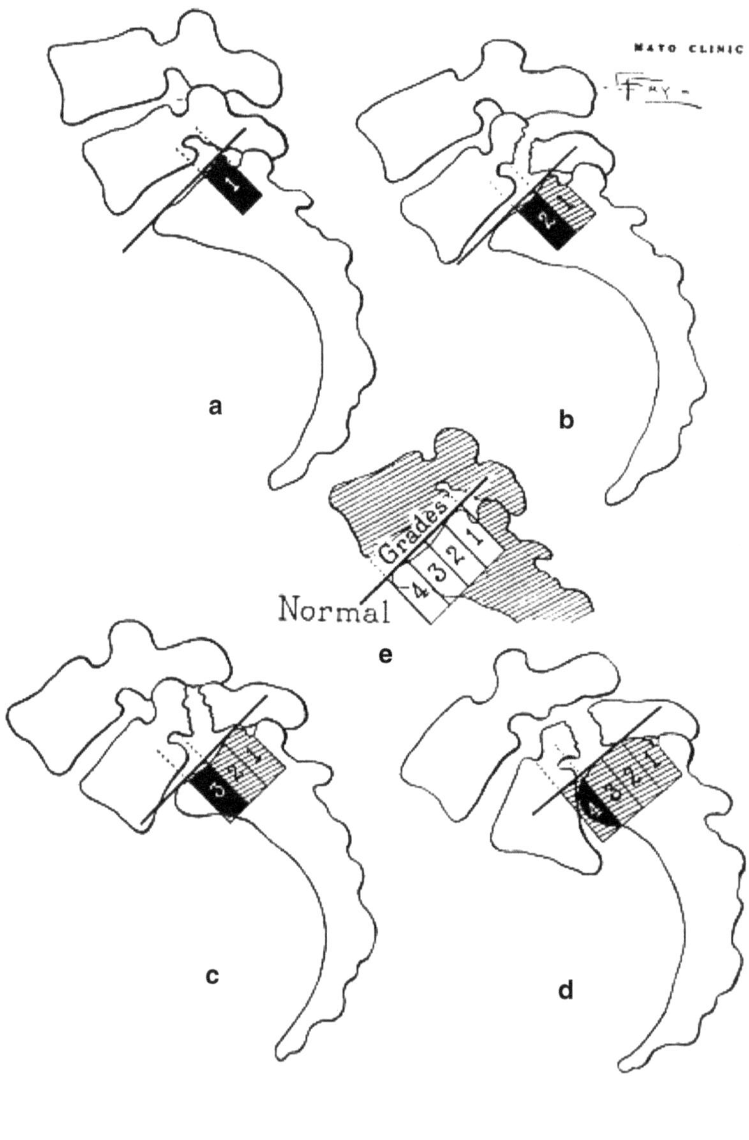

Fig. 7.1 Meyerding classification. [Reprinted from Meyerding HW. Spondylolisthesis. Surg Gynecol Obstet 1932;54:371–377. With permission from American College of Surgeons.]

remember and apply. Although he did not give any more information than a way to describe the severity of slippage, it set the foundation for important, large-scale studies involving spondylolisthesis [2–12] which eventually gave us surgical outcomes data based on his grading system. To date, there has not been a study evaluating the reliability of the Meyerding classification system.

Wiltse Classification

The Wiltse classification categorizes spondylolisthesis based on etiology. The five main categories are dysplastic, isthmic, degenerative, traumatic, and pathological [13, 14]. Isthmic is then subdivided into lytic, elongated, and acute fracture. This system is very widely used as a first step in describing the pathology exhibited on X-ray. Unfortunately, outside of placing the defect into a category, it does not assist in formulating a management plan. Also, as with many of the other earlier classification systems, the overall sagittal balance of the patient is not considered. Despite these shortcomings, the Wiltse classification system has remained one of the more important methods of categorizing spondylolisthesis. Table 7.2 summarizes this system.

Type 1, Dysplastic, describes cases where there is a congenital defect of the upper sacrum or the arch of L5 creating a situation where the forward thrust of the spinal column cannot be opposed and the slip progresses. The pars is usually normal but, if not, it is not the main pathology. There is a high association with spina bifida occulta (94 %) [14].

Table 7.2 Wiltse classification

Type	Description
I	*Dysplastic*—Congenital abnormalities of upper sacrum or L5 arch allows listhesis
II	*Isthmic*—defect in the pars interarticularis
IIA	Lytic—fatigue fracture of the pars
IIB	Elongated but intact pars
IIC	Acute fracture
III	*Degenerative*—results from longstanding intersegmental instability
IV	*Traumatic*—acute fractures in posterior elements exclusive of pars
V	*Pathologic*—destruction of posterior elements from generalized or localized disease of bone
VI	*Post surgical*

Type 2, Isthmic, involves a primary defect in the pars articularis from a failed neural arch. Approximately one-third are associated with spina bifida occulta and can be seen on 5–20 % of spine X-rays [15]. The three subcategories are lytic, elongated, and acute fracture. Lytic involves the fatigue fracture of the pars. This type is commonly found in the pediatric population, especially in athletes. This injury may reflect repetitive trauma or worsening of a pre-existing condition. The elongation subtype is similar to the lytic subtype but the pars is left intact. It is thought to be the result of multiple rounds of microfractures and healing, resulting in an elongated pars and slippage of vertebral body. The acute fracture subtype is caused by trauma and involves fracture of the pars and its resulting incompetence.

Type 3 is Degenerative. Longstanding intersegmental instability causes remodeling of the facets. This particular subtype occurs most commonly at L4–5, especially when L5 is sacralized. This subtype usually occurs in patients over the age of 50, and the slippage is usually less than 30 %. The pars remains intact [16].

Type 4 is Traumatic. An acute fracture of any part of the posterior element that keeps the spine from slipping forward will compromise its ability to maintain proper alignment.

Type 5 is Pathological. Bone disease, local or generalized, may prevent the posterior elements from opposing the forward slip of the spine. For example, Albers-Schönberg disease can cause pars fractures [13]. Other diseases such as arthrogryposis [16] and Paget's disease can cause systemic bone disease and result in spondylolisthesis.

Marchetti and Bartolozzi Classification

The Marchetti and Bartolozzi classification [17, 18] is one of the most commonly followed classification systems for spondylolisthesis.

Table 7.3 Marchetti and Bartolozzi classification

Developmental	Acquired
High dysplastic	Traumatic
With lysis	Acute fracture
With elongation	Stress fracture
Low dysplastic	Postsurgical
With lysis	Direct
With elongation	Indirect
	Pathologic
	Local
	Systemic
	Degenerative
	Primary
	Secondary

This is an etiology based system. The original classification proposed in 1982 classified spondylolisthesis into two broad categories: Developmental and Acquired (Table 7.3). The acquired type includes iatrogenic, traumatic, and pathologic subdivisions. This system was updated and modified by Marchetti and Bartolozzi in 1994 and sub-classified the developmental type into high and low dysplastic subtypes. The acquired type was expanded to include a traumatic subtype, and the term "postsurgical" was used to replace the iatrogenic subtype [18].

Developmental Spondylolisthesis

Developmental spondylolisthesis is further categorized into two types: high and low dysplastic, depending on the severity of dysplastic changes at L5 or S1 posterior elements. High and low dysplastic changes represent the morphological changes at the lumbosacral junction with different degrees of expression. Each of these dysplastic types is sub-classified with regard to the changes in the pars: elongation or lysis.

Dysplastic features commonly seen in both variants include dysplastic facet joints and spina bifida. Significant dysplastic features may be present at initial presentation or may develop secondarily in the high dysplastic variant. These include significant lumbosacral kyphosis, sacral dome rounding, vertical sacrum, trapezoidal vertebral body of L5, and hypoplastic transverse process. Severe dysplastic features in the high dysplastic type predispose the young spine for significant slippage, progression of deformity, and significant sagittal malalignment. Common low dysplastic features include preserved shape of the L5 vertebral body and sacral dome and relatively normal lumbosacral profile. Low dysplastic type has a lesser chance of significant progression of slippage. However, this variant can progress to the high dysplastic type with growth and morphological changes and needs to be followed carefully for any signs of progression.

Acquired Spondylolisthesis

Acquired spondylolisthesis includes traumatic, postsurgical, pathologic, and degenerative types. All of these types are subdivided as per the specific etiology and/or the chronicity of the etiological factors (Table 7.3). The stress fracture variant of traumatic acquired spondylolisthesis is distinct from the spondylolytic dysplastic type. It is seen commonly in athletes, particularly gymnasts [19, 20] and occurs secondary to repetitive stress or fatigue (flexion and extension) at the pars interarticularis without any other dysplastic feature. Postsurgical spondylolisthesis develops commonly after excessive resection of posterior elements without adequate stabilization.

This classification system was the first to use developmental class with high and low dysplastic variants. This classification helped to emphasize the role of dysplastic changes as an etiopathological factor for spondylolisthesis and its significance for progression of the deformity.

The limitations of this classification system include lack of clear definition of dysplastic types [21], inadequate distinction amongst high and low dysplastic types [22], and lack of consideration of spinopelvic alignment in classification [22, 23].

Herman Classification

Herman and Pizzutillo [24] proposed a new classification system for spondylolysis and spondylolisthesis specifically for the adolescent and

Table 7.4 Herman classification

Type	Description
I	Dysplastic
II	Developmental
III	Traumatic
IIIA	Acute
IIIB	Chronic
	Stress reaction
	Stress fracture
	Spondylotic defect (nonunion of pars)
IV	Pathologic

pediatric populations. This classification system is based on clinical presentation and spinal morphology (Table 7.4) and combines the basic classification elements of the Wiltse classification [13] and the Marchetti and Bartolozzi classification [18]. This classification system aims to provide treatment and management guidelines, including nonoperative care, which are relevant to children and adolescents.

This system classifies spondylolisthesis in pediatric patients into 4 main types: dysplastic, developmental, traumatic, and pathologic. Traumatic is subcategorized into acute and chronic groups. The chronic subgroup is further subcategorized into stress reaction, stress fracture, and spondylolytic defect (pars nonunion).

Type I, dysplastic, is similar to the dysplastic class of Wiltse and includes all congenital or developmental posterior elements defects except for pars. Progressive deformity and variable neurologic involvement, including radiculopathy and bladder/bowel changes, are usually seen in this class [24]. Close follow-up is recommended for children in this class, and operative intervention is indicated in cases of neurological presentation or progressive deformity irrespective of the severity.

Type II, developmental, includes spondylolysis and spondylolisthesis secondary to an incidentally diagnosed pars defect. These patients develop a defect secondary to genetic predisposition in most of the cases; sports activity or athletic overuse is generally not a causative factor [24, 25]. Progression is uncommon in this class, and conservative treatment and follow-up is recommended.

Type III includes traumatic defect of pars interarticularis and is subdivided as acute traumatic (high energy trauma) and chronic, or slowly evolving pars defect. Treatment recommendations for this type include conservative management in the initial stages, but most patients with type IIIB high grade spondylolisthesis require surgical intervention. Failure to respond to conservative treatment in 3 months is a surgical indication regardless of the subtype and grade of translation [24].

The Type IV (pathologic) variant includes defect of pars, lamina, and pedicle secondary to a pathologic process like tumors, infection, or osteogenesis imperfecta. Treatment is individualized in this category but includes surgical intervention in most cases.

While this system is valuable in that it differentiates traumatic and developmental isthmic spondylolisthesis, it does not consider patients with pars/isthmic defects or the degree of dysplasia. Mainly, this classification is used to guide non-surgical management.

Mac-Thiong Classification

In 2006, Mac-Thiong and Labelle proposed a new classification system designed to compensate for the shortcomings of the previous systems [21] (Table 7.5). The criticism of the Marchetti and Bartolozzi system is that while differentiation between high and low dysplastic subtypes is important, there were no criteria set forth to help categorize into these groups. Also, Herman's system does not consider the degree of dysplasia or include patients with pars defects or elongation. In particular, none of these systems are able to guide surgical management of this complex disease process. Therefore, Mac-Thiong and Labelle developed a new system with specific goals in mind. First, this system was meant to guide surgical treatment. Second, it was to be used to grade the severity of spondylolisthesis. Third, the criteria for defining high and low dysplastic spondylolisthesis were delineated. Finally, the concept of sagittal spinopelvic balance was incorporated to help guide surgical planning. This system was developed by identifying 92 articles that

Table 7.5 Mac-Thiong classification

Grade	Degree of dysplasia	Sacropelvic balance	Suggested treatment
Low-grade (1 or 2)	*Low-dysplastic* • Minimal lumbosacral kyphosis • Nearly rectangular L5 • Minimal sacral doming • Relatively normal sacrum • Minimal dysplasia of posterior elements • Relatively normal transverse processes	Low PI/low SS (*nutcracker type*) • Sacral slope ≤40	Grade 1: pars repair Grade 2: in situ L5–S1 PLF ± instrumentation ± reduction
		High PI/high SS (*shear type*) • Sacral slope >40	In situ L5–S1 PLF ± instrumentation ± reduction for Grade 2
	High-dysplastic • Lumbosacral kyphosis • Trapezoidal L5 • Sacral doming • Sacral dysplasia and kyphosis • Dysplasia of posterior elements • Small transverse processes	Low PI/low SS (*nutcracker type*) • Sacral slope ≤40	In situ L5–S1 PLF ± instrumentation ± reduction for Grade 2
		High PI/high SS (*shear type*) • Sacral slope >40	In situ L5–S1 PLF and instrumentation ± L4 and pelvic fixation ± reduction for Grade 2
High grade (3 or 4)	*Low-dysplastic* • Minimal lumbosacral kyphosis • Nearly rectangular L5 • Minimal sacral doming • Relatively normal sacrum • Minimal dysplasia of posterior elements • Relatively normal transverse processes	High SS/low PT (*balanced pelvis*) • Balanced sacrum • Sacral slope ≥50 • Pelvic tilt ≤35	In situ L4–S1 PLF and instrumentation ± pelvic fixation ± partial reduction
		Low SS/high PT (*retroverted pelvis*) • Vertical sacrum • Sacral slope <50 • Pelvic tilt ≥25	Partial reduction and L4–S1-pelvic instrumentation and PLF ± L5–S1 IF
	High-dysplastic • Lumbosacral kyphosis • Trapezoidal L5 • Sacral doming • Sacral dysplasia and kyphosis • Dysplasia of posterior elements • Small transverse processes	High SS/low PT (*balanced pelvis*) • Balanced sacrum • Sacral slope ≥50 • Pelvic tilt ≤35	Partial reduction and L4–S1-pelvic instrumentation and PLF ± L5–S1 IF
		Low SS/high PT (*retroverted pelvis*) • Vertical sacrum • Sacral slope <50 • Pelvic tilt ≥25	Partial reduction and L4–S1-pelvic instrumentation and PLF ± L5–S1 IF
Spondyloptosis	*High-dysplastic*		Circumferential fusion, instrumentation ± reduction

PI, pelvic incidence; SS, sacral slope; PT, pelvic tilt; PLF, posterior/posterolateral lumbar fusion; IF, interbody fusion

discussed classification, risk factors for progression, spinopelvic balance, sacropelvic morphology, dysplastic changes, and surgical management of spondylolisthesis.

The risk factors for progression identified by the authors include female gender, young age at presentation, slip severity at presentation, non-isthmic type, high slip angle, and high degree of dysplasia [21]. Of these, the quantifiable measures of severity serve as objective indicators that first, describe the deformity, and second, guide the degree of surgical intervention. The status of spinopelvic alignment was recognized as an element that predicts progression. A slip angle >55° (normal: −10–0°) and a lumbosacral angle of <100° (normal: 90–110°) were found to be predictive of progression. As seen in Fig. 7.2, the slip angle was defined as the angle formed by the lines along the inferior endplate of L5 and the superior endplate of S1. The lumbosacral angle as described by Dubousset is formed by the line along the superior endplate of L5 and the line along the posterior aspect of the S1 body [26].

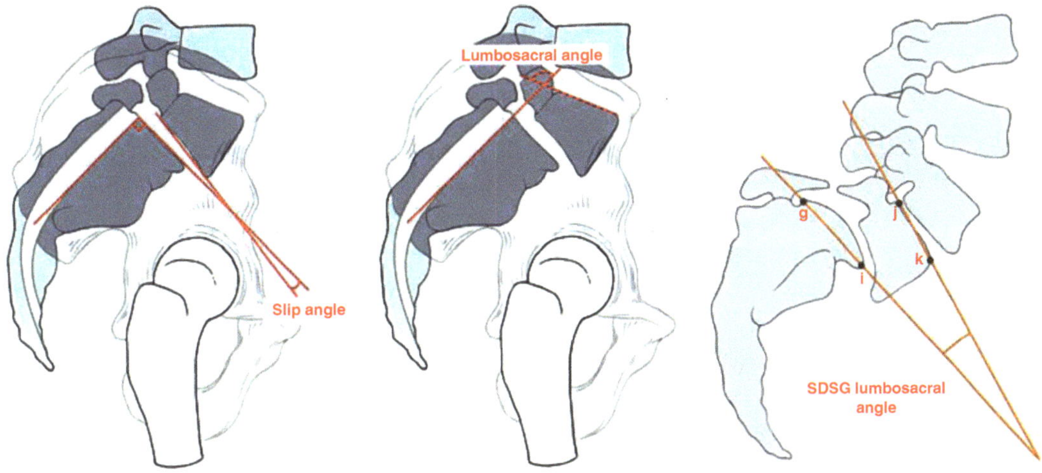

Fig. 7.2 Various spinosacral angles. [Reprinted from Mac-Thiong JM, Labelle H. A proposal for a surgical classification of pediatric lumbosacral spondylolisthesis based on current literature. Eur Spine J. 2006;15(10):1425–35. With permission from Springer Verlag.]

Degree of dysplasia also contributes significantly to the progression of spondylolisthesis, and this is highlighted in the Marchetti and Bartolozzi system [18]. They subcategorized developmental spondylolisthesis into low and high dysplastic groups depending on the morphology of the lumbosacral junction. Significant dysplasia can not only contribute to progression, but several studies have described unfavorable surgical outcomes and non-fusion due to the incompetence of the posterior elements in maintaining proper alignment. Secondary wedging and doming of the S1 level can be an indicator of its severity.

The orientation of the spinopelvic junction is an important determinant of the development and progression of spondylolisthesis because as the pattern of mechanical stress changes along the L5–S1 junction, the adaptive changes made by the body along with growth patterns in the case of adolescents can distort the way the spine cooperates with the sacrum. The orientation of the pelvis is most commonly described by using parameters defined by the Spine Deformity Study Group, or SDSG [27]. The pelvic incidence is a unique morphological descriptor of an individual's pelvis independent of its orientation in space (Fig. 7.3). It is described as the angle formed by the line drawn from the midpoint of the S1 superior endplate and the center of the femoral head and a perpendicular line bisecting the S1 endplate. The pelvic incidence (PI) is related to the positional parameters sacral slope (SS) and pelvic tilt (PT) by PI = PT + SS. The PT is described as the angle of the line connecting the center of the femoral head and the midpoint of the sacral endplate from vertical. The sacral slope is the angle of the sacral endplate from horizontal. PT and SS are defined in relation to vertical and horizontal, respectively, and, therefore, are dependent on the position of the pelvis. Studies have shown that not only is the PI different between normal patients and those with spondylolisthesis but the severity of the deformity is linearly related to the PI [28–30]. The various patterns of high or low PI and high or low SS will affect the biomechanics at the lumbosacral junction in different ways. Roussouly et al. discussed the increased shear stress in patients with a high PI associated with a high SS (>40°) which would stress the L5 pars as compared to patients with lower PI and SS [31]. In the patients with lower shear stress, the lytic defect would be the result of repetitive trauma of L4 and S1 on L5 during extension (nutcracker effect). With respect to low grade spondylolisthesis (Meyerding grade 1 or 2), Roussouly and colleagues used cluster analysis to demonstrate the existence of these two distinct populations of patients, with the high PI/high SS group representing the shear type and the low

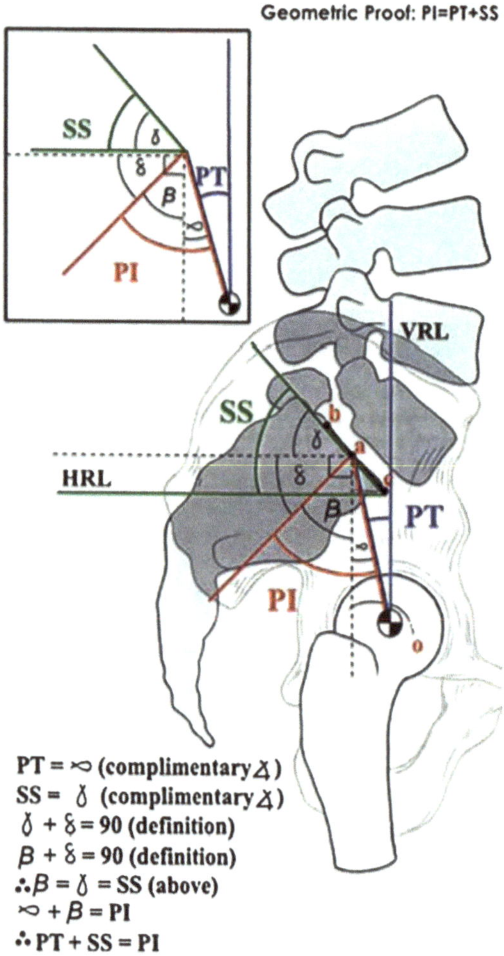

Fig. 7.3 Pelvic incidence. [Reprinted from Mac-Thiong JM, Labelle H. A proposal for a surgical classification of pediatric lumbosacral spondylolisthesis based on current literature. Eur Spine J. 2006;15(10):1425–35. With permission from Springer Verlag.]

PI/low SS group representing the nutcracker type [32]. Similarly, Hresko et al. used cluster analysis to define two subsets of subjects with high grade spondylolisthesis (Meyerding grade 3 or 4) [33]. Patients with high SS/low PT have a relatively balanced sacropelvic relationship, and patients with low SS/high PT have a retroverted pelvis and vertical sacrum along with lumbosacral kyphosis and sacropelvic imbalance. The mechanism of compensation for various degrees of lumbosacral imbalance depends on the severity of the imbalance. As imbalance develops, an increase in lumbar lordosis maintains the center of gravity over the hips. However, as the maximal lordosis is attained, the pelvis must be retroverted to keep the center of gravity over the hips. The relationship PI = SS + PT dictates that with the decrease in SS, the PT must increase to maintain balance. According to Mac-Thiong and Labelle, once the anatomic limit of these mechanisms is reached, sagittal imbalance results, forcing the subject to lean forward [21]. The types of sagittal spinopelvic configurations are depicted in Fig. 7.4.

The significance of the Mac-Thiong classification is that it provides treatment options based on grade [21]. In general, those with low grade spondylolisthesis are best served by an in situ posterolateral fusion with a favorable fusion rate regardless of instrumentation [34, 35]. For high grade spondylolisthesis, in situ posterolateral fusion affords less consistent results with up to 50 % progression [36, 37]. Additionally, patients with highly dysplastic posterior elements may not provide the surface area necessary to attain adequate fusion [38]. Evidence supports circumferential fusion, especially when reduction is performed [38–40]. Reduction, while providing decompression of the nerve roots and improving sagittal balance, is controversial at best.

Applying the classification system is based on three characteristics determined from imaging studies. The degree of slip is simply determined according to Meyerding on a lateral X-ray. Low grade is 0, 1, and 2. High grade is 3 or 4, and the final category is spondyloptosis. Then, dysplasia is described as low if two or fewer criteria are met or high if three or more are met. The dysplastic features considered are lumbosacral kyphosis, L5 vertebral body wedging, doming of the sacral endplate, dysplastic posterior elements, transverse process surface area, L5/S1 disc, and bone and connective tissue abnormalities. Finally, the sagittal spinopelvic balance is considered as described by Roussouly et al. [31] and Hresko et al. [33]. The low grade subtype is classified as low PI/low SS (nutcracker type) or high PI/low SS (shear type) with SS of 40° being the point of division. The high grade subtype is classified as high SS/low PT (balanced pelvis), or low SS/high PT (retroverted pelvis) (Fig. 7.5) depending on where they lie on Hresko's cluster plot. Each

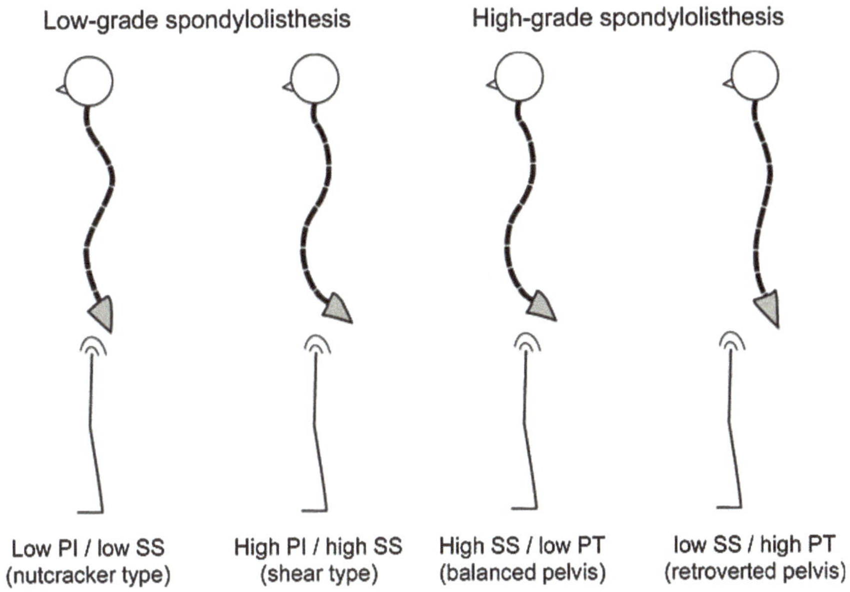

Fig. 7.4 Sagittal spinopelvic balance. [Reprinted from Mac-Thiong JM, Labelle H. A proposal for a surgical classification of pediatric lumbosacral spondylolisthesis based on current literature. Eur Spine J. 2006;15(10):1425–35. With permission from Springer Verlag.]

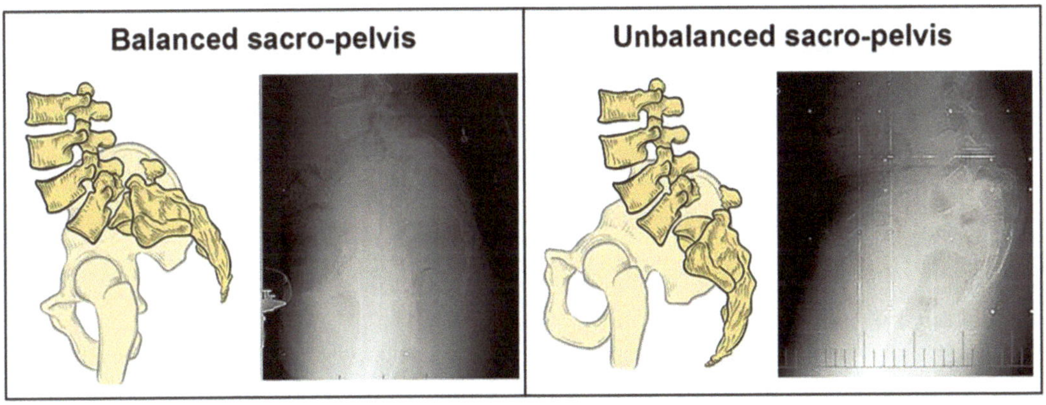

Fig. 7.5 Sacropelvic balance. [Reprinted from Mac-Thiong JM, Labelle H, Parent S, Hresko MT, Deviren V, Weidenbaum M. Reliability and development of a new classification of lumbosacral spondylolisthesis. Scoliosis. 2008;3:19. With permission from BioMed Central, Ltd.]

category has a corresponding surgical treatment recommendation. These options will be discussed further in another chapter in this volume.

In this study, Mac-Thiong and Labelle recognized the importance of the degree of slip, the spinopelvic relationship, and dysplastic morphology in redefining spondylolisthesis. It was an important step in the understanding of spondylolisthesis and a significant step in bringing together the treatment algorithms found in the literature. Unfortunately, in a subsequent reliability study, Mac-Thiong et al. discovered that while the intraobserver reliability was high, the interobserver reliability was only moderate because of the difficulty in classifying the degree of dysplasia [41]. In so doing, the SDSG introduced a new classification based on a modification of the Mac-Thiong system.

SDSG Classification

The key to developing a surgical classification system depends on simplicity and reliability. If it is difficult to apply, the inappropriate surgical management strategy may be recommended. The Mac-Thiong system, while comprehensive in scope and surgical management strategies, was difficult to apply. The interobserver reliability was only moderate in a follow-up reliability study, and this was due mostly to the classification of dysplasia [41]. Also, there was a modification of sacropelvic parameters for patients with low grade spondylolisthesis. In a cluster analysis of PI, SS, and PT, these subjects were divided into two separate groups. There was one group with normal or near normal PI (<60°) and another group with high PI (>60°) [42]. In addition, global sagittal alignment was included after recognition that it plays an important part of health-related quality of life in patients with spinal deformity. These modifications in the newly revised SDSG classification system for spondylolisthesis recognize five types (Table 7.6). The grading system is based on the slip grade, sacropelvic balance, and the global spinopelvic balance. Application of the system has been simplified when compared to the previous version. First, determine whether the slip is low grade (Meyerding 1 or 2) or high grade (Meyerding 3 or 4). Next, measure the sacropelvic parameters of SS and PT, and calculate PI. For low grade spondylolisthesis, two subgroups are divided at PI value of 60°. For high grade spondylolisthesis, the Hresko et al. [42] method is applied. Patients are separated into these categories based on the threshold line defined in the cluster analysis. Above the line, the patient is classified as having a balanced sacropelvis (high SS/low PT) and below the line, the patient is categorized to the unbalanced group (low SS/high PT). The global spinopelvic balance is also easily determined. If the C7 plumb line falls over or posterior to the femoral head, the spine is balanced. However, if it lies anterior to the femoral heads, the spine is unbalanced. Usually if the sacropelvis is balanced, the patient displays global spinal balance regardless of the grade [41]. However, this may not be the case in patients with high grade spondylolisthesis with an unbalanced pelvis. A reliability study was performed on this system as well. Using a computer assisted method of identifying anatomic landmarks, the group was able to demonstrate high reliability in both inter- and intraobserver reliability [43].

Table 7.6 SDSG classification

Slip grade	Sacropelvic balance	Spinopelvic balance	Spondylolisthesis type
Low grade	Normal PI	–	Type 1
	High PI	–	Type 2
High grade	Balanced	–	Type 3
	Unbalanced	Balanced	Type 4
		Unbalanced	Type 5

Significantly, the surgical recommendations were eliminated from this system. While the ideal system would help guide management, the high reliability of the SDSG system provides a strong base from which future questions about spondylolisthesis management can be answered. Classification systems will continue to evolve as new treatment strategies and insights into the disease process emerge. Surgical management of spondylolisthesis will be discussed in other chapters of this volume.

Conclusion

Classification systems serve to give us a frame of reference when thinking about a disease process. For spondylolisthesis, various methods have been developed that categorize according to etiology, degree of deformity, and different radiographic parameters. While there are advantages and disadvantages to each system, they can also complement each other. For example, the Meyerding classification system was utilized in the Mac-Thiong and SDSG classification systems. Also, the latest iteration by the SDSG is a modification of the previous system based on reliability studies. It is important to realize that if a system is too difficult to apply with reproducible results, its utility is limited, especially if one is trying to develop a surgical treatment strategy based on its categorization. In this chapter we explored the different classification schemes for spondylolisthesis and discussed their strengths and weaknesses. While some were for historical interest, the others framed this disease based on their categories and provided insight into the etiology and progression of this deformity. Knowledge of the classification systems of spondylolisthesis is a prerequisite to successful diagnosis and management of this disease.

References

1. Meyerding HW. Spondylolisthesis. Surg Gynecol Obstet. 1932;54:371–7.
2. Radcliff K, Hwang R, Hilibrand A, Smith HE, Gruskay J, Lurie JD, et al. The effect of iliac crest autograft on the outcome of fusion in the setting of degenerative spondylolisthesis: a subgroup analysis of the Spine Patient Outcomes Research Trial (SPORT). J Bone Joint Surg Am. 2012;94(18):1685–92.
3. Rihn JA, Radcliff K, Hilibrand AS, Anderson DT, Zhao W, Lurie J, et al. Does obesity affect outcomes of treatment for lumbar stenosis and degenerative spondylolisthesis? Analysis of the Spine Patient Outcomes Research Trial (SPORT). Spine (Phila Pa 1976). 2012;37(23):1933–46.
4. Smorgick Y, Park DK, Baker KC, Lurie JD, Tosteson TD, Zhao W, et al. Single versus multilevel fusion for single-level degenerative spondylolisthesis and multilevel lumbar stenosis: four-year results of the spine patient outcomes research trial. Spine (Phila Pa 1976). 2013;38(10):797–805.
5. Riouallon G, Lachaniette CH, Poignard A, Allain J. Outcomes of anterior lumbar interbody fusion in low-grade isthmic spondylolisthesis in adults: a continuous series of 65 cases with an average follow-up of 6.6 years. Orthop Traumatol Surg Res. 2013;99(2):155–61.
6. Marchi L, Abdala N, Oliveira L, Amaral R, Coutinho E, Pimenta L. Stand-alone lateral interbody fusion for the treatment of low-grade degenerative spondylolisthesis. Sci World J. 2012;2012:456346.
7. Farrokhi MR, Rahmanian A, Masoudi MS. Posterolateral versus posterior interbody fusion in isthmic spondylolisthesis. J Neurotrauma. 2012; 29(8):1567–73.
8. Yuan JD, Wang J, Zhou HB, Fu Q, Chen ZM, Zhao J. Analysis of results on minimum 4-year follow-up of modified posterior lumbar interbody fusion for the treatment of isthmic spondylolisthesis. Zhongguo Gu Shang. 2010;23(7):519–22.
9. Pearson AM, Lurie JD, Blood EA, Frymoyer JW, Braeutigam H, An H, et al. Spine patient outcomes research trial: radiographic predictors of clinical outcomes after operative or nonoperative treatment of degenerative spondylolisthesis. Spine (Phila Pa 1976). 2008;33(25):2759–66.
10. Weinstein JN, Lurie JD, Tosteson TD, Hanscom B, Tosteson AN, Blood EA, et al. Surgical versus nonsurgical treatment for lumbar degenerative spondylolisthesis. N Engl J Med. 2007;356(22):2257–70.
11. Swan J, Hurwitz E, Malek F, van den Haak E, Cheng I, Alamin T, et al. Surgical treatment for unstable low-grade isthmic spondylolisthesis in adults: a prospective controlled study of posterior instrumented fusion compared with combined anterior-posterior fusion. Spine J. 2006;6(6):606–14.
12. Ekman P, Moller H, Hedlund R. The long-term effect of posterolateral fusion in adult isthmic spondylolisthesis: a randomized controlled study. Spine J. 2005; 5(1):36–44.
13. Wiltse LL, Newman PH, Macnab I. Classification of spondylolisis and spondylolisthesis. Clin Orthop Relat Res. 1976;117:23–9.
14. Wynne-Davies R, Scott JH. Inheritance and spondylolisthesis: a radiographic family survey. J Bone Joint Surg Br. 1979;61-B(3):301–5.
15. Frymoyer JW. Back pain and sciatica. N Engl J Med. 1988;318(5):291–300.
16. Petajan JH, Momberger GL, Aase J, Wright DG. Arthrogryposis syndrome (Kuskokwim disease) in the Eskimo. JAMA. 1969;209(10):1481–6.
17. Marchetti PG, Binazzi R, Briccoli A, Vaccari V, Borelli P, De Zerbi M, et al. The surgical treatment of spondylolisthesis. Chir Organi Mov. 1994;79(1): 85–91.
18. Bridwell K, editor. Textbook of spinal surgery. Philadelphia, PA: Lippincott-Raven; 1997.
19. Jackson DW, Wiltse LL, Cirincoine RJ. Spondylolysis in the female gymnast. Clin Orthop Relat Res. 1976; 117:68–73.
20. Letts M, Smallman T, Afanasiev R, Gouw G. Fracture of the pars interarticularis in adolescent athletes: a clinical-biomechanical analysis. J Pediatr Orthop. 1986;6(1):40–6.
21. Mac-Thiong JM, Labelle H. A proposal for a surgical classification of pediatric lumbosacral spondylolisthesis based on current literature. Eur Spine J. 2006; 15(10):1425–35.
22. Kasliwal MK, Smith JS, Kanter A, Chen CJ, Mummaneni PV, Hart RA, et al. Management of high-grade spondylolisthesis. Neurosurg Clin N Am. 2013;24(2):275–91.
23. Lamartina C, Zavatsky JM, Petruzzi M, Specchia N. Novel concepts in the evaluation and treatment of high-dysplastic spondylolisthesis. Eur Spine J. 2009; 18(Suppl)1:133–42.
24. Herman MJ, Pizzutillo PD. Spondylolysis and spondylolisthesis in the child and adolescent: a new classification. Clin Orthop Relat Res. 2005;434:46–54.
25. Haun DW, Kettner NW. Spondylolysis and spondylolisthesis: a narrative review of etiology, diagnosis, and conservative management. J Chiropr Med. 2005;4(4): 206–17.

26. Dubousset J. Treatment of spondylolysis and spondylolisthesis in children and adolescents. Clin Orthop Relat Res. 1997;337:77–85.
27. O'Brien MF, Kuklo TR, Blanke KM. Spinal Deformity Study Group – radiographic measurement manual. Memphis: Medtronic Sofamor Danek; 2004.
28. Hanson DS, Bridwell KH, Rhee JM, Lenke LG. Correlation of pelvic incidence with low- and high-grade isthmic spondylolisthesis. Spine (Phila Pa 1976). 2002;27(18):2026–9.
29. Jackson RP, Phipps T, Hales C, Surber J. Pelvic lordosis and alignment in spondylolisthesis. Spine (Phila Pa 1976). 2003;28(2):151–60.
30. Labelle H, Roussouly P, Berthonnaud E, Transfeldt E, O'Brien M, Chopin D, et al. Spondylolisthesis, pelvic incidence, and spinopelvic balance: a correlation study. Spine (Phila Pa 1976). 2004;29(18):2049–54.
31. Roussouly P, Gollogly S, Berthonnaud E, Labelle H, Weidenbaum M. Sagittal alignment of the spine and pelvis in the presence of L5-S1 isthmic lysis and low-grade spondylolisthesis. Spine (Phila Pa 1976). 2006;31(21):2484–90.
32. Labelle H, Roussouly P, Transfeldt E, Hresko MT, O'Brien M, Berthonnaud E. The importance of spinopelvic balance after spinal instrumentation for high grade developmental spondylolisthesis. In: Scoliosis Research Society annual meeting, September 10–13, Quebec City, Quebec, Canada; 2003.
33. Hresko MT, Labelle H, Roussouly P, editors. High grade spondylolisthesis: correlations between pelvic version and spine balance. In: Pediatric Orthopaedic Society of North America annual meeting, May 13–15, Ottawa, Ontario, Canada; 2005.
34. Askar Z, Wardlaw D, Koti M. Scott wiring for direct repair of lumbar spondylolysis. Spine (Phila Pa 1976). 2003;28(4):354–7.
35. Bradford DS, Iza J. Repair of the defect in spondylolysis or minimal degrees of spondylolisthesis by segmental wire fixation and bone grafting. Spine (Phila Pa 1976). 1985;10(7):673–9.
36. Grzegorzewski A, Kumar SJ. In situ posterolateral spine arthrodesis for grades III, IV, and V spondylolisthesis in children and adolescents. J Pediatr Orthop. 2000;20(4):506–11.
37. Lenke LG, Bridwell KH, Bullis D, Betz RR, Baldus C, Schoenecker PL. Results of in situ fusion for isthmic spondylolisthesis. J Spinal Disord. 1992; 5(4):433–42.
38. Molinari RW, Bridwell KH, Lenke LG, Ungacta FF, Riew KD. Complications in the surgical treatment of pediatric high-grade, isthmic dysplastic spondylolisthesis. A comparison of three surgical approaches. Spine (Phila Pa 1976). 1999;24(16): 1701–11.
39. Mardjetko S, Albert T, Andersson G, Bridwell K, DeWald C, Gaines R, et al. Spine/SRS spondylolisthesis summary statement. Spine (Phila Pa 1976). 2005;30(6 Suppl):S3.
40. Molinari RW, Bridwell KH, Lenke LG, Baldus C. Anterior column support in surgery for high-grade, isthmic spondylolisthesis. Clin Orthop Relat Res. 2002;394:109–20.
41. Mac-Thiong JM, Labelle H, Parent S, Hresko MT, Deviren V, Weidenbaum M. Reliability and development of a new classification of lumbosacral spondylolisthesis. Scoliosis. 2008;3:19.
42. Hresko MT, Labelle H, Roussouly P, Berthonnaud E. Classification of high-grade spondylolistheses based on pelvic version and spine balance: possible rationale for reduction. Spine (Phila Pa 1976). 2007;32(20):2208–13.
43. Mac-Thiong JM, Duong L, Parent S, Hresko MT, Dimar JR, Weidenbaum M, et al. Reliability of the Spinal Deformity Study Group classification of lumbosacral spondylolisthesis. Spine (Phila Pa 1976). 2012;37(2):E95–102.

Role of the Pelvis in the Diagnosis and Management of L5-S1 Spondylolisthesis

8

Hubert Labelle and Jean-Marc Mac-Thiong

The Pelvis: From Quadrupeds to Humans

Posture is defined as the alignment or orientation of body segments while maintaining an upright position. The posture of a human standing subject can be viewed as a set of mutually articulating body sections: the head is balanced on the trunk by the cervical spine, the trunk and thoracolumbar spine articulate on the pelvis which, in turn, articulates with the lower limbs at the hip joints, in order to maintain a stable posture and to expend a minimum of energy. There is a narrow range in which the body can remain balanced without external support and with minimal effort. Human posture is relatively simple to understand in the frontal plane, with a normal vertical straight spine delineating an axis that passes through the middle of the head, sacrum, and pelvis, with the limbs symmetrically distributed on each side (Fig. 8.1). The situation is much more complex in the sagittal plane: the spine has multiple curves and the pelvis plays a unique role in this equation by virtue of its shape, which can be conceptualized as a circle in which the lower limbs articulate on the acetabulums and on which the spine articulates eccentrically on the sacrum, creating an asymmetric configuration and potentially unstable situation when compared to the frontal plane (Fig. 8.1).

Evolution from the quadrupedal to the bipedal posture in primates and humans has been allowed by progressive and very significant changes in the shape and position of the pelvis and spine and of their supporting ligaments and muscles (Fig. 8.2). A quadruped has no lumbar lordosis and a more longitudinal and narrow shaped pelvis, such as in the skeleton illustrated in Fig. 8.2. In sharp contrast, a human has a well-developed lumbar lordosis and a much "rounder" pelvic shape, a situation which has gradually evolved in primates along with the transition to the bipedal posture. As discussed in the following section, Pelvic Incidence is a simple measurement that characterizes the shape of the pelvis, and this angle has increased significantly from quadruped to bipeds. These changes in shape and morphology of the pelvis are crucial to the understanding and management of L5-S1 spondylolisthesis, a disorder which does not occur in quadrupeds, but which is frequently associated with activities involving a lordotic effect on the lumbar spine in bipeds, such as gymnastics. It is therefore very important to have a basic understanding of the role of the pelvis in normal human posture and spondylolisthesis, so the goal of this chapter is to review current knowledge on this topic.

H. Labelle, M.D. (✉)
J.-M. Mac-Thiong, M.D., Ph.D.
Department of Surgery, Ste-Justine University Center Hospital/University of Montreal, 3175 Cote Ste-Catherine, Montreal, QC, Canada H3T 1C5
e-mail: hubert.labelle@umontreal.ca; macthiong@gmail.com

A.L. Wollowick and V. Sarwahi (eds.), *Spondylolisthesis: Diagnosis, Non-Surgical Management, and Surgical Techniques*, DOI 10.1007/978-1-4899-7575-1_8,

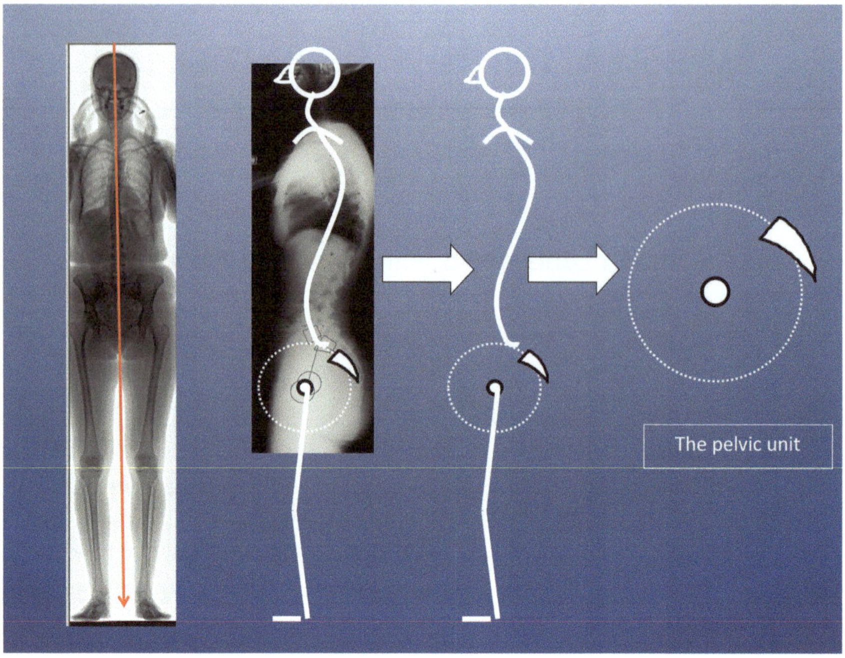

Fig. 8.1 Spino-pelvic alignment in the frontal and sagittal planes

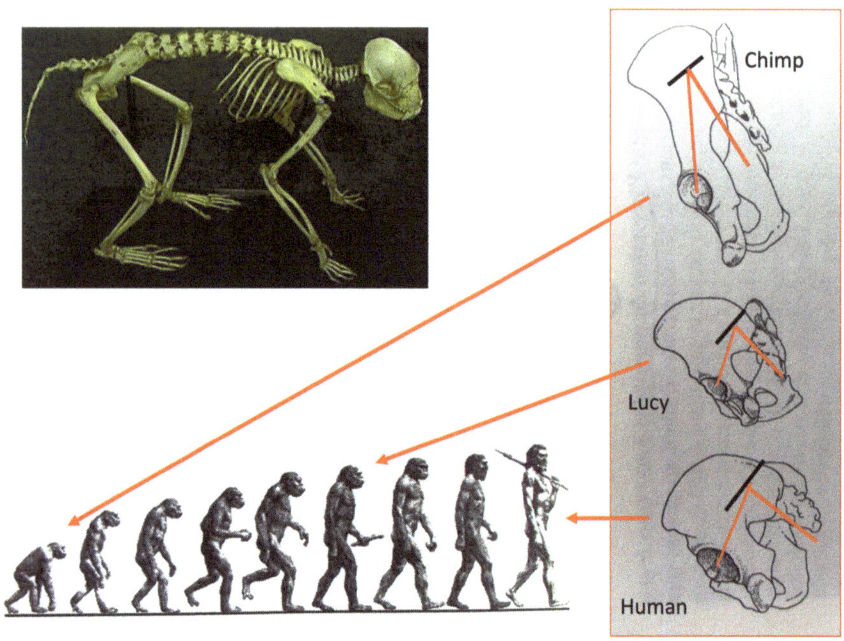

Fig. 8.2 Evolution from the quadrupedal to the bipedal posture in primates and humans

Spino-Pelvic Measures and Their Variations in Normal Humans

How can the shape/morphology of the pelvis be quantified in a simple but useful way for clinicians? Different parameters have been used to describe pelvic morphology based on standing lateral radiographs [1], but our preference goes to pelvic incidence (PI), a simple measurement introduced by Duval-Beaupère et al. [2, 3] PI is a fundamental pelvic anatomic parameter that is specific and constant for each individual and determines pelvic orientation as well as the size of

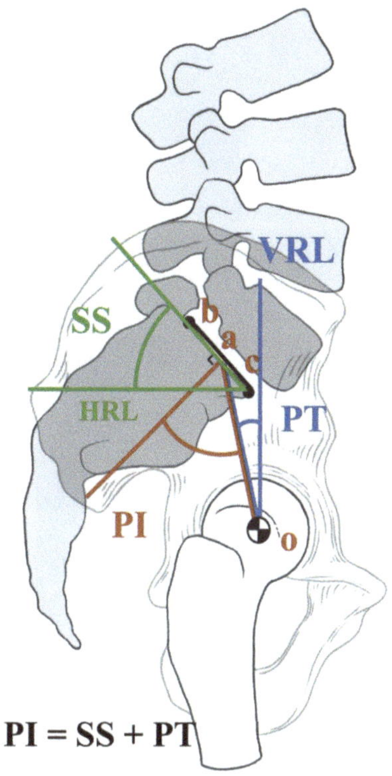

Fig. 8.3 Mathematical relationship between pelvic incidence (*PI*), sacral slope (*SS*), and pelvic tilt (*PT*). Horizontal reference line (*HRL*); vertical reference line (*VRL*). [Reprinted from Berthonnaud E, Dimnet J, Labelle H, et al. Spondylolisthesis. In : O'Brien MF, Kuklo TR, Blanke KM, Lenke LG (eds). Spinal Deformity Study Group. Radiographic Measurement Manual. Memphis, TN: Medtronic Sofamor Danek, 2004:95–108. With permission from Orthopaedic Research and Education Center.]

lumbar lordosis (LL). PI remains relatively constant before walking age and thereafter, it increases significantly during childhood and adolescence until reaching its maximum and thereafter constant value in adulthood [4, 5]. PI is defined as the angle between a line perpendicular to the sacral plate and a line joining the sacral plate to the center of the axis of the femoral heads (Fig. 8.3). It is important to understand that PI is a descriptor of pelvic morphology and not of pelvic orientation: therefore, its angular value is unaffected by changes in human posture and will remain the same whether a subject is standing, sitting, or lying down, with the assumption that there is no significant motion occurring at the sacroiliac joints. In contrast, the pelvic tilt (PT) and the sacral slope (SS) are position-dependent variables, and are very useful to characterize the spatial orientation of the pelvis. SS is defined as the angle between the sacral endplate and the horizontal line (Fig. 8.3), while PT is defined as the angle between the vertical line and the line joining the middle of the sacral endplate and the axis of the femoral heads (Fig. 8.3). Because they are measured with respect to the horizontal and to the vertical, respectively, SS and PT describe the orientation of the pelvis in the sagittal plane and not its morphology. PI, SS, and PT are particularly useful because it can be demonstrated that PI is the arithmetic sum of the sacral slope (SS)+pelvic tilt (PT), the two position-dependent variables that determine pelvic orientation in the sagittal plane (Fig. 8.3). Because of this mathematical association between PI, SS, and PT, the morphology of the pelvis, as quantified by PI, is therefore a strong determinant of the spatial orientation of the pelvis in the standing position: the greater PI, the greater has to be SS, PT, or both. PI, PT, and SS are best measured from a standing lateral radiograph of the entire spine including the pelvis when evaluating the global sagittal balance.

Vaz et al. [6] have studied and reported the association and ranges of PI, PT, SS, Lumbar Lordosis (LL), and Thoracic Kyphosis (TK) in 100 young normal adult volunteers and have shown that all these parameters are closely linked and balance themselves, by muscular activity, to maintain the global axis of gravity over the femoral heads. The pelvic shape, best quantified by the PI angle, determines the position of the sacral end. The spine reacts to this position by adapting through LL, the amount of lordosis increasing as the SS increases to balance the trunk in the upright position (Fig. 8.4). Berthonnaud et al. [7], in a review of 160 normal adult volunteers, have shown that the pelvis and spine in the sagittal plane can be considered as a linear chain linking the head to the pelvis where the shape and orientation of each anatomic segment are closely related and influence the adjacent segment, to maintain a stable posture with a minimum of energy expenditure. Changes in shape or orientation at one level will have a direct influence on the adjacent segment. Knowledge of these normal

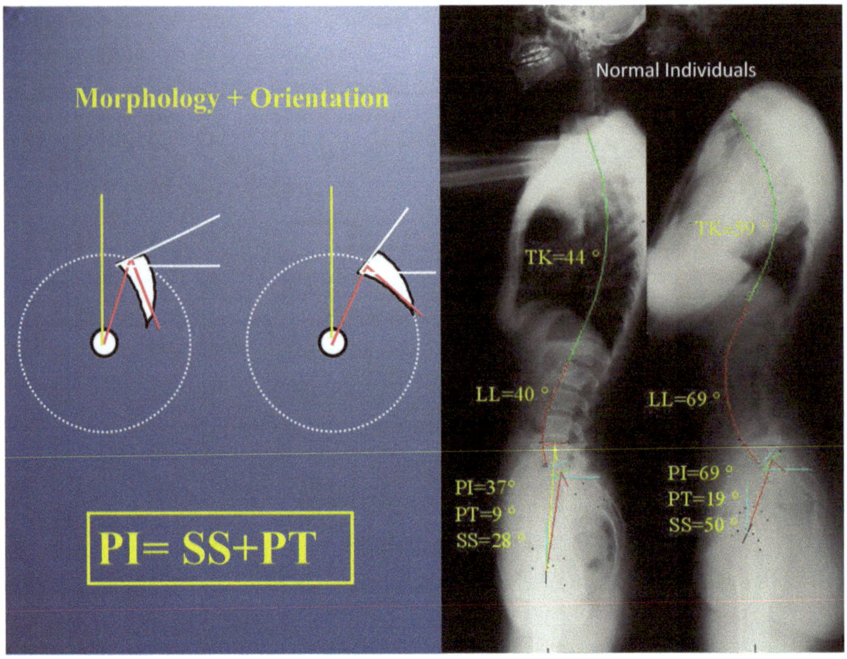

Fig. 8.4 The relationship between morphology (PI) and orientation (SS, PT) of the pelvis, with the resulting shapes of the spine in two normal individuals, one with a low PI, and one with a high PI

relationships is of prime importance for the comprehension of sagittal balance in normal and pathologic conditions of the spine and pelvis. Mac-Thiong et al. [8, 9] have reported similar results in a reference pediatric and adolescent population of 180 subjects aged 4–18 years.

A balanced pelvis and spine results in a global spino-pelvic balance that is typically maintained within a narrow range of values in normal individuals. As shown by Mac-Thiong et al. [9, 10], the C7-plumbline of 85 % of normal adults and children aged >10 years stands behind the hip axis. In order to maintain an adequate global spino-pelvic balance (with minimum energy expenditure) throughout life despite ongoing degenerative changes, adjusting pelvic orientation is the key. Accordingly, a small increase in PT and a reciprocally small decrease in SS can occur with aging, thereby causing retroversion of the pelvis in an effort to prevent forward displacement of C7-plumbline [11]. Similarly in conditions that will tend to move the C7-plumbline forward, such as in spondylolisthesis or post-traumatic kyphosis, retroversion of the pelvis can also decrease the incidence of global sagittal imbalance. In addition, young patients with healthy discs and muscles also can increase their lordosis in an attempt to prevent the forward displacement of the C7-plumbline.

The Pelvis in L5-S1 Spondylolisthesis

Sagittal sacro-pelvic morphology and orientation modulate the geometry of the lumbar spine and consequently, the mechanical stresses at the lumbo-sacral junction. In L5-S1 spondylolisthesis, it has been clearly demonstrated over the past decade that sacro-pelvic morphology is frequently abnormal and that combined with the presence of a local lumbo-sacral deformity and dysplasia, it can result in an abnormal sacro-pelvic orientation as well as in a disturbed global sagittal balance of the spine. These findings have important implications for the evaluation and treatment of patients with spondylolisthesis, and especially for those with a high-grade slip.

When compared with normal populations, PI is significantly higher [12–14] in spondylolisthesis and the difference in PI tends to increase in a direct linear fashion as severity of the spondylolisthesis increases [13]. The cause–effect relationship between pelvic morphology and spondylolisthesis remains to be clarified. Other measures of spino-pelvic balance are also significantly different in control populations compared to subjects with L5-S1 spondylolisthesis (Table 8.1).

In static standing position, the way SS and PT balance refers to the concept of *sacro-pelvic balance*. Members of the Spinal Deformity Study Group (SDSG) have specifically investigated sacro-pelvic balance in low-grade and high-grade spondylolisthesis (HGS). Roussouly et al. [15] proposed two different subgroups of sacro-pelvic balance observed in subjects with low-grade spondylolisthesis, that could be related to the etiology. In their opinion, patients with high PI and SS have increased shear stresses at the lumbosacral junction, causing more tension on the pars interarticularis at L5, and ultimately a pars defect (Fig. 8.5). On the opposite, patients with a low PI and a smaller SS have impingement of the posterior elements of L5 between L4 and S1 during extension, thereby causing a "nutcracker" effect on the pars interarticularis at L5 until lysis occurs (Fig. 8.5). On the basis of K-means cluster analysis, Labelle et al. [16] have confirmed the existence of these two distinct subgroups of sacro-pelvic balance in a larger SDSG cohort of low-grade isthmic spondylolisthesis: a subgroup

Table 8.1 Normal values of spino-pelvic alignment from the literature [7, 9, 11, 19, 21, 29]

	3–9 years	10–18 years	≥18 years	Low-grade spondylolisthesis	High-grade spondylolisthesis
PI (°)	43.7°±9.0°	46.9°±11.4°	52.6°±10.4°	61.0°±12.9°	73.0°±12.8°
PT (°)	5.5°±7.6°	7.7°±8.3°	13.0°±6.8°	6.4°±12.3°	27.4°±9.0°
SS (°)	38.2°±7.7°	39.1°±7.6°	39.6°±7.9°	50.0°±10.8°	46.2°±10.8°
L5-S1 angle (°)	−23°±8°	−25°±6°	−24°±6°	−11.5°±7.5°	36.6°±24.0°
LL (°)[a]	−42.3°±13.1°	−45.6°±12.5°	−42.7°±5.4°	−54.7°±14.5°	−86.4°±16.2°
TK (°)	42.0°±10.6°	45.8°±10.4°	47.5°±4.8°	41.7°±9.7°	30.4°±13.6°
C7 plumbline (mm)[b]	18±46	−5±42	0±24	15.2±28.3	50.5±42.4

[a]Lumbar lordosis measured down to L5
[b]Center of C7 vertebral body vs. postero-superior corner of S1 vertebral body

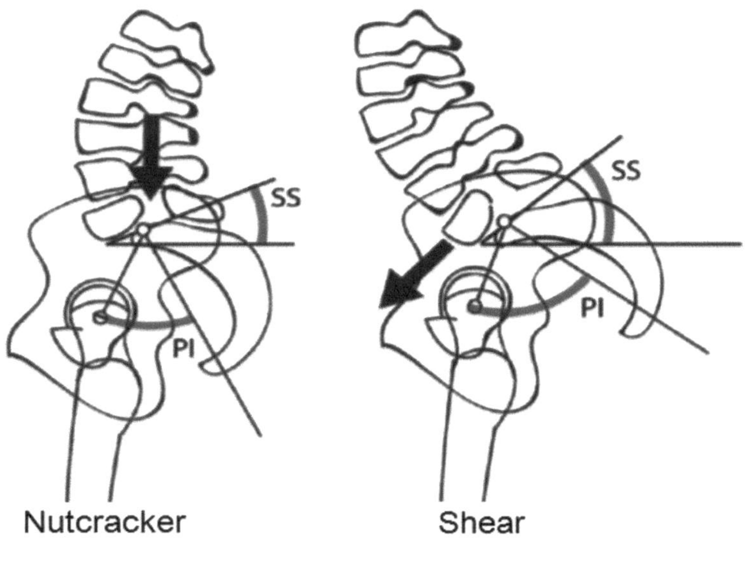

Fig. 8.5 The two subgroups of sacro-pelvic balance observed in subjects with low-grade spondylolisthesis. [Reprinted from Roussouly P, Gollogly S, Berthonnaud É, et al. Sagittal alignment of the spine and pelvis in the presence of L5-S1 isthmic lysis and low-grade spondylolisthesis. Spine 2006;31:2484–2490. With permission from Wolters Kluwer Health.]

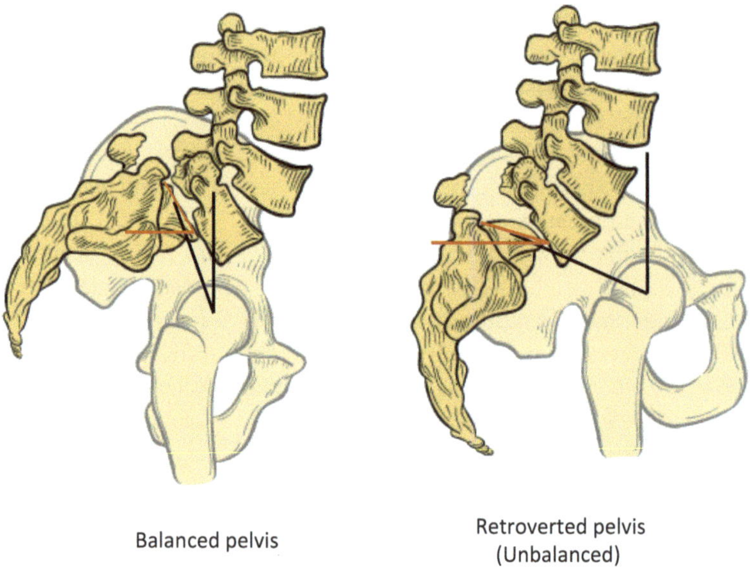

Fig. 8.6 The two subgroups of sacro-pelvic balance observed in subjects with high-grade spondylolisthesis. [Reprinted from Hresko MT, Labelle H, Roussouly P, et al. Classification of high-grade spondylolisthesis based on pelvic version and spine balance: possible rationale for reduction. Spine 2007; 32:2208-2213. With permission from Wolters Kluwer Health.]

with normal PI (between 45° and 60°) or low PI (<45°), and a subgroup with high PI (>60°). The clinical relevance of these findings is that since PI is always much greater than normal in HGS [13], it is assumed that the risk of progression in the low-grade subgroup with a normal PI is much lower than in the subgroup with an abnormally high PI value. It is hypothesized that the subgroup with normal PI corresponds to acquired traumatic cases with an acute or stress fracture (Marchetti and Bartolozzi [17] classification) in subjects with a normal sacro-pelvic morphology, whereas the other subgroup with high PI is associated with more dysplastic cases, but this assumption remains to be verified. As for HGS, Hresko et al. [18] have identified two subgroups of patients: balanced versus unbalanced pelvis (Fig. 8.6). The "balanced" group includes patients standing with a high SS and a low PT, a posture similar to normal individuals with high PI, whereas the "unbalanced" group includes patients standing with a retroverted pelvis and a vertical sacrum, corresponding to a low SS and a high PT. Each new subject with HGS can be easily classified by simply using the raw SS and PT values or, in borderline cases, by using the nomogram provided by Hresko et al. [18].

In static standing position, the way the spine and the pelvis balance themselves refers to the concept of *spino-pelvic balance*. By using a postural model of spino-pelvic balance showing the relationships between parameters of each successive anatomical segment from the thoracic spine to the sacro-pelvis, Mac-Thiong et al. [19] have observed that a relatively normal posture is maintained in low-grade spondylolisthesis, whereas posture is clearly abnormal in HGS. In HGS, the spino-pelvic balance is particularly disturbed in the subgroup with an unbalanced sacro-pelvis, as described by Hresko et al. [18]. They also reported that for most patients with spondylolisthesis (low grades and balanced high grades), the global spino-pelvic balance (position of C7 vertebral body over the femoral heads) was relatively constant with the C7-plumbline projecting behind the femoral heads, regardless of the local lumbo-sacral deformity and particularly of the alignment of C7-plumbline with respect to S1, indicating the predominant influence of the sacro-pelvis in the achievement of a normal global spino-pelvic balance.

Recent studies have correlated spino-pelvic and sacro-pelvic balance with health related quality of life (HRQoL) measures. Tanguay et al. [20] have demonstrated that increased lumbo-sacral kyphosis (LSK) has a significant association with a decrease in the physical aspect of the quality of life for patients with adolescent L5-S1 spondylolisthesis. The effect of LSK is particularly important for patients with HGS, independent of the slip percentage. Therefore, LSK values should be included in the routine evaluation of patients with spondylolisthesis, in order to fully appreciate the severity of the deformity and its clinical impact on the quality of life of patients. Harroud et al. [21], in a cohort of subjects with HGS, have noted that an increasing positive sagittal alignment was related to a poorer SRS-22 total score, especially when the C7-Plumbline is in front of the hip axis. Global sagittal alignment should therefore always be assessed in patients with HGS.

L5-S1 Spondylisthesis Classification Based on Sagittal Posture and Its Clinical Relevance

The findings described in the previous section have stimulated a renewed interest for the radiological evaluation and classification of spino-pelvic alignment in L5-S1 spondylolisthesis. The commonly used classification systems from Wiltse et al. [22] and from Marchetti and Bartolozzi [17] are useful to identify the underlying pathology, but they are of little help to guide surgical treatment. Recently, the SDSG has proposed a classification system [16, 23] in six different sagittal postures, based on the radiographic measurement of slip grade and spino-pelvic alignment (pelvic incidence, sacro-pelvic and spinal balance). Figure 8.7 summarizes the classification. The rationale of the classification was derived from the analysis of a multi-center radiological database of patients with L5-S1 developmental or acquired stress fracture spondylolisthesis, containing standing lateral radiographs of the spine and pelvis of 816 subjects with grade 1–5 spondylolisthesis, aged between 10–40 years and collected from 43 spine surgeons in North America and Europe. The classification is now based on four important characteristics that can be assessed on standing

Slip	Pelvic Balance	Spinal Balance	Type
Low Grade Slip<50%	PI<45°	-	1
	PI=45-60°	-	2
	PI≥60°	-	3
High Grade Slip≥50%	Balanced Pelvis	-	4
	Unbalanced Pelvis	Balanced Spine	5 5A (LSK≥80°) 5B (LSK<80°)
	Unbalanced Pelvis	Unbalanced Spine	6

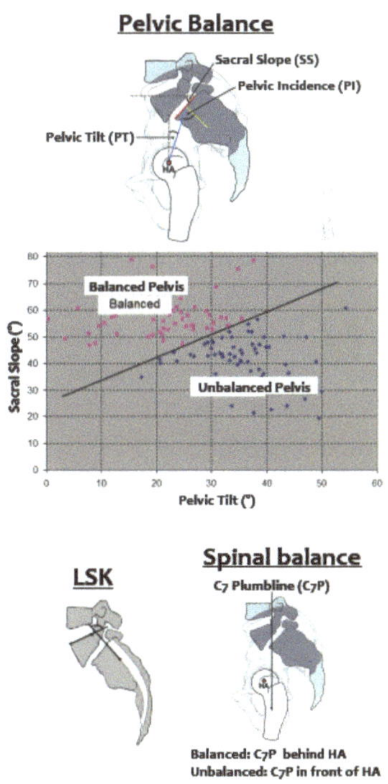

Fig. 8.7 Classification of pediatric lumbo-sacral spondylolisthesis. [Reprinted from Labelle H, Mac-Thiong JM, Roussouly P. Spino-pelvic sagittal balance of spondylolisthesis: a review and classification. Eur Spine J. 2011 Sep; 20(5):641-6. With permission from Springer-Verlag.]

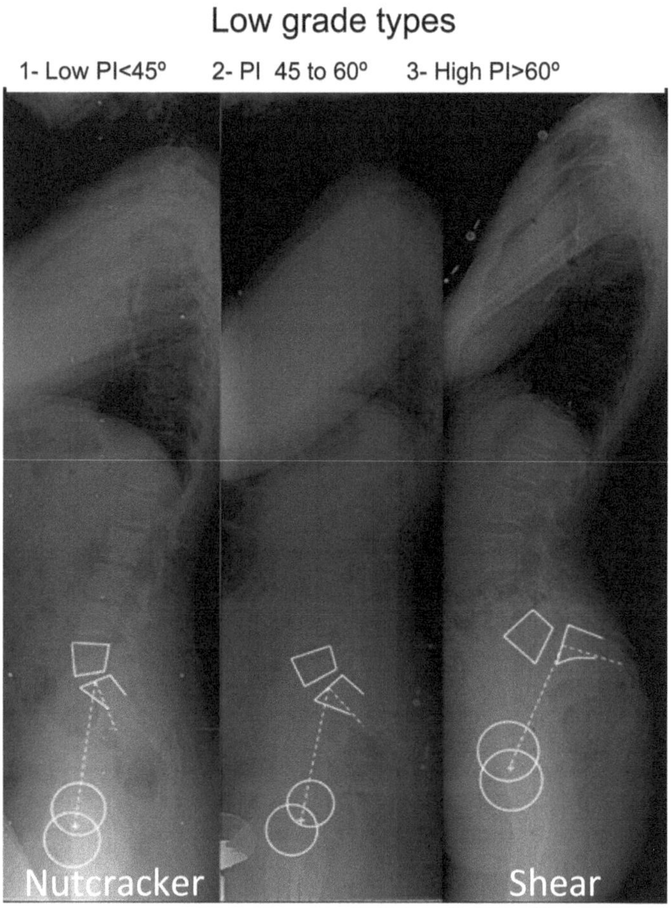

Fig. 8.8 The three types of spino-pelvic posture in low-grade spondylolisthesis. [Reprinted from Labelle H, Mac-Thiong JM, Roussouly P. Spino-pelvic sagittal balance of spondylolisthesis: a review and classification. Eur Spine J. 2011 Sep; 20(5):641-6. With permission from Springer-Verlag.]

sagittal radiographs of the spine and pelvis: (1) the grade of slip (low or high), (2) the pelvic incidence (low, normal or high), (3) the spino-pelvic balance (balanced or unbalanced), and (4) the lumbo-sacral kyphosis (low or high LSK). Accordingly, six different sub-types can be identified (Figs. 8.8 and 8.9).

To classify a patient, the degree of slip is quantified first from the lateral standing radiograph, in order to determine if it is low-grade (grades 0, 1, and 2, or <50 % slip) or high-grade (grades 3, 4, and spondyloptosis, or ≥50 % slip). Next, the sagittal balance is measured by determining sacro-pelvic and spino-pelvic alignment, using measurements of PI, SS, PT, and the C7 plumbline. For low-grade spondylolisthesis, three types of sacro-pelvic balance can be found (Fig. 8.8): type 1, the nutcracker type, a subgroup with low PI (<45°), type 2, a subgroup with normal PI (between 45° and 60°), and type 3, the shear type, a subgroup with high PI (>60°). For HGS, three types are also found (Fig. 8.9). Each subject is first classified as having a balanced or an unbalanced sacro-pelvis using raw PT and SS values or the nomogram provided by Hresko et al. [18]. When SS is greater than PT, or when SS and PT are located above the threshold line, the subject is classified as high SS/low PT. On the other hand, when SS is lower than PT or when SS and PT are located below the threshold line, the subject is classified as low SS/high PT. Next, spino-pelvic balance is determined using the C7 plumbline. If this line falls over or behind the femoral heads, the spine is balanced, while if it lies in front of the femoral heads, the spine is unbalanced. In our experience, the spine is almost always balanced in low-grade and in HGS with a balanced sacro-pelvis and therefore,

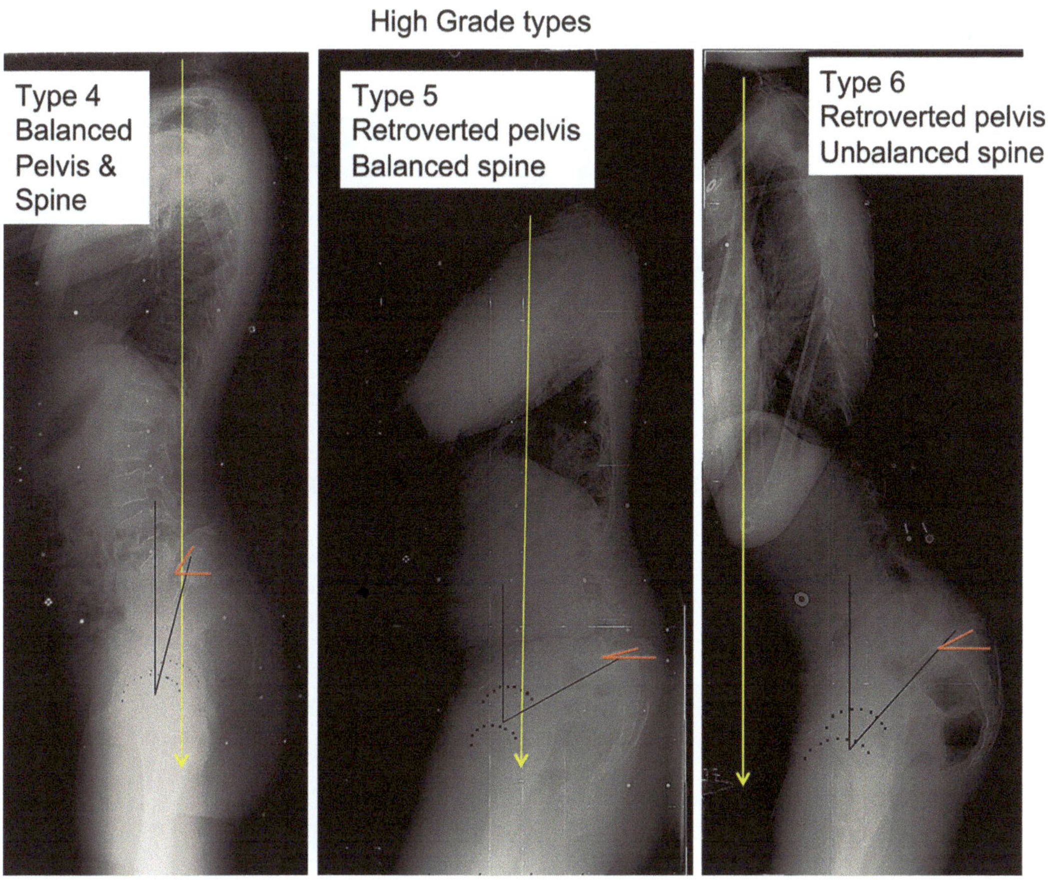

Fig. 8.9 The 3 types of spino-pelvic posture in high grade spondylolisthesis. [Reprinted from Labelle H, Mac-Thiong JM, Roussouly P. Spino-pelvic sagittal balance of spondylolisthesis: a review and classification. Eur Spine J. 2011 Sep; 20(5):641-6. With permission from Springer-Verlag.]

spinal balance needs to be measured mainly in high-grade deformities with an unbalanced pelvis (types 5 and 6). Therefore, the three types in HGS are: type 4 balanced pelvis, type 5 retroverted pelvis with balanced spine, and type 6 retroverted pelvis with unbalanced spine. Figures 8.8 and 8.9 illustrate clinical examples of these six basic postures. More recently, following the demonstration that increased lumbo-sacral kyphosis (LSK) is associated with a decrease in HRQoL in HGS [20], two sub-types of type 5 posture have been recognized: Type 5a, associated with a normal or low lumbo-sacral kyphosis (as measured by Dubousset's lumbo-sacral angle ≥80°) [23], and type 5b, associated with high lumbo-sacral kyphosis (as measured by Dubousset's lumbo-sacral angle <80°) [24]. Figure 8.10 illustrates the two type 5 sub-types. In a recent clinical assessment of this refined version of the classification system, Mac-Thiong et al. [25] found improved and substantial intra- and inter-observer reliability similar to other currently used classifications for spinal deformity, with an overall intra- and inter-observer agreements of 80 % (kappa: 0.74) and 71 % (kappa: 0.65), respectively.

The proposed classification emphasizes that subjects with L5-S1 spondylolisthesis are a heterogeneous group with various adaptations of their posture and that clinicians need to keep this fact in mind for evaluation and treatment. Abnormal spino-pelvic balance alters the biomechanical stresses at the lumbo-sacral junction and the compensation mechanisms used to maintain

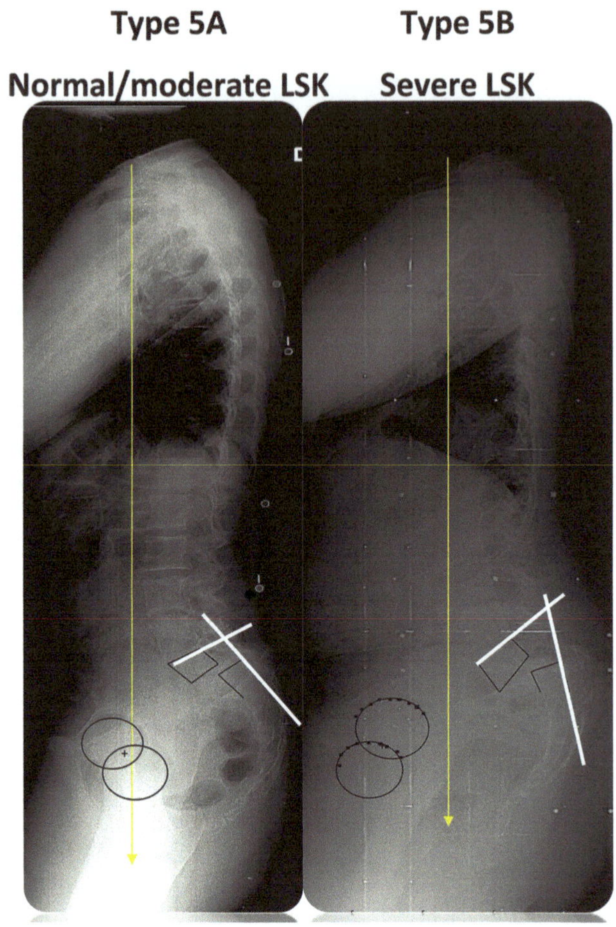

Fig. 8.10 The two sub-types of type 5 spino-pelvic posture

an adequate posture. The clinical relevance of this classification can be summarized as follows:

Since PI is always much greater than normal in HGS, this suggests that the risk of progression in skeletally immature subjects with types 1 and 2 with lower or normal PI may be lower than in the shear type 3 with abnormally high PI and SS values imposing higher shear stresses at the L5-S1 junction. In these subjects as well as those with type 4 alignment, there is an increased lumbar lordosis in order to keep the center of gravity and C7 plumbline behind the hips to maintain a balanced posture. This first compensation mechanism occurs by increasing the intervertebral segmental lordosis and/or by including more vertebrae in the lordotic segment. For each patient, there is a maximal attainable lumbar lordosis beyond which the patient will then attempt to maintain a balanced posture by progressive retroversion of the pelvis. This second compensation mechanism corresponds to the abnormal posture found in types 5 and 6 with a retroverted pelvis/vertical sacrum. Because each patient has a fixed pelvic incidence, since it is an anatomic parameter, SS decreases along with the retroversion of the pelvis and PT increases as the sacrum becomes vertical. When the limit of these two compensation mechanisms is reached, the patient develops sagittal trunk imbalance, most often characterized either by compensatory hip flexion, by forward leaning of the trunk with positive sagittal imbalance of the spine, or a combination of both, as seen in type 6 posture. Finally, in immature subjects, increased LSK combined with the anterior slipping of L5 induces higher pressure on the anterior part of the S1 growth plate, which itself leads to decreased growth of the anterior sacrum according to Hueter-Volkmann Law, inducing progressive rounding of the sacrum and the so-called sacral dome deformity often seen in high grade spondylolisthesis.

Although more outcome studies are needed before a definitive treatment algorithm can be established for each subtype, it is suggested that for subjects with a type 4 spino-pelvic posture, forceful attempts at reduction of the deformity may not be required and that instrumentation and fusion after simple postural reduction by prone positioning of patients under anesthesia on the operating table, may be all that is necessary to maintain adequate sagittal alignment, since adequate sagittal spino-pelvic alignment is already present in these subjects. For subjects with a type 5 posture, reduction and realignment procedures should preferably be attempted, but in subtype 5a, instrumentation and fusion after postural reduction may also be sufficient to achieve adequate sagittal alignment, since spinal alignment is maintained and lumbo-sacral kyphosis is within normal limits. Reduction and realignment procedures would appear mandatory in types 5b and 6 deformities where sagittal alignment is severely disturbed. While the need for reduction in the surgical treatment of L5-S1 spondylolisthesis is still debated, many studies published in the last decade support the value of this classification for the decision-making process [16, 17, 26–28].

References

1. Labelle H, Roussouly P, Berthonnaud E, et al. The importance of spino-pelvic balance in L5-S1 developmental spondylolisthesis: a review of pertinent radiologic measurements. Spine. 2005;30:S27–34.
2. Duval-Beaupère G, Schimdt C, Cosson P. A Barycentremetric study of the sagittal shape of spine and pelvis: the conditions required for an economic standing position. Ann Biomed Eng. 1992;20: 451–62.
3. Legaye J, Duval-Beaupère G, Hecquet J, et al. Pelvic incidence: a fundamental pelvic parameter for 3D regulation of spinal sagittal curves. Eur Spine J. 1998;7:99–103.
4. Mangione P, Gomez D, Senegas J. Study of the course of the incidence angle during growth. Eur Spine J. 1997;6:163–7.
5. MacThiong JM, Labelle H, Berthonnaud E, et al. Sagittal alignment of the spine and pelvis during growth. Spine. 2004;29:1642–7.
6. Vaz G, Roussouly P, Berthonnaud E, et al. Morphology and equilibrium of pelvis and spine. Eur Spine J. 2002;11:80–7.
7. Berthonnaud E, Dimnet J, Roussouly P, et al. Analysis of the sagittal balance of the spine and pelvis using shape and orientation parameters. J Spinal Disord Tech. 2005;18:40–7.
8. Mac-Thiong J-M, Labelle H, Berthonnaud É, et al. Sagittal spinopelvic balance in normal children and adolescents. Eur Spine J. 2007;16:227–34.
9. Mac-Thiong J-M, Labelle H, Roussouly P. Pediatric sagittal alignment. Eur Spine J. 2011;20:S586–90.
10. Mac-Thiong J-M, Roussouly P, Berthonnaud É, Guigui P. Sagittal parameters of global spinal balance: normative values from a prospective cohort of seven hundred nine Caucasian asymptomatic adults. Spine. 2010;35:E1193–8.
11. Mac-Thiong J-M, Roussouly P, Berthonnaud É, Guigui P. Age- and sex-related variations in sagittal sacropelvic morphology and balance in asymptomatic adults. Eur Spine J. 2011;20:S572–7.
12. Curylo LJ, Edwards C, DeWald RW. Radiographic markers in spondyloptosis: implications for spondylolisthesis progression. Spine. 2002;27:2021–5.
13. Labelle H, Roussouly P, Berthonnaud É, et al. Spondylolisthesis, pelvic incidence, and spinopelvic balance: a correlation study. Spine. 2004;29: 2049–954.
14. Whitesides Jr TE, Horton WC, Hutton WC, et al. Spondylotic spondylolisthesis: a study of pelvic and lumbosacral parameters of possible etiologic effect in two genetically and geographically distinct groups with high occurrence. Spine. 2005;30(6S):S12–21.
15. Roussouly P, Gollogly S, Berthonnaud É, et al. Sagittal alignment of the spine and pelvis in the presence of L5-S1 isthmic lysis and low-grade spondylolisthesis. Spine. 2006;31:2484–90.
16. Labelle H, Roussouly P, Berthonnaud E, et al. Spondylolisthesis classification based on spinopelvic alignment. Presented at the Scoliosis Research Society Annual Meeting; September 2009; San Antonio, TX.
17. Marchetti PC, Bartolozzi P. Classification of spondylolisthesis as a guideline for treatment. In: Bridwell KH, DeWald RL, Hammerberg KW, et al., editors. The textbook of spinal surgery. 2nd ed. Philadelphia, PA: Lippincott-Raven; 1997. p. 1211–54.
18. Hresko MT, Labelle H, Roussouly P, et al. Classification of high-grade spondylolisthesis based on pelvic version and spine balance: possible rationale for reduction. Spine. 2007;32:2208–13.
19. Mac-Thiong J-M, Wang Z, de Guise JA, et al. Postural model of sagittal spino-pelvic alignment and its relevance for lumbosacral developmental spondylolisthesis. Spine. 2008;33(21):2316–25.
20. Tanguay F, Labelle H, Wang Z, Joncas J, de Guise JA, Mac-Thiong JM. Clinical significance of lumbosacral

kyphosis in adolescent spondylolisthesis. Spine. 2012;37(4):304–8.

21. Harroud A, Labelle H, Joncas J, Mac-Thiong JM. Global sagittal alignment and health-related quality of life in lumbosacral spondylolisthesis. Eur Spine J. 2013;22(4):849–56.
22. Wiltse LL, Newman PH, Macnab I. Classification of spondylolysis and spondylolisthesis. Clin Orthop. 1976;117:23–9.
23. Labelle H, Mac-Thiong JM, Roussouly P. Spino-pelvic sagittal balance of spondylolisthesis: a review and classification. Eur Spine J. 2011;20(5):641–6.
24. Glavas P, Mac-Thiong J-M, Parent S, et al. Assessment of lumbosacral kyphosis in spondylolisthesis: a computer assisted reliability study of six measurement techniques. Eur Spine J. 2009;18(2):212–7.
25. Mac-Thiong JM, Duong L, Parent S, Hresko MT, Dimar 2nd JR, Weidenbaum M, Labelle H. Reliability of the SDSG Classification of lumbosacral spondylolisthesis. Spine (Phila Pa 1976). 2012;37(2): E95–102.
26. Labelle H, Roussouly P, Chopin D, Berthonnaud E, Hresko T, O'Brien M. Spino-pelvic alignment after surgical correction for developmental spondylolisthesis. Eur Spine J. 2008;17:1170–6.
27. Agabegi SS, Fischgrund JS. Contemporary management of isthmic spondylolisthesis: pediatric and adult. Spine J. 2010;10(6):530–43. Epub 2010 Apr 8.
28. Martiniani M, Lamartina C, Specchia N. "In situ" fusion or reduction in high-grade high dysplastic developmental spondylolisthesis (HDSS). Eur Spine J. 2012;21 Suppl 1:S134–40.
29. Kuntz IV C, Shaffrey CI, Ondra SL, Durrani AA, Mummaneni PV, Levin LS, Pettigrew DB. Spinal deformity: a new classification derived from neutral upright spinal alignment measurements in asymptomatic juvenile, adolescent, adult, and geriatric individuals. Neurosurgery. 2008;63:A25–39.

9 Non-operative Treatment of Spondylolisthesis

Benjamin D. Roye, Michael Vitale, and Farah Hameed

Introduction

Spondylolisthesis is the anterior slippage of a vertebra on its subjacent, or caudal, neighbor. This condition most commonly occurs in the lumbar spine with L5 being the single most commonly affected vertebra, with frequency decreasing with ascending lumbar levels. This condition has never been described in infants [1], but spondylolysis, a pre-slip problem, occurs in approximately 4.4 % of 6 year olds and 6 % of adolescents. This would seem to indicate a mechanical component in the development of this condition [2]. Spondylolisthesis may be diagnosed incidentally or during a workup for low back pain. Symptoms can vary from mild low back pain to severe pain with radicular symptoms and rarely, in severe slips, problems with bowel and bladder function.

B.D. Roye, M.D., M.P.H.
Department of Orthopedic Surgery, Morgan Stanley Children's Hospital of New York, 3959 Broadway, 8th Floor, North, New York, NY 10032, USA
e-mail: bdr5@columbia.edu

M. Vitale, M.D., M.P.H. (✉)
Columbia University Medical Center, 3959 Broadway, 8 North, New York, NY 10032, USA
e-mail: mgv166@gmail.com

F. Hameed, M.D.
Department of Rehabilitation and Regenerative Medicine, Columbia University Medical Center, 180 Fort Washington, HP 1-199, New York, NY 10032, USA
e-mail: FH2z8z@columbia.edu

Natural History

The natural history of spondylolisthesis is not fully understood, a fact that complicates treatment decisions. The few natural history studies in existence are relatively small and are almost impossible to reproduce in this day and age. However, there are many reports in the literature documenting the intermediate and long-term outcomes of treatment for spondylolisthesis [2–7]. One must have some understanding of the natural history in order to verify the effectiveness of any intervention, surgical or otherwise.

One of the largest and longest natural history studies for spondylolisthesis was published by Beutler et al. in 2003. In the 1950s, 500 asymptomatic elementary school children from a single school system in Pennsylvania were screened radiographically for spondylolysis and spondylolisthesis. From this cohort, 30 subjects were identified and tracked for over 45 years from the time of diagnosis (either in childhood or early adulthood) until study completion. In this population, all the slips were low grade at presentation (Meyerding 1 or 2) and no slip progressed to a high grade (Meyerding 3–5) [2]. While some slips showed progression over time, the rate of

A.L. Wollowick and V. Sarwahi (eds.), *Spondylolisthesis: Diagnosis, Non-Surgical Management, and Surgical Techniques*, DOI 10.1007/978-1-4899-7575-1_9,

slip progression slowed with each decade from 7 % over the first decade down to 2 % in the fourth decade. The presence of back pain or radicular leg symptoms was not associated with the slip percentage. In fact, the incidence and severity of back pain in this population *mirrored the general population* and there was no statistical association between pain and other factors including age at presentation, slip percentage, and lumbar index.

An early study out of Rochester, MN identified 114 children and adolescents (9–19 years of age) with spondylolysis and had variable follow-up of 1–9 years [1]. 85 % of their patients had grade 1 or 2 slips, and in these patients 82 % complained of back pain, 5 % presented with complaints about a postural change (from a parent), and 13 % had an incidental diagnosis (typically from a pre-employment radiograph). None of these patients treated without surgery had progression of their slip angle.

Nachamson and Frennered published their average 7-year follow-up of 47 patients diagnosed with spondylolysis or spondylolisthesis before the age of 16 in 1991 [4]. They found that only 4 % of patients with low-grade spondylolisthesis progressed (there were no high-grade slips in their cohort), none progressed to a Meyerding 3 or 4 slip, and there was no correlation between progression with age, sex, slip angle, lumbar index, or disc height. Of those treated non-operatively, 83 % continued normal activities of daily living without restriction. They also found that at last follow-up pain scores *did not differ significantly when compared to age matched norms*. Interestingly surgically treated patients had *more* progression of slip angle at last follow-up than non-surgical patients, a finding mirrored in other studies [8]. Nachamson concluded that low-grade spondylolisthesis has a benign course.

While there are no natural history studies for untreated high-grade spondylolisthesis (Meyerding grade 3 and 4 slips), there are several outcome studies in the literature, although the populations tend to be small as these slips are much less common. Harris and Weinstein compared long-term outcomes of non-operative and operative management of Meyerding grade 3–4 spondylolisthesis in young patients (age 10–25 at diagnosis) [9]. Of their 11 patients treated non-operatively, after an average 18-year follow-up, 36 % were symptom free, 55 % had mild symptoms, and only one had significant symptoms. Symptoms were associated with the presence of scoliosis, lateral listhesis, tight hamstrings, limited spinal motion, progression of the spondylolisthesis, obesity, weak abdominal muscles, and positive neurological findings. Symptoms were not associated with the severity of the slip. All of the patients led an active life, 45 % worked as manual laborers, and only one required minor adjustments in their lifestyle.

Specifically in the younger pediatric and adolescent age group (skeletally immature patients), those patients with high-grade spondylolisthesis seem to be much less likely to have successful outcomes on long-term follow-up with conservative management. Pizzutillo et al. retrospectively followed 82 adolescent patients (aged 6–21 years) with spondylolisthesis for 1–14.3 years [10]. Twelve of these patients had a high-grade 3 or 4 slippage, and only one improved with non-operative treatment. The rest (92 %) required operative treatment to control symptoms. However, 67 % of patients with grade 1 or 2 spondylolisthesis had significant improvement with non-operative treatments. It seems that in a younger population, a high-grade slip at presentation combined with an increased risk for progression with continued growth, spondylolisthesis is much more likely to become more symptomatic and requires surgical intervention to effectively treat symptoms.

Interestingly, thoughts on the impact of disk degeneration at the level of the spondylolisthesis have been evolving. Many authors have supposed that the degenerative process of the disc occurring at the level of the spondylolisthesis, as well as the levels above, predisposes to progression of the slippage and over time may become a pain generator [11]. However, there has been recent speculation in the literature (supported by the natural history data) that progression of spondylolisthesis often *does not* occur, especially in those who have finished growing and have low grades of slip at presentation. With these cases, there may actually be a loss of mobility and *inherent stabilization* at that segment as the disc degenerates, therefore *decreasing* the risk of progression at that level. Seitsalo, a proponent of this concept, has published long-term studies showing minimal progression and/or stability of the disc at the level of the spondylolisthesis in children with low-grade spondylolisthesis over a 10 to 15-year follow-up [8, 12]. His data is supported by the natural history data of Beutler [2] as well as other outcome studies [4].

Risk Factors for Progression

For spondylolysis to exist, by definition there must be some insufficiency or incompetency of the posterior elements. As indicated in the Wiltse classification scheme, the problem can be either traumatic (isthmic) or developmental (dysplastic) (it has never been noted congenitally). Of note, family history has been implicated in developing spondylolysis, and this condition occurs in 15–70 % of first degree relatives of individuals with the disorder [13]. The pars injury (spondylolysis) that occurs in the isthmic form of spondylolisthesis is always bilateral, as unilateral lesions have never been observed to progress to a slip [1, 2, 14]. There are clearly certain activities that place increased stress on the posterior elements of the spine and predispose to this problem including sports and dance activities that require repetitive hyperlordosis/extension of the lumbar spine or repetitive loading and unloading of the lumbar spine.

Several long-term outcome studies have shown that most slips demonstrate little, if any progression; 80–90 % of the ultimate slip percentage is present at the time of diagnosis and only 44 % of patients, athletes, and non-athletes alike, demonstrate any additional progression [14, 15, 16]. However, there are factors that seem to be associated with an increased risk of slip progression including increasing slip percentage (greater than 20–30 % slippage on presentation), skeletal immaturity, and the presence of a dysplastic (as opposed to isthmic) spondylolysis [17].

Furthermore, there is research to suggest several sagittal plane radiographic parameters, including the lumbar index, sacral inclination and slip angle, may be helpful in predicting which patients will progress, although findings are conflicting [18, 19]. The lumbar index looks at the relative wedging of lumbar vertebrae and is defined as the ratio of anterior vertebral height to posterior vertebral height. The sacral inclination is the angle formed between a line tangential to the posterior border of the sacrum and perpendicular to the floor, and thus measures of how vertical or horizontal the sacrum is in space. The slip angle measures the orientation of the slipped vertebra relative to the sacrum and is defined as the angle between the superior endplate of the slipped vertebra (usually L5) and a perpendicular drawn from a line parallel to the posterior border of S1. Individuals with increased sacral inclination and slip angles have increased sheer forces across their spondylolysis and can lead to worsening sagittal imbalance at the level of the slip [20]. The forward displacement of the lumbar vertebral body creates a lumbosacral kyphosis and displaces the center of gravity anteriorly in relation to the sacrum, thus producing a positive sagittal balance. The body compensates with hyperlordosis of the lumbar spine and thoracic hypokyphosis, which can initially help restore this balance. However it has been postulated that a larger lumbosacral kyphosis at diagnosis may constitute a risk factor for further progression due to the inability of these compensatory mechanisms to accommodate and maintain the center of gravity in the setting where a slip continues to progress [7, 19]. Pelvic incidence (PI), a non-modifiable measurement intrinsic to a pelvis (e.g., it does not change as the position of the pelvis changes in space), measures the relationship of the center of the hips to the sacrum with larger values indicating the hips are more anterior to the sacrum. It has been shown that individuals with spondylolisthesis have a higher PI than do individuals without slips [21].

Treatment Options

Given the benign natural history of low grade spondylolisthesis, non-operative interventions should represent the mainstay of treatment. As the natural history studies have shown us, there is no role for treating asymptomatic low-grade spondylolisthesis. Even most high-grade lesions can initially be treated conservatively. Treatment options for low-grade spondylolisthesis in children and adolescents include pain medications, bracing, activity restriction, and therapeutic exercises. The treatment of spondylolisthesis focuses primarily on pain management, although prevention of further slippage may be a consideration as well [22]. While many cases of congenital (dysplastic) spondylolisthesis are asymptomatic [3, 22] and discovered incidentally, children and adolescents are often diagnosed with spondylolisthesis during a workup for pain [2]. The pain may be in the lower back, radicular (with symptoms radiating into the buttock, thigh, leg, or foot) or both [14]. The pain generator may be due to slippage, dynamic motion/instability, pars fracture/elongation, or from the intervertebral disc [3, 23, 24].

Medical Treatment

Pain control can be facilitated in some cases with medications such as nonsteroidal anti-inflammatories and acetaminophen in conjunction with activity modification. For patients presenting with radicular or neuropathic pain, medications such as gabapentin, pregabalin, or amitryptiline can be effective in diminishing symptoms related to nerve irritation [25–28]. A full neurologic evaluation should be performed at the time of presentation to rule out any neurologic abnormalities, as well as any change in bowel or bladder function. At times, stronger pain medications such as tramadol or narcotics can be used if there is severe pain, especially at rest, but typically activity modification and over-the-counter pain medications or anti-inflammatories are adequate to improve symptoms [3, 23, 24].

Modalities

Modalities such as ice, heat, and massage are thought to help with any related myofascial pain and spasm from the underlying bony pathology. Ultrasound may be used to deliver medications or ionic compounds into the muscles to help reduce symptoms in the low back. Other modalities such as electrical muscle stimulation or transcutaneous electrical nerve stimulation may also be helpful to decrease pain in the low back musculature, although these have not been specifically studied in the setting of spondylolisthesis. Acupuncture, while not specifically studied for the pediatric population with spondylolisthesis, maybe a helpful adjunct to decrease pain in the acute phase and possibly for chronic symptoms. Bone stimulators, electromagnetic stimulation, and pulsed electromagnetic fields have been used effectively in case reports for patients with spondylolysis, persistent pain, and evidence of nonunion, but has not been studied in a controlled way on patients with spondylolisthesis [22, 29].

Physical Therapy

Physical therapy is the central part of initial treatment in all patients with symptomatic spondylolisthesis, even for those with high-grade slips and/or radicular symptoms. Physical therapy plays a critical role in improving the stabilization of the lumbar spine and decreasing pain. Unfortunately, there are very few controlled studies evaluating specific exercise regimens, and most studies with a non-surgical group do not specify their treatment protocol. In general, a neutral spine strengthening and stabilization protocol is recommended, with avoidance of hyperextension of the lumbar spine.

O'Sullivan et al. produced the only randomized controlled trial studying the efficacy of a lumbar stabilization protocol to control symptoms of chronic low back pain in spondylolisthesis. Their population of subjects with low-grade spondylolisthesis underwent a 10-week treatment program strengthening the deep abdominal muscles (including the transversus abdominus and internal obliques) and the lumbar multifidi muscles [30]. These muscles surrounding the lumbar spine primarily contribute to dynamic segmental stabilization. Once the patient was able to activate these muscles without substitution of the larger core muscles (such as the external oblique and rectus abdominus) the patient was asked to incorporate this muscular co-contraction into their day-to-day activities that would typically provoke symptoms. The goal was to train the neuromuscular system in order to provide dynamic stability at the level of symptoms. Those who underwent the specific exercise program showed a statistically significant reduction in pain intensity and functional disability levels after the 10-week program, which was *maintained at a 30-month follow-up*.

A Finnish study in 1990 by Seitsalo followed 149 patients with low-grade spondylolisthesis (slip < 30 %) who presented before age 20 [8]. Seventy-two of their patients were treated non-operatively with rest and physical therapy which included core stabilization, although a specific regimen was not specified. After an average follow-up was 15.3 years, 75 % had no complaints of pain, no patient elected to have surgery and, also of note, no patient had progression of their slip after skeletal maturity.

Other physical therapy goals include decreasing hamstring tightness and spasm, which is felt to extend the pelvis, leading to increased lumbar lordosis and stress on the posterior elements of the spine. Hamstring stretching can improve this lordosis and stress on the posterior elements of the lumbar spine. Additionally, stretching of the thoracodorsal and lumbodorsal fascia can also help to reduce the lordotic alignment and improve pain and function [3, 31, 32].

Bracing

Bracing for acute presentation of spondylolisthesis has been a standard treatment used by many practitioners to alleviate pain symptoms. It's important to remember that the goal of brace treatment is not to heal the spondylolytic defect, but rather to control symptoms and possibly prevent progression of the injury [10, 22, 31, 33–40]. An anti-lordotic TLSO or soft spinal corset to limit the spinal motion has been shown to be effective in reducing pain and may help facilitate progression of early rehabilitation intervention. Bracing regimens vary widely and there is no consensus as to their most appropriate use, or even if they are required at all. In fact, there are no controlled studies showing that brace treatment is superior to rest/activity modification and therapy alone. Some studies advocate bracing for not more than 6 weeks [24], while other studies recommend bracing for 6 months or more [10, 22, 31, 33–40]. Early studies showed that anti-lordotic bracing for spondylolysis or low-grade spondylolisthesis in addition to physical therapy produced improvement in the non-operatively treated patients, however in this same study patients also did well who were treated without a brace [1].

Similar results were discovered for symptomatic patients with spondylolysis or low-grade spondylolisthesis by Steiner and Micheli [31]. In this study, a modified Boston brace was worn for 23 h/day for 6 months, followed by a 6-month weaning period. Participation in sports was allowed, however the patient was required to wear the brace and be pain free while playing. Physical therapy was introduced once pain control was achieved and was coupled with bracing to prevent further progression of the spondylolysis to spondylolisthesis. Excellent results were found in 78 % of patients at average follow-up of 2.5 years. Bell et al. studied a small group of symptomatic patients with low-grade spondylolisthesis with a brace for on average 25 months, coupled with physical therapy. He found that all the patients had improvement in pain symptoms, and no patient had progression of the slip [34]. Unfortunately, none of these studies have a control group without bracing, so it is still unclear if bracing is better than activity restriction and therapy alone. Multiple studies have shown that low-grade slips do not regularly progress, even without brace treatment [1, 2, 41]. This fact is reinforced by a recent meta-analysis that compared the progression of spondylolysis or grade 1 spondylolisthesis in 15 observational studies. Their primary conclusions were that in the context of at least 1 year follow-up, children and young adults treated non-operatively were able to return to pain-free or near pain-free, unrestricted activities 84 % of the time. Additionally, there was no significant difference in clinical outcomes between patients treated with and without bracing [41].

Treatment Protocols

In much of the literature cohorts of patients with spondylolisthesis and spondylolysis are combined, making it difficult to make specific evidence based treatment recommendations for the spondylolisthetic patient. Several authors have published treatment recommendations based on their research and experience, although they do not represent original research per se. Most of our understanding in regard to natural history and progression of spondylolisthesis is based on observational studies, and to our knowledge, there are no controlled studies evaluating non-operative treatments as described above.

In 2003, McTimoney and Micheli proposed management recommendations for a first-time diagnosis of low-grade spondylolysis and/or spondylolisthesis [22]. Once diagnosis has been established, their recommendations include a Boston brace at neutral (without lordosis) for 23 h/day. Additionally the patient should work with physical therapy. Follow-up should first be done at 4 weeks, and once pain free, the patient can be permitted to return to sports with the brace. They will likely need trimming of the brace to allow them to return to sporting activities, but they should continue to avoid any extension of the spine with sports. At the 6-month visit, a lateral X-ray should be performed to evaluate for any progression. At that time if there has been no progression the brace should be weaned over a period of 6 months. The last step should be returning to sports without the brace, especially if they have a great deal of extension in their sport.

Some practitioners propose much less strict guidelines for return to play with athletes with a first-time diagnosis of spondylolisthesis. This is due to the studies that suggest that progression of low-grade spondylolisthesis is rare, especially in patients who are skeletally mature. Bracing has not always been recommended due to cost as well as the cumbersome effects of it on the child's day to day activities. Bracing has been proposed by some to be initiated only if activity modification and physical therapy are not improving pain. The goal of bracing for these practitioners is to improve pain and help facilitate progression of physical therapy. In this population, bracing rarely exceeds a duration of 6–8 weeks [3].

Author's Recommendations

The authors have developed a protocol to treat the child or adolescent who presents with a painful, low-grade spondylolisthesis. Setting expectations upfront is very important—the family needs to be aware that the duration of treatment can take up to 6–12 months, and even longer in rare instances. The diagnosis is confirmed based on radiographs taken at presentation, typically as part of an evaluation for back pain. An MRI scan may be obtained to evaluate the posterior elements, as well as the nerve roots in cases of radicular symptoms. Initial treatment includes activity modification and rest; specifically, any activity that reproduces their pain is to be avoided, especially in athletes. Based on physical exam findings, physical therapy is prescribed; we utilize a neutral spine stabilization and strengthening program. The goals of physical therapy are two pronged: (1) improved flexibility (especially of the hamstrings and the thoracodorsal and lumbodorsal fascia); and (2) strengthening through abdominal/core and anti-lordotic low back exercises. Bracing is not recommended for the patient who is asymptomatic with activity modification and physical therapy. However, for the child having continued pain with daily activities, the rapidly growing child, the child who is non-compliant with activity restrictions, or in those for whom quick return to sport is desired, anti-lordotic bracing can improve pain, function and allow for return to activity. Once initiated, the anti-lordotic lumbosacral brace is to be worn full time while the patient is upright. However, the brace may be removed for sleeping and physical therapy sessions. Brace wear continues until the patient has demonstrated improved strength and flexibility, and no longer has pain on exam with routine activities of daily living.

A follow-up visit should be arranged a few weeks after initiating physical therapy to review the child's home exercise program and ascertain improvements in strength and flexibility. After a minimum of 6 weeks of therapy, if the patient demonstrates significant gains towards their therapy goals, as well as diminution of symptoms, then a gradual return to sport and other physical activities can be discussed. Avoidance of hyperextension until fully pain free through a complete range of motion is essential. It's critical that the parent and child understand the importance of continuing of their home exercise program once pain free in order to maintain the strength and flexibility achieved with physical therapy.

In terms of follow-up imaging, we recommend lateral radiographs every 12 months in a skeletally mature patient. During periods of rapid growth, a follow-up lateral radiograph should be obtained at 6 and 12 months after presentation to ensure no progression is occurring. If progression is occurring, closer follow-up is indicated.

If the patient is unable to have pain free return to sport/activity, anti-lordotic bracing can be attempted to help with symptoms, with gradual weaning of the brace over 3–6 months as tolerated by the patient. However, if symptoms persist and PT goals have not been fully met, therapy and activity restrictions should continue. Alternatively, at times a change in sport activity (e.g., change of position or event) can provide a good compromise to the overachieving athlete who does not wish to abandon athletic activities. If pain continues after 6–12 months, despite compliance with the outlined treatment plan, other treatments including surgery can be considered.

High-grade slips in the actively growing child have a poor prognosis in the authors' experience, similar to the findings of Pizzutillo and Boxall et al., and most of these patients progress to surgery [10, 42]. However, the above treatment regimen is still initiated (activity restriction, bracing and therapy), unless there are obvious neurologic impairments identified that might require more acute surgical management. Our management of these patients differs from those with low-grade slips in that we will be more likely to initiate brace treatment, and we recommend lateral radiographs every 3 months to monitor for progression. Additionally, avoidance of contact sports or sports with hyperextension is essential to minimize risk of pain symptoms and/or progression. For those who do not improve with more conservative treatments, or those with neurologic impairments, surgical treatment is considered.

Conclusion

In summary, children and adolescents with low-grade (grade 1 or 2) spondylolisthesis have an excellent prognosis, and the child will not likely need restricted activity in the long term. Activity modification and physical therapy focusing on spine stabilization exercises and hamstring and thoraco/lumbodorsal flexibility are typically sufficient to control symptoms. With long-term follow-up studies to help guide our counseling and conversations, we understand that very few patients progress in their amount of slippage, and there is not a significantly increased risk of pain long term. In growing children, follow-up radiographs should be performed every 6 months until skeletal maturity to evaluate for further slippage. Bracing can be considered if symptoms are more severe or the patient is a growing athlete or under pressure to return quickly to sport. For those patients with high grade spondylolisthesis (grade 3 or 4) on presentation, non-surgical outcomes have been proven to be less successful, especially in the actively growing child, and surgery should be considered if the slip is progressing or if pain is not improving with conservative interventions.

References

1. Turner RH, Bianco Jr AJ. Spondylolysis and spondylolisthesis in children and teen-agers. J Bone Joint Surg Am. 1971;53(7):1298–306.
2. Beutler WJ, Fredrickson BE, Murtland A, Sweeney CA, Grant WD, Baker D. The natural history of spondylolysis and spondylolisthesis: 45-year follow-up evaluation. Spine (Phila Pa 1976). 2003;28(10):1027–35. doi:10.1097/01.brs.0000061992.98108.a0. discussion 1035.
3. Cavalier R, Herman MJ, Cheung EV, Pizzutillo PD. Spondylolysis and spondylolisthesis in children and adolescents: I. Diagnosis, natural history, and nonsurgical management. J Am Acad Orthop Surg. 2006;14(7):417–24.
4. Frennered AK, Danielson BI, Nachemson AL. Natural history of symptomatic isthmic low-grade spondylolisthesis in children and adolescents: a seven-year follow-up study. J Pediatr Orthop. 1991;11(2):209–13.
5. Lonstein JE. Spondylolisthesis in children. Cause, natural history, and management. Spine (Phila Pa 1976). 1999;24(24):2640–8.

6. Osterman K, Schlenzka D, Poussa M, Seitsalo S, Virta L. Isthmic spondylolisthesis in symptomatic and asymptomatic subjects, epidemiology, and natural history with special reference to disk abnormality and mode of treatment. Clin Orthop Relat Res. 1993;297: 65–70.
7. Tsirikos AI, Garrido EG. Spondylolysis and spondylolisthesis in children and adolescents. J Bone Joint Surg Br. 2010;92(6):751–9. doi:10.1302/0301-620x.92b6.23014.
8. Seitsalo S. Operative and conservative treatment of moderate spondylolisthesis in young patients. J Bone Joint Surg Br. 1990;72(5):908–13.
9. Harris IE, Weinstein SL. Long-term follow-up of patients with grade-III and IV spondylolisthesis. Treatment with and without posterior fusion. J Bone Joint Surg Am. 1987;69(7):960–9.
10. Pizzutillo PD, Hummer 3rd CD. Nonoperative treatment for painful adolescent spondylolysis or spondylolisthesis. J Pediatr Orthop. 1989;9(5): 538–40.
11. Schlenzka D, Poussa M, Seitsalo S, Osterman K. Intervertebral disc changes in adolescents with isthmic spondylolisthesis. J Spinal Disord. 1991;4(3): 344–52.
12. Seitsalo S, Schlenzka D, Poussa M, Osterman K. Disc degeneration in young patients with isthmic spondylolisthesis treated operatively or conservatively: a long-term follow-up. Eur Spine J. 1997;6(6):393–7.
13. Albanese M, Pizzutillo PD. Family study of spondylolysis and spondylolisthesis. J Pediatr Orthop. 1982;2(5):496–9.
14. Seitsalo S, Osterman K, Hyvarinen H, Tallroth K, Schlenzka D, Poussa M. Progression of spondylolisthesis in children and adolescents. A long-term follow-up of 272 patients. Spine (Phila Pa 1976). 1991;16(4):417–21.
15. Fredrickson BE, Baker D, McHolick WJ, Yuan HA, Lubicky JP. The natural history of spondylolysis and spondylolisthesis. J Bone Joint Surg Am. 1984;66(5): 699–707.
16. Muschik M, Hahnel H, Robinson PN, Perka C, Muschik C. Competitive sports and the progression of spondylolisthesis. J Pediatr Orthop. 1996;16(3): 364–9.
17. McPhee IB, O'Brien JP, McCall IW, Park WM. Progression of lumbosacral spondylolisthesis. Australas Radiol. 1981;25(1):91–5.
18. Dubousset J. Treatment of spondylolysis and spondylolisthesis in children and adolescents. Clin Orthop Relat Res. 1997;337:77–85.
19. Tanguay F, Labelle H, Wang Z, Joncas J, de Guise JA, Mac-Thiong JM. Clinical significance of lumbosacral kyphosis in adolescent spondylolisthesis. Spine (Phila Pa 1976). 2012;37(4):304–8. doi:10.1097/BRS.0b013e31821cc558.
20. Hosoe H, Ohmori K. Degenerative lumbosacral spondylolisthesis: possible factors which predispose the fifth lumbar vertebra to slip. J Bone Joint Surg Br. 2008;90(3):356–9. doi:10.1302/0301-620x.90b3.19606.
21. Labelle H, Roussouly P, Berthonnaud E, Transfeldt E, O'Brien M, Chopin D, et al. Spondylolisthesis, pelvic incidence, and spinopelvic balance: a correlation study. Spine (Phila Pa 1976). 2004;29(18):2049–54.
22. McTimoney CA, Micheli LJ. Current evaluation and management of spondylolysis and spondylolisthesis. Curr Sports Med Rep. 2003;2(1):41–6.
23. Herman MJ, Pizzutillo PD. Spondylolysis and spondylolisthesis in the child and adolescent: a new classification. Clin Orthop Relat Res. 2005;434:46–54.
24. Herman MJ, Pizzutillo PD, Cavalier R. Spondylolysis and spondylolisthesis in the child and adolescent athlete. Orthop Clin North Am. 2003;34(3):461–7. vii.
25. Baron R, Freynhagen R, Tolle TR, Cloutier C, Leon T, Murphy TK, Phillips K. The efficacy and safety of pregabalin in the treatment of neuropathic pain associated with chronic lumbosacral radiculopathy. Pain. 2010;150(3):420–7. doi:10.1016/j.pain.2010.04.013.
26. Kasimcan O, Kaptan H. Efficacy of gabapentin for radiculopathy caused by lumbar spinal stenosis and lumbar disk hernia. Neurol Med Chir (Tokyo). 2010;50(12):1070–3.
27. Khoromi S, Cui L, Nackers L, Max MB. Morphine, nortriptyline and their combination vs. placebo in patients with chronic lumbar root pain. Pain. 2007;130(1–2):66–75. doi:10.1016/j.pain.2006.10.029.
28. Yildirim K, Deniz O, Gureser G, Karatay S, Ugur M, Erdal A, Senel K. Gabapentin monotherapy in patients with chronic radiculopathy: the efficacy and impact on life quality. J Back Musculoskelet Rehabil. 2009;22(1):17–20. doi:10.3233/bmr-2009-0210.
29. Stasinopoulos D. Treatment of spondylolysis with external electrical stimulation in young athletes: a critical literature review. Br J Sports Med. 2004;38(3): 352–4.
30. O'Sullivan PB, Phyty GD, Twomey LT, Allison GT. Evaluation of specific stabilizing exercise in the treatment of chronic low back pain with radiologic diagnosis of spondylolysis or spondylolisthesis. Spine (Phila Pa 1976). 1997;22(24):2959–67.
31. Steiner ME, Micheli LJ. Treatment of symptomatic spondylolysis and spondylolisthesis with the modified Boston brace. Spine (Phila Pa 1976). 1985;10(10):937–43.
32. Sys J, Michielsen J, Bracke P, Martens M, Verstreken J. Nonoperative treatment of active spondylolysis in elite athletes with normal X-ray findings: literature review and results of conservative treatment. Eur Spine J. 2001;10(6):498–504.
33. Anderson K, Sarwark JF, Conway JJ, Logue ES, Schafer MF. Quantitative assessment with SPECT imaging of stress injuries of the pars interarticularis and response to bracing. J Pediatr Orthop. 2000;20(1):28–33.
34. Bell DF, Ehrlich MG, Zaleske DJ. Brace treatment for symptomatic spondylolisthesis. Clin Orthop Relat Res. 1988;236:192–8.
35. Blanda J, Bethem D, Moats W, Lew M. Defects of pars interarticularis in athletes: a protocol for nonoperative treatment. J Spinal Disord. 1993;6(5):406–11.

36. d'Hemecourt PA, Gerbino PG 2nd, Micheli LJ. Back injuries in the young athlete. Clin Sports Med. 2000;19(4):663–79.
37. d'Hemecourt PA, Zurakowski D, Kriemler S, Micheli LJ. Spondylolysis: returning the athlete to sports participation with brace treatment. Orthopedics. 2002;25(6):653–7.
38. Debnath UK, Freeman BJ, Grevitt MP, Sithole J, Scammell BE, Webb JK. Clinical outcome of symptomatic unilateral stress injuries of the lumbar pars interarticularis. Spine (Phila Pa 1976). 2007;32(9): 995–1000. doi:10.1097/01.brs.0000260978.10073.90.
39. El Rassi G, Takemitsu M, Woratanarat P, Shah SA. Lumbar spondylolysis in pediatric and adolescent soccer players. Am J Sports Med. 2005;33(11):1688–93. doi:10.1177/0363546505275645.
40. Letts M, Smallman T, Afanasiev R, Gouw G. Fracture of the pars interarticularis in adolescent athletes: a clinical-biomechanical analysis. J Pediatr Orthop. 1986;6(1):40–6.
41. Klein G, Mehlman CT, McCarty M. Nonoperative treatment of spondylolysis and grade I spondylolisthesis in children and young adults: a meta-analysis of observational studies. J Pediatr Orthop. 2009;29(2): 146–56. doi:10.1097/BPO.0b013e3181977fc5.
42. Boxall D, Bradford DS, Winter RB, Moe JH. Management of severe spondylolisthesis in children and adolescents. J Bone Joint Surg Am. 1979;61(4):479–95.

Non-surgical Management of Spondylolisthesis in Adults

10

Joseph M. Zavatsky, David C. Briski, and Richard Frisch

Introduction

Spondylolisthesis is defined as the non-physiologic translation of a proximal vertebra in relation to its caudal segment. Numerous classification systems have been created to describe not only the etiology but also the severity of spondylolisthesis. The Wiltse–Newman classification is the most widely used [1]. It describes five primary etiologies of spondylolisthesis. Four of these etiologies are acquired: isthmic, degenerative, traumatic, and pathologic, with the fifth consisting of congenital or dysplastic anomalies. Iatrogenic spondylolisthesis, as a result of surgery, can additionally be classified as its own entity.

Spondylolisthesis in adults more commonly has an isthmic or degenerative etiology, according to the Wiltse–Newman classification, and their non-operative treatment options will be the focus of this chapter.

J.M. Zavatsky, M.D. (✉)
Spine, Scoliosis and Deformity Institute, Florida Orthopaedic Institute, 10908 North Ridgedale Rd., Tampa, FL 33617, USA
e-mail: josephzavatsky@yahoo.com

D.C. Briski, M.D.
Department of Orthopaedic Surgery, Ochsner Medical Center, 1514 Jefferson Hwy, New Orleans, LA 70121, USA
e-mail: dcbriski@gmail.com

R. Frisch, M.D.
Southeastern Spine Institute, 1106 Chuck Dawley Boulevard, Mount Pleasant, SC 29464, USA

Treatment

Patients with suspected spondylolisthesis require detailed clinical and radiographic examinations. This includes taking a detailed history, performing a thorough physical examination, and obtaining appropriate imaging studies to establish the severity of disease. The comprehensive evaluation of the spondylolisthesis patient is reviewed in other chapters. However, once the evaluation is complete, the clinical and radiographic examinations must correlate with the patient's complaints and guide possible treatment options.

While no randomized studies have been reported to date that delineate a non-operative treatment algorithm, a multi-dimensional approach is advocated. All patients should be educated about the benefits of practicing healthy back care with proper lifting and bending techniques and understanding ergonomics, along with avoiding prolonged periods of sitting and driving. Smoking cessation, along with weight loss to obtain an ideal body weight should be emphasized as risk factors that the patient can control in an attempt to reduce or eliminate their back pain. Additionally, activity modification can reduce environmental pain generators, along with various physical therapy (PT) modalities with attention to

A.L. Wollowick and V. Sarwahi (eds.), *Spondylolisthesis: Diagnosis, Non-Surgical Management, and Surgical Techniques*, DOI 10.1007/978-1-4899-7575-1_10,

core strengthening, flexion and extension exercises, aerobic conditioning for weight loss, and the occasional utilization of bracing.

Non-narcotic medications including the use of non-steroidal anti-inflammatory drugs (NSAIDs) should also be part of the initial conservative treatment plan. Steroid injections including interlaminar, transforaminal, pars inter-articularis, as well as facet injections can also be therapeutic and offer diagnostic value. Additionally, chiropractic spinal manipulation and acupuncture are alternative treatment modalities. When patients do not improve with these non-operative treatment options, surgery may be indicated.

Physical Therapy

Conservative therapy must be specific to the disease being treated. As part of most PT programs, low-impact aerobic activity is encouraged for weight loss. The use of a stationary bike is promoted because the flexed posture of the lumbar spine, and leaning forward theoretically opens the central canal and neural foramen, potentially alleviating neurologic symptoms in patients with stenosis. Exercises focused upon stability of the trunk should be implemented when seeking to treat spondylolisthesis through conservative modalities. Flexion-based PT exercise regimens appear to be superior to extension-based programs in achieving symptomatic relief.

Flexion exercises have been shown to yield favorable results in the few randomized studies published. Sinaki et al. reported on 48 patients with symptomatic low back pain secondary to spondylolisthesis who were treated conservatively and followed for 3 years after initial examination to compare the outcomes of two exercise programs [2]. The patients were divided into two groups: those doing flexion abdominal exercises and those doing extension back strengthening exercises. All patients received instructions on posture, lifting techniques, and the use of heat for relief of symptoms. After 3 months, only 27 % of patients who were instructed to perform flexion exercises had moderate or severe pain, and only 32 % were unable to work or had limited their work. Of the patients who were instructed in extension exercises, 67 % had moderate or severe pain, and 61 % were unable to work or had limited their work. At 3-year follow-up, only 19 % of the flexion group had moderate or severe pain and 24 % were unable to work or had limited their work. The respective figures for the extension group were 67 and 61 %. The overall recovery rate after 3 months was 58 % for the flexion group and 6 % for the extension group. At 3 years these figures improved to 62 % for the flexion group and dropped to 0 % for the extension group. Based on these findings, the authors suggested that if a conservative treatment program is prescribed, flexion or isometric back strengthening exercises should be considered.

Gramse et al. reported on 47 patients with symptomatic back pain secondary to spondylolisthesis who were not surgical candidates and treated with a physical therapy program [3]. Twenty-eight patients were treated with flexion exercises of the lumbar spine. Nineteen patients were treated with extension-type exercises, in addition to flexion exercises. At follow-up, 7 of the 28 patients (25 %) in the flexion exercise group rated their pain as moderate to severe, whereas 13 (68 %) of 19 in the extension group rated their pain as moderate to severe. In the flexion group, 23 patients (82 %) reported less pain, and 5 (18 %) rated their pain as unchanged or worse, whereas patients in the extension group, 7 (37 %) rated their pain as less, and 12 (63 %) as unchanged or worse. In addition to having less pain, the flexion exercise group did not modify their work and leisure activities as much, had less dependence on lumbar bracing, and a greater chance of recovery.

O'Sullivan performed a randomized, controlled trial, using a test–retest design by mailing questionnaires at 3, 6, and 30-months follow-up to determine the efficacy of a specific exercise intervention in the treatment of patients with chronic low back pain and the diagnosis of spondylolysis or spondylolisthesis [4]. Forty-four patients with this condition were assigned randomly to 2 treatment groups. The study group underwent a 10-week exercise treatment program involving the specific training of the deep abdominal muscles, with co-activation of the lumbar multifidus proximal to the pars defects. The control group underwent treatment as directed by their treating practitioner. After intervention, the study group who participated in the specific exercise treatment program showed a statistically significant reduction in pain intensity and functional disability levels, which was maintained at the 30-month follow-up. The control group showed no significant change in these parameters at no time point throughout the study. The authors concluded that a "specific exercise" treatment approach appears more effective than other commonly prescribed conservative treatment programs in patients with chronically symptomatic spondylolysis or spondylolisthesis.

Predicting treatment response to physical therapy can be difficult when implementing physical therapy exercises. Hicks et al. prospectively sought to determine predictors for successful treatment of low back pain through stabilization exercises in patients with lumbar segmental instability [5]. They were able to report on a total of 54 patients over a 1-year period. Patients underwent an 8-week biweekly program with additional home exercises verified via self-logs. The program was designed to specifically assess core stabilizers of the spine including rectus abdominus, transversus abdominus, internal oblique abdominals, erector spinae and multifidus muscles. Success of treatment was defined as greater than 50 % improvement from baseline to post-therapy symptoms assessed by Oswestry disability questionnaires (ODQ). Eighteen patients (33 %) were considered successes, 21 (38.9 %) patients observed improvement, while 15 (27.8 %) patients experienced less than a 6-point improvement based upon their ODQ and were quantified as failures. The authors identified four key variables as predictors of successful treatment, which included age less than 40 years old (3.7 higher odds of success), average straight leg raise at baseline, the presence of aberrant movement during lumbar range of motion, and a positive prone instability test.

Bracing

The implementation of bracing has been studied to a limited degree in adults, and most data has been published in the pediatric population. Steiner and Micheli reported on 67 young adult patients with symptomatic spondylolysis or grade 1 spondylolisthesis who were treated with modified Boston bracing [6]. The average follow-up was 2.5 years. Following treatment, 52 persons (78 %) had either an excellent or good result with no pain and returned to their full activities. Nine (13 %) continued to have mild symptoms, and 6 patients (9 %) subsequently required in situ fusion. Twelve of the patients showed radiographic evidence of healing of their pars defect(s). This group and those with the best overall results tended to be men with spondylolysis and relatively acute onset of symptoms. Clinical age, delay in treatment, occurrence of spina bifida, and bone scan result did not correlate with the ultimate clinical result.

Spratt et al. evaluated the efficacy of bracing along with flexion and extension exercises for low back pain in adult patients with retrodisplacement, spondylolisthesis, and normal sagittal translation [7]. The authors set out to determine if non-operative treatment involving bracing, exercise, and education, controlling for either flexion or extension postures would result in a distinctive pattern of favorable or unfavorable results depending on the type of radiographic instability. Fifty-six patients were randomized into one of three bracing treatment groups (flexion, extension, and control). The flexion treatment group was designed to minimize lumbar extension or lordosis and each patient was fitted with a Raney Flexion Jacket and instructed by a physical therapist in proper techniques for performing a series of lumbar flexion exercises. The extension treatment group was designed to maintain lumbar extension or lordosis and was fitted a Camp hyperextension brace and instructed by a physical therapist in proper techniques for performing a series of McKenzie-type extension exercises. The control group was not provided with any information regarding flexion or extension posture and was given a Velcro wrap corset without a thermoplastic mold and was seen by a physical therapist with no specific exercise program. Patients were assessed at admission and at 1-month follow-up. The sample was relatively evenly divided between men (46 %) and women (54 %), and by age. Brace treatments were not shown to reduce patient range of motion or lessen trunk strength. Improvements were seen in VAS scores for patients braced in extension compared to those braced in flexion and in the control groups. The authors concluded that clinicians should consider extension-bracing treatment, along with complimentary education and exercise programs. This regimen may represent a relatively powerful modality and viable conservative treatment approach even for patients with chronic low back pain.

Non-narcotic Medications

The utilization of NSAID medications has long been established as a first-line short-term therapy for the treatment of lower back pain. As a class of medication, they comprise the most commonly prescribed medication for the treatment of low back pain regardless of the specific etiology. Few studies have been published directly assessing their utilization for the treatment of spondylolisthesis. Van Tulder et al. completed a systemic review of double-blinded, randomized trials implementing NSAIDs for the treatment of low back pain [8]. Their review encompassed 51 trials totaling 6,057 patients. The authors concluded that while NSAIDs as a class were effective for the short-term relief of low back pain, in many cases paracetamol (acetaminophen) was equally as effective. In addition, it was noted that sufficient evidence advocating the use of NSAIDs for long-term therapy was not available at the time of publication.

Corticosteroid Injections

Epidural corticosteroid injections (ESIs) have been shown to yield viable short-term management results for patients with lumbar back pain secondary to multiple etiologies [9, 10]. The short and long-term outcomes secondary to epidural steroid injections have been assessed in multiple other lumbar pathologies. Amongst all the data available on ESIs, Cuckler et al. specifically evaluated ESIs for the treatment of patients with lumbar radicular pain [11]. They enrolled 73 patients in a prospective, randomized, double-blinded fashion. At the conclusion of the study no statistical significance was observed between the control and experimental groups after 23 months.

To date, only one study has been identified, which directly assesses the use of ESIs for the treatment of isolated spondylolisthesis. Kraiwattanapong et al. reviewed 33 patients undergoing transforaminal ESIs over a period of 12 months [12]. Their findings correlated with the historical literature, in which ESIs offered only short-term efficacy in the relief of patients symptoms, with a plateau and even failure long-term.

Alternative Therapy

Chiropractic manipulation of the spine provides the mainstay of alternative treatment for symptomatic spondylolisthesis. No randomized studies evaluating the outcomes of manipulation have been published to date. In 1987 Mierau et al. assessed the therapeutic outcomes secondary to spinal manipulation of 285 patients with and without spondylolisthesis [13]. Of the 285 patients included in the study, 25 patients had the diagnosis of spondylolisthesis. They failed to demonstrate a difference in outcomes between the groups with and without spinal manipulation.

Lee et al. designed a prospective randomized controlled pilot trial evaluating the efficacy of acupuncture for the treatment of spondylolisthesis. As this trial has only recently been approved in 2014, the data is unavailable for review [14]. However, given the historically mixed success of acupuncture as a viable alternative therapy, the authors remain cautiously optimistic as to the success of this modality.

Conservative Management vs. Surgery

There are a limited number of studies that have compared conservative vs. surgical management of low-grade spondylolisthesis in adults. Two major systemic reviews assessed the current literature discussing the conservative medical management of spondylolisthesis. Kalichman and Hunter reviewed all related literature from 1950 to 2007, while Garet et al. reviewed all pertinent literature from 1966 to 2012 [15, 16]. Both reviews demonstrated a deficiency of recommendations and objective data regarding both the standardization and success of medical management for the treatment of spondylolisthesis. Garet et al. did cite both the SPORT [17] and Möller's prospective randomized controlled trial (PRCT) [18] trials as the highest level of evidence at the time of publication as they are both level-I, prospective, randomized, controlled trials. The SPORT trail evaluated the treatment of degenerative spondylolisthesis, while Möller's PRCT trial evaluated isthmic spondylolisthesis in adults.

Spine Patient Outcomes Research Trial

The Spine Patient Outcomes Research Trial (SPORT) study evaluated the surgical and conservative management of patients with adult degenerative spondylolisthesis [17]. The study enrolled 304 patients in the prospective randomized control arm and 303 patients, who refused randomization, into the observational cohort. The intent-to-treat analysis of the randomized cohort, which was limited by non-adherence to the assigned treatment, demonstrated that surgery had no significant advantage over non-operative treatment. At the 3 and 4-year follow-up visits, non-operative treatment showed a slight but non-significant advantage. But there was significant crossover of patients in the two treatment arms, which was a major limitation of the study. Additionally, there was lack of randomization and control for the surgical group because there was heterogeneity in the surgical procedures received for treatment.

Non-operative treatments used during the SPORT included physical therapy (43 % [176 of 412]), epidural steroid injections (47 % [192 of 412]), NSAIDs (54 % [224 of 412]), and opioids (35 % [146 of 412]). The non-operative treatments were similar in the randomized cohort and the observational cohort, although more patients in the randomized cohort than in the observational cohort reported: visits to a surgeon (48 % [122 of 252] compared with 38 % [60 of 160], $p=0.04$); receiving injections (51 % [128 of 252] compared with 40 % 64 of 160], $p=0.04$); and opioid use (40 % [100 of 252] compared with 29 % [46 of 160], $p=0.03$).

Of the 159 patients who were randomized to the surgery group, 105 (66 %) underwent surgery and were available for 4-year follow-up. One hundred forty-five patients were randomized to conservative care, but of the 99 patients who were available for follow-up at 4 years, 79 (54 %) had crossed over and underwent surgery. Because of the patient crossover, the as-treated analysis yielded the most useful data, and the cohort who was surgically treated was found to have significant improvements in: their neurogenic intermittent claudication (NIC) pain ($p=0.006$), NIC function (PCS $p=0.047$; ODI $p=0.002$), patient satisfaction, and self-rated progress over 4 years when compared with the group treated conservatively. The non-operative treatment group demonstrated only modest improvement over time.

Möller's Prospective Randomized Controlled Trial

Möller's PRCT compared the surgical and conservative management in the treatment of isthmic spondylolisthesis in adults [18]. In this study, 111 patients were randomized into one of three treatment arms: group I, posterior lumbar fusion (PLF); group II, PLF with instrumentation; and group III, exercise program. There were 106 patients (93 %) included in the 2-year follow-up data. Seventy-seven patients underwent surgery and 34 patients enrolled in an exercise program.

The 34 patients randomized to the exercise program were referred to a physiotherapist with a special interest in spondylolisthesis. The exercise program was based on strength and postural training, with the emphasis on back and abdominal muscle exercises where 12 different exercises were performed. To allow for exercises at home, 8 of the 12 exercises did not include specific training equipment. Four exercises included a pulley machine and a leg press machine. The patients exercised three times a week for the first 6 months, and twice a week between months 6–12. The exercise program was supervised by a physiotherapist and required approximately 45 min to complete all the exercises. After 1 year, the patients were instructed to continue PT with a home exercise program, which consisted of the eight exercises that did not need special equipment. Two-thirds of the patients complied with the full program during the first year. After the first year, it was not known to what extent the patients continued with the recommended exercises.

Surgical management resulted in better functional outcomes, assessed using the disability rating index (DRI), and decreased pain ($p<0.01$). The patients in the exercise treatment group demonstrated no functional improvement and the DRI did not change, but the pain decreased slightly ($p<0.02$).

In patients who fail conservative modalities, both the SPORT and the Möller PRCT studies provide strong evidence to support the surgical management of adult low-grade degenerative and isthmic spondylolisthesis, respectively.

Other Studies

Matsudaira et al. reviewed 53 patients with spinal stenosis and degenerative spondylolisthesis treated with decompressive laminectomy with PLF ($n=19$), decompression alone with laminoplasty ($n=18$), and non-operative management ($n=13$) in a cohort that refused surgery [19]. There was no improvement over the 2-year follow-up for the group treated non-operatively. When the non-operative group was compared with the two surgical groups, a level of significance was achieved ($p<0.0001$) for improvement in the decompression with PLF, and laminoplasty groups. Although deformity progression was observed in the non-instrumented groups, there were no significant differences identified between the decompression with PLF groups and the laminoplasty groups. The authors recommended laminoplasty over decompression with PLF, stating that motion preservation may potentially lower the incidence of adjacent-level disease.

Anderson et al. analyzed interspinous process decompression (IPD) using the X-STOP as an alternative to conservative care in the treatment of low-grade degenerative spondylolisthesis [20]. In this level-I PRCT, 75 patients were randomized to either X-STOP spacer placement ($n=42$) or the control group ($n=33$). At the 2-year follow-up, only 12.9 % of the patients in the control group who were treated conservatively demonstrated significant improvement in pain and function vs. 63.4 % of the patients in the X-STOP group.

Recommendations

The initial non-surgical treatment of low-grade spondylolisthesis is similar to the non-operative management of other mechanical lumbar spinal disorders. Frymoyer in fact proposed a comprehensive conservative management plan in 1994 for the treatment of spondylolisthesis. The recommendations placed forward mirror the aforementioned modalities and included PT, aerobic activity via a stationary bicycle, weight loss, NSAIDs, careful management of the patient's osteoporosis, as well as the avoidance of prolonged bed rest [21]. However, no standardized method is currently accepted for the conservative management of spondylolisthesis despite prior recommendations.

Parker et al. recently reported on a prospective study that sought to evaluate the 2-year quality of life outcomes for patients with lumbar spine pathology as well as the financial implications of their conservative treatment [22]. In addition to spondylolisthesis, the study also evaluated patients with spinal stenosis and disc herniation. Fifty patients were in each subpopulation and enrolled in a comprehensive medical management program that included physical therapy, NSAIDs, spinal epidural steroid injections, muscle relaxants, and oral narcotic agents. After the 2-year period, 18 of the original 50 spondylolisthesis patients (36 %) required surgical management due to lack of significant improvement.

The overall mean cost for treating each patient conservatively was $6,606.00. Despite the relatively low conversion of enrolled patients towards definitive surgical management, the authors advocated surgical intervention as opposed to medical management citing both the high risk of failure to improve and the financial implications.

The utilization of bracing has been demonstrated to be effective. To avoid decompensation or atrophy of the abdominal and paraspinal musculature, bracing may be optimized when used in conjunction with core strengthening exercises [7]. Therefore, bracing may be advocated if the patient obtains favorable results from its use as part of a multi-disciplinary approach. NSAIDs may provide short-term pain relief, but the surgeon must be aware of the gastro-intestinal complications, and plan for their avoidance accordingly when prescribing NSAID medications. Epidural steroid injections can also be effective especially in the short-term. ESIs may not only provide short-term pain relief, but they can also be of diagnostic value. Muscle relaxants may be helpful in some patients with greater pain and muscle spasm, but caution should be exercised, especially in elderly patients. Narcotic analgesics should only be used sparingly and for short durations in cases of severe pain.

Authors Approach

A non-operative treatment algorithm for patients with spondylolisthesis does not exist currently. Although there are no data supporting one non-operative treatment over another, the authors recommend a patient-centered, multi-disciplinary approach when undertaking conservative treatment for spondylolisthesis.

Patient education is paramount and all patients are informed about the benefits of practicing healthy back care with proper ergonomics, lifting and bending techniques. Patients are also counseled about the deleterious effects of smoking and obesity and how these factors can influence their prognosis. Additionally, patients are informed to avoid environmental pain generators through activity modification.

The mainstay of prescribed non-operative treatment includes PT with core strengthening, flexion exercises, and NSAID therapy. If the patient's body habitus permits, and they are compliant with participating in PT, a brace is prescribed.

Transforaminal ESIs, facet, and pars interarticularis injections are implemented at the pathologic lumbar level as an adjunct if initial therapy fails to provide significant relief. Injections are repeated so long as the patient obtains more than 2–3 months of relief in an attempt to avoid surgery. Injections are also advocated due to their diagnostic value. Although patients may only obtain hours to weeks of relief of their back or leg pain with the injections, this provides information and confirmation that the pathologic level injected is the cause of the patient's symptoms, especially in a patient with multi-level spinal pathology. If these non-operative treatment modalities fail to provide significant long-term relief and the patient's pain is affecting their activities of daily living, surgery is advocated so long as the prescribed injections are diagnostic.

The patient's symptomatology should provide the tactical approach to treatment in the short-term, and clear long-term goals should be developed with the patient at the onset of treatment so patient expectations are realistic and achievable. Those patients who fail an initial 6-month trial of conservative care are less likely to improve and surgical management may result in improved outcomes when compared with continued non-operative management.

Conclusion

The spine surgeon must consider the natural progression of spondylolisthesis when formulating a treatment plan. With only 1/3 of patient's slippage progressing on average, those patients suffering from adult low-grade spondylolisthesis will likely respond to non-operative management consisting of activity modification, physical therapy, and NSAIDs. Conversely those patients who present at onset with neurologic symptoms are more at risk to fail conservative treatment [23].

The lack of standardized treatment protocols and level-I evidence presents a challenge to the spine surgeon when contemplating which non-operative treatment options are optimal, in addition to determining who will benefit from surgical intervention for spondylolisthesis. However, the surgeon must invariably work with each patient as the head of a multi-disciplinary team for non-operative management to be effective while maintaining clear objectives to define both success and failure of such management.

References

1. Wiltse LL, Newman PH, Macnab I. Classification of spondylolisis and spondylolisthesis. Clin Orthop Relat Res. 1976;117:23–9.
2. Sinaki M, Lutness MP, Ilstrup DM, Chu CP, Gramse RR. Lumbar spondylolisthesis: retrospective comparison and three-year follow-up of two conservative treatment programs. Arch Phys Med Rehabil. 1989;70(8):594–8.
3. Gramse RR, Sinaki M, Ilstrup DM. Lumbar spondylolisthesis: a rational approach to conservative treatment. Mayo Clin Proc. 1980;55(11):681–6.
4. O'Sullivan PB. Lumbar segmental 'instability': clinical presentation and specific stabilizing exercise management. Man Ther. 2000;5(1):2–12.
5. Hicks GE, Fritz JM, Delitto A, McGill SM. Preliminary development of a clinical prediction rule for determining which patients with low back pain will respond to a stabilization exercise program. Arch Phys Med Rehabil. 2005;86(9):1753–62.
6. Steiner ME, Micheli LJ. Treatment of symptomatic spondylolysis and spondylolisthesis with the modified Boston brace. Spine. 1985;10(10):937–43.
7. Spratt KF, Weinstein JN, Lehmann TR, Woody J, Sayre H. Efficacy of flexion and extension treatments incorporating braces for low-back pain patients with retrodisplacement, spondylolisthesis, or normal sagittal translation. Spine. 1993;18(13):1839–49.
8. Van Tulder MW, Scholten RJ, Koes BW, Deyo RA. Nonsteroidal anti-inflammatory drugs for low back pain: a systematic review within the framework of the Cochrane Collaboration Back Review Group. Spine. 2000;25(19):2501–13.
9. Riew KD, Yin Y, Gilula L, Bridwell KH, Lenke LG, Lauryssen C, et al. The effect of nerve-root injections on the need for operative treatment of lumbar radicular pain. A prospective, randomized, controlled, double-blind study. J Bone Joint Surg Am. 2000;82-A(11):1589–93.
10. Vibert BT, Sliva CD, Herkowitz HN. Treatment of instability and spondylolisthesis: surgical versus nonsurgical treatment. Clin Orthop Relat Res. 2006;443:222–7.
11. Cuckler JM, Bernini PA, Wiesel SW, Booth Jr RE, Rothman RH, Pickens GT. The use of epidural steroids in the treatment of lumbar radicular pain. A prospective, randomized, double-blind study. J Bone Joint Surg Am. 1985;67(1):63–6.
12. Kraiwattanapong C, Wechmongkolgorn S, Chatriyanuyok B, Woratanarat P, Udomsubpayakul U, Chanplakorn P, et al. Outcomes of fluoroscopically guided lumbar transforaminal epidural steroid injections in degenerative lumbar spondylolisthesis patients. Asian Spine J. 2014;8(2):119–28.
13. Mierau D, Cassidy JD, McGregor M, Kirkaldy-Willis WH. A comparison of the effectiveness of spinal manipulative therapy for low back pain patients with and without spondylolisthesis. J Manipulative Physiol Ther. 1987;10(2):49–55.
14. Lee HJ, Seo JC, Kwak MA, Park SH, Min BM, Cho MS, et al. Acupuncture for low back pain due to spondylolisthesis: study protocol for a randomized controlled pilot trial. Trials. 2014;15:105.
15. Kalichman L, Hunter DJ. Diagnosis and conservative management of degenerative lumbar spondylolisthesis. Eur Spine J. 2008;17(3):327–35.
16. Garet M, Reiman MP, Mathers J, Sylvain J. Nonoperative treatment in lumbar spondylolysis and spondylolisthesis: a systematic review. Sports Health. 2013;5(3):225–32.
17. Weinstein JN, Lurie JD, Tosteson TD, Zhao W, Blood EA, Tosteson AN, et al. Surgical compared with non-operative treatment for lumbar degenerative spondylolisthesis. Four-year results in the Spine Patient Outcomes Research Trial (SPORT) randomized and observational cohorts. J Bone Joint Surg Am. 2009;91(6):1295–304.
18. Möller H, Hedlund R. Surgery versus conservative management in adult isthmic spondylolisthesis—a prospective randomized study: part 1. Spine. 2000; 25(13):1711–5.
19. Matsudaira K, Yamakazi T, Seichi A, Takeshita K, Hoshi K, Kishimoto J, Nakamura K. Spinal stenosi in grade I degenerative lumbar spondylolisthesis: a comparative study of outcomes following laminoplasty and laminectomy with instrumented spinal fusion. J Orthop Sci. 2005;10:270–6.
20. Anderson PA, Tribus CB, Kitchel SH. Treatment of neurogenic claudication by interspinous decompression: application of the X STOP device in patients with lumbar degenerative spondylolisthesis. J Neurosurg Spine. 2006;4(6):463–71.
21. Frymoyer JW. Degenerative spondylolisthesis: diagnosis and treatment. J Am Acad Orthop Surg. 1994;2(1):9–15.
22. Parker SL, Godil SS, Mendenhall SK, Zuckerman SL, Shau DN, McGirt MJ. Two-year comprehensive medical management of degenerative lumbar spine disease (lumbar spondylolisthesis, stenosis, or disc herniation): a value analysis of cost, pain, disability, and quality of life: clinical article. J Neurosurg Spine. 2014;21(2):143–9.
23. Matsunaga S, Ijiri K, Hayashi K. Nonsurgically managed patients with degenerative spondylolisthesis: a 10- to 18-year follow-up study. J Neurosurg. 2000;93(2 Suppl):194–8.

Part II

Surgical Techniques

Surgical Techniques: Spondylolysis Repair

11

Leok-Lim Lau and Suken A. Shah

Introduction

Lumbar spondylolysis is a bony defect in the pars interarticularis, which is the bony bridge that adjoins the superior and inferior articular processes without slippage of the adjacent vertebra. It can occur unilaterally or bilaterally in the pars. The defect can be unilaterally incomplete or complete, unilaterally complete with contralateral incomplete, or bilaterally complete. A report of three defects involving both pars and the center of the right lamina has been described [1]. A bilateral incomplete defect has not been previously described [2]. By far the most common type of defect is bilaterally complete.

Lower lumbar vertebrae are commonly affected, particularly at L5, and with decreasing frequency at L4, L3, and L2. The usual presentation is single level vertebra involvement. It can affect two levels of vertebrae in continuity or incontiguously (Fig. 11.1). Up to three levels of contiguous vertebrae involvement has been reported [3]. Multiple-level spondylolysis are rare. Fifteen percent of affected patients with spondylolysis may progress to spondylolisthesis. The slippage is unlikely to be more than 40 % [4].

The reported incidence in the general population varies depending on the age group. Lumbar spondylolysis in newborn is rarely described [5]. It is reported in 4.4 % of preschool children. This increases to 6 % in adulthood [4]. A higher incidence of up to 15 % is noted among young athletes. Males are twice as commonly affected compared to females. This ratio becomes 1:1 in the symptomatic populations suggesting a higher proportion of females may become symptomatic. The underlying reason, however, is not well understood; it may reflect the more active participation in sports among young women. It represents the most common organic cause of low back pain in children, adolescents, and young adults. The rate of spontaneous healing with bone is thought to be extremely low, but fibrous unions can result in long-term pain relief without instability.

The pars interarticularis is normally an area under great stress posteriorly in a normal vertebra given its small area and frequent impaction with the inferior articular process at the level above in a lordotic lumbar spine in an erect position [6]. Acute trauma or chronic repetitive microtrauma, particularly hyperextension, is believed to place pathological shear stresses at the pars and results in

L.-L. Lau, M.B.Ch.B., F.R.C.S. (Orth.)
University Orthopaedics, Hand and Reconstructive Microsurgery Cluster, National University Health System, 5 Lower Kent Ridge Road, Singapore 119074, Singapore
e-mail: leok_lim_lau@nuhs.edu.sg

S.A. Shah, M.D. (✉)
Department of Orthopaedics, Nemours/Alfred I. duPont Hospital for Children, 1600 Rockland Road, Wilmington, DE 19803, USA
e-mail: sshah@nemours.org

A.L. Wollowick and V. Sarwahi (eds.), *Spondylolisthesis: Diagnosis, Non-Surgical Management, and Surgical Techniques*, DOI 10.1007/978-1-4899-7575-1_11,

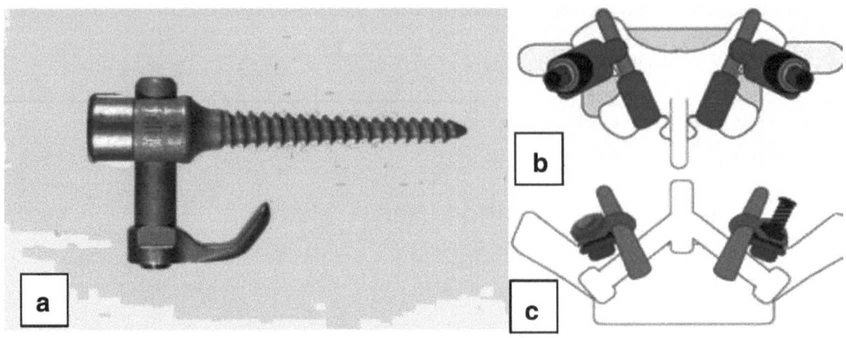

Fig. 11.1 Pedicle screw, rod, and laminar hook construct. (**a**) The lateral view of the construct. The appearance of the construct at the posterior view (**b**) and inferior view (**c**) of the vertebra

lumbar spondylolysis [7, 8]. This probably explains the absence of such pathology in non-ambulatory adults and the higher incidence noted in young athletes involved in sports with repetitive hyperextension activities like gymnastics, diving, football, and now more commonly, soccer.

Many children and adolescents with spondylolysis are asymptomatic. The most common presentation is activity-related back pain, particularly in extension. The postulated causes of pain in spondylolysis include rich nociceptive nerve endings within the defect, hypermobility of the loose posterior arch with stimulation of the nerve endings within the defect, relative instability of the vertebral body, and excessive stress on the underlying disc. It is thus important to ascertain the primary pain generators prior to surgical intervention.

Diagnostic Imaging

Patients with suspected lumbar spondylolysis are investigated with an erect posterior–anterior (PA) and lateral radiographs of the lumbosacral spine. Some patients may have spinal bifida occulta associated with the pars defects. This has implications during the surgical approach. Oblique radiographs have increased X-rays exposure and have not been shown to add additional information [9]. The authors have virtually abandoned oblique X-rays and bone scans in favor of advanced imaging that is more diagnostic. Thin cut computed tomography (CT) with reverse gantry alignment to lumbar lordosis is recommended in cases that spondylolysis is suspected but not well demonstrated in radiographs to confirm the diagnosis [10]. Pre-operative CT scan is indicated to evaluate the size of the pars defect and degree of bony sclerosis (i.e., atrophic or hypertrophic non-union). Magnetic resonance imaging (MRI) is indicated for patients with an atypical presentation or with neurological symptoms. It may show a pre-lysis stage in patients with normal CT scan, by showing signal intensity in the pars or pedicle. It can also prognosticate the healing ability of a defect after a trial of conservative treatment. High signal intensity around the pedicle reveals remaining potential for bony union to occur [11]. MRI is performed pre-operatively to assess discal health at the spondylolytic segment.

Table 11.1 Factors affecting patient selection in pars repair

Factors
• Duration of symptoms/adequacy of non-operative treatment
• Concordance of pars injection with temporary symptom resolution
• Age
• Segmental instability
• Lumbar disc health
• Unilateral or bilateral involvement

Indications for Pars Repair

Careful patient-selection yields a better outcome: a few factors influence the decision to repair the pars (Table 11.1).

Unremitting Pain/Increasing Pain Attributed to the Pars Defect

Non-operative treatment without adversely affecting quality of life is the mainstay of the management. More than 80 % of children and adolescents respond to this with near resolution of symptoms, or occasional recurrence of pain. Return to sports after rest and rehabilitation with core strengthening and flexibility exercises can be expected.

Generally, if recurrent pain with sports precludes their return, or patients have failed 6 months or more of non-operative treatment, then surgical repair can be an option. The non-responders who are considered for surgery should undergo a diagnostic injection with pars infiltration. This is done by injection of small volume of local anesthetic (e.g., bupivacaine) and a corticosteroid into the spondylolytic pars interarticularis under CT guidance. A concordant result in the pars injection should be at least 70 % improvement in pain and is a prognostic feature of good functional outcome postoperatively [12–14].

Age

The correlation between age and clinical outcome is conflicting. Most authors state that patients in the age range of 20–30 years have worse clinical results than younger patients [8, 15–17]. A more recent study did not find an association between patient's age and post-operative VAS score [13]. The compounding factors in these studies include:

1. Higher prevalence of disc degeneration in the population with spondylolysis at an age of more than 25 years compared to the normal control population [18]
2. Functional outcome does not correlate with bony union [8]

Ideal patients for pars repair are younger than 20 years old. One should proceed with caution in an older patient.

Segmental Instability and Degenerative Disc

Better outcome is observed with fusion when compared to direct pars repair in patients with spondylolisthesis [19]. Up to grade 1 (<25 % slippage) spondylolisthesis is amenable for pars repair. Fixation can be used to compress the defect and reduce the slip, but results are variable.

Disc degeneration at the level below the spondylolytic segment may result in an independent pain generator and is a contraindication to pars repair. The disc degeneration does not correlate with the grade of vertebral slip [20]. The degeneration is demonstrated by structural changes, signal change, and height loss of the discs as classified by the Pfirrmann classification on MRI [21] (see Table 11.2). Pfirrmann grade 1 or 2 is an ideal indication; grade 3 or above is contraindicated for pars repair, and may benefit from fusion.

Unilateral vs. Bilateral Pars Defects

An acute unilateral pars defect has a good prognosis and may heal spontaneously. Longer conservative treatment is recommended prior to surgical intervention.

Table 11.2 Classification of disc degeneration (Pfirrmann)

Grade	Structure	Distinction of nucleus and annulus	Signal intensity	Height of intervertebral disc
I	Homogeneous, bright white	Clear	Hyperintense, isointense to cerebrospinal fluid	Normal
II	Inhomogeneous with or without horizontal bands	Clear	Hyperintense, isointense to cerebrospinal fluid	Normal
III	Inhomogeneous, gray	Unclear	Intermediate	Normal to slightly decreased
IV	Inhomogeneous, gray to black	Lost	Intermediate to hypointense	Normal to moderately decreased
V	Inhomogeneous, black	Lost	Hypointense	Collapsed disc space

Surgical Treatment

The Evolution

The surgical strategy has evolved over time. Earlier surgical procedures involved arthrodesis of the motion segment by posterolateral or interbody fusion techniques. These procedures sacrificed the mobility of the involved motion segment and placed excessive mechanical stress at the adjacent levels, both of which are undesirable and potentially harmful in younger patients.

In 1968, Kimura described a direct repair of the isthmic defect of the pars interarticularis without instrumentation, as an alternative to segmental fusion [22]. This technique had the advantage of preserving segmental motion. Scott began using a wiring technique as a tension band with bone graft to augment the lytic defect in 1968. Many authors used the Scott wiring method, whereas others have modified the technique to include pedicle screws or cable instead of wire [23, 24].

In 1970, Buck [25] documented the use of a lag screw across the lytic defect, and many other authors have described their outcomes following this technique. In 1984, Morscher et al. [26] reported that the Buck technique of using a 3.5-mm lag screw did not work well with a thin or dysplastic lamina, and advocated using laminar fixation with a hook screw device specially made for this purpose. The major problem of this technique was screw placement and facet joint violation. A screw placement analysis showed that in 15 % of cases, there was screw penetration into the inferior articular process of the superior vertebra. Other authors have reported using pedicle screws to secure the lamina with either a rod-hook construct [27] or a U- or V-shaped rod under the spinous process [7, 28].

Other common contemporary techniques of pars repair are direct repair using a laminar/pars compression screw through the fractured pars (modified Buck's technique) and compression of the fracture fragments using a pedicle screw, rod, and laminar hook construct within the same segment. They are shown to have the least amount of motion across the defect during flexion, extension, and rotation compared to the Scott wiring technique [29]. Adjacent segment mobility is not increased compared to untreated spondylolysis or pedicle screw-rod motion segment fixation in segmental arthrodesis [30]. These two constructs represent the most ideal anatomical constructs biomechanically and a relatively straightforward once the surgeon addresses the pseudarthrosis at the pars.

Surgical Technique

Positioning

Patient is placed prone on a radiolucent operating table with four posts (e.g., flat Jackson table or AMSCO table). All the pressure areas are adequately padded including the chest, anterior superior iliac spine and patella. The abdomen is hung free which otherwise would impede venous return and increase bleeding at the surgical site. Prophylactic antibiotics are administered according to the local guidelines.

Direct Laminar/Pars Compression Screw Fixation

Intra-operative fluoroscopy is used for localization prior to skin incision (Figs. 11.2, 11.3 and Table 11.3). A paraspinal approach, similar to

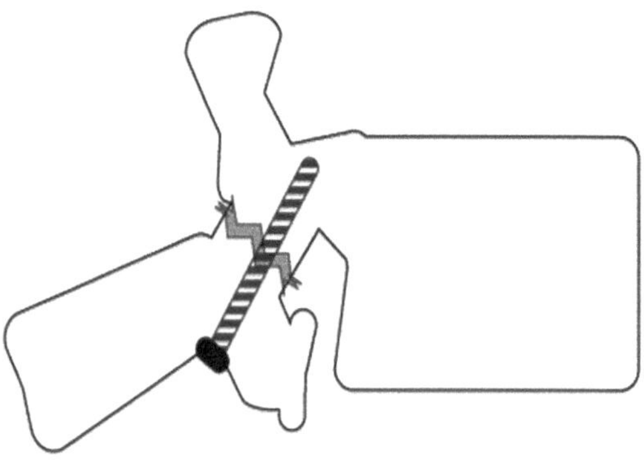

Fig. 11.2 Direct laminar/pars compression screw fixation after excision of the fibrocartilaginous tissue and bone graft at the pars defect

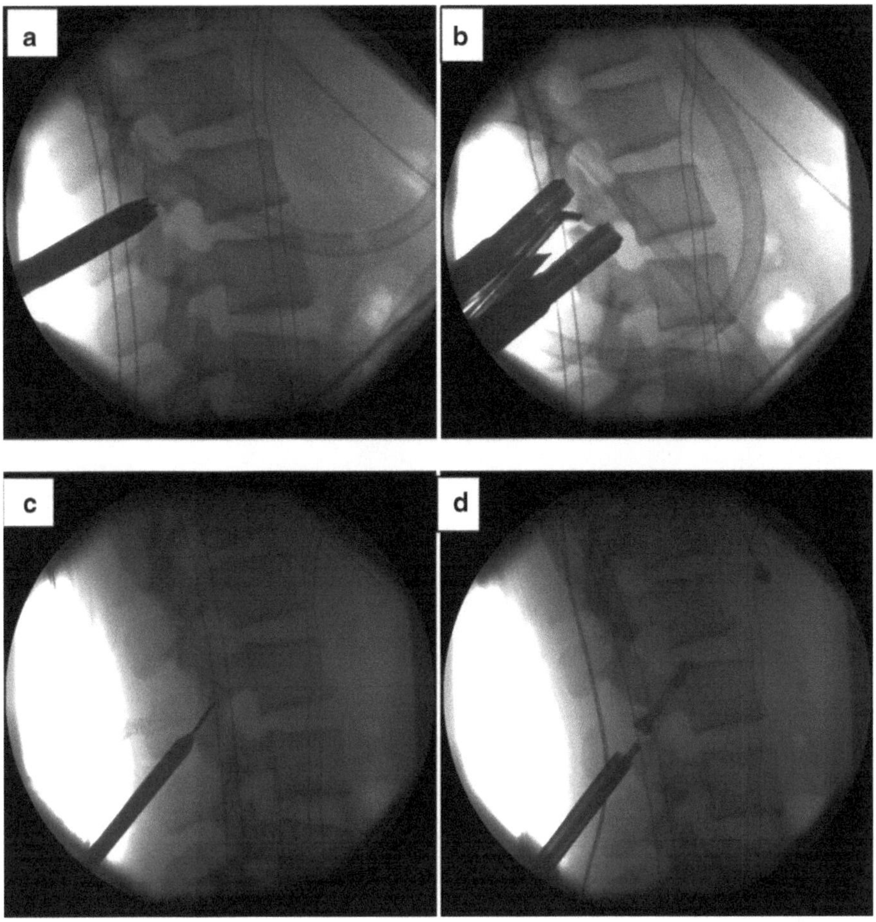

Fig. 11.3 (**a**) A minimal invasive expandable retractor is sited at the pars defect. (**b**) The fibrocartilaginous tissue at the pars defect is rongeured. (**c**) K-wire is placed across the pars defect. (**d**) A cannulated 4.5 mm titanium screw is placed across the pars defect

Table 11.3 Steps in direct laminar/pars compression screw fixation

1. Intra-operative fluoroscopy for level localization
2. Wiltse muscle-sparing approach
3. Expandable retractor over the pars interarticularis
4. Localization of the defect and fibrocartilaginous tissue around the defect is removed
5. Fracture site preparation, removal of sclerotic surface using burr until bleeding subchondral bone seen
6. Entry point of the screw identified (caudal margin of the lamina lateral to the base of the spinous process)
7. 1 guidewire is placed across each defect to the junction of the pars, transverse process, and pedicle cortex
8. Position guided and confirmed by fluoroscopy or CT navigation
9. Over drill the guidewire with 3.2 mm drill
10. An appropriately sized 4.5 mm titanium cortical screw is inserted but not tightened
11. Place the autologous cancellous bone graft into and over the defect
12. The screw is tightened completely to obtain cortical purchase and compression

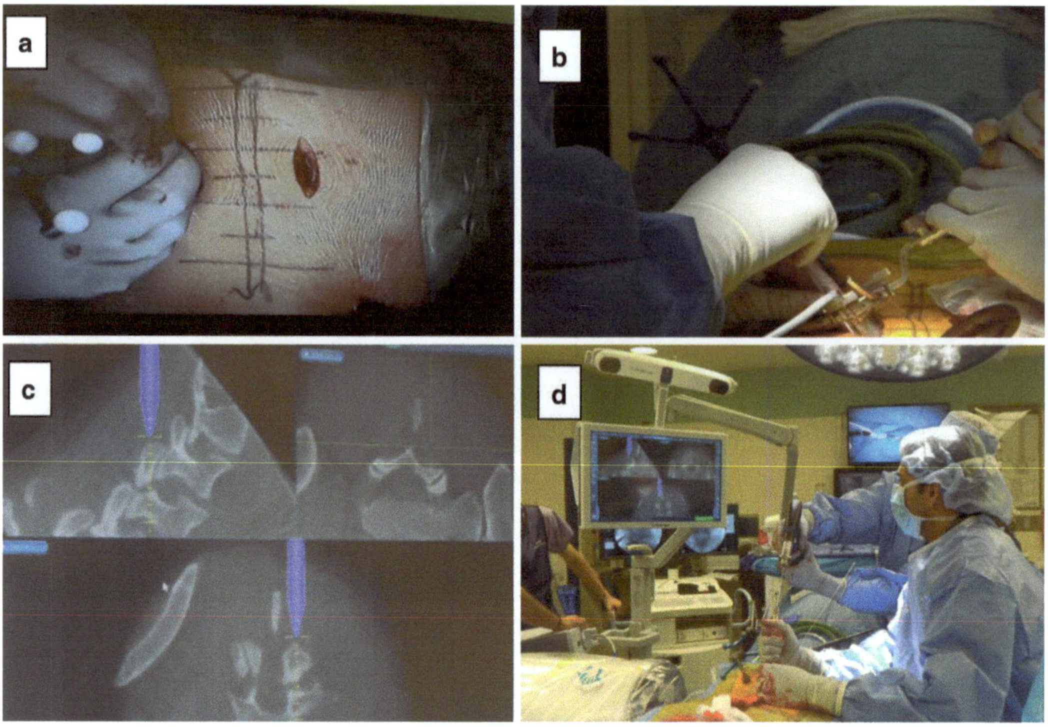

Fig. 11.4 (**a**) Wiltse-like approach is shown. (**b**) Using a CT guided navigation probe to determine the entry point of lamina screw. (**c**) The entry point of laminar screw is determined. Ideal trajectory is perpendicular to the defect and at the axis of the lamina to accommodate a 4.5 mm cannulated screw intra-osseously. (**d**) The setup of CT guided navigation system is shown

Wiltse is employed for fascial incision. The longissimus–multifidus muscle interval is bluntly dissected with a finger in order to preserve the vascularity and prevent unnecessary tissue damage. A minimally invasive expandable retractor is used, and through this retractor, the pars interarticularis is subperiosteally dissected, leaving the adjacent facet capsules intact. The defect is located, and the fibrous tissue in the defect is removed with pituitary rongeurs. The sclerotic surfaces are prepared with a high-speed burr until bleeding bone surface is seen, but care is taken not to resect too much bone—this results in enlarging the defect. Gross motion is noted through the pars fracture. Great care is taken not to disrupt the joint capsule bilaterally. The entry point of the screw is made by creating a notch in the caudal margin of the lamina 10 mm lateral to the base of the spinous process. Then, using the Discovery or F2 cannulated screw system for facet fusion (DePuy Synthes Spine, Raynham, MA, USA), two guidewires are placed to provide adequate fixation across the pars defects from an ipsilateral infralaminar approach into the junction of the pars and transverse processes and pedicle cortex. The guidewire placement is confirmed via fluoroscopy in multiple planes. Alternatively, the guidewire placement could be aided by CT navigation (Fig. 11.4). The guidewire is then over drilled, and a cannulated screw is placed over the guidewire, providing compression and fixation across the defect. A 3.2-mm drill bit is used to drill the path of the screw with the trajectory angled 30° lateral to the sagittal plane, toward the ipsilateral pedicle, crossing the lytic defect. An appropriately sized, 4.5-mm titanium cortical screw is inserted along the path across the defect, but not tightened completely. Then cancellous bone graft obtained from the posterior iliac crest is packed in the lytic defect, and the screw is tightened completely to obtain a good purchase in the solid bone of the ipsilateral

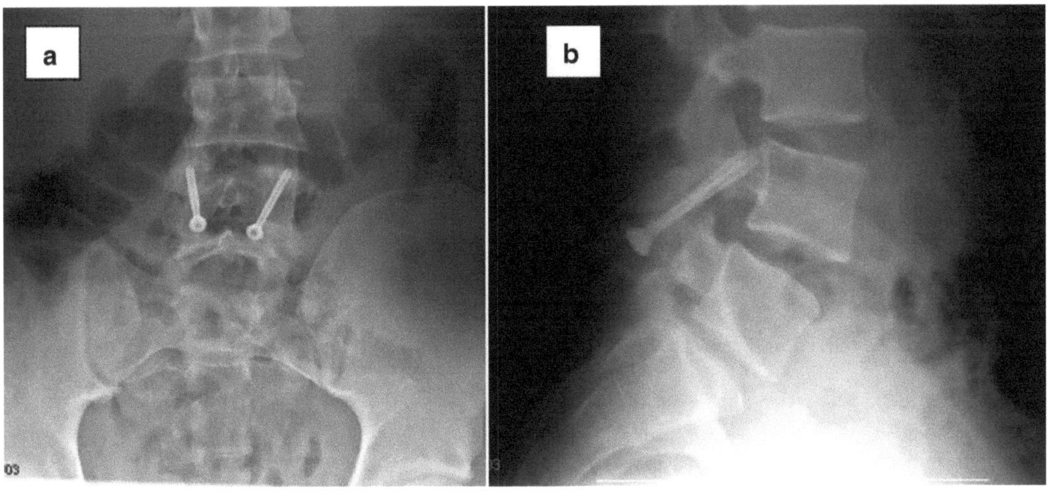

Fig. 11.5 (**a**, **b**) AP and lateral radiographs after direct laminar/pars compression screw fixation

pedicle and compression across the defect. Radiographic AP and lateral views of the lumbar spine are taken (Fig. 11.5).

Pedicle Screw, Rod, and Laminar Hook Construct

A midline incision is made and the paraspinal musculature is elevated laterally to expose the lamina, pars, and base of the transverse process (Fig. 11.7 and Table 11.4). The spinous process, lamina, pars, superior articular process, and transverse process are carefully and meticulously exposed in their entirety. Care is taken not to injure the facet joint capsule. Then using a burr, the fibrocartilaginous defect is debrided down to bleeding subchondral bone. Anatomic landmarks or fluoroscopy are then used to determine the pedicle screw starting point, preferably slightly inferior and lateral to avoid facet violation. A starting hole is burred, and a pedicle finder is used to enter the pedicle. The walls and floor of the created tract are assessed with a ball-tipped probe, and the hole is tapped and prepared for a multiaxial pedicle screw.

Bone graft is harvested from the iliac crest and placed in the defect before screw insertion. The inferior lamina of the involved vertebra is prepared to accept an infralaminar hook. Once the hook is inserted and impacted, a small rod is introduced into the screw head. The construct is then loaded with compression and tightened. Radiographic AP and lateral views of the lumbar spine are taken (Fig. 11.6).

Table 11.4 Steps in pedicle screw, rod, and laminar hook construct

1.	Intra-operative fluoroscopy for level localization
2.	A midline skin incision with paraspinal muscle elevation
3.	Expose spinous process, lamina, pars, superior articular process, and transverse process while preserving the facet joint capsule
4.	Localization of the defect and fibrocartilaginous tissue around the defect is removed
5.	Defect site preparation, removal of sclerotic surface using burr until bleeding subchondral bone seen
6.	Pedicle screw starting point is identified, burred, and cannulated with a pedicle finder
7.	Pedicle track is tapped after checking for breach on the walls and floor with a ball-tip probe
8.	Autologous bone graft is placed in and over the defect
9.	Appropriate sized polyaxial pedicle screw is inserted
10.	Inferior lamina of the vertebra is prepared to accept an infralaminar hook. The hook is inserted and impacted
11.	Small rod is introduced into the screw head
12.	The construct is loaded with compression and tightened

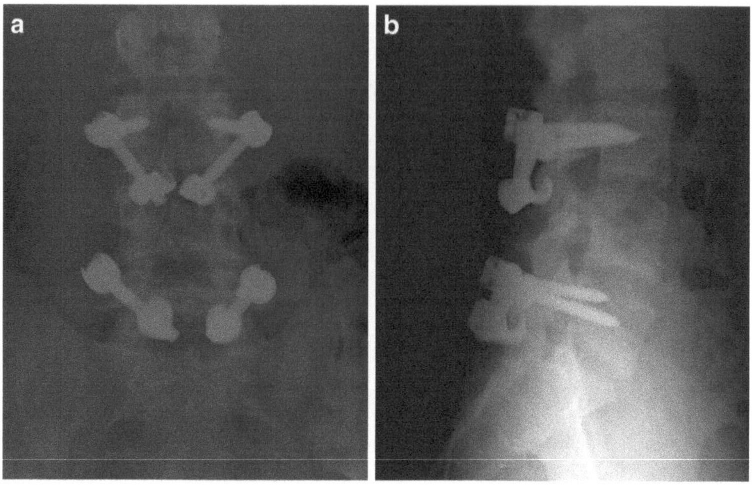

Fig. 11.6 (**a**, **b**) AP and lateral radiographs of lumbar spine after 2 incontiguous vertebral level pars repair bilaterally using pedicle screw, rod, and laminar hook construct

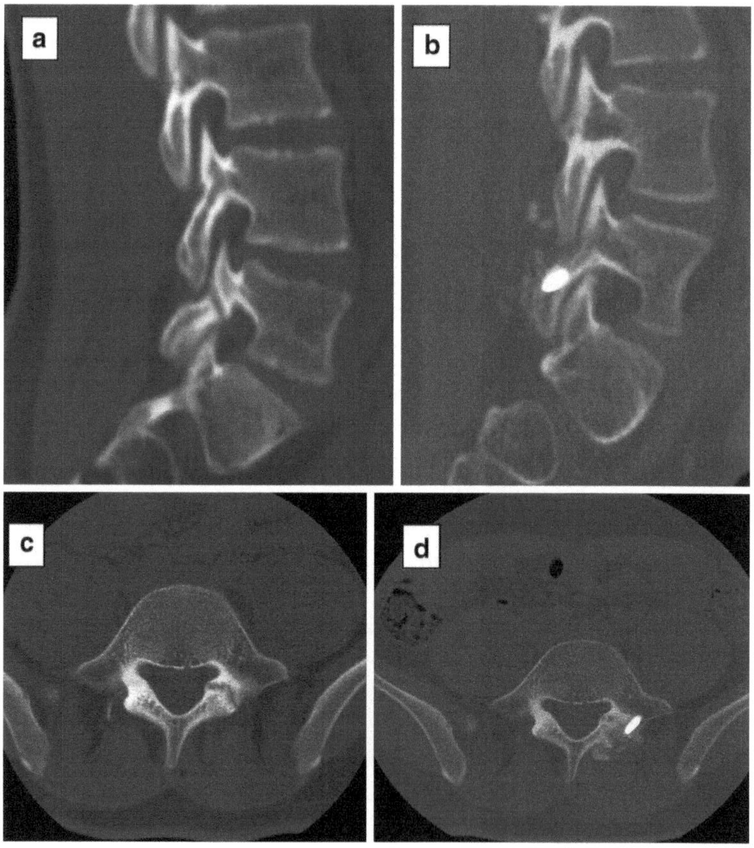

Fig. 11.7 (**a**, **b**) The sagittal view of a CT scan showing pars defect before and after direct laminar/pars compression screw fixation. (**c**, **d**) Axial view of the CT scan showing left pars defect before and after surgery. Bony union is achieved

Postoperative Care

The patients are allowed to sit and ambulate with a lumbosacral orthosis (LSO) with single leg extension on the first postoperative day. The brace is recommended for a period of 6 weeks. After 6 weeks, the brace is shortened to an LSO for 6 more weeks. Physical therapy is used to increase flexibility and isometrically strengthen the core muscles and stabilize the spine at 6–12 weeks. Patients are cleared for full physical activity at 4–6 months after confirmation of healing (Fig. 11.7).

Surgical Outcome

With a careful patient selection, majority of the patients has a good to excellent outcome. Overall successful outcome is expected in 90 % of the cases in our experience [13, 31].

Karatas et al. further found that 7 of 15 patients were able to return to competitive sports. Another seven resumed recreational or club sports activities. Bony union was achieved in all cases. We reported no complications in the group with direct pars repair using laminar screws. One patient had a mild sensory deficit in the L5 nerve distribution and two superficial wound infections were noted in the group with a pedicle screw, rod, and hook construct. There were no events of dislodged implants, loosening, breakage, or reoperation at a mean follow-up of 23 months [31].

Menga et al. reported a mean 5.8 point improvement in VAS score at a minimum of 2 years follow-up. 76 % of the athletes returned to competitive sports. Two of the 31 patients had unilateral intralaminar screw fracture at L5. Conversion to segmental fusion was reported at 2/31 (6 %). One patient had a deep wound infection [13].

The best surgical technique is under debate, but pars repair should be considered in young patients with symptomatic defects who have failed non-operative treatment but have healthy discs, facets, and minimal to no listhesis. A few studies have compared pedicle screw with hook constructs and direct pars screw fixation in a cohort of 47 patients and concluded that pars screw fixation was superior to the pedicle screw universal hook system in relation to operative time, blood loss, hospital stay, healing rate, and clinical outcome [31, 32].

References

1. Ariyoshi M, et al. Spondylolysis at three sites in the same lumbar vertebra. Int J Sports Med. 1999;20(1):56–7.
2. Chen MR, et al. Anatomic variability of 120 L5 spondylolytic defects. Global Spine J. 2013;3(4):243–8.
3. Sharifi G, et al. Bilateral three-level lumbar spondylolysis repaired by hook-screw technique. Global Spine J. 2012;2(1):51–6.
4. Beutler WJ, et al. The natural history of spondylolysis and spondylolisthesis: 45-year follow-up evaluation. Spine (Phila Pa 1976). 2003;28(10):1027–35. discussion 1035.
5. Borkow SE, Kleiger B. Spondylolisthesis in the newborn. A case report. Clin Orthop Relat Res. 1971;81: 73–6.
6. Inceoglu S, Mageswaran P. Multi-scale finite element modelling at the posterior lumbar vertebra: analysis of pedicle stresses due to pars fracture. Comput Methods Biomech Biomed Eng. 2014;17(7):787–91.
7. Gillet P, Petit M. Direct repair of spondylolysis without spondylolisthesis, using a rod-screw construct and bone grafting of the pars defect. Spine (Phila Pa 1976). 1999;24(12):1252–6.
8. Hioki A, et al. Repair of pars defects by segmental transverse wiring for athletes with symptomatic spondylolysis: relationship between bony union and postoperative symptoms. Spine (Phila Pa 1976). 2012; 37(9):802–7.
9. Beck NA, et al. Do oblique views add value in the diagnosis of spondylolysis in adolescents? J Bone Joint Surg Am. 2013;95(10):e65.
10. Saifuddin A, et al. Orientation of lumbar pars defects: implications for radiological detection and surgical management. J Bone Joint Surg Br. 1998;80(2): 208–11.
11. Sairyo K, Sakai T, Yasui N. Conservative treatment of lumbar spondylolysis in childhood and adolescence: the radiological signs which predict healing. J Bone Joint Surg Br. 2009;91(2):206–9.
12. Suh PB, Esses SI, Kostuik JP. Repair of pars interarticularis defect. The prognostic value of pars infiltration. Spine (Phila Pa 1976). 1991;16(8 Suppl):S445–8.
13. Menga EN, et al. Clinical results and functional outcomes after direct intralaminar screw repair of spondylolysis. Spine (Phila Pa 1976). 2014;39(1):104–10.
14. Wu SS, Lee CH, Chen PQ. Operative repair of symptomatic spondylolysis following a positive response to diagnostic pars injection. J Spinal Disord. 1999;12(1):10–6.
15. Dai LY, et al. Direct repair of defect in lumbar spondylolysis and mild isthmic spondylolisthesis by bone grafting, with or without facet joint fusion. Eur Spine J. 2001;10(1):78–83.
16. Smith JA, Hu SS. Management of spondylolysis and spondylolisthesis in the pediatric and adolescent population. Orthop Clin North Am. 1999;30(3):487–99. ix.
17. Nicol RO, Scott JH. Lytic spondylolysis. Repair by wiring. Spine (Phila Pa 1976). 1986;11(10):1027–30.
18. Szypryt EP, et al. The prevalence of disc degeneration associated with neural arch defects of the lumbar spine assessed by magnetic resonance imaging. Spine (Phila Pa 1976). 1989;14(9):977–81.
19. Schlenzka D, et al. Direct repair for treatment of symptomatic spondylolysis and low-grade isthmic spondylolisthesis in young patients: no benefit in comparison to segmental fusion after a mean follow-up of 14.8 years. Eur Spine J. 2006;15(10):1437–47.
20. Dai LY. Disc degeneration in patients with lumbar spondylolysis. J Spinal Disord. 2000;13(6):478–86.

21. Pfirrmann CW, et al. Magnetic resonance classification of lumbar intervertebral disc degeneration. Spine (Phila Pa 1976). 2001;26(17):1873–8.
22. Kimura M. My method of filing the lesion with spongy bone in spondylolysis and spondylolistesis. Seikei Geka. 1968;19(4):285–96.
23. Salib RM, Pettine KA. Modified repair of a defect in spondylolysis or minimal spondylolisthesis by pedicle screw, segmental wire fixation, and bone grafting. Spine (Phila Pa 1976). 1993;18(4):440–3.
24. Giudici F, et al. Long-term results of the direct repair of spondylolisthesis. Eur Spine J. 2011;20 Suppl 1:S115–20.
25. Buck JE. Direct repair of the defect in spondylolisthesis. Preliminary report. J Bone Joint Surg Br. 1970;52(3):432–7.
26. Morscher E, Gerber B, Fasel J. Surgical treatment of spondylolisthesis by bone grafting and direct stabilization of spondylolysis by means of a hook screw. Arch Orthop Trauma Surg. 1984;103(3):175–8.
27. Tokuhashi Y, Matsuzaki H. Repair of defects in spondylolysis by segmental pedicular screw hook fixation. A preliminary report. Spine (Phila Pa 1976). 1996;21(17):2041–5.
28. Altaf F, et al. Repair of spondylolysis using compression with a modular link and screws. J Bone Joint Surg Br. 2011;93(1):73–7.
29. Fan J, et al. Direct repair of spondylolysis by TSRH's hook plus screw fixation and bone grafting: biomechanical study and clinical report. Arch Orthop Trauma Surg. 2010;130(2):209–15.
30. Mihara H, et al. The biomechanical effects of spondylolysis and its treatment. Spine (Phila Pa 1976). 2003;28(3):235–8.
31. Karatas AF, et al. Comparison of direct pars repair techniques of spondylolysis in pediatric and adolescent patients: pars compression screw versus pedicle screw-rod-hook. J Spinal Disord Tech. 2012 PMID: 23075858.
32. Shin MH, et al. Direct pars repair surgery using two different surgical methods: pedicle screw with universal hook system and direct pars screw fixation in symptomatic lumbar spondylosis patients. J Korean Neurosurg Soc. 2012;51(1):14–9.

Decompression and Spinal Fusion in Low Grade Spondylolisthesis

12

John R. Dimar II, Calvin C. Kuo, and Andrew J. Cordiale

Introduction

Spondylolisthesis may become symptomatic due to the development of compressive neuropathies, progressive slippage and/or instability, acquired degenerative disc disease, or more commonly a combination of these factors. The neurologic symptoms result from the spinal stenosis that most often presents as specific nerve root involvement or more rarely with spinal claudication symptoms. The compression is produced by the degeneration of the disc resulting narrowing of the disc space with resultant forminal stenosis, protrusion of the disc into the canal, hypertrophy of the ligamentum flavum, degeneration of the facet joints resulting in osteophytes and facet synovial cysts (Fig. 12.1: synovial cyst + spondylolisthesis), all of which collectively narrow the canal producing "static" stenosis. The addition of "dynamic" anterolisthesis of the vertebra results in additional stenosis that produces the classic symptoms of low back pain, buttock pain, along with classic radicular symptoms that include numbness, tingling that radiates down the legs. While most patients with a symptomatic degenerative spondylolisthesis present with neurogenic pain and no low back pain, some may develop concurrent mechanical low back pain. The back pain is frequently mechanical in nature being made worse with prolonged standing, walking, bending, lifting, and twisting. The patient may also experience catching, clunking, popping, or the feeling of instability when the spondylolisthesis moves forward and then reduces due to instability. This may be particularly evident in an advanced degenerative L4–5 spondylolisthesis or upper level sports related isthmic spondylolisthesis. The radicular symptoms are worsened by standing, walking and may become constant being present even with sitting and lying especially in the morning when arising. These patients will classically get "relief" by sitting down and flexing the spine forward, which opens up the spinal canal relieving the nerve compression. As with spinal stenosis patients, they will exhibit the classic "shopping cart sign" where they find relief of neurogenic pain when they lean forward and push the shopping cart. The pathophysiology of neurogenic claudication is believed to be secondary to loss of blood flow to the lumbar dorsal root ganglions and nerves secondary to the stenosis producing compression of the epidural vessels, which is made worse by weight-bearing [1, 2]. Classically, a

J.R. Dimar II, M.D. (✉)
Department of Orthopaedic Surgery, University of Louisville School of Medicine, Louisville, KY, USA

Norton Leatherman Spine Center, 210 East Gray Street, Suite 900, Louisville, KY 40202, USA
e-mail: jdimar2@aol.com

C.C. Kuo, M.D. • A.J. Cordiale, D.O., M.S.
Norton Leatherman Spine Center, 210 East Gray Street, Suite 900, Louisville, KY 40202, USA
e-mail: calvin.kuo@gmail.com; drcordiale@gmail.com

A.L. Wollowick and V. Sarwahi (eds.), *Spondylolisthesis: Diagnosis, Non-Surgical Management, and Surgical Techniques*, DOI 10.1007/978-1-4899-7575-1_12,

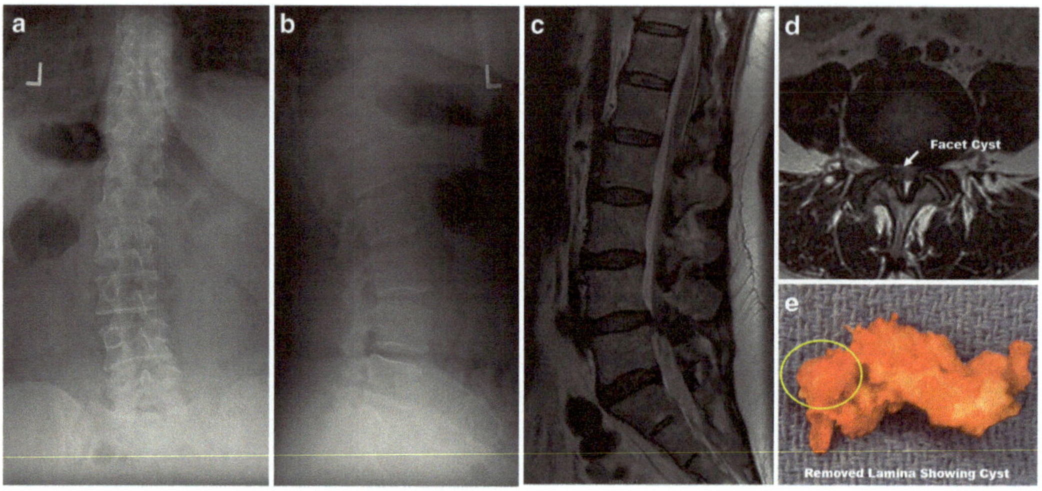

Fig. 12.1 Sixty-five-year-old female presented with 3 months of low back pain and right L5 radicular symptoms who was treated conservatively and required surgery. (**a**, **b**) Anterior–posterior and lateral plain radiographs of a *grade I L4–5 degenerative spondylolisthesis* with 4 mm of anterolisthesis. (**c**–**e**) T2 sagittal and coronal MRI image showing spinal stenosis and right facet joint internal cyst and intra-operative picture showing the actual cyst removed with the lamina during decompression

degenerative spondylolisthesis will present with radiculopathy of the transversing L5 nerve root due to lateral recess stenosis while severe foraminal stenosis may result in compression of the exiting L4 nerve root [3] (Fig. 12.2: L4–5 foraminal stenosis due to facet hypertrophy). An L5–S1 isthmic spondylolisthesis will also present with L5 radiculopathy caused by narrowing of the L5–S1 foramen compressing the exiting L5 nerve root along with some compression of the root on the superior corner of the sacrum on a higher grade spondylolisthesis. Additionally, the L5 nerve root that passes under the pars articularis defect may become compressed by the fibrocartilagenous hypertrophy that occurs secondary to motion circumferentially around the defect (Fig. 12.3: L5–S1 oblique view of the forminal and pars defect fibrocartilagenous hypertrophy causing stenosis). Seated flexion and extension plain radiographs may demonstrate this dynamic instability as anterolisthesis and reduction of the spondylolisthesis with the patient's movement. The same finding is frequently observed following anesthetic relaxation and positioning of the patient on the operating room table in the prone position [4].

Indications for Surgical Treatment

The high incidence of radiculopathy demonstrates the importance of the need for thorough decompression. The *strong indications* for surgery include: progressive neurological deficits such as severe radiculopathy, weakness, intractable pain, the loss of bowel/bladder control, or rarely acute cauda equina syndrome. The *relative indications* include intractable back pain, sagittal imbalance, failure of 3–6 months of conservative care, intolerable radiculopathy, or severe interference with the activities of daily living that affect the patient's quality of life. If surgery is decided upon there are a variety of procedures available including decompression, decompression with/without dynamic stabilization, or decompression with fusion. There is evidence to support that the addition of a fusion to the decompression improves outcomes when surgically treating a spondylolisthesis. There are a wide variety of options available to fuse a spondylolisthesis following decompression including posterolateral, TLIF, anterior, and direct lateral, and all can be combined with various forms of cages and pedicular

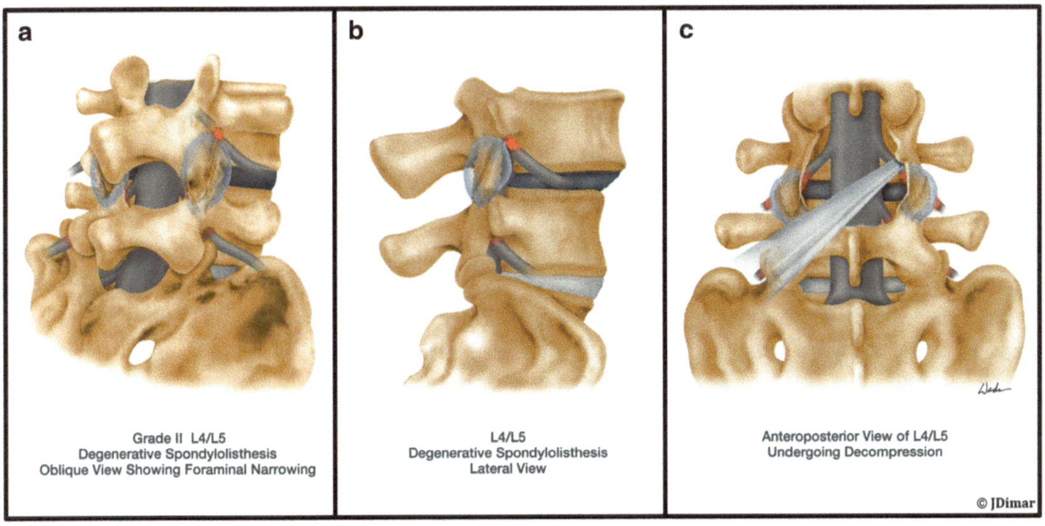

Fig. 12.2 Drawing of L4–5 facet stenosis. Illustration of a grade 2 L4–5 degenerative spondylolisthesis. (**a**) *Oblique view* of a *grade 2 L4–5 degenerative spondylolisthesis* demonstrating facet spondylosis, capsular hypertrophy, and foraminal narrowing that can affect both the exiting nerve root (L4) and the transversing nerve root (L5) is severe enough and associated with concurrent central stenosis. (**b**) *Lateral view* of L4–5 foraminal stenosis affecting the L4 and L5 nerve roots. (**c**) *Posterior view* showing wide decompression addressing bilateral foraminal stenosis and any central stenosis of all four potential nerve root compressive pathology. The restoration of the central canal and foraminal size is assisted by reduction of the spondylolisthesis by a variety of methods

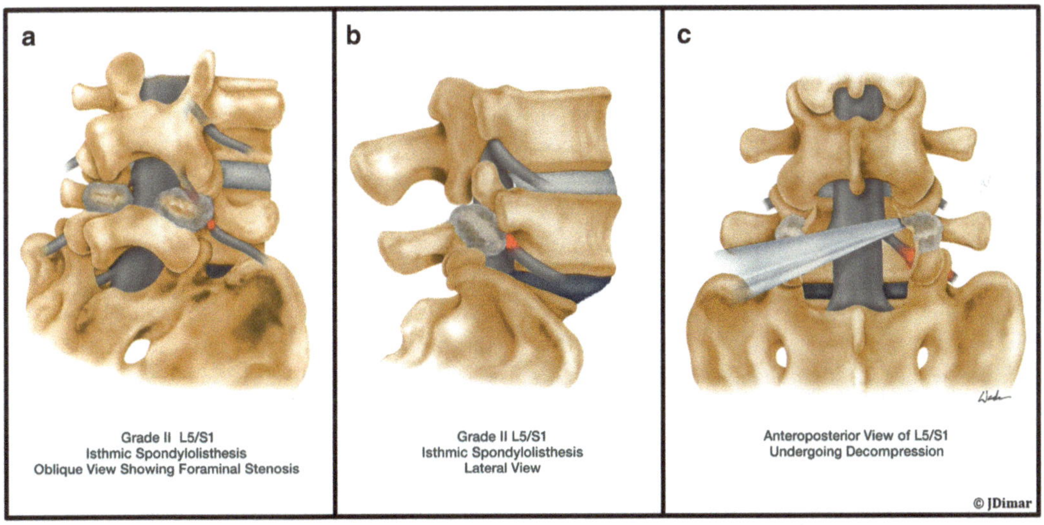

Fig. 12.3 Drawing of L5–S1 spondylolisthesis. Illustration of a grade 2 L5–S1 isthmic spondylolisthesis. (**a**) *Oblique view* of a *grade 2 L5–S1 isthmic spondylolisthesis* demonstrating *acquired* facet spondylosis, capsular hypertrophy, and foraminal narrowing that affects the exiting L5 nerve and is often associated with concurrent central stenosis. (**b**) *Lateral view* of L5–S1 foraminal stenosis affecting the L5 nerve root. (**c**) *Posterior view* showing a wide decompression addressing bilateral foraminal stenosis and any central stenosis causing potential nerve root compressive pathology. The decompression needs to be carried out *laterally along the entire path of the L5 nerve root to decompress any extra-foraminal stenosis*. The restoration of the central canal and foraminal size is also assisted by reduction of the spondylolisthesis by a variety of methods

instrumentation to improve the fusion rates and the durability of the outcomes of the procedures. There also are various inter-spinous process devices available to distract the lamina and concurrently the foramen thus improving radicular symptoms [4–13]. Finally, there are a wide variety of currently available materials available to facilitate the fusions including autograft, allograft, ceramics, and the bone morphogenetic proteins since a successful fusion remains critical to the success of the surgery. This chapter focuses on decompression and fusion without and with instrumentation.

In 1991, Herkowitz led the way with the first prospective, randomized study comparing an L3–4 or L4–5 degenerative spondylolisthesis with stenosis undergoing a decompressive laminectomy compared to a laminectomy with arthrodesis in 50 patients. The study showed that the patients whom demonstrated inter-transverse process fusion had superior outcomes when back and leg pain was evaluated [5]. A follow-up study by Fischgrund comparing fusion success in degenerative spondylolisthesis with and without instrumentation found that of the 67/76 patients available at 2-year follow-up fusion occurred in 82 % of instrumented cases as compared to only 45 % of non-instrumented cases ($P=0.0015$). However, clinical outcome was excellent or good in 76 % of patients with instrumentation and 85 % without instrumentation ($P=0.45$). The authors concluded that instrumentation significantly improves fusions but not necessarily patient outcomes [6]. One shortcoming of the study is that the 2-year follow-up period in this study may not be significantly long enough to delineate long-term clinical outcomes benefit of using instrumentation to improve the fusion rate. However, a review of Fischgrund's original series with an average of a 7.8-year follow-up by Kornblum et al. [14] showed those with single-level spondylolisthesis and spinal stenosis treated with posterior decompression and fusion using autograft showed a solid fusion in only 46 % of the patients (22/47). In contrast, the clinical outcome data of the 86 % of the patients who had a solid fusion were good or excellent while those with a pseudarthrosis had only 56 % reporting good or excellent result. This study showed that a solid fusion provides improved outcomes and longer lasting results. Since instrumentation increases a fusion success most surgeons recommended using instrumentation concurrently with a posterolateral fusion to improve the long-term results. Although instrumentation raises the success of a lumbar spinal fusion certain factors have been identified that decrease the fusion rate even with instrumentation including high disc spaces and segmental kyphosis [15].

The question of whether or not to reduce a degenerative spondylolisthesis by indirect or direct means was evaluated in a study by Montgomery where the pre- and post-operative standing lateral lumbosacral radiographs were compared following the indirect, passive correction of 25 patients with single-level spondylolisthesis following positioning on the operating table. The percentage slip decreased from 24 to 15 to 6 % on standing flexion, extension, and intra-operative lateral radiographs, respectively ($P<0.001$). In both instances, standing and operative positioning, the reduction was not dependent on grade of slip, slip angle, or degenerative disc disease (DDD) [4].

Spine Patient Outcomes Research Trial (SPORT) was a prospective evaluation of patients with degenerative spondylolisthesis that has reported 2-year [16] and 4-year outcomes [17]. The study was critiqued for allowing severely symptomatic patients in the conservative treatment group to cross over to the surgical treatment group, producing both an intent-to-treat and as-treated analysis of the data. In the as-treated analysis, SPORT demonstrated that patients who underwent decompression and concurrent fusion achieved substantially greater improvement in pain and function compared to those treated non-operatively at 2- and 4-year follow-up periods. The study has shown durability of improvements with surgical treatment in patients with lumbar disc herniations at 8-year follow-up [18], and analysis of patients with degenerative spondylolisthesis with 8-year follow-up is pending.

Surgical Techniques

Decompression

Patients who have a degenerative spondylolisthesis with symptomatic spinal stenosis that have not improved with medical/interventional treatment are potential candidates for decompression surgery [19]. Although rarely employed as an isolated procedure, decompression alone is also a viable procedure in certain populations including a stable spondylolisthesis that exhibits ankylosis or in older individuals who have serious co-morbidities where a more extensive surgical fusion would potentially be contraindicated. However, there is always the risk in a younger patient that they may develop further slippage or have worse long-term outcomes if they are not fused [5, 14, 16] (Fig. 12.4: Post-decompression worsening of slippage).

The standard surgical technique is an open posterior decompression that is performed with the patient lying in the prone position either on a Wilson frame or on a Jackson table with all bone prominences well padded. Ensure that the abdomen hangs freely to allow blood to pool in the abdominal cavity. The use of the Jackson table will frequently result in postural reduction of mobile spondylolisthesis and will help minimize the venous congestion and blood pooling into the surgical field. A standard posterior mid-line incision is made through the skin, sub-cutaneous fat, fascia and muscle is carried down to the lamina. Regardless of which procedure is performed, laminectomy, laminotomy, most stenotic patients will improve as long as they are adequately decompressed [8]. The supraspinous ligaments, inter-spinous, and facet capsules should be preserved to maintain stability following the decompression. Once the levels of the decompressive laminotomies are verified with plain radiographs or fluoroscopy the hypertrophied inter-spinous and ligamentum flavum can be resected along with part of the lamina and any overgrown portion of the facet into the foramen. The central canal and foramen should be palpated with an appropriate probe to ensure the decompression is adequate. When necessary the decompression can be expanded to a complete laminectomy from pedicle to pedicle to adequately restore the spinal canal dimensions. However, this will tend to destabilize the spinal segment [7].

Dural tears can be a frequent complication during decompression of a degenerative spondylolisthesis when trying to enter into the spinal canal. The increased risk of dural tears is due to the narrowed canal and frequent adhesions that form between the juxtafacet cysts to the dura, which is itself commonly thinned in degenerative spondylolisthesis patients. There are four anatomical zones of dissection where dural tears are likely to occur: the caudal margin of the cranial lamina, cranial margin of the caudal lamina, herniated disc level, and medial aspect of the facet joint adjacent to the insertion of the hypertrophic ligamentum flavum [20]. The authors' preference is to repair all dural tears primarily and have fibrin glue applied while with extensive tearing a dural patch can be employed. Although rarely employed as an isolated procedure in a patient with a degenerative spondylolisthesis, decompression is effective in stable slips where a full decompression and fusion is contraindicated due to significant co-morbidities.

Decompression with Fusion Without Instrumentation

A decompression and fusion has been shown to offer better clinical outcomes compared with decompression alone in spondylolisthesis patients [19, 21]. However, the fusion technique employed has been shown to have no difference in outcome over the other after 4-year follow-up [22]. In addition to the exposure for decompression, the paraspinal muscles are reflected out to the transverse process tips and the facet capsules removed and then decorticated. It is necessary to ensure there is a clear, unencumbered path from one transverse process to the other along the inter-transverse

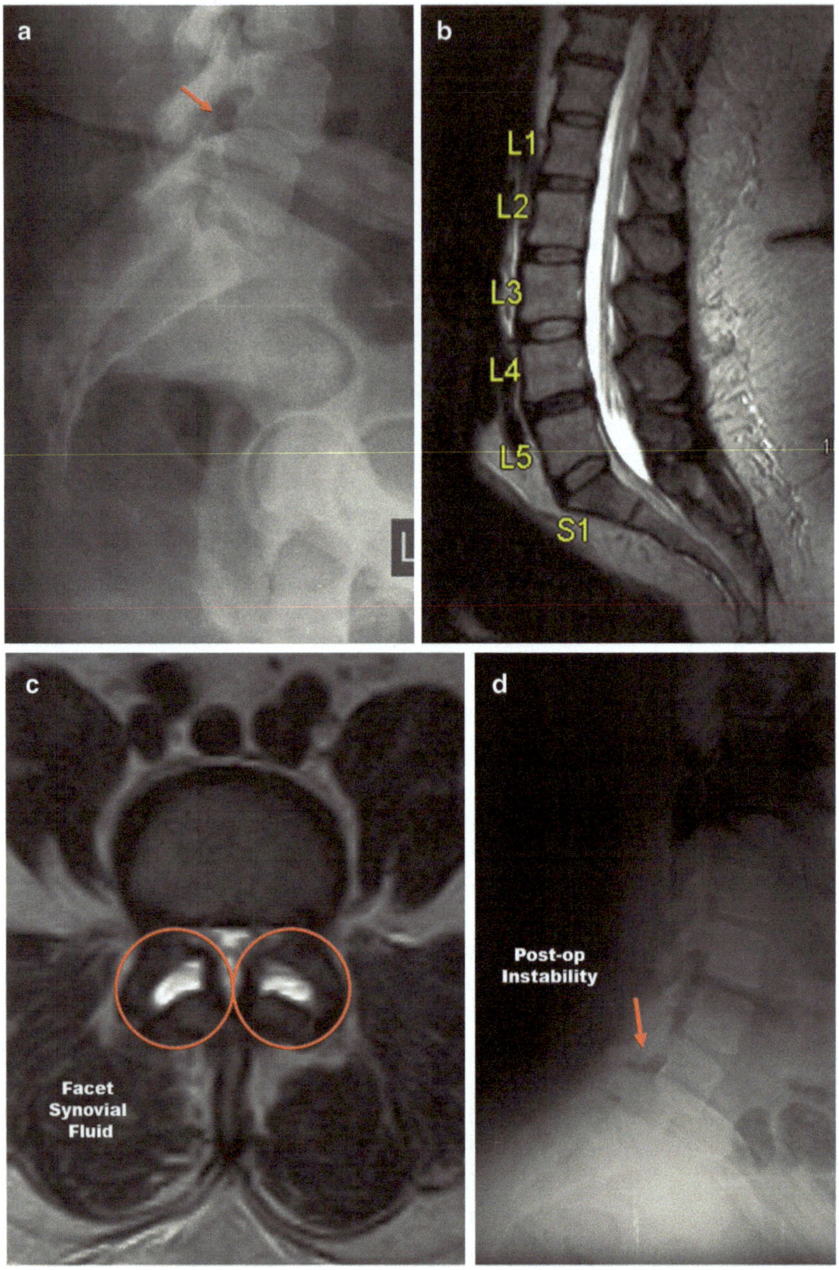

Fig. 12.4 Fifty-two-year-old female presented with severe low back pain and bilateral L5 radicular symptoms following a "Minimally Invasive Decompression." (**a**, **b**) Lateral plain radiograph taken prior to index surgery with a *grade I L4–5 degenerative spondylolisthesis* with 1–2 mm of anterolisthesis and a recumbent MRI that deceptively shows a degenerative disc at L4–5 and no spondylolisthesis due to postural reduction. (**c**, **d**) T2 axial MRI image showing inflammatory bilateral facet synovial fluid and joint widening following the MIS procedure and a lateral plain radiograph showing post-operative iatrogenic L4–5 instability with a marked increase in anterolisthesis to 14 mm

ligament. The proper preparation of this area is critical to obtaining a solid intra-transverse process fusion. Take care not to penetrate anterior to the inter-transverse ligament, as this will bring you into the retroperitoneal space and create a hole that your bone graft may fall into. During the dissection the facet artery should be cauterized at the decorticated facet and care must be taken not to disrupt the cephalad facets and their corresponding neurovascular bundles since they innervate a portion of the paraspinal muscles that will atrophy if denervated. Once the soft tissues have been adequately stripped free from the fusion surfaces, decorticate the remaining exposed bony surfaces of the transverse processes, pars, and facets and to the lower level transverse process and lay the bone graft material of choice along these surfaces and packed into the facets. Primary grafting material includes local products of decompression, iliac crest bone graft (ICBG), allograft, demineralized bone matrix (DBM), and biologics such as BMP-2 or 7 [23, 24]. Each of these has its benefits and drawbacks as far as effectiveness, complications, fusion success and cost profile and are frequently used in various combinations.

Decompression with Fusion and Instrumentation

To achieve a higher rate of fusion, pedicle screws and rod instrumentation are often recommended [6, 19]. The use of an interbody device for fusion and sagittal alignment is presented later in the book.

The first consideration for posterior decompression and instrumentation with fusion is the type of surgical table to use. The authors prefer the Jackson table with an instrumented fusion due to its versatility, lordosing effect on the spine, and the ability to have improved intra-operative radiographic and image guidance capabilities. Following standard prone positioning the posterior mid-line approach is utilized and a facet and posterior-lateral fusion technique may be utilized as described above. Pedicular instrumentation begins with identifying and preparing the entrance point of the pedicle and it is the authors' preferred practice and recommendation to use continuous neuromonitoring during the process of spinal instrumentation. The location may vary slightly depending upon individual patients' anatomy, but in the lumbar spine, generally the entrance to the pedicle will be at the inferior-lateral border of the facet. Ensure that there is not an overgrown facet osteophyte since it will tend to push the starting point too far laterally. The facet osteophyte can be easily removed with a broad rongeur, burr or curette to restore normal anatomy. Alternately, following decompression the inner border of the curved pedicle can be palpated to assist in targeting the pedicle probing.

The usual starting point for pedicle screw insertion is at the confluence of the transverse process (cephalocaudal positioning), the pars (medial border), and the lateral border of the facet. It is good practice to review the patient's imaging to adjust for normal variations that occur when spanning multiple levels and variations from patient to patient. The entrance point can be started with a number of instruments, commonly with the burr or a spiked awl. Fluoroscopy, image guidance, and intra-operative CT scanning techniques may also be used and have been shown to improve pedicle screw placement [25]. Then, a pedicle probe of choice is oscillated as mild axial load is applied. A neuromonitoring stimulated pedicle probe may be useful during this process. It is the authors' preferred practice to stimulate every screw with neuromonitoring since it has a high sensitivity of detecting a medial breach [26]. Initial probing is done to a depth of 20 mm, which represents the average length of the adult lumbar pedicle and once this measurement is reached during the pedicle probing process, it is good measure to lean back on the handle of the probe to direct the tip medially, particularly when using a curved probe. Due to normal anatomical variations in the shape of the pedicles and their level in the spine, the process of pedicle sounding is slightly different in the upper and lower lumbar spine. When using a curved probe (a straight one is less likely to need this particular maneuver) the upper lumbar spine (L1–L2), start with curved pedicle probe angled outward to approximately 20 mm, then rotate the probe 180° and lean back and continue to desired depth. And in the lower half of the lumbar spine (L3–L5), begin with the curve facing medial and advance again until 20 mm and then lean back and continue to depth. Always ensure to use two hands, one that operates the probe, while the other acts as a control to keep your angulation on target and as a stop measure to ensure controlled advancement.

If any resistance is met, it is good practice to double check the selected starting point and angle of approach. Additionally, a ball tip (feeler) probe should be used during the process to palpate all four walls of the pedicle and its floor following probing and tapping, unless self-tapping screws are used. Once the screws are placed, final EMG stimulation should be done. Screws that stimulate below the acceptable threshold of the neuromonitoring system should be removed and the pedicle inspected, then redirected and replaced, or abandoned as needed.

Decompression is performed as necessary. The decompression is partially accomplished by postural reduction by opening the spinal canal, improving the *dynamic* stenosis of the slippage. The *static* stenosis is addressed by direct surgical decompressive techniques of the canal narrowing secondary to the acquired chances of facet and disc degeneration. The facets differ in their orientation from L2/3 to L5–S1 with the upper levels being more sagittally oriented with the facets become progressively more coronally oriented the further down the spine until they reach their maximum coronal orientation at L5–S1. Because of this orientation the amount of facet resection differs with the level that is decompressed. Excessive resection of the facets, particularly in the upper segments of the spine, results in a greater chance of further destabilizing the spondylotic segment. Often it is necessary to resect a substantial portion of the facet joint to adequately decompress the nerve root that the spinal segment is rendered unstable leading to the need for a concurrent fusion. Decompression of the forminal stenosis applies primarily to a *degenerative spondylolisthesis* (typically L4–5), which partially occurs due to the facet hypertrophy where the spondylosis narrows the exiting foramen (Fig. 12.5: L5–S1 degenerative spondylolisthesis). This is somewhat different from the etiology of nerve root compression that occurs in an *isthmic type spondylolisthesis* (L5–S1) where the compression occurs beneath the pars defect due to fibrocartilagenous hypertrophy that narrows the foramen resulting in the compression of the exiting L5 nerve root. Therefore, when addressing a degenerative spondylolisthesis it is important to thoroughly decompress the nerve roots in their respective foramen where the disc degeneration and overgrowth of the facet and capsule results in four zones of stenosis: central, subarticular, foraminal, and extra-foraminal stenosis. The nerve must be also followed out along its entire course to ensure that there is no residual compression. This point is particularly important when addressing an L5–S1 isthmic spondylolisthesis. Inadequate decompression along the L5 nerve root lateral to the foramen is a frequent cause of residual stenosis and persistent radiculopathy. The vertebral body may compress the nerve in the foraminal zone, which is improved by the concurrent reduction maneuvers during instrumentation or with resection of anterolateral discal osteophytes during the discectomy (Fig. 12.6: Isthmic L5–S1 spondylolisthesis). Dural tears should be addressed with primary repair, fibrin glue, and dural grafting if necessary.

During the decompression meticulous attention should be paid to hemostasis since the decompression, if difficult can result in significant blood loss. The epidural venous plexus should be cauterized with the bipolar electrocautery to keep the field dry and improve visualization. Gel foam and thrombin (powderized with 1 % epinephrine), hemostatic agents, bone wax, and cottonoids can also be used to control bleeding. Once the decompression and instrumentation is finished meticulous bone grafting is done.

There are many available bone grafting materials that have shown variable success in achieving a solid fusion which is critical to the long-term success of the surgery. The gold standard remains iliac crest bone graft (ICBG), but various combinations of ICBG, local bone graft, ceramics, demineralized bone matrixes, various

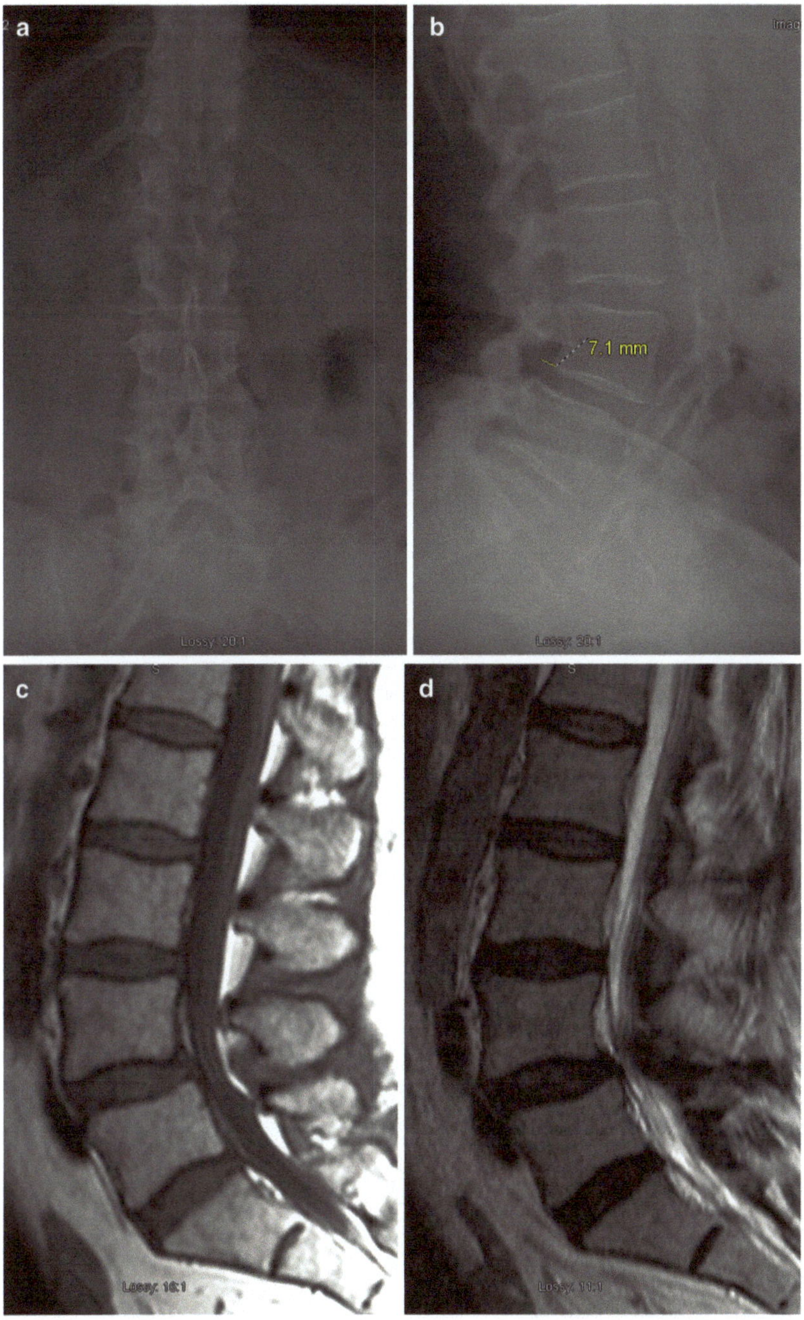

Fig. 12.5 Fifty-three-year-old female presented with 2 years of persistent right L5 radicular symptoms already treated with NSAIDs, physical therapy, and epidural blocks. She was treated with an L4–5 decompression, posterolateral fusion using iliac crest and local bone graft. (**a**, **b**) Anterior–posterior and lateral radiographs of *grade I L4–5 degenerative spondylolisthesis* with 7 mm of anterolisthesis. (**c**, **d**) T1 and T2 sagittal MRI images showing the L4–5 spondylolisthesis with spontaneous postural reduction in the recumbent position. (**e**, **f**) T2 axial view showing severe central stenosis, facet fluid sign and intra-operative lateral radiograph showing slip reduction. (**g**, **h**) Two-year post-operative anterior–posterior and lateral radiographs following L4–5 solid posterior-lateral fusion

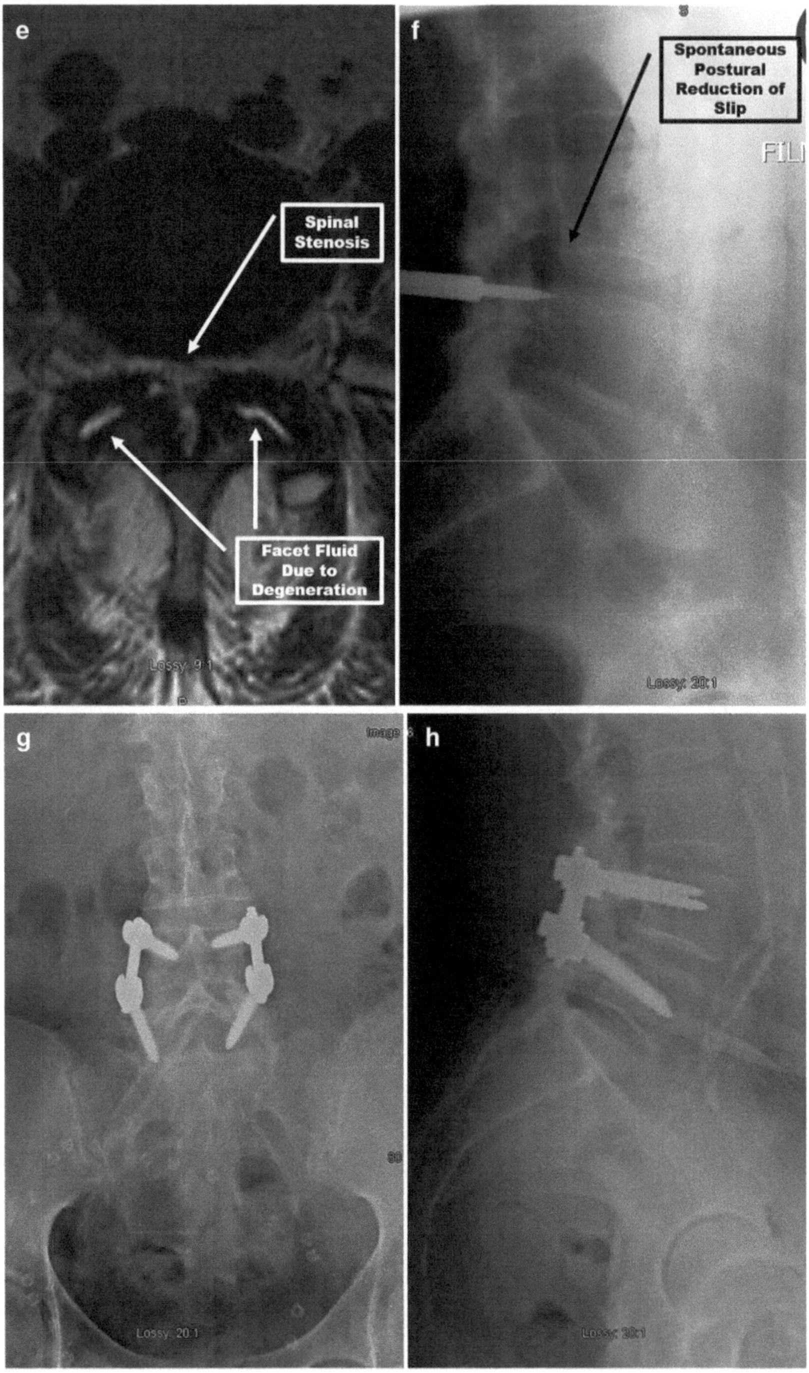

Fig. 12.5 (continued)

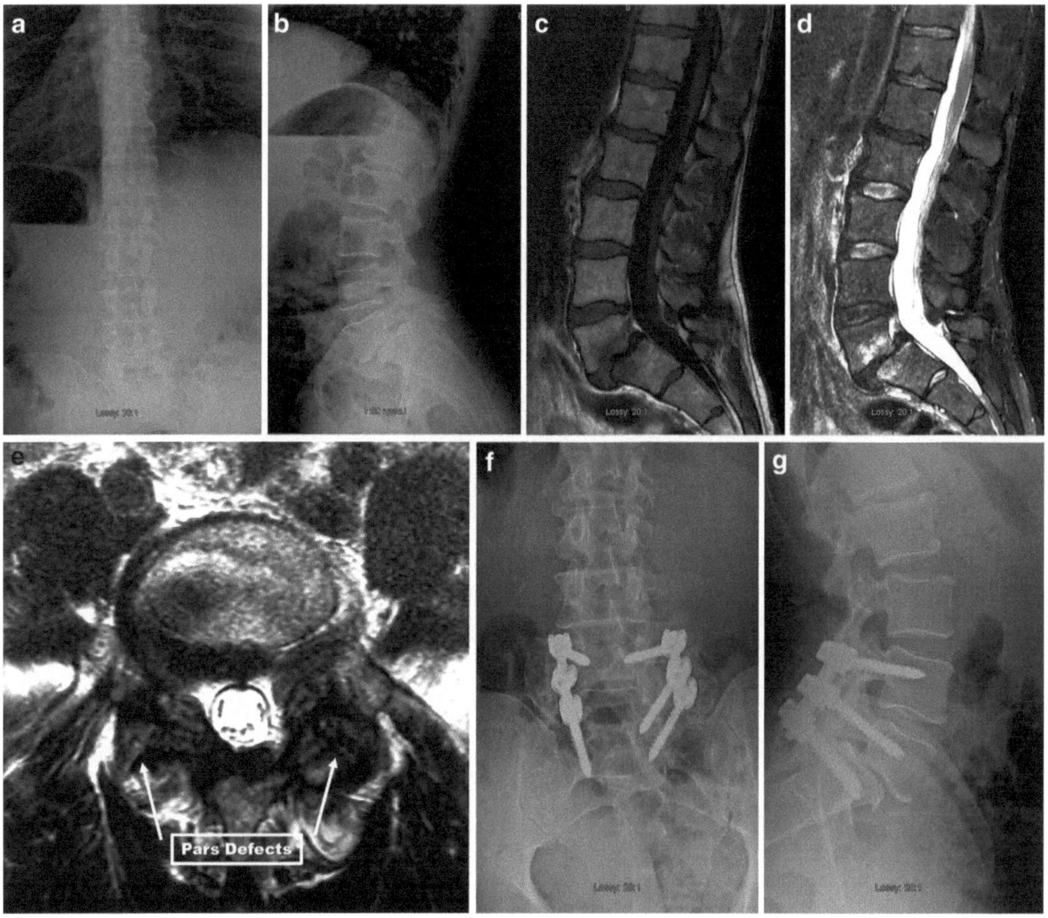

Fig. 12.6 Fifty-two-year-old male presented with many years of mechanical low back pain, now has persistent bilateral L5 radicular symptoms refractory to NSAIDs, physical therapy and epidural blocks. He was treated with an L4–5–S1 decompression, posterolateral fusion using iliac crest and local bone graft. (**a**, **b**) Anterior–posterior and lateral radiographs showing a *grade II isthmic spondylolisthesis*. (**c**, **d**) T1 and T2 sagittal MRI images showing the L5–S1 spondylolisthesis with modic changes and a degenerative disc at L4–5. (**e**) T2 axial view showing pars defect. (**f**, **g**) Two-year post-operative anterior-posterior and lateral radiographs following L4-5-S1 solid posterior-lateral fusion

allograft materials, and bone morphogenetic protein (BMP) have been used for bone grafting. Recent studies have shown reliable fusions and a low rate in BMP related complications when used in posterior fusions but some complication have been observed including: symptomatic seroma, ectopic bone, osteolysis, cage subsidence, wound problems and a possible cancer risk increase [27]. However, a recent analyses of the Medicare data base of patients undergoing fusion with the use of BMP demonstrated no detectable increase in risk of cancer [28, 29]. Once the fusion environment and requirements have been assessed for each particular patient the bone grafting material of choice can then be placed in the lateral gutters precisely to ensure an intra-transverse process fusion (Fig. 12.7: Picture of proper ICBG technique). Crosslinks are recommended in cases of short instrumentation constructs, cases where an anterior release is performed or where the laminae have been completely removed to restore rotational stability. Final anteroposterior and lateral radiographs to confirm the proper level of surgery and the instrumentation placement should be done prior to standard closure.

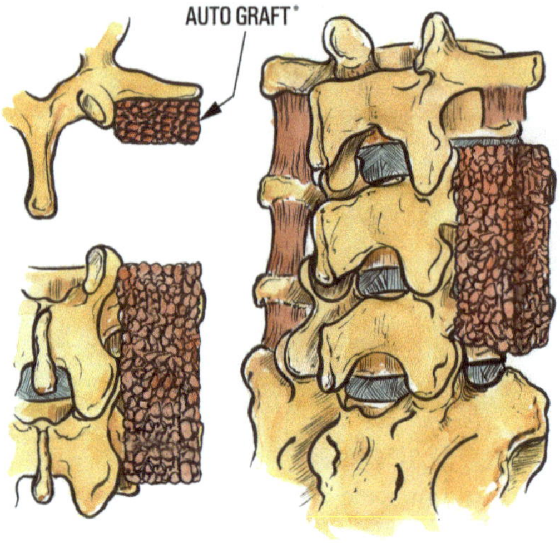

Fig. 12.7 Picture demonstrating the use of autograft to obtain an intra-transverse process fusion following thorough decortication of the transverse processes. Meticulous attention must always be paid to the fusion, instrumentation, although important, is secondary to long-term fusion success

Summary

Operative treatment of spondylolisthesis is based on the need to decompress nerve root compression and stabilize, reduce or restore balance, and obtain a successful fusion. Sufficient decompression is critical to relieve neurologic symptoms. Some studies suggest that patients do better when decompression is accompanied with fusion. While the recent use of instrumentation allows the fusion to be more robust and solid, the incremental benefits of instrumentation on clinical outcome are not clear. When instability is evident on preoperative radiographs or during the intraoperative period, instrumentation can provide stability while the fusion matures and solidifies.

References

1. Takahashi K, Miyazaki T, Takino T, Matsui T, Tomita K. Epidural pressure measurements. Relationship between epidural pressure and posture in patients with lumbar spinal stenosis. Spine. 1995;20(6):650–3.
2. Takahashi K, Kagechika K, Takino T, Matsui T, Miyazaki T, Shima I. Changes in epidural pressure during walking in patients with lumbar spinal stenosis. Spine. 1995;20(24):2746–9.
3. Sengupta D, Herkowitz H. Degenerative spondylolisthesis: review of current trends and controversies. Spine. 2005;30(6 Suppl):S71–81.
4. Montgomery D, Fischgrund J. Passive reduction of spondylolisthesis on the operating room table: a prospective study. J Spinal Disord. 1994;7(2):167–72.
5. Herkowitz H, Kurz L. Degenerative lumbar spondylolisthesis with spinal stenosis. A prospective study comparing decompression with decompression and intertransverse process arthrodesis. J Bone Joint Surg Am. 1991;73(6):802–8.
6. Fischgrund J, Mackay M, Herkowitz H, Brower R, Montgomery D, Kurz L. 1997 Volvo Award winner in clinical studies. Degenerative lumbar spondylolisthesis with spinal stenosis: a prospective, randomized study comparing decompressive laminectomy and arthrodesis with and without spinal instrumentation. Spine. 1997;22(24):2807–12.
7. Nakanishi K, Tanaka N, Fujimoto Y, Okuda T, Kamei N, Nakamae T, et al. Medium-term clinical results of microsurgical lumbar flavectomy that preserves facet joints in cases of lumbar degenerative spondylolisthesis: comparison of bilateral laminotomy with bilateral decompression by a unilateral approach. J Spinal Disord Tech. 2013;26(7):351–8.
8. Matsudaira K, Yamazaki T, Seichi A, Takeshita K, Hoshi K, Kishimoto J, et al. Spinal stenosis in grade I degenerative lumbar spondylolisthesis: a comparative study of outcomes following laminoplasty and laminectomy with instrumented spinal fusion. J Orthop Sci. 2005;10(3):270–6.
9. Davis R, Errico T, Bae H, Auerbach J. Decompression and Coflex interlaminar stabilization compared with decompression and instrumented spinal fusion for spinal stenosis and low-grade degenerative spondylolisthesis: two-year results from the prospective, randomized, multicenter, Food and Drug Administration Investigational Device Exemption trial. Spine. 2013;38(18):1529–39.
10. Gomleksiz C, Sasani M, Oktenoglu T, Ozer A. A short history of posterior dynamic stabilization. Adv Orthop. 2012;2012:629698.
11. Harris E, Sayadipour A, Massey P, Duplantier N, Anderson D. Mini-open versus open decompression and fusion for lumbar degenerative spondylolisthesis with stenosis. Am J Orthop. 2011;40(12):E257–61.
12. Boissiere L, Perrin G, Rigal J, Michel F, Barrey C. Lumbar-sacral fusion by a combined approach using interbody PEEK cage and posterior pedicle-screw fixation: clinical and radiological results from a prospective study. Orthop Traumatol Surg Res. 2013;99(8):945–51.
13. Anderson P, Tribus C, Kitchel S. Treatment of neurogenic claudication by interspinous decompression: application of the X STOP device in patients with lumbar degenerative spondylolisthesis. J Neurosurg Spine. 2006;4(6):463–71.

14. Kornblum M, Fischgrund J, Herkowitz H, Abraham D, Berkower D, Ditkoff J. Degenerative lumbar spondylolisthesis with spinal stenosis: a prospective long-term study comparing fusion and pseudarthrosis. Spine. 2004;29(7):726–33.
15. Suda K, Ito M, Abumi K, Haba H, Taneichi H, Kaneda K. Radiological risk factors of pseudoarthrosis and/or instrument breakage after PLF with the pedicle screw system in isthmic spondylolisthesis. J Spinal Disord Tech. 2006;19(8):541–6.
16. Weinstein J, Lurie J, Tosteson T, Hanscom B, Tosteson A, Blood E, et al. Surgical versus nonsurgical treatment for lumbar degenerative spondylolisthesis. N Engl J Med. 2007;356(22):2257–70.
17. Weinstein J, Lurie J, Tosteson T, Zhao W, Blood E, Tosteson A, et al. Surgical compared with nonoperative treatment for lumbar degenerative spondylolisthesis. four-year results in the Spine Patient Outcomes Research Trial (SPORT) randomized and observational cohorts. J Bone Joint Surg Am. 2009;91(6):1295–304.
18. Lurie JD, Tosteson TD, Tosteson AN, Zhao W, Morgan TS, Abdu WA, et al. Surgical versus nonoperative treatment for lumbar disc herniation: eight-year results for the spine patient outcomes research trial. Spine. 2014;39(1):3–16.
19. Wr W, Bono C, Gilbert T, Kreiner D, Mazanec D, Shaffer W, et al. An evidence-based clinical guideline for the diagnosis and treatment of degenerative lumbar spondylolisthesis. Spine J. 2009;9(7):609–14.
20. Takahashi Y, Sato T, Hyodo H, Kawamata T, Takahashi E, Miyatake N, et al. Incidental durotomy during lumbar spine surgery: risk factors and anatomic locations: clinical article. J Neurosurg Spine. 2013;18(2):165–9.
21. Martin C, Gruszczynski A, Braunsfurth H, Fallatah S, O'Neil J, Wai E. The surgical management of degenerative lumbar spondylolisthesis: a systematic review. Spine. 2007;32(16):1791–8.
22. Abdu W, Lurie J, Spratt K, Tosteson A, Zhao W, Tosteson T, et al. Degenerative spondylolisthesis: does fusion method influence outcome? Four-year results of the spine patient outcomes research trial. Spine. 2009;34(21):2351–60.
23. Vaccaro A, Lawrence J, Patel T, Katz L, Anderson D, Fischgrund J, et al. The safety and efficacy of OP-1 (rhBMP-7) as a replacement for iliac crest autograft in posterolateral lumbar arthrodesis: a long-term (>4 years) pivotal study. Spine. 2008;33(26): 2850–62.
24. Hurlbert R, Alexander D, Bailey S, Mahood J, Abraham E, McBroom R, et al. rhBMP-2 for posterolateral instrumented lumbar fusion: a multicenter prospective randomized controlled trial. Spine. 2013;38(25):2139–48.
25. Santos E, Sembrano J, Mueller B, Polly D. Optimizing iliac screw fixation: a biomechanical study on screw length, trajectory, and diameter. J Neurosurg Spine. 2011;14(2):219–25.
26. Glassman S, Dimar J, Puno R, Johnson J, Shields C, Linden R. A prospective analysis of intraoperative electromyographic monitoring of pedicle screw placement with computed tomographic scan confirmation. Spine. 1995;20(12):1375–9.
27. Singh K, Ahmadinia K, Park D, Nandyala S, Marquez-Lara A, Patel A, et al. Complications of spinal fusion with utilization of bone morphogenic protein. A systematic review of the literature. Spine. 2014;39:91–101.
28. Kelly MP, Savage JW, Bentzen SM, Hsu WK, Ellison SA, Anderson PA. Cancer risk from bone morphogenetic protein exposure in spinal arthrodesis. J Bone Joint Surg Am. 2014;96(17):1417–22.
29. Cooper GS, Kou TD. Risk of cancer after lumbar fusion surgery with recombinant human bone morphogenic protein-2 (rh-BMP-2). Spine. 2013;38(21):1862–8.

13 Surgical Techniques: Posterior Lumbar Interbody Fusion

Louis F. Amorosa, Jeffrey A. Rihn, and Todd J. Albert

Introduction

Posterior lumbar interbody fusion (PLIF) is a type of interbody fusion technique used in lumbar fusion surgery. It is one of several possible interbody fusion techniques in the lumbar spine. PLIF technique was first described over 60 years ago by Cloward who reported overall excellent results with over an 85 % success rate achieving fusion and pain control in a series of 321 patients [1]. The technique of PLIF has remained largely unchanged since its original description with few modifications to the discectomy technique and endplate preparation [2]. Instead of iliac crest strut autograft, there are now many other interbody bone graft alternatives. While Cloward had low complication rates with the PLIF and high fusion rates, others have not universally been able to replicate his results, especially without the concurrent use of pedicle screw instrumentation [3]. The introduction of pedicle screws in conjunction with the procedure adds immediate internal stability to the PLIF, which increases the likelihood of successful fusion [4].

Standard fusion alternatives to PLIF include anterior lumbar interbody fusion (ALIF), transforaminal interbody fusion (TLIF), and lateral interbody fusion (XLIF or DLIF). Indications for one interbody technique over another still have yet to be completely elucidated from the available evidence in the literature. In fact, the necessity of using an interbody fusion technique over posterolateral fusion alone has yet to be completely validated in the literature. This chapter will attempt to help the surgeon better understand the indications for PLIF over alternative fusion procedures, the surgical technique for the procedure, the complications associated with the PLIF and how best to avoid them, and the available evidence from the literature on outcomes using PLIF as the fusion procedure of choice.

L.F. Amorosa, M.D. (✉)
Department of Orthopaedic Surgery, Westchester Medical Center, New York Medical College, Hawthorne, NY, USA
e-mail: amorosal@wcmc.edu

J.A. Rihn, M.D.
Department of Orthopaedic Surgery, The Rothman Institute, Thomas Jefferson University Hospital, 925 Chestnut Street 5th Floor, Philadelphia, PA 19107, USA
e-mail: jrihno16@yahoo.com

T.J. Albert, M.D.
Hospital for Special Surgery, 535 E 70th Street, New York, NY 10021, USA

Indications for PLIF

Interbody Fusion Versus Posterolateral Fusion Alone

Interbody fusions in general are indicated for circumferential fusion of the spinal motion segment, in conjunction with posterolateral pedicle

A.L. Wollowick and V. Sarwahi (eds.), *Spondylolisthesis: Diagnosis, Non-Surgical Management, and Surgical Techniques*, DOI 10.1007/978-1-4899-7575-1_13,

screw instrumentation with or without bone grafting. With the use of modern pedicle screw instrumentation and autogenous bone graft, posterolateral fusion alone results in reported fusion rates of 90–100 % [5–7]. Fusion rates with PLIF vary in the literature, but earlier studies from proponents of the procedure reported fusion rates of 98–100 % [8, 9]. Studies comparing functional outcomes from posterolateral fusion alone to PLIF have also not shown a significant benefit to performing the PLIF procedure [10, 11]. Relatively high rates of complications and secondary surgeries due to these complications with the use of both PLIF and TLIF are well documented in the literature [12]. Therefore, in a new healthcare environment in which cost and benefits are increasingly more scrutinized, the indications for PLIF over posterolateral fusion alone may become more difficult to justify.

Evidence for the use of interbody fusion in general and the PLIF specifically in the setting of spondylolisthesis and degenerative scoliosis remains equivocal. While it found fusion to have better outcomes than nonoperative treatment, a systematic review of the literature failed to identify the superiority of one fusion technique over the other when comparing posterolateral fusion alone to PLIF or ALIF in the setting of isthmic spondylolisthesis [13]. In general, we typically use an interbody fusion in the setting of collapsed disc space, in association with a spondylolisthesis and kyphotic collapse [10], or when the disc space is asymmetrically collapsed, resulting in a degenerative scoliosis [14]. Using the interbody device to prop open the disc space results in an indirect decompression of the exiting nerve roots and restores coronal alignment in the setting of scoliosis or lateral listhesis. Using the interbody also can help restore saggital alignment by increasing the amount of lumbar lordosis in the setting of spondylolisthesis [15]. Though the evidence from the literature is lacking, we believe that better sagittal alignment may improve long-term outcomes and decrease the likelihood of adjacent segment degeneration (ASD). A PLIF can also be performed in the case of a recurrent disc herniation after previous discectomy refractory to conservative measures with a significant amount of associated back pain [16].

Contraindications to PLIF

At and above the level of the conus medullaris, the PLIF procedure should not be used as the spinal cord does not tolerate retraction. Other contraindications that have been proposed include epidural fibrosis, which would limit safe access to the disc space, active infection, conjoined nerve roots which also limit access to the disc space, severe ankylosis, and severe osteoporosis [12].

We avoid performing surgery for back pain in the setting of degenerative disc disease in the absence of instability or deformity. The results of operative treatment for back pain and degenerative disc disease have not been shown to be significantly better than nonoperative treatments and have a higher complication rate [17, 18]. When surgery is performed for degenerative disc disease and back pain, the results of interbody fusion and posterolateral fusion as opposed to posterolateral fusion alone are equivocal and do not show any major clinical benefit to performing the PLIF procedure and add significant length of surgery and risk of complications [19].

PLIF Versus Other Forms of Interbody Fusion

vs. ALIF

When to perform a PLIF versus other forms of interbody fusion are largely based on surgeon preferences and experience, although each interbody fusion technique has certain advantages and disadvantages over the others. In most cases, when two or more levels are indicated to undergo interbody fusion, as is often the case with degenerative scoliosis, ALIF typically is our technique of choice as multiple levels can be addressed with one surgical approach. A small retrospective comparative study found a 95 % fusion rate and good functional outcomes with a two-level PLIF for degenerative spondylolisthesis compared to a matched single-level PLIF group [20]. Using the PLIF at greater than two levels to restore a degenerative scoliosis has been described though it is technically demanding and increases the risk of complications [21].

We generally avoid ALIF when the patient has had multiple prior abdominal surgeries, which can make a retroperitoneal or transperitoneal approach much more challenging with a higher risk of bowel perforation and great vessel injury. A recent study comparing 42 matched ALIF patients to 42 TLIF patients who underwent the procedures as part of a degenerative scoliosis decompression and fusion surgery found that patients who underwent ALIF had better restoration of their lumbar lordosis and saggital alignment, while TLIF patients had a better correction of their scoliosis [22]. While it is difficult to extrapolate data such as this from studies devoted to TLIF to the PLIF, we can assume that PLIF would show similar results as the TLIF. A study which compared the ALIF to PLIF in 48 patients with spondylolisthesis found a higher incidence of ASD in the PLIF group ($p=0.008$) with high clinical success in both groups [23].

vs. XLIF/DLIF

Lateral retroperitoneal transpsoas approach, also called Direct or Extreme Lateral interbody Fusion, referred to as DLIF or XLIF, is a retroperitoneal approach to the lumbar vertebrae that can be performed in a minimally invasive fashion utilizing specialized retractors and neuromonitoring probes. The lateral interbody has similar indications as ALIF. Multiple interbody motion segments can be addressed via the same surgical approach. For anatomical reasons which will be addressed in more detail in another chapter, this approach becomes technically challenging at L4–5 due to danger to the branches of the lumbar plexus passing within the psoas major and generally contraindicated at L5–S1 due to the iliac crest blocking a direct lateral approach [24, 25]. As the lateral retroperitoneal transpsoas approach becomes more widely used and indications more appropriately defined, there should be more studies comparing it to other interbody fusion techniques. However, we generally will consider this procedure for multilevel interbody fusion at L1–4, typically in degenerative scoliosis patients. More evidence is necessary before this procedure is a common alternative to standard interbody techniques at these levels. Our empiric observation is that the XLIF procedure fails to restore lordosis as well as the alternatives, which may in part be due to technical errors during the procedure.

vs. TLIF

Transforaminal lumbar interbody fusion is a technique very similar to the PLIF procedure and performed through the same posterior incision as the PLIF. It is an adaptation of the PLIF procedure and was originally described by Harms and Rollinger [26]. In the TLIF procedure the disc space is approached posterolaterally via the neuroforamen with osteotomy of the pars interarticularis and removal of the inferior articular facet of the superior vertebrae. With PLIF, on the other hand, the disc space is approached from a directly posterior direction and part of the pars interarticularis and the facet joint is preserved. The TLIF has the advantage in that the neural elements, namely the dural sac and the exiting nerve root, require minimal retraction in order to perform the procedure, which may result in a lower complication rate.

While both PLIF and TLIF have been widely used for decades, there are no Level I or II studies comparing complications and clinical outcomes between the two procedures. In cadaveric studies, the PLIF and TLIF procedures have similar biomechanical characteristics. In one study, the TLIF showed increased stability at the interbody-endplate interface but higher pedicle screw stress [27].

We typically perform the TLIF procedure over the PLIF procedure as it avoids more than minimal retraction on the dural sac. However, in most cases, depending on the surgeon's training and experience, a PLIF may be preferred over a TLIF and indications to use one over the other are generally the same. The one case in which TLIF is preferred to PLIF is the presence of a far lateral disc herniations when fusion is indicated such as in degenerative scoliosis, spondylolisthesis, or lateral listesis. In these cases, a TLIF procedure would be the fusion procedure of choice as the disc herniation is directly decompressed via the neuroforamen once the osteotomy is performed.

Surgical Technique

The PLIF is performed with the patient in the prone position. An Andrews frame can be used or a flat Jackson table. Some surgeons prefer to perform the PLIF on the Andrews frame as it has the benefit of allowing the interlaminar space to be widened, which makes it technically easier to enter the spinal canal, decompress it, and perform the discectomy and PLIF. The Andrews frame also allows the abdominal vessels to be completely free, decreasing venous distension in the spinal canal, and may result in less bleeding during the procedure. It is important to remember though that the patient is in less lordosis with the Andrews frame and therefore after the PLIF has been performed and prior to final tightening of the pedicle screw-rod construct, the operating table or the patient's position may need to be modified to add lordosis to the motion segment to be fused. A postero-anterior radiograph is also not possible with the Andrews frame and therefore it typically should not be used in degenerative scoliosis cases where the amount of correction in the coronal plane is desired to be evaluated intraoperatively. For these technical reasons, in most cases we prefer a standard Jackson table—it allows or improves upon lordosis and allows for biplanar orthogonal fluoroscopy and or radiographs (Fig. 13.1).

An arterial line is used in interbody fusion procedures as it allows for instantaneous blood pressure monitoring. An acute drop in blood pressure not accounted for by anything else and not responding to fluids suggests a possible disruption of the anterior longitudinal and retroperitoneal great vessel rupture. In this catastrophic situation, the wound should be quickly closed and the patient flipped supine at which time an emergent exploratory laparatomy to repair the injured vessel versus a CT angiogram if the patient is stable enough to have this test obtained. This is a rare complication of the PLIF but due to the catastrophic nature of the event, it should always be a concern during the procedure [28–30].

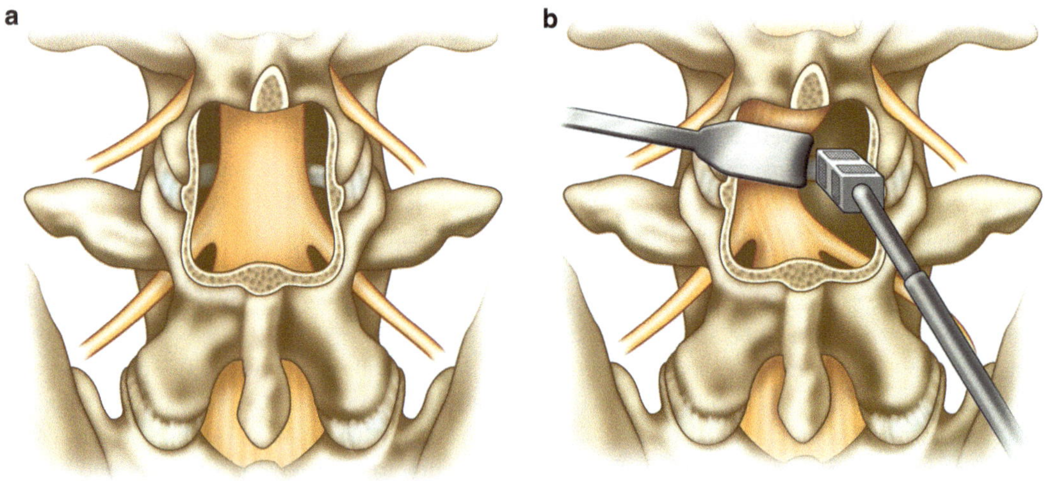

Fig. 13.1 PLIF at the L4–5 level. (**a**) A laminectomy is performed. The interspinous ligament between L4 and L5 spinous processes are removed and the caudal part of the spinous process of L4 and the cephalad half of the spinous process of L5 is removed. A lamina spreader may be placed in between L4 and L5 spinous processes to facilitate ligamentum flavum removal and lateral recess and foraminal decompression. Part of the pars of L5 and facet joints of L4–5 are preserved to promote stability and midline direct posterior interbody fusion. (**b**) The dural sac is retracted and an annuolotomy is performed. A total discectomy is then performed. In most situations, this is repeated bilaterally to ensure complete discectomy and bilateral interbody placement for greater biomechanical stability and greater surface area to promote fusion. After complete cartilaginous removal of the end plates and trialing, an interbody graft is tamped into place. The interbody should sit anteriorly in the disc space to promote restoration of lordosis and limit the likelihood of posterior cage migration into the spinal canal. We typically use a cage device although a piece of structural iliac crest bone graft can also be used

We typically utilize neuromonitoring including SSEPs and EMGs during all lumbar surgical procedures involving pedicle screw instrumentation or interbody fusion. While there is little high level evidence to support the use of neuromonitoring in the lumbar spine, the medicolegal implications of not utilizing are high.

For the open PLIF procedure, a standard midline incision is used. We always perform bilateral pedicle screw instrumentation and therefore both sides of the spine should be exposed. The facet joint of the most proximal pedicle being exposed should not be violated in order to decrease the likelihood of iatrogenic destabilization and ASD. All levels to be fused should be exposed out to the transverse processes. It is helpful to coordinate with the anesthesiologist to provide relaxation during the exposure as this allows for easier stripping and lateral retraction of the paraspinal muscles off of the posterior elements.

The order and specific of the decompression, instrumentation, and interbody fusion can vary based on surgeon preference and training. We typically cannulate the pedicles for instrumentation first using anatomic landmarks. However, if preferred in patients with significant deformity or small pedicles, the pedicles can be cannulated using lateral fluoroscopy. Alternatively, the medial wall of the pedicles can be palpated from within in the spinal canal and then cannulated once the laminectomy has been performed.

The decompression is begun with removal of the interspinous ligament and full or partial laminectomy depending on the pathology seen on MRI. Part of the spinous processes at the level of the PLIF can be preserved at least temporarily. By preserving them, a laminar spreader can be used to distract across the desired disc space of the PLIF in order to facilitate decompression of the spinal canal, lateral recess, and foramina. The distraction from the lamina spreader also allows for distraction across the disc space which helps with placement of a larger interbody and restoration of the collapsed disc space height.

In the PLIF procedure, at least part of the pars interarticularis is preserved and up to half of the medial facet joints can be removed to obtain adequate decompression. The discectomy and subsequent PLIF are performed from a directly posterior direction. The dural sac and the traversing caudal nerve root are retracted medially in order to allow for passage of scalpel for annulotomy, curettes, distracters, shavers, trial, and finally the interbody fusion device itself. With a significant degree of stenosis or a large disc herniation often present in PLIF procedures, it is important to identify and protect the traversing nerve root prior to beginning the discectomy because the nerve root can often be crushed and mistaken for an epidural vessel or disc space. If this is the case, the surgeon may inadvertently injure the nerve root with bipolar cuatery or by cutting it believing it to the pathologic disc.

In order to most safely retract the dural sac and nerve root, as much ligamentum flavum and adhesions as necessary should be removed. The inferior pedicle should be palpated with a woodson or other blunt instrument. The disc space should be superior to the pedicle in close proximity to it. Often there is an epidural leash of vessels or other fibrotic adhesions which should be cauterized with bipolar cuatery. A penfield 4 or other small blunt instrument should be used to free the adhesions and bipolar cautery used to coagulate any epidural vessels overlying the disc space. This is important as it allows mobilization and excursion of the dura and nerve root, which makes it less likely for excessive dural and nerve root retraction, which can cause durotomy or radiculitis. A blunt nerve root retractor is then used to gently retract the dural sac and inferior nerve root.

At this point, with adequate visualization of the disc space and distraction provided by the laminar spreader, the discectomy and interbody placement is performed. A 15 blade scalpel is used to perform an annulotomy over the disc space. The cut should be from medial to lateral in order to avoid cutting the dura or nerve root. A small pituitary is then used to remove the disc followed by curettes, shavers, and other instruments. Throughout the procedure, the surgeon and assistant who is retracting the dural sac should take care to retract gently while at the same time preventing any instrument from injuring the dural sac or nerve root.

Trials are used and the proper height decided based upon the fit of the trial. It is at this time that the lamina spreader may be temporarily removed to get a better sense of the fit of the trial. It can be placed back into position prior to final placement of the interbody device. By trialing and placing the interbody device with the lamina spreader in place, we feel that proper disc height is more closely restored while at the same time providing an indirect decompression of the formina. However, one must be careful so as not to over-distract the disc space, which may result in over-stuffing the disc space with an interbody too large longitudinally, resulting in either a traction injury to the traversing nerve roots and/or point loading and graft subsidence into the end plate. Typically, modern interbody cages have a threaded hole which allows an insertion device to impact them into the disc space with a mallet, and then can be unscrewed to easily disengage from the impacted interbody without disrupting the tight fit obtained with impaction.

Once the PLIF procedure has been performed, pedicle screws are placed through the previously cannulated pedicle screw holes. Alternatively, pedicle screws can be placed prior to the PLIF procedure and can be used for distraction of the disc space. However, in older and osteoporotic patients, we avoid using pedicle screws for distraction of the disc space or for reduction of a spondylolisthesis out of concern for loosening of the screws and weakening their pullout strength with these maneuvers [31].

Reduction of Spondylolisthesis and Deformity Correction Using the PLIF

Spondylolisthesis, if significant, can be reduced or fused in situ. No definitive evidence exists for better functional outcomes with reduction versus fusion in situ and in most situations, a grade 1 spondylolisthesis can be left in situ. However, if the surgeon desires reduction of a grade 2 degenerative or high grade isthmic spondylolisthesis, which may benefit the overall sagittal balance of the patient, various reduction maneuvers have been described. Reduction can be obtained with simple prone positioning on the table. It can also be obtained by various pedicle screw construct maneuvers with rods or plates. The reduction can also be obtained by performing the PLIF procedure with an insert and rotate method of distraction [32, 33] (Fig. 13.2).

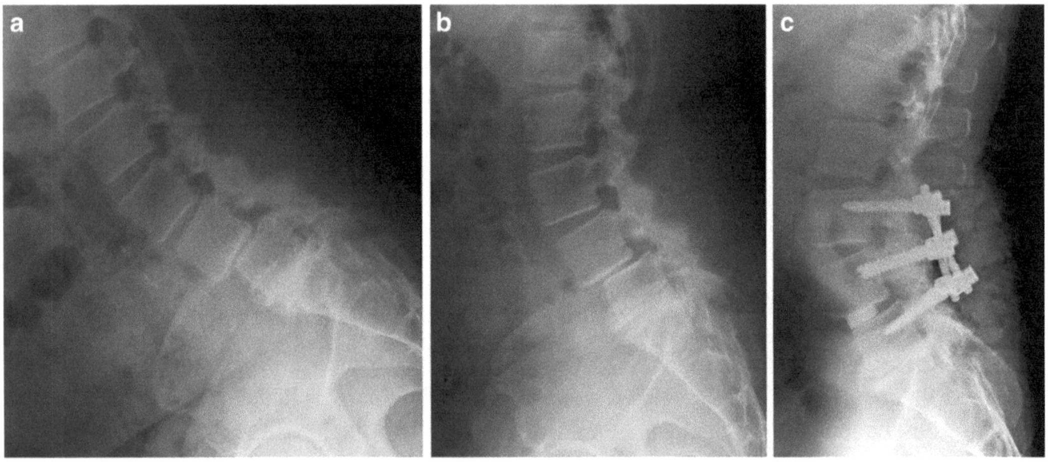

Fig. 13.2 A 55-year-old male presented with neuroclaudication in the legs and severe back pain after having failed nonoperative treatment. (**a**, **b**) Flexion and extension radiographs showed an L4–5 degenerative spondylolisthesis with kyphotic collapse as well as a slight spondylolisthesis at L3–4 with fluid in the L3–4 facet joints on preoperative MRI. (**c**) The patient underwent posterior lumbar decompression and fusion from L3–5 with PLIF at L4–5. PLIF trialing and insertion successfully reduced the L4–5 spondylolisthesis and restored lordosis. His back pain and leg symptoms resolved subsequently

In terms of coronal deformity correction, we typically elect to perform a TLIF over a PLIF, as removing the entire inferior facet of the cepahalad vertebrae helps to mobilize the spinal motion segment best. If a unilateral PLIF is performed, it should be performed on the side of the concavity of the curve. Techniques which can be used to distract a collapsed disc space include using a lamina spreader across the spinous processes; temporary rod placement on the pedicle screws to hold the disc space distracted while the PLIF is performed; custom distracters which attach to the pedicle screws and are available with most modern pedicle screw systems; disc space distracters once the annulotomy and discectomy is performed [22]. Caution should be used when using pedicle screws for distraction or reduction purposes in osteoporotic individuals [31].

Depth

The depth of the PLIF should be carefully followed. The distance of most lumbar disc endplates from posterior to anterior is approximately 30 mm. However, it is always a good idea to measure the distance of the disc space from posterior to anterior on preoperative axial MRI or CT scan. Modern interbody instrumentation systems have etchings which allow the surgeon to be aware of the depth of the instrumentation at all times during the procedure. While as much disc material as possible should be removed to promote a solid fusion, depth penetration of greater than 30 mm from the posterior longitudinal line to anterior risks violation of the anterior longitudinal ligament (ALL) and retroperitoneal great vessel injury.

While not wanting to violate the ALL, the goal should be to place the interbody as anteriorly as possible within the disc space in order to restore the sagittal alignment and normal lordosis of the intervertebral level [15]. Placing the interbody anteriorly also decreases the likelihood of the graft migrating posteriorly into the spinal canal.

Unilateral Versus Bilateral PLIF

Depending on the clinical scenario, bilateral PLIF procedures may be indicated. If the patient has a degenerative scoliosis due to asymmetric disc space collapse, the surgeon may elect to place a unilateral PLIF on the collapsed side, which acts as a shim to prop open the collapsed space and correct the curve due to it.

If the disc space is completely and symmetrically collapsed, there may be a benefit to performing bilateral PLIF procedures. By performing bilateral PLIFs, a more thorough discectomy can be performed as the disc is removed from both sides of the posterior canal. Also bilateral PLIFs provide greater end plate interbody surface area. Using bilateral PLIFs theoretically increases the likelihood of fusion and lessens the likelihood of graft subsidence due to point loading; however, there is very little evidence from the literature to support this view. A retrospective study comparing 88 cases of unilateral PLIF to 99 cases of bilateral PLIF found no significant differences in visual analog scale, Oswestry disability index, lumbar lordosis, lumbar scoliotic angles, fusion level scoliotic angles, or fixation stabilities [34]. However, the unilateral PLIF group had a significantly lower operative time than the bilateral PLIF group. Molinari et al. retrospectively compared unilateral to bilateral PLIF in a military population and found no difference in hospital stay, fusion rates, pain levels, functional outcomes, or patient satisfaction [35]. However, the bilateral procedure resulted in a higher incidence of dural tears and an average increased cost of $1,728 per patient.

When electing to perform a unilateral PLIF, we chose to perform the PLIF on the most symptomatic side in terms of leg pain, which should correlate to the more stenotic side on MRI. Also, if there is asymmetric disc space collapse, the PLIF is placed on the collapsed side. When the patient has severe bilateral leg symptoms and the disc space is symmetrically collapsed, a bilateral procedure with interbody cages may be elected.

Cage Selection and the Use of RhBMP2

The choice of the type of interbody graft to use is largely surgeon dependent. Various materials have been used for the interbody device to promote fusion. These include iliac crest bone graft, other forms of autograft including the spinous process and lamina, allograft bone, titanium cages, threaded cages (e.g., Bagby and Kuslich [BAK]), polymeric rectangular cages (e.g. Brantigan cage), and various synthetic ceramic and polymeric cages. While autologous structural iliac crest is considered the gold standard, it is typically no longer used except in the case of revision or infection due to the donor site morbidity. Studies have shown varying success with multiple different materials without one definitively better bone graft alternative [36]. More studies are needed to elucidate the best form of interbody graft; however, we feel that proper discectomy and endplate preparation may be more important in promoting fusion than the type of bone graft or bone graft equivalent used.

The use of RhBMP-2 has become common in spinal fusion surgery based largely on industry sponsored studies. However, higher levels of evidence and systematic critical reviews of the existing literature have failed to show a benefit of RhBMP-2 and increased complication rates with its use. Complications associated with RhBMP-2 include endplate osteolysis, radiculitis, ectopic bone formation, and carcinogenic risk when used in high doses [37, 38]. Therefore, we do not recommend the use of RhBMP2 in the cage construct. Instead we pack local decompressed cancellous autologous bone graft into the interbody cage.

In addition to the type of interbody, the shape of the interbody is important to consider. A wedge-shaped interbody has been shown to restore lumbar lordosis and sagittal alignment better than a rectangular-shaped alternative [39]. In terms of other dimensions, bullet-shaped and banana-shaped cages are also available. A biomechanical study comparing different cage shapes in the setting of TLIF did not find a difference in construct stability when used in conjunction with pedicle screw fixation [40]. This would seem to apply to cage shapes for PLIF as well. Another biomechanical study comparing two small posterolateral cages, one small anterior banana cage, and one central rectangular cage found no significant differences in failure forces across the endplates or the stiffness of the motion segment in compression [41]. However, banana-shaped cages typically have a greater surface area and are better suited for a TLIF as they can span the disc space when inserted from a posterolateral position and allow for greater surface area to promoted fusion. When performing a PLIF, a straight cage is used typically and if greater surface area to promote fusion is desired, then consideration should be given to performing bilateral PLIF procedures.

Complications: Prevention and Management

Great Vessel Injury

Great vessel injury is an extremely rare but devastating injury that the surgeon should be aware of during the PLIF procedure. The incidence of great vessel injury during lumbar discectomy is unknown due to underreporting of complications and specifically those resulting in death, but it is estimated to 0.01 and 2.4 % of lumbar discectomies [28–30]. Case reports exist of uncontrolled hemorrhage and death with great vessel injury specifically during the PLIF procedure [42]. If anterior penetration of the ALL occurs, there is a risk of injury to the great vessels depending on the level being fused. This is why it is extremely important to be aware of the depth of the instruments being used to perform the discectomy and modern day instrumentation systems have markings on them to better judge their depth. As a general rule, one should not penetrate further than 30 mm from the posterior to anterior disc space to avoid ALL disruption.

The key to patient survival and recovery when a great vessel injury is early recognition of the injury and emergent vascular surgery evaluation. In some situations, injury to a retroperitoneal great vessel may be somewhat obvious, recognizable by hemorrhage in the disc space or acute sudden hypotension intraoperatively. It also may be recognized immediately postoperatively when the patient is flipped and becomes hypotensive with a distended abdomen. In other situations, the injury may result in an arteriovenous fistula or pseudoaneurysm not recognized until months later. Treatment of vascular injury involves either open repair via a retroperitoneal approach or angiography and endovascular repair, depending on the preferences of the vascular team and stability of the patient [43].

Adjacent Segment Degeneration

Whether or not ASD is a complication of interbody fusion and spinal arthrodesis in general or is rather part of the natural history of disc degeneration and arthritis has yet to be fully elucidated from the literature [44]. The overall incidence of ASD after a PLIF procedure was shown in one study to be 33 % at 2 years postoperatively with a 29 % incidence of radiographic progression and a 4 % incidence of both radiologic and clinical ASD [45]. Multiple studies have shown that ASD is due to multiple factors including age-related disc degeneration as well as disruption of surrounding segmental stabilizing structures during the decompression and fusion procedure. Cadaveric biomechanical studies have shown that the ALIF, which is typically larger and has more surface area in contact with the endplates, better restores the natural stress distribution pattern of adjacent levels than the PLIF [46]. One clinical study found a statistically significant higher incidence of ASD after the PLIF procedure than the ALIF procedure [23]. Total disc arthroplasty was developed as an alternative to fusion with this in mind in order to preserve or lessen the degree of stiffness and adjacent level stresses. A systematic review of the literature found weak evidence to support the effectiveness of total disc arthroplasty compared to arthrodesis to prevent ASD; however, increasing patient age also had a strong effect on ASD [47]. We do not view total disc arthroplasty in the lumbar spine as a viable alternative to arthrodesis based on the evidence from the literature.

One study retrospectively examined risk factors for ASD after the PLIF procedure in 87 patients with a history of L4–5 degenerative spondylolisis at 2 years postoperatively [45]. In 58 patients (67 %), there was no progression of ASD. In 25 patients (29 %), there was progression of ASD at L3–4 but no neurologic decline. In four patients (4 %), there was progression of ASD and neurologic decline at that level and subsequent surgery. No preoperative radiologic signs could be identified as risk factors for radiologic ASD. L3 laminar horizontalization and L3/4 facet tropism were identified as risk factors for clinically significant ASD, although it is difficult to draw any conclusions from a group of only four patients. While ASD may be accelerated by the use of arthrodesis and interbody fusion, it may also be part of the natural history and should not prevent the surgeon and patient from considering an interbody fusion or PLIF specifically. The best surgeon-controlled technique of preventing ASD is to not violate the adjacent level facet joints, which are not part of the planned fusion levels.

Neurologic Injury

Neurologic injury from a PLIF procedure is an uncommon but serious adverse complication. Often referred to as a "battered nerve root syndrome," it is believed to result from excessive or prolonged retraction on the nerve root during discectomy procedures, including PLIF [48]. One argument for the use of TLIF and other interbody techniques over the PLIF procedure is that minimal to no retraction of the dural sac or nerve roots is necessary with these alternatives. Evidence from the literature does show a trend toward a higher incidence of neurologic injury with the PLIF compared to other interbody procedures although it is equivocal. For instance, in one retrospective comparative study comparing 39 patients who underwent ALIF to 35 patients who underwent PLIF, one patient who underwent the ALIF suffered a neurologic injury due to the type of interbody used, while no patients in the PLIF group suffered neurologic injuries [49]. The XLIF has its own concerns for neurologic injury not to nerve roots but the lumbar plexus.

Many argue that the TLIF is a better procedure than the PLIF based on a lower incidence of neurologic injury, and the evidence from the literature, while not a high level, points to this being true. In a retrospective study comparing 40 patients who underwent TLIF to 34 patients who underwent PLIF, there were four cases (11.8 %) of neurologic injury in the PLIF group versus no cases of neurologic injury in the TLIF group [50]. The authors did not report on whether or not this was a statistically significant difference or whether the neurologic injuries were transient or permanent [50]. In another retrospective comparative study, 76 patients who underwent PLIF were compared to 43 patients who underwent TLIF. While there was a trend toward a higher incidence of iatrogenic nerve root dysfunction in the PLIF group versus the TLIF group (6 [7.8 %] versus 1 [2 %] respectively), this difference did not reach statistical significance [51]. Furthermore, in all patients who suffered nerve root dysfunction, the morbidity was transient and resolved by 3 months postoperatively.

It is believed that neurologic injury during the procedure may be a result of excessive and/or prolonged retraction on the nerve root. In a study of 31 patients who underwent posterior lumbar discectomy, a pressure transducer was used to measure the amount of retraction on the traversing nerve root as well as the length of retraction [52]. In the four of 31 patients with the highest retraction pressure, all had transient sensory changes postoperatively in the distribution of the retracted nerve root. The time of retraction was also longer by greater than 4 min on average in this group than in the rest of the patients. The study supports the assertion that nerve root dysfunction is likely the result of excessive and/or prolonged retraction on the nerve root during the procedure. Therefore, in order to prevent neurologic injury, the discectomy and interbody placement should be performed as quickly but as safely as possible to limit the amount of nerve root retraction.

Durotomy

Durotomy during the PLIF procedure can occur with either the decompressive laminectomy and medial facetectomy or during the discectomy and interbody placement. It is not at all certain that a well-repaired durotomy has any short- or long-term clinically adverse effects. In an analysis of 389 patients with degenerative spondylolisthesis from the spine patient outcomes research trial (SPORT) who underwent decompressive laminectomy with or without fusion, there was a 10.5 % incidence of durotomy [53]. The authors found no difference in incidence of nerve root injury, mortality, additional surgeries, SF-36 body pain and physical function, or Oswestry Disability Index at 1, 2, 3, and 4 years postoperatively. While the clinical consequences of a repaired durotomy are equivocal, the medicolegal ramifications are not: incidental durotomy was reported as the second leading cause of lawsuits in spine surgery [54].

Much like neurologic injury, it is believed durotomy is more common with the PLIF procedure than other interbody procedures, including the TLIF, because less dural sac and nerve root manipulation is required with the TLIF procedure. However, high levels of evidence from the literature are sparse on this topic. In a retrospective study comparing 40 patients who underwent TLIF to 34 patients who underwent PLIF, there was a higher incidence of durotomy in the PLIF group compared to TLIF group (13 [17 %] versus 4 [9 %]), though this was not a statistically significant difference [51].

While durotomy is often attributable to multiple factors, including epidural fibrosis, revision surgery, ossification of the ligamentum flavum, and synovial cysts, meticulous surgical technique should help minimize the risk of durotomy [55]. The dural sac should be as freely mobile as possible prior to retraction. That is, the epidural leash that is typically present ventrally in the spinal canal should be carefully cauterized with bipolar cuatery without cauterizing the dura or nerve roots, and then gently and bluntly swept away with a penfield 4 or other blunt instrument. This should be freed over the disc space as well as cephalad and cuadad to it. If performed appropriately, the dural sac should be more easily mobilized for safe retraction, otherwise there is a risk of tearing the dural sac either dorsally or ventrally, which is extremely challenging to repair. This careful but thorough cauterization also helps to control hemostasis from epidural bleeding during the discectomy and interbody placement.

If an incidental durotomy does occur during any portion of the procedure, the most important thing is to recognize and address it adequately. While the clinical consequences of a durotomy recognized and repaired intraoperatively are debatable, unrepaired or inadequately repaired durotomies may lead to persistence of cerebrospinal fluid leakage, pseudomeningocele, arachnoiditis, meningitis, and sepsis [56–58].

When recognized intraoperatively, the durotomy should undergo a direct repair if repairable. We advocate suture repair with 6-0 goretex, as well as duragen, fat graft, and fibrin glue sprayed over the repair at the end of the case. Traditional recommendations are that the patient should be on bedrest for at least 24 h postoperatively. A retrospective comparative study of 61 patients repaired with fibrin glue did not show any difference in complication rate between patients mobilized on postoperative day one, two, or three, and advocated mobilization as quickly as possible to decrease length of hospital stay and length of care [59]. We agree that as long as a good repair is achieved, the patient can be mobilized on postoperative day one and monitored for spinal headache, which if does occur, mobilization should be slowed.

Ventral dural tears may be technically challenging or nearly impossible to repair. Various techniques of addressing them have been described, including a pull through repair, indirect repair with overlying free fat graft and overlying muscle, or covering with fibrin glue [60]. In cases such as these when a direct repair cannot be performed, we recommend that the patient be kept flat for at least 24 h postoperatively and then closely monitored with mobilization for any sign of spinal headache.

Interbody Migration

Although rare, the exact incidence of implant migration varies by study. While anterior migration of the interbody has been described in a case report [61], the much more common complication related to cage migration is posterior migration. Early posterior cage migration results in loss of the lumbar lordosis obtained with the procedure, and if cage migration into the spinal canal occurs, can result in neurologic compromise due to dural sac or nerve root impingement. Cage migration also suggests that the spinal motion segment is not rigidly stabilized. One retrospective study of 118 patients who underwent bilateral PLIF using paired BAK cages at a single level found three patients who experienced cage migration [62]. All patients with cage migration had undergone uninstrumented fusion and no patients who underwent instrumented fusion with pedicle screws experienced cage migration. The study confirms that well-placed pedicle screw fixation used concurrently provides immediate stability to the motion segment and may prevent movement of the cage. In another study of 1,070 patients, posterior cage migration with the PLIF procedure occurred in nine patients (0.008 % incidence) [63]. The authors noted the risk of posterior migration was associated with PLIF at L5–S1, a higher disc height, and a pear shaped disc space.

In the early postoperative period, cage migration suggests construct instability and poor pressfit impaction of the interbody graft. If the cage has migrated into the spinal canal, we recommend revision surgery with removal of the PLIF and placement of a larger graft. If the patient is asymptomatic, the options should be discussed, including revision surgery and observation to see if they fuse without pain or neurologic deficit.

Pseudarthrosis/Failure of Fusion

The PLIF procedure has fusion rates that are reported to be between 90 and 100 % [8–10, 21, 51, 64]. We consider pseudarthrosis to be failure of fusion by 6 months postoperatively seen radiographically. Pseudarthrosis should be suspected by lack of visible bridging bone of the graft endplate interface, movement of the fused motion segment on flexion/extension films or pedicle screw loosening or implant failure on radiographs, and should be confirmed by CT scan, which will show no evidence of bridging callus. Because a posterolateral fusion is performed in conjunction with the PLIF, we consider a construct to have successfully fused if any of the three fusion interfaces has bridging callus. Even if the PLIF fails to fuse if one or both posterolateral fusions have healed, the construct is considered fused and stable. Risk factors for pseudarthrosis include smoking, diabetes, and steroid and non-steroidal usage [65].

No high level evidence exists for standard treatment recommendations, and the choice of operative treatment is dictated by the clinical scenario. Radiographic evidence of pseudarthrosis without evidence of pedicle screw or rod failure, and no sign of interbody migration can be managed with observation. However, if the patient has significant back pain, implant loosening or failure, or interbody migration, operative intervention with fusion exploration and revision surgery is indicated [66]. A metabolic workup should be performed and infection should be ruled out with MRI and inflammatory laboratory markers. Assuming no sign of infection, we perform an ALIF procedure through a retroperitoneal approach to remove the PLIF cage, debride the disc space of fibrous tissue, scrape the endplates to bleeding bone, and place structural iliac crest autograft into the disc space. By performing this through the anterior approach, epidural fibrosis and scarring from the prior PLIF path may be avoided. If the pedicle screw constructs are loose or broken, we then turn the patient prone and revise the pedicle screw construct with larger screws and if necessary extend the construct to the pelvis in order to obtain stable fixation. We use cancellous iliac crest bone graft in the posterolateral gutters if fusion has failed in these locations.

Infection

Infected interbody fusions are uncommon but extremely challenging to treat. One large retrospective study of posterior fusions of the thoracolumbar spine found an infection rate of 3.5 % (26 of 737 patients) [67]. Nineteen patients had early postoperative infections and the remaining seven had late onset infection. In order to reduce the risk of infection, we irrigate the wound with 3 L of bacitracin-injected normal saline at the end of the procedure and prior to bone graft application of the posterolateral gutters. We then place vancomycin powder (1 g) in the wound at the end of the case as studies have shown it to decrease the risk of postoperative infection [68].

Oftentimes, signs of infection are obvious, with draining wound or erythema, fever, chills, increased back pain, or florid sepsis. In a septic patient with purulent drainage from the wound, the patient should be taken for irrigation and debridement emergently, serial debridements and possible implant removal if infection persists. Cultures should be taken at the time of initial debridement and intravenous antibiotics tailored to the isolated organisms for at least 6 weeks.

There is no high level evidence from the literature to guide the treatment of infected pseudarthroses. Ha and Kim retrospectively reported on a series of ten patients with infected PLIF pseudarthroses [69]. They all underwent anterior retroperitoneal removal of the interbody with disc space debridement and structure iliac crest autograft as well as removal of posterior implants and serial debridements. Five of ten patients were infected with methicillin resistant *Staphylococcus aureus* (MRSA). In all ten patients the infection was cleared through this treatment and in nine of ten the pseudarthrosis went on to fuse. However, another retrospective study of 111 patients who underwent the PLIF procedure found eight patients (7.2 %) who were treated for a deep infection. In six of eight patients the PLIF cage was left in place and in two of eight patients the cage was revised from a posterior approach [70]. All eight patients went on to clear the infection with long-term antibiotics and heal their fusion.

Infection can occur with hematogenous seeding several months to years after the operation. Late infection with a successful fusion having already occurred entails implants removal and thorough debridement of infected and necrotic tissue followed by long-term antibiotics [67].

In cases of infected pseudarthrosis, where the fusion failed to heal and infection is present, management entails initial debridement followed by serial debridements, removal of the interbody device if not fused, typically from an anterior retroperitoneal approach at which structural autologous iliac crest can be placed into the disc space; followed by removal and exchange of all metal implants, with extension of the fusion if fixation is poor. Typically this involves extension to the pelvis in the case of an L5–S1 interbody fusion. Not only does the anterior retroperitoneal approach enable a thorough disc space and endplate debridement and PLIF removal, but if a concomitant paraspinal psoas abscess exists, which is often the case, this can be directly debrided through the same approach.

Depending on the state of the soft tissues, multiple irrigation and debridements should be performed prior to final implant placement. Negative pressure wound therapy (vacuum-assisted closure device) may be used for wounds left open between debridements and in some cases may be used to allow the wound to heal by secondary intention depending on the state of the soft tissues [71]. The vacuum sponge should not be placed directly over the dura, and it should be carefully monitored for high output or significant blood loss in the canister [72]. Plastic surgery may be consulted to create paraspinal muscle flaps to ensure a good closure with vascularized muscle, which has been found to have good results in a retrospective study [73].

Conclusion

The PLIF procedure is a technically demanding procedure with defined and limited indications. It is indicated at lumbar levels below the level of the conus medullaris in the setting of degenerative scoliosis to restore coronal and sagittal balance and promote fusion, some cases of degenerative spondylolisthesis or isthmic spondylolisthesis to indirectly reduce foraminal compression and restore sagittal balance, and may be indicated as a procedure for recurrent disc herniation. The TLIF procedure can also be used for any of these indications, and the decision to perform a TLIF versus a PLIF is largely based on surgeon preference. The PLIF may have a higher complication rate in terms of dural tear and neurologic nerve root injury due to greater retraction on the dural sac. However, fusion rates in the PLIF procedure are historically high and if complications can be avoided and managed, long-term patient satisfaction may be achieved.

References

1. Cloward RB. The treatment of ruptured lumbar intervertebral discs by vertebral body fusion. I. Indications, operative technique, after care. J Neurosurg. 1953; 10:154–68.
2. Lin PM. A technical modification of Cloward's posterior lumbar interbody fusion. Neurosurgery. 1977;1:118–24.
3. Elias WJ, Simmons NE, Kaptain GJ, Chadduck JB, Whitehill R. Complications of posterior lumbar interbody fusion when using a titanium threaded cage device. J Neurosurg. 2000;93:45–52.
4. Steffee AD, Sitkowski DJ. Posterior lumbar interbody fusion and plates. Clin Orthop Relat Res. 1988;227: 99–102.
5. Schnee CL, Freese A, Ansell LV. Outcome analysis for adults with spondylolisthesis treated with posterolateral fusion and transpedicular screw fixation. J Neurosurg. 1997;86:56–63.
6. Schwab FJ, Nazarian DG, Mahmud F, Michelsen CB. Effects of spinal instrumentation on fusion of the lumbosacral spine. Spine. 1995;20:2023–8.
7. Wood 2nd GW, Boyd RJ, Carothers TA, et al. The effect of pedicle screw/plate fixation on lumbar/lumbosacral autogenous bone graft fusions in patients

with degenerative disc disease. Spine. 1995;20: 819–30.
8. Brantigan JW, Steffee AD, Lewis ML, Quinn LM, Persenaire JM. Lumbar interbody fusion using the Brantigan I/F cage for posterior lumbar interbody fusion and the variable pedicle screw placement system: two-year results from a Food and Drug Administration investigational device exemption clinical trial. Spine. 2000;25:1437–46.
9. Brantigan JW, Neidre A, Toohey JS. The lumbar I/F cage for posterior lumbar interbody fusion with the variable screw placement system: 10-year results of a Food and Drug Administration clinical trial. Spine J. 2004;4:681–8.
10. Dehoux E, Fourati E, Madi K, Reddy B, Segal P. Posterolateral versus interbody fusion in isthmic spondylolisthesis: functional results in 52 cases with a minimum follow-up of 6 years. Acta Orthop Belg. 2004;70:578–82.
11. Ekman P, Moller H, Tullberg T, Neumann P, Hedlund R. Posterior lumbar interbody fusion versus posterolateral fusion in adult isthmic spondylolisthesis. Spine. 2007;32:2178–83.
12. Chrastil J, Patel AA. Complications associated with posterior and transforaminal lumbar interbody fusion. J Am Acad Orthop Surg. 2012;20:283–91.
13. Jacobs WC, Vreeling A, De Kleuver M. Fusion for low-grade adult isthmic spondylolisthesis: a systematic review of the literature. Eur Spine J. 2006; 15:391–402.
14. Wu CH, Wong CB, Chen LH, Niu CC, Tsai TT, Chen WJ. Instrumented posterior lumbar interbody fusion for patients with degenerative lumbar scoliosis. J Spinal Disord Tech. 2008;21:310–5.
15. Kwon BK, Berta S, Daffner SD, et al. Radiographic analysis of transforaminal lumbar interbody fusion for the treatment of adult isthmic spondylolisthesis. J Spinal Disord Tech. 2003;16:469–76.
16. Chitnavis B, Barbagallo G, Selway R, Dardis R, Hussain A, Gullan R. Posterior lumbar interbody fusion for revision disc surgery: review of 50 cases in which carbon fiber cages were implanted. J Neurosurg. 2001;95:190–5.
17. Brox JI, Sorensen R, Friis A, et al. Randomized clinical trial of lumbar instrumented fusion and cognitive intervention and exercises in patients with chronic low back pain and disc degeneration. Spine. 2003; 28:1913–21.
18. Mirza SK, Deyo RA. Systematic review of randomized trials comparing lumbar fusion surgery to nonoperative care for treatment of chronic back pain. Spine. 2007;32:816–23.
19. Fritzell P, Hagg O, Wessberg P, Nordwall A, Swedish Lumbar Spine Study Group. Chronic low back pain and fusion: a comparison of three surgical techniques: a prospective multicenter randomized study from the Swedish lumbar spine study group. Spine. 2002;27: 1131–41.
20. Sakaura H, Yamashita T, Miwa T, Ohzono K, Ohwada T. Outcomes of 2-level posterior lumbar interbody fusion for 2-level degenerative lumbar spondylolisthesis. J Neurosurg Spine. 2013;19(1):90–4.
21. Enker P, Steffee AD. Interbody fusion and instrumentation. Clin Orthop Relat Res. 1994;300:90–101.
22. Dorward IG, Lenke LG, Bridwell KH, et al. Transforaminal versus anterior lumbar interbody fusion in long deformity constructs: a matched cohort analysis. Spine. 2013;38(12):E755–62.
23. Min JH, Jang JS, Lee SH. Comparison of anterior- and posterior-approach instrumented lumbar interbody fusion for spondylolisthesis. J Neurosurg Spine. 2007;7:21–6.
24. Banagan K, Gelb D, Poelstra K, Ludwig S. Anatomic mapping of lumbar nerve roots during a direct lateral transpsoas approach to the spine: a cadaveric study. Spine. 2011;36:E687–91.
25. Ahmadian A, Deukmedjian AR, Abel N, Dakwar E, Uribe JS. Analysis of lumbar plexopathies and nerve injury after lateral retroperitoneal transpsoas approach: diagnostic standardization. J Neurosurg Spine. 2013; 18:289–97.
26. Harms J, Rolinger H. A one-stager procedure in operative treatment of spondylolistheses: dorsal traction-reposition and anterior fusion (author's transl). Z Orthop Ihre Grenzgeb. 1982;120:343–7.
27. Xu H, Tang H, Guan X, et al. Biomechanical comparison of posterior lumbar interbody fusion and transforaminal lumbar interbody fusion by finite element analysis. Neurosurgery. 2013;72:21–6.
28. Goodkin R, Laska LL. Vascular and visceral injuries associated with lumbar disc surgery: medicolegal implications. Surg Neurol. 1998;49:358–70. discussion 70–2.
29. Papadoulas S, Konstantinou D, Kourea HP, Kritikos N, Haftouras N, Tsolakis JA. Vascular injury complicating lumbar disc surgery. A systematic review. Eur J Vasc Endovasc Surg. 2002;24:189–95.
30. Szolar DH, Preidler KW, Steiner H, et al. Vascular complications in lumbar disk surgery: report of four cases. Neuroradiology. 1996;38:521–5.
31. Paik H, Kang DG, Lehman Jr RA, Gaume RE, Ambati DV, Dmitriev AE. The biomechanical consequences of rod reduction on pedicle screws: should it be avoided? Spine J. 2013;13(11):1617–26.
32. Jaslow IA. Intercorporal bone graft in spinal fusion after disc removal. Surg Gynecol Obstet. 1946;82: 215–8.
33. Sears W. Posterior lumbar interbody fusion for degenerative spondylolisthesis: restoration of sagittal balance using insert-and-rotate interbody spacers. Spine J. 2005;5:170–9.
34. Lee JH, Lee JH, Yoon KS, Kang SB, Jo CH. Comparative study of unilateral and bilateral cages with respect to clinical outcomes and stability in instrumented posterior lumbar interbody fusion. Neurosurgery. 2008;63:109–13. discussion 13–4.
35. Molinari RW, Sloboda J, Johnstone FL. Are 2 cages needed with instrumented PLIF? A comparison of 1 versus 2 interbody cages in a military population. Am J Orthop. 2003;32:337–43. discussion 43.

36. Rihn JA, Kirkpatrick K, Albert TJ. Graft options in posterolateral and posterior interbody lumbar fusion. Spine. 2010;35:1629–39.
37. Haid Jr RW, Branch Jr CL, Alexander JT, Burkus JK. Posterior lumbar interbody fusion using recombinant human bone morphogenetic protein type 2 with cylindrical interbody cages. Spine J. 2004;4:527–38. discussion 38–9.
38. Carragee EJ, Hurwitz EL, Weiner BK. A critical review of recombinant human bone morphogenetic protein-2 trials in spinal surgery: emerging safety concerns and lessons learned. Spine J. 2011;11: 471–91.
39. Godde S, Fritsch E, Dienst M, Kohn D. Influence of cage geometry on sagittal alignment in instrumented posterior lumbar interbody fusion. Spine. 2003;28: 1693–9.
40. Cho W, Wu C, Mehbod AA, Transfeldt EE. Comparison of cage designs for transforaminal lumbar interbody fusion: a biomechanical study. Clin Biomech (Bristol, Avon). 2008;23:979–85.
41. Lam FC, Alkalay R, Groff MW. The effects of design and positioning of carbon fiber lumbar interbody cages and their subsidence in vertebral bodies. J Spinal Disord Tech. 2012;25:116–22.
42. Postacchini R, Cinotti G, Postacchini F. Injury to major abdominal vessels during posterior lumbar interbody fusion. A case report and review of the literature. Spine J. 2013;13:e7–11.
43. van Zitteren M, Fan B, Lohle PN, et al. A shift toward endovascular repair for vascular complications in lumbar disc surgery during the last decade. Ann Vasc Surg. 2013;27(6):810–9.
44. Helgeson MD, Bevevino AJ, Hilibrand AS. Update on the evidence for adjacent segment degeneration and disease. Spine J. 2013;13:342–51.
45. Okuda S, Iwasaki M, Miyauchi A, Aono H, Morita M, Yamamoto T. Risk factors for adjacent segment degeneration after PLIF. Spine. 2004;29:1535–40.
46. Kumar N, Judith MR, Kumar A, Mishra V, Robert MC. Analysis of stress distribution in lumbar interbody fusion. Spine. 2005;30:1731–5.
47. Harrop JS, Youssef JA, Maltenfort M, et al. Lumbar adjacent segment degeneration and disease after arthrodesis and total disc arthroplasty. Spine. 2008; 33:1701–7.
48. Bertrand G. The "battered" root problem. Orthop Clin North Am. 1975;6:305–10.
49. Madan SS, Boeree NR. Comparison of instrumented anterior interbody fusion with instrumented circumferential lumbar fusion. Eur Spine J. 2003;12: 567–75.
50. Humphreys SC, Hodges SD, Patwardhan AG, Eck JC, Murphy RB, Covington LA. Comparison of posterior and transforaminal approaches to lumbar interbody fusion. Spine. 2001;26:567–71.
51. Mehta VA, McGirt MJ, Garces Ambrossi GL, et al. Trans-foraminal versus posterior lumbar interbody fusion: comparison of surgical morbidity. Neurol Res. 2011;33:38–42.
52. Matsui H, Kitagawa H, Kawaguchi Y, Tsuji H. Physiologic changes of nerve root during posterior lumbar discectomy. Spine. 1995;20:654–9.
53. Desai A, Ball PA, Bekelis K, et al. Surgery for lumbar degenerative spondylolisthesis in spine patient outcomes research trial: does incidental durotomy affect outcome? Spine. 2012;37:406–13.
54. Goodkin R, Laska LL. Unintended "incidental" durotomy during surgery of the lumbar spine: medicolegal implications. Surg Neurol. 1995;43:4–12. discussion 12–4.
55. Epstein NE. The frequency and etiology of intraoperative dural tears in 110 predominantly geriatric patients undergoing multilevel laminectomy with noninstrumented fusions. J Spinal Disord Tech. 2007;20:380–6.
56. Eismont FJ, Wiesel SW, Rothman RH. Treatment of dural tears associated with spinal surgery. J Bone Joint Surg Am. 1981;63:1132–6.
57. Koo J, Adamson R, Wagner Jr FC, Hrdy DB. A new cause of chronic meningitis: infected lumbar pseudomeningocele. Am J Med. 1989;86:103–4.
58. Cammisa Jr FP, Girardi FP, Sangani PK, Parvataneni HK, Cadag S, Sandhu HS. Incidental durotomy in spine surgery. Spine. 2000;25:2663–7.
59. Low JC, von Niederhausern B, Rutherford SA, King AT. Pilot study of perioperative accidental durotomy: does the period of postoperative bed rest reduce the incidence of complication? Br J Neurosurg. 2013;27(6):800–2.
60. Lin PM. Posterior lumbar interbody fusion technique: complications and pitfalls. Clin Orthop Relat Res. 1985;193:90–102.
61. Proubasta IR, Vallve EQ, Aguilar LF, Villanueva CL, Iglesias JJ. Intraoperative antepulsion of a fusion cage in posterior lumbar interbody fusion: a case report and review of the literature. Spine. 2002;27:E399–402.
62. Chen L, Yang H, Tang T. Cage migration in spondylolisthesis treated with posterior lumbar interbody fusion using BAK cages. Spine. 2005;30:2171–5.
63. Kimura H, Shikata J, Odate S, Soeda T, Yamamura S. Risk factors for cage retropulsion after posterior lumbar interbody fusion: analysis of 1070 cases. Spine. 2012;37:1164–9.
64. Musluman AM, Yilmaz A, Cansever T, et al. Posterior lumbar interbody fusion versus posterolateral fusion with instrumentation in the treatment of low-grade isthmic spondylolisthesis: midterm clinical outcomes. J Neurosurg Spine. 2011;14:488–96.
65. Larsen JM, Capen DA. Pseudarthrosis of the lumbar spine. J Am Acad Orthop Surg. 1997;5:153–62.
66. Fogel GR, Toohey JS, Neidre A, Brantigan JW. Fusion assessment of posterior lumbar interbody fusion using radiolucent cages: X-ray films and helical computed tomography scans compared with surgical exploration of fusion. Spine J. 2008;8:570–7.
67. Sierra-Hoffman M, Jinadatha C, Carpenter JL, Rahm M. Postoperative instrumented spine infections: a retrospective review. South Med J. 2010;103:25–30.
68. Sweet FA, Roh M, Sliva C. Intrawound application of vancomycin for prophylaxis in instrumented

thoracolumbar fusions: efficacy, drug levels, and patient outcomes. Spine. 2011;36:2084–8.
69. Ha KY, Kim YH. Postoperative spondylitis after posterior lumbar interbody fusion using cages. Eur Spine J. 2004;13:419–24.
70. Mirovsky Y, Floman Y, Smorgick Y, et al. Management of deep wound infection after posterior lumbar interbody fusion with cages. J Spinal Disord Tech. 2007; 20:127–31.
71. Mehbod AA, Ogilvie JW, Pinto MR, et al. Postoperative deep wound infections in adults after spinal fusion: management with vacuum-assisted wound closure. J Spinal Disord Tech. 2005;18:14–7.
72. Jones GA, Butler J, Lieberman I, Schlenk R. Negative-pressure wound therapy in the treatment of complex postoperative spinal wound infections: complications and lessons learned using vacuum-assisted closure. J Neurosurg Spine. 2007;6: 407–11.
73. Dumanian GA, Ondra SL, Liu J, Schafer MF, Chao JD. Muscle flap salvage of spine wounds with soft tissue defects or infection. Spine. 2003;28:1203–11.

Anterior Lumbar Interbody Fusion

14

Johnny Zhao, Jeffrey L. Gum, John R. Dimar II, and Jacob M. Buchowski

Abbreviations

ALIF	Anterior lumbar interbody fusion
HRQOL	Health related quality of life
PLIF	Posterior lumbar interbody fusion
RE	Retrograde ejaculation
rhBMP-2	Recombinant human bone morphogenetic protein-2
TLIF	Transforaminal lumbar interbody fusion

J. Zhao, M.D., M.S. • J.M. Buchowski, M.D., M.S. (✉)
Department of Orthopaedic Surgery, Center for Spinal Tumors, BJC Institute of Health, Washington University in St. Louis, 425 South Euclid Avenue, Campus Box 8233, St. Louis, MO 63110, USA
e-mail: buchowskij@wudosis.wustl.edu

J.L. Gum, M.D.
Adult and Pediatric Spine Surgeon, Norton Leatherman Spine Center, 210 East Gray Street, Suite 900, Louisville, KY 40202, USA
e-mail: jlgum001@gmail.com

J.R. Dimar II, M.D.
Department of Orthopaedic Surgery, University of Louisville School of Medicine, Norton Leatherman Spine Center, 550 South Jackson Street, First Floor ACB, Campus Box 8233, Louisville, KY 40205, USA
e-mail: John.Dimar@nortonhealthcare.org

History

In 1906, the German surgeon W. Muller reported the first attempted anterior access to the lumbar spine via a transperitoneal approach [1]. Although his patient did well, subsequent attempts revealed significant complications which delayed widespread acceptance of the approach. The first reports of an anterior approach for lumbar spinal fusion were later reported by Capener [2] in 1932 and by Burns [3] in 1933. Both Capener and Burns utilized a transperitoneal approach. It was not until over a decade later, in 1944, that Iwahara utilized the retroperitoneal approach for a lumbar spine fusion [4]. Shortly thereafter, other surgeons adopted and expanded the anterior lumbar interbody fusion (ALIF) to treat an increasing number of disorders. Lane and Moore reported treating degenerative disc diseases with ALIF in 1948 [5]. Two years later, a retroperitoneal ALIF was used to treat sciatica caused by lumbar disc protrusion [6].

In the 1950s and 1960s, much progress was made with regard to bone grafting techniques for ALIF. Hodgson and Stock were among the first to experiment with various bone grafting materials [7]. While he performed posterior-approach surgeries, Cloward [8] introduced the dowel technique for anterior cervical fusions, which was then adopted for the ALIF. With these rapid developments, published reports of fusion rates for ALIFs in this era were as high as 96 % [9, 10].

A.L. Wollowick and V. Sarwahi (eds.), *Spondylolisthesis: Diagnosis, Non-Surgical Management, and Surgical Techniques*, DOI 10.1007/978-1-4899-7575-1_14,

The next major development in ALIF was the incorporation of instrumentation. Cylindrical cages were the first of these devices and were initially used on humans in 1992 [11]. Once the Food and Drug Administration (FDA) approved the Bagby–Kuslich (BAK) cage in the lumbar spine in 1997, the interbody options exploded [12]. Modifications to the cages including shape, material, delivery method, surface design, and graft processing have been quick to market. Although the technology has certainly advanced, the number of spine surgeons utilizing ALIF procedures over the past 10–20 years has declined. Increased recognition of complications, debatable indications, the current medicolegal environment, and the increasing reliance on vascular access surgeons are all likely contributing to this decline. The predominant factor is most likely the evolution of posterior-only surgery and 3-column fixation with pedicle screws [13].

Preoperative Evaluation

Patients with spondylolisthesis that may potentially undergo an ALIF must be carefully evaluated. Plain radiographs including anterior–posterior (AP) and lateral views are a minimum requirement. Oblique views and coned-down or "spot" views are sometimes helpful to evaluate the foramen and target levels, respectively. Additionally, dynamic radiographs such as flexion and extension views are helpful to identify instability. Patients with gross instability evident on dynamic radiographs are likely to benefit most from a fusion-type procedure as the instability can be a significant source of pathology. Identification of disc degeneration and/or collapse is also important. Significant collapse can make insertion of a large interbody device and bone graft difficult. Advanced imaging such as computed tomography (CT) or magnetic resonance imaging (MRI) can be helpful as well, although not absolutely necessary. These modalities can help identify foraminal narrowing, central or lateral recess stenosis, or hypertrophied ligamentum flavum. Except for the use of indirect techniques, some of these are not possible to address via anterior surgery and must be carefully considered.

It is critical to identify comorbidities that may complicate the approach. Previous abdominal surgery with transperitoneal or retroperitoneal adhesions can be disastrous if not impossible to navigate. Vascular complications are the most common complication and thus, a detailed preoperative evaluation is imperative. Known calcific arterial disease can make repair difficult if needed and interferes with mobilization which is necessary depending on level to be accessed. Previous vascular procedures must be noted as well as any vascular anomalies. Attention to obesity is also important, especially abdominal-type obesity. Increased operative time, blood loss, complications, and difficulty with access are all well documented [14–16].

Retrograde ejaculation (RE) is a known complication of any anterior approach to the lumbar spine. Although RE is more common [17] via a transperitoneal approach, it still occurs after retroperitoneal access and therefore must be discussed with every male patient. Alternative conception plans can be utilized if discussed prior to this complication.

Identification of patients who are at high risk for pseudarthrosis (smokers, revision, infection, etc.) is critical as well. Anterior approaches have the advantage of direct visualization of the disc space. This provides a theoretical advantage of improved disc space preparation, which can in turn improve fusion rates.

Currently, there is debate regarding the use of an ALIF without some form of posterior fixation (stand-alone), particularly in cases where spinal instability may be present such as in patients with spondylolysis and/or spondylolisthesis. Circumferential fixation and fusion is biomechanically more desirable in such cases and can be clinically advantageous. In general, however, although revision rates as high as 31 % have been reported with stand-alone modern cages [18], more recent and larger studies dispute the necessity of a second surgery requiring posterior fixation reporting no difference in outcomes or revision rate [11, 19].

Surgical Technique

The surgical approach for an ALIF typically is divided into thoracolumbar (T12-L2), mid-lumbar (L2-L5), and lumbosacral (L5-S1). As previously described, spondylolisthesis more commonly occurs in the lower lumbar levels and thus, we will focus on mid-lumbar and lumbosacral approaches. Currently, the retroperitoneal approach (versus transperitoneal) is more commonly utilized. It offers an avascular plan and decreased manipulation of the bowel, which results in a lower complication rate. Recent reports describe laparoscopic access via a transperitoneal approach, but this method is correlated with increased risk of vascular injury combined with extended operative times and is therefore not discussed in this chapter. Most commonly, the transperitoneal approach is utilized in the setting of revision anterior surgery as the retroperitoneal adhesions are difficult to navigate.

Lumbar and Lumbosacral Retroperitoneal Approach

The patient can be positioned supine (most common) or lateral on a bean bag. For either position, it is important to use a radiolucent table and a table that can control the amount of lumbar lordosis with a break in the operating table, kidney rest, or inflatable bladder (Fig. 14.1). This helps hyperextend the lumbar spine facilitating anterior opening of the disc space once accessed. Although midline longitudinal and horizontal incisions (Fig. 14.2) have been described, a left vertical paramedian incision is typically utilized (Fig. 14.3). This avoids the more prominent and thin-walled common iliac vein or vena cava on the right and directs the dissection towards the aorta (L2-5) or left iliac (L5-S1). If vascular injury does occur, repair of the left iliac artery or aorta is less technically demanding compared to the common iliac vein or vena cava. Identification of the bony landmarks including the symphysis pubis, anterior superior iliac spine, superior portion of the iliac crest, and the 12th rib is helpful. The L4-L5 disc space is located at the level of the umbilicus and the superior iliac crest. The L5-S1 disc space is typically equidistant between the umbilicus and the superior margin of the symphysis pubis. The skin incision is carried through the subcutaneous layer until the external oblique fascia is encountered. A vertical incision is used to enter the anterior rectus sheath and mobilize the rectus muscle belly (Fig. 14.4). Access to the posterior rectus sheath is obtained by mobilizing the muscle belly toward the midline. The arcuate or semilunar line can be visualized at this point. Blunt dissection of the peritoneum from the deep surface of the posterior rectus sheath is achieved by a lateral to medial sweeping motion of the fingers. The peritoneal sac and its contents can be bluntly dissected off the psoas muscle and retracted medially. The left ureter is identified and retracted with the peritoneal sac.

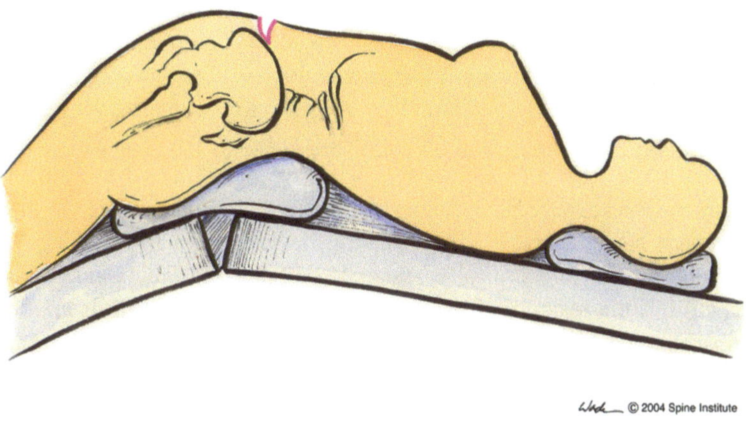

Fig. 14.1 Schematic drawing of a patient positioned supine on a radiolucent table and a break at the level of the lumbar spine. This allows for hyperlordosis with easier exposure and access to the target disc once exposed (Courtesy of John R. Dimar II, MD © 2004 Spine Institute/Leatherman Spine Center)

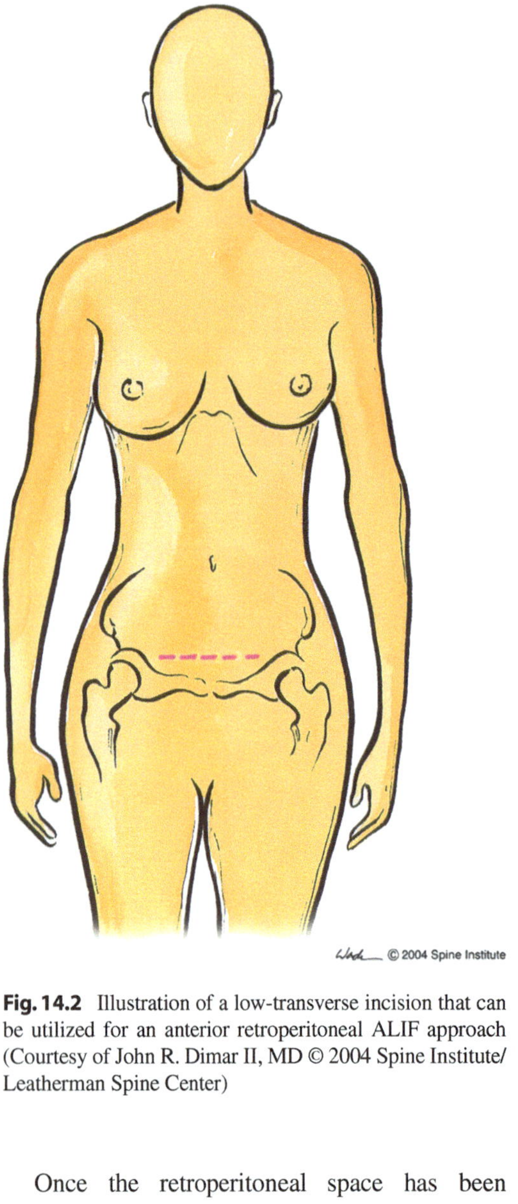

Fig. 14.2 Illustration of a low-transverse incision that can be utilized for an anterior retroperitoneal ALIF approach (Courtesy of John R. Dimar II, MD © 2004 Spine Institute/ Leatherman Spine Center)

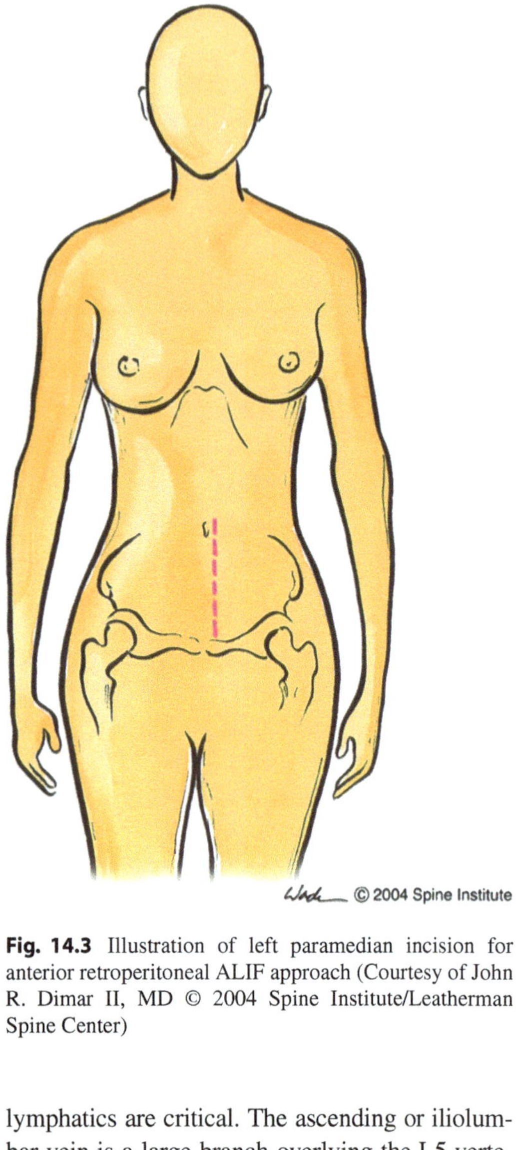

Fig. 14.3 Illustration of left paramedian incision for anterior retroperitoneal ALIF approach (Courtesy of John R. Dimar II, MD © 2004 Spine Institute/Leatherman Spine Center)

Once the retroperitoneal space has been exposed, a radiolucent self-retaining retractor is usually utilized to help retract and protect the retroperitoneal structures. Moist laps rolled into cigar-like cylinders can be used to protect the tips of the blades and provide more surface area for retraction to keep the peritoneum from protruding between blades. Several adjustments of the self-retaining setup are typically required, but this completes the majority of the approach. The left iliac vein and artery are retracted and any segmental vessels are divided laterally. Segmental vessel control and avoidance of lumbar sympathetics and lymphatics are critical. The ascending or iliolumbar vein is a large branch overlying the L5 vertebral body and can restrict mobilization of the iliac vein preventing access to the L4-5 disc space. We recommend ligating this branch to avoid excessive traction on the left iliac vein. The sacral promontory is usually palpable and dissection should be directed towards this. The middle sacral vessels are exposed and ligated to allow proper mobilization of overlying soft tissue (Fig. 14.5).

The anterior longitudinal ligament is incised sharply. It is important to limit electrocautery use at this point during the procedure. Injury to the sympathetic plexus can cause retrograde ejaculation, which can be devastating to young males.

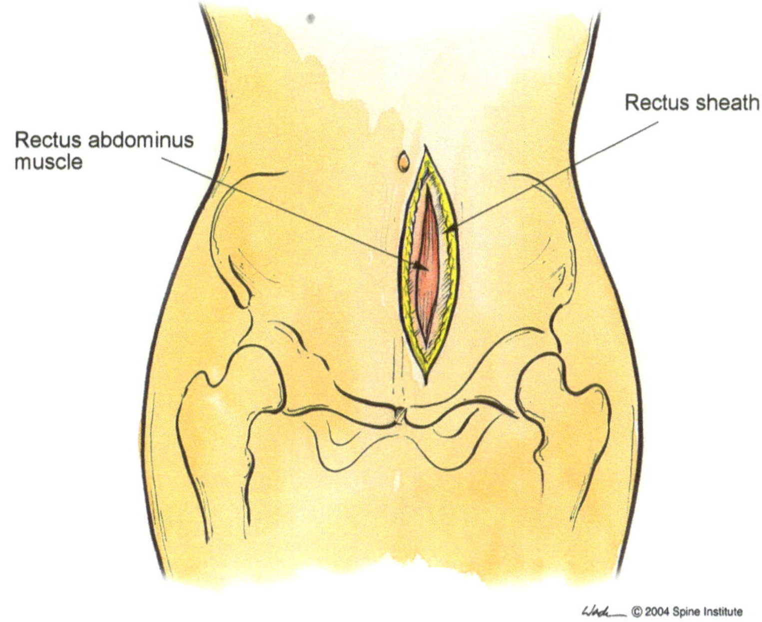

Fig. 14.4 Illustration showing dissection through the subcutaneous layer and identification of the rectus abdominus muscle (Courtesy of John R. Dimar II, MD © 2004 Spine Institute/Leatherman Spine Center)

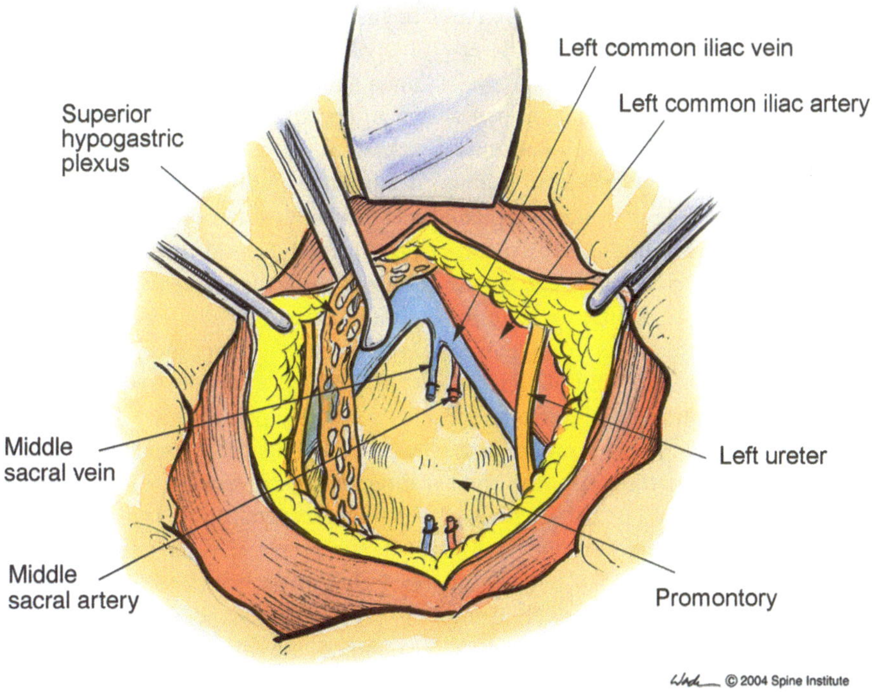

Fig 14.5 Illustration showing the ligation of the middle sacral vein and artery and identification of the sacral promontory. Careful mobilization of the superior hypogastric plexus is critical (Courtesy of John R. Dimar II, MD © 2004 Spine Institute/Leatherman Spine Center)

Blunt dissection using Kittner sponges are preferred. Radiographic confirmation is recommended to avoid wrong-level surgery. Recently at our center, disc penetration with needle localization has been minimized in anterior cervical discectomy and fusion procedures to avoid inadvertent promotion of disc degeneration. We follow the same principle when localizing the target disc space for an ALIF. The discectomy is then performed. The goal is to remove all the disc fragments and cartilaginous endplates to obtain an adequate cancellous surface optimized for fusion. Any remaining disc material or cartilage fragments have the potential to inhibit fusion. Too much destruction of the endplates can lead to graft subsidence, construct instability, regional angular malalignment, and ultimate failure. Once the endplates have been adequately prepared, the interbody graft or device can be inserted.

Lumbar Transperitoneal Approach

Positioning and the bony landmarks are similar to those in a retroperitoneal approach. It is recommended to utilize a bowel preparation to flatten the bowel and decrease contamination if a perforation is encountered. Longitudinal, transverse, or low-transverse (Pfannenstiel) incisions can be utilized. Appropriate preoperative planning is critical as there are limitations to expanding the transverse incisions to adjacent levels. The superficial dissection is similar to the retroperitoneal approach. The peritoneum is elevated with clamps or forceps to elevate off of underlying bowel to prevent unintentional perforation. For more proximal levels in the lumbar spine, the small bowel can be mobilized to the right and the sigmoid colon to the left. Alternatively, the peritoneum can be incised at the lateral reflection (white line of Toldt) and both small bowel and colon mobilized to the right. Bony palpation of the sacral promontory will approximate the appropriate level before incising the retroperitoneum. Radiographic confirmation is then recommended.

Interbody Graft

The primary goals of interbody fusion are to treat the patients' pain and to stabilize the target spinal levels. An ideal interbody graft for an ALIF needs to provide good surface area for fusion and restore segmental alignment while providing structural stability. Biomechanically, increasing disc space height indirectly decompresses the neural foramen and the degenerative disc space is stabilized. Both of these target pain generators and, in theory, help relieve the patient of their symptoms.

The first interbody fusion for the treatment of spondylolisthesis [3] utilized an autogenous tibial dowel. Autogenous graft remained the mainstay for the interbody choice for several decades and even today is considered the "gold standard," although it is not the most common interbody structural support used. Donor site morbidity and unacceptable pseudarthrosis rates, when used as a stand-alone construct, pushed for development of newer interbody options [20]. After approval of the BAK cage in 1997, a surge in interbody options was observed. Even with evolving technology, there is no current agreed upon graft design or material.

Allografts in the form of femoral rings, fibular struts, or iliac crest are seeing a resurgence. Traditionally, allograft was the answer to donor site morbidity. Graft subsidence was common but instrumentation with either anterior plates or posterior fixation has improved this technique. Graft dissolution, especially with the use of recombinant human bone morphogenetic protein-2 (rhBMP-2), is a concern with allograft. Although very low, the potential for disease transmission must be considered when choosing to use allograft. Improvements in screening protocols have greatly reduced this potential. Additionally, different preparation methods are now available including fresh-frozen or freeze-dried allografts. A prospective, randomized, single-site study examined the difference between frozen and freeze-dried allograft when used as part of a circumferential ALIF [21]. They compared 100 patients with a minimum 24 month follow-up and found that although the fresh-frozen graft took longer to incorporate, freeze-dried graft had a higher pseudarthrosis rate. Biomechanical studies have shown that fresh-frozen allograft fails at an average load 50 % less than freeze-dried, but this appears to not be clinically significant [22].

The first metal cage was developed to treat race horses with cervical stenosis. The BAK titanium cage (Zimmer Spine, Warsaw, IN) was a threaded cylinder that was screwed into the disk space. The Ray Fusion Cage (Stryker Spine, Allendale, NJ), a second generation titanium cage, was a lower profile threaded cylinder that allowed more bone graft to be inserted. As a third generation design, the LT-CAGE (Medtronic Sofamer Danek, Memphis, TN) quickly became the most utilized interbody cage in North America. The cage offered a trapezoidal lordotic design that increased surface area for improved fusion rates. Composite designs such as polyetheretherketone (PEEK) were developed to help reduce artifact and to mimic biomechanical properties of cortical bone. The ability to machine PEEK into any shape or size makes it desirable.

rhBMP-2 stimulates bone growth and was first found in the extracellular matrix surrounding bone. rhBMP-2 delivered on an absorbable collagen sponge (ACS) was first approved by the FDA for ALIF procedures in 2002 following the results of a prospective, randomized, multi-center clinical trial [23]. In this study, 279 patients who underwent ALIF for lumbar degenerative disc disease were divided into the experimental rhBMP-2/ACS group and the control autogenous iliac crest bone graft group. At 24 months postoperatively, the rate of fusion as determined by plain radiographs and computed tomography (CT) was higher for the experimental group (94.5 %) than for the control (88.7 %). One study found that rhBMP-2, when used in allograft femoral rings, significantly improved the fusion rates at 6, 12, and 24 month follow-up compared to allograft femoral rings alone [24]. In addition to the higher rate of fusion, the acceptance of rhBMP-2 use for ALIF was an important development because it gave surgeons an alternative that does not have the complications associated with harvesting autogenous or allograft bone [25]. In the years following FDA approval, rates of rhBMP-2 use rose dramatically from 0.69 % of all spinal fusions in 2002 to 24.9 % in 2006 [26]. The potential side-effects of rhBMP-2 use in ALIF are heavily debated [23–28] and further discussed later in the chapter.

Outcomes

Historically, failure or success of an ALIF was defined by the treating surgeon's interpretation of whether spinal fusion was achieved. Studies have typically reported acceptable fusion rates between 47 % [29] and 96 % [10]. These fluctuations may be reflective of differing patient populations, individual surgeon technique, and fusion assessment technique. It is generally agreed that ALIF results in excellent restoration of disc height and lumbar lordosis [30]. The majority of published outcomes focus on spondylolisthesis at the L4-L5 and L5-S1 levels, as these are the most common levels affected. It has been noted that patients undergoing ALIF at more cephalad spinal levels tend to do worse [31], although this may be related to worse pathology rather than just characteristics intrinsic to the level or the approach to it. Here, a multivariate regression analysis of 242 patients undergoing ALIF demonstrated that level was an independent risk factor.

While more recent studies continue to report fusion rates and radiographic results, there has been a trend in the literature to focus on patient-perceived outcomes, especially within the last decade. Health related quality of life (HRQOL) questionnaires are used to assess pain reduction, patient function, and improvements in quality of life. This type of information more accurately measures how much patients benefit from the procedure than radiographic results alone. However, among all the various tools [e.g., Oswestry Disability Index (ODI), Visual Analog Scale, Short Form-36] that have been utilized, no one is used universally across all studies.

The Spinal Patient Outcomes Research Trial (SPORT) found that patients undergoing surgery experienced significantly greater improvements in pain, function, satisfaction, and progress measured by SF-36 over a 4-year time period than those who received non-operative treatment [32].

Furthermore, the treatment effect of surgery for spondylolisthesis was greater than for lumbar spinal stenosis and lumbar disc herniation [33, 34]. Although there were limitations to the study and not all surgical candidates underwent ALIF for the treatment of spondylolisthesis specifically, these results further highlight the important role of surgery in management of spondylolisthesis.

There have been several studies with long-term follow-up that demonstrate good outcomes for ALIF for both degenerative and isthmic spondylolisthesis. Takahashi et al. [35] followed 39 degenerative spondylolisthesis patients who underwent ALIF for a maximum of 30 years postoperatively, with a mean follow-up of 12.5 years. The authors stated that 76 % of patients had satisfactory results for 10 years post-operatively, 60 % for 20 years, and 52 % for 30 years. A "satisfactory result" was defined as at least 25 out of 29 points on the Japanese Orthopaedic Association index, a patient self-report which measures low back pain, leg pain, gait disturbance, and activities of daily living. This study concluded that at ultra-long-term follow-up, ALIF is a viable treatment option for spondylolisthesis. More recently, Riouallon et al. [36] described their study of 65 patients undergoing ALIF for low-grade isthmic spondylolisthesis with an average follow-up of 6.6 years. Their fusion rate was 91 %. Lumbar pain and radicular pain either completely disappeared or regressed in 69 and 85 % of patients, respectively, according to the Visual Analog Scale. Together, these two studies further reinforce the strength of ALIF for treatment of spondylolisthesis.

Comparison between ALIF and other lumbar fusion procedures can be dichotomized between interbody comparison (ALIF, PLIF, or TLIF) and stand-alone ALIF versus posterolateral fusion only. One study of 46 Japanese patients with degenerative spondylolisthesis at L4 compared non-instrumented (stand-alone) ALIF to posterolateral fusion and found that ALIF reduced back pain significantly more than posterolateral fusion, but that ALIF also required longer hospital stay and bed rest [37]. Interbody delivery options consist of anterior (ALIF), posterior (PLIF), and transforaminal (TLIF) approaches. Currently, there is debate to which delivery method is preferred, as several studies demonstrate they have similar radiographic and clinical outcomes [38]. Kim et al. [39] reported a comparison of ALIF and TLIF in 128 patients with low-grade isthmic spondylolisthesis. They found that functional scores for the ODI improved more in patients undergoing TLIF, but restoration of sagittal balance based on radiographs was more common in patients who underwent ALIF. They recommended TLIF at the L4-5 level and ALIF at the L5-S1 level.

The increased consistency in the use of patient-reported HRQOL outcomes has been instrumental in developing a platform for cost analysis. Although no study has directly looked at cost-comparison or cost-effectiveness of ALIF, several studies include patients undergoing ALIF in the analysis. Polly et al. [40] examined pooled SF-36 data on 1,826 lumbar spinal fusion cases, of which 935 were ALIF. They found a cost–benefit ratio comparable to other well-accepted medical interventions such as total hip replacement. Cost-effectiveness of the SPORT data also reported that surgery was good value for treating degenerative spondylolisthesis over a 4-year time period [41]. In the SPORT study, 46 of 372 patients underwent interbody fusion. Overall, these types of analysis are essential in an increasingly cost-conscious era.

Complications

Although ALIF is considered to be a safe procedure, complications can be devastating. Vascular complications are the most frequently encountered. The great vessels, bifurcation of the abdominal aorta into the iliac vessels, and numerous veins reside in the L4-S1 region. A recent review by Inamasu et al. [42] reported that the incidence of vascular injury is between 0 and 18.1 %. Vessel injuries occur more often in surgeries involving the L4-L5 level rather than those at L5-S1, due to the anatomic location of the major vessels. Venous injury is much more common than arterial injury. This occurs most commonly during vein retraction, but can also occur as a result of discectomy or graft placement [42]. The critical veins in this region are the left common iliac vein, the inferior vena cava, and the iliolumbar vein. If perforation of a vein occurs, manual compression followed by primary repair is effective in most scenarios.

The aorta and iliac arteries tend to be more elastic and can be retracted more readily than their corresponding veins, so injuries are less common. However, there is a potential for left iliac artery thrombosis after prolonged periods of retraction. Emergency thrombectomy or bypass surgery is needed immediately if this occurs [43]. The patient may have unclear symptoms, which include pain and motor/sensory deficits in the lower left extremity, and these are often mistaken for nerve root irritation. It has been suggested to periodically release the left iliac artery during surgery or to use a pulse oximeter on the left great toe in order to prevent or detect this complication [44].

A particular point that has been in discussion is the role of a vascular or general surgeon for anterior access. One argument says that the "access" surgeon has had more training and is more experienced in the abdominal cavity than a spine surgeon, particularly those who were trained in neurosurgery. This would seem practical in order to better avoid and address, if they occur, any complications. The current medicolegal climate likely plays a role in the decision to utilize an access surgeon as well. However, it has been reported [45] that there is no significant difference between ALIF surgeries undertaken by spine surgeons alone or with the help of an "access" surgeon. Other studies have indicated that procedures performed by only a spinal surgeon actually involve fewer complications [46]. This may be due to greater familiarity of the spinal surgeons specifically with respect to the approach required for ALIF. However, it should be noted that some surgeons, while undertaking ALIFs alone and effectively resolving vascular complications in the vast majority of cases, still retain the option to call on their vascular colleagues. In one instance, surgeons who performed 304 anterior lumbar spine surgeries "without the assistance of a vascular access surgeon in all cases" nonetheless required vascular surgeon aid in 9 (3 %) cases for complication management [47].

There is also a risk of direct injury to the viscera, most often involving the ureter, peritoneum, and bowel. In particular, attention should be paid to identify and mobilize the ureter and its surrounding tissue. One review of 471 cases of ALIF reported only one instance of ureter damage [48]. Peritoneal damage and bowel perforation are most frequently found in patients undergoing revision surgery or who have had previous abdominal surgery [49]. If bowel injury occurs, immediate repair must be completed and the surrounding area must be irrigated well to prevent infection. Ileus is a well-known complication of ALIF. The condition is important to note because it is a critical component of hospital length of stay postoperatively. The reported incidence rate of ileus is between 0.6 and 5.6 % [50]. In general, patients respond well to medical management; most cases resolve and do not require excessively lengthy hospital stay. Other bowel complications include acute colonic pseudoobstruction, toxic megacolon, and large bowel obstruction. The primary concern in these cases is perforation, which has a high mortality rate. Conservative management for these conditions involves correction of metabolic anomalies and regular enemas, while neostigmine and surgical intervention are applicable in more serious cases [43].

A recent controversial topic is the incidence of retrograde ejaculation in male patients undergoing ALIF. The identified and well-documented cause of retrograde ejaculation is damage to the sympathetic nerves of the superior hypogastric plexus. Although retrograde ejaculation has been noted in the past as a possible complication of ALIF [29], with an incidence ranging from 4.1 to 11.6 % [17, 51], Carragee et al. [52] published a study which suggested that rhBMP-2 was associated with increased risk of retrograde ejaculation in ALIF patients. 7.2 % of patients in the rhBMP-2 group, compared to 0.6 % of patients in the control group, developed retrograde ejaculation, although one of the non-rhBMP-2 patients with RE was excluded for diabetic neuropathy. Also, rhBMP-2 was used with femoral ring allografts, which is off-label. More recently, another group compared retrograde ejaculation rates between patients undergoing ALIF with rhBMP-2 use and those undergoing an artificial disc replacement [53]. They found no significant difference in retrograde ejaculation rate between the two groups. Their method was relevant because artificial disc replacement also uses an anterior approach to the spine. This evidence suggests that retrograde ejaculation is associated with the approach itself rather than with rhBMP-2 use. The conflicting evidence has led to a large controversy regarding the future of rhBMP-2 in ALIF for spondylolisthesis [54–56].

Injuries can also occur to the sympathetic trunk and somatic nerves in the region. The chief complaint of sympathetic trunk damage is typically a cold foot contralateral to the side of the damage, although in reality the ipsilateral foot is warm due to unopposed parasympathetic vasodilation [49]. Care must be taken to rule out arterial thrombosis by checking the dorsalis pedis and posterior tibial pulses. In one study [57], the incidence of sympathetic trunk damage was 6 %, although most patients' symptoms resolved by 6 months postoperatively.

Perioperative wound infection is a major source of morbidity and mortality in hospitals. In studies of complications of ALIF, the combined infection rate (superficial and deep) has been reported to be between 3 and 4.3 % [45, 47]. There is no direct comparison of infection rates between ALIF and the other interbody fusion methods. However, one study which looked at infection rates for combined ALIF/PLIF procedures found that infections were more common at the posterior site than at the anterior site [58].

Another article evaluated the rate of complications of lumbar interbody fusion devices when used from either an anterior or posterior approach [59]. The authors found that the relative risk of having a perioperative complication was 4.75 times higher in the PLIF group than in the ALIF group. Additionally, the risk of having a major postoperative complication was 6.8 times higher in the PLIF patients. However, the authors themselves do point out a number of issues with their own study, such as patient demographics differing between the two groups and inconsistencies in device usage. Overall, ALIF procedures involve a number of very serious potential complications. It is important to recognize these when they occur and to adequately treat them.

References

1. Gjessing MH. Osteoplastic anterior fusion of the lower lumbar spine in spondylolisthesis, localized spondylosis, and tuberculous spondylitis. Acta Orthop. 1951; 20(3):200–13.
2. Capener N. Spondylolisthesis. Br J Surg. 1932;19(75): 374–86.
3. Burns B. An operation for spondylolisthesis. Lancet. 1933;1:1233–9.
4. Iwahara T. A new method of vertebral body fusion. Surg Jpn. 1944;8:271–87.
5. Lane JD, Moore ES. Transperitoneal approach to the intervertebral disc in the lumbar area. Ann Surg. 1948;127(3):537–51.
6. Harmon PH. Results from the treatment of sciatica due to lumbar disc protrusion. Am J Surg. 1950; 80(6):829–40.
7. Hodgson AR, Stock FE. Anterior spinal fusion a preliminary communication on the radical treatment of pott's disease and pott's paraplegia. Br J Surg. 1956;44(185):266–75.
8. Cloward RB. Lesions of the intervertebral disks and their treatment by interbody fusion methods. The painful disk. Clin Orthop Relat Res. 1963;27:51–77.
9. Crock HV. Anterior lumbar interbody fusion: indications for its use and notes on surgical technique. Clin Orthop Relat Res. 1982;165:157–63.
10. Fujimaki A, Crock HV, Bedbrook GM. The results of 150 anterior lumbar interbody fusion operations performed by two surgeons in Australia. Clin Orthop Relat Res. 1982;165:164–7.
11. Kuslich SD, Ulstrom CL, Griffith SL, Ahern JW, Dowdle JD. The Bagby and Kuslich method of lumbar interbody fusion. History, techniques, and 2-year follow-up results of a United States prospective, multicenter trial. Spine. 1998;23(11):1267–78. Discussion 1279.
12. Lekovic GP, Han PP, Kenny KJ, Dickman CA. Bone dowels in anterior lumbar interbody fusion. J Spinal Disord Tech. 2007;20(5):374–9.
13. Bridwell KH, Dewald RL. The textbook of spinal surgery. Philadelphia: Wolters Kluwer/Lippincott Williams & Wilkins Health; 2011.
14. Djurasovic M, Bratcher KR, Glassman SD, Dimar JR, Carreon LY. The effect of obesity on clinical outcomes after lumbar fusion. Spine. 2008;33(16):1789–92.
15. Mogannam A, Bianchi C, Chiriano J, Patel S, Teruya TH, Lum SS, et al. Effects of prior abdominal surgery, obesity, and lumbar spine level on anterior retroperitoneal exposure of the lumbar spine anterior retroperitoneal exposure of the spine. Arch Surg. 2012; 147(12):1130–4.
16. Patel N, Bagan B, Vadera S, Maltenfort MG, Deutsch H, Vaccaro AR, et al. Obesity and spine surgery: relation to perioperative complications. J Neurosurg Spine. 2007;6(4):291–7.
17. Sasso RC, Kenneth Burkus J, LeHuec J-C. Retrograde ejaculation after anterior lumbar interbody fusion: transperitoneal versus retroperitoneal exposure. Spine. 2003;28(10):1023–6.

18. O'Dowd J, Mullholland R, Harris M. BAK cage: Nottingham results. San Francisco: North American Spine Society; 1998.
19. Ray CD. Threaded titanium cages for lumbar interbody fusions. Spine. 1997;22(6):667–79. Discussion 679–680.
20. Stauffer RN, Coventry MB. Anterior interbody lumbar spine fusion analysis of mayo clinic series. J Bone Joint Surg Am. 1972;54(4):756–68.
21. Thalgott JS, Fogarty ME, Giuffre JM, Christenson SD, Epstein AK, Aprill C. A prospective, randomized, blinded, single-site study to evaluate the clinical and radiographic differences between frozen and freeze-dried allograft when used as part of a circumferential anterior lumbar interbody fusion procedure. Spine. 2009;34(12):1251–6.
22. Brantigan JW, Cunningham BW, Warden K, McAfee PC, Steffee AD. Compression strength of donor bone for posterior lumbar interbody fusion. Spine. 1993;18(9):1213–21.
23. Burkus JK, Gornet MF, Dickman CA, Zdeblick TA. Anterior lumbar interbody fusion using rhBMP-2 with tapered interbody cages. J Spinal Disord Tech. 2002;15(5):337–49.
24. Slosar PJ, Josey R, Reynolds J. Accelerating lumbar fusions by combining rhBMP-2 with allograft bone: a prospective analysis of interbody fusion rates and clinical outcomes. Spine J. 2007;7(3):301–7.
25. McKay WF, Peckham SM, Badura JM. A comprehensive clinical review of recombinant human bone morphogenetic protein-2 (INFUSE® bone graft). Int Orthop. 2007;31(6):729–34.
26. Cahill KS, Chi JH, Day A, Claus EB. Prevalence, complications, and hospital charges associated with use of bone-morphogenetic proteins in spinal fusion procedures. JAMA. 2009;302(1):58–66.
27. Lubelski D, Abdullah KG, Steinmetz MP, Alvin MD, Amy SN, Chakka S, et al. Adverse events with the use of rhBMP-2 in thoracolumbar and lumbar spine fusions: a nine year institutional analysis. J Spinal Disord Tech. 2013;1.
28. Mroz TE, Wang JC, Hashimoto R, Norvell DC. Complications related to osteobiologics use in spine surgery: a systematic review. Spine. 2010;35(9 Suppl):S86–104.
29. Christensen FB, Bünger CE. Retrograde ejaculation after retroperitoneal lower lumbar interbody fusion. Int Orthop. 1997;21(3):176–80.
30. Jiang S-D, Chen J-W, Jiang L-S. Which procedure is better for lumbar interbody fusion: anterior lumbar interbody fusion or transforaminal lumbar interbody fusion? Arch Orthop Trauma Surg. 2012;132(9):1259–66.
31. Kalb S, Perez-Orribo L, Kalani MYS, Snyder LA, Martirosyan NL, Burns K, et al. The influence of common medical conditions on the outcome of anterior lumbar interbody fusion. J Spinal Disord Tech. 2013;1
32. Weinstein JN, Lurie JD, Tosteson TD, Zhao W, Blood EA, Tosteson AN, Birkmeyer N, Herkowitz H, Longley M, Lenke L, Emery S, Hu SS. Surgical compared with nonoperative treatment for lumbar degenerative spondylolisthesis. Four-year results in the spine patient outcomes research trial (SPORT) randomized and observational cohorts. J Bone Joint Surg Am. 2009;91(6):1295.
33. Weinstein JN, Lurie JD, Tosteson TD, Tosteson AN, Blood E, Abdu WA, et al. Surgical versus nonoperative treatment for lumbar disc herniation: four-year results for the spine patient outcomes research trial (SPORT). Spine. 2008;33(25):2789.
34. Weinstein JN, Tosteson TD, Lurie JD, Tosteson A, Blood E, Herkowitz H, et al. Surgical versus nonoperative treatment for lumbar spinal stenosis four-year results of the spine patient outcomes research trial. Spine. 2010;35(14):1329–38.
35. Takahashi K, Kitahara H, Yamagata M, Murakami M, Takata K, Miyamoto K, et al. Long-term results of anterior interbody fusion for treatment of degenerative spondylolisthesis. Spine. 1990;15(11):1211–5.
36. Riouallon G, Lachaniette C-H-F, Poignard A, Allain J. Outcomes of anterior lumbar interbody fusion in low-grade isthmic spondylolisthesis in adults: a continuous series of 65 cases with an average follow-up of 6.6years. Orthop Traumatol Surg Res. 2013; 99(2):155–61.
37. Ohtori S, Koshi T, Yamashita M, Takaso M, Yamauchi K, Inoue G, et al. Single-level instrumented posterolateral fusion versus non-instrumented anterior interbody fusion for lumbar spondylolisthesis: a prospective study with a 2-year follow-up. J Orthop Sci. 2011; 16(4):352–8.
38. Min J-H, Jang J-S, Lee S-H. Comparison of anterior- and posterior-approach instrumented lumbar interbody fusion for spondylolisthesis. J Neurosurg Spine. 2007;7(1):21–6.
39. Kim J-S, Lee K-Y, Lee S-H, Lee H-Y. Which lumbar interbody fusion technique is better in terms of level for the treatment of unstable isthmic spondylolisthesis? Clinical article. J Neurosurg Spine. 2010; 12(2):171–7.
40. Polly Jr DW, Glassman SD, Schwender JD, Shaffrey CI, Branch C, Burkus JK, et al. SF-36 PCS benefit-cost ratio of lumbar fusion comparison to other surgical interventions: a thought experiment. Spine. 2007;32(11):S20–6.
41. Tosteson ANA, Tosteson TD, Lurie JD, Abdu W, Herkowitz H, Andersson G, et al. Comparative effectiveness evidence from the spine patient outcomes research trial: surgical versus nonoperative care for spinal stenosis, degenerative spondylolisthesis, and intervertebral disc herniation. Spine. 2011;36(24): 2061–8.
42. Inamasu J, Guiot BH. Vascular injury and complication in neurosurgical spine surgery. Acta Neurochir (Wien). 2006;148(4):375–87.
43. Than KD, Wang AC, Rahman SU, Wilson TJ, Valdivia JM, Park P, et al. Complication avoidance and management in anterior lumbar interbody fusion. Neurosurg Focus. 2011;31(4):E6.

44. Brau SA, Delamarter RB, Schiffman ML, Williams LA, Watkins RG. Left iliac artery thrombosis during anterior lumbar surgery. Ann Vasc Surg. 2004; 18(1):48–51.
45. Quraishi NA, Konig M, Booker SJ, Shafafy M, Boszczyk BM, Grevitt MP, et al. Access related complications in anterior lumbar surgery performed by spinal surgeons. Eur Spine J. 2013;22 Suppl 1: S16–20.
46. Smith MW, Rahn KA, Shugart RM, Belschner CD, Stout KS, Cheng I. Comparison of perioperative parameters and complications observed in the anterior exposure of the lumbar spine by a spine surgeon with and without the assistance of an access surgeon. Spine J. 2011;11(5):389–94.
47. Quraishi NA, Konig M, Booker SJ, Shafafy M, Boszczyk BM, Grevitt MP, et al. Access related complications in anterior lumbar surgery performed by spinal surgeons. Eur Spine J. 2012;22(S1):16–20.
48. Sasso RC, Best NM, Mummaneni PV, Reilly TM, Hussain SM. Analysis of operative complications in a series of 471 anterior lumbar interbody fusion procedures. Spine. 2005;30(6):670–4.
49. Czerwein Jr JK, Thakur N, Migliori SJ, Lucas P, Palumbo M. Complications of anterior lumbar surgery. J Am Acad Orthop Surg. 2011;19(5):251–8.
50. Santos ERG, Pinto MR, Lonstein JE, Denis F, Garvey TA, Perra JH, et al. Revision lumbar arthrodesis for the treatment of lumbar cage pseudoarthrosis: complications. J Spinal Disord Tech. 2008;21(6):418–21.
51. Schwender JD, Casnellie MT, Perra JH, Transfeldt EE, Pinto MR, Denis F, et al. Perioperative complications in revision anterior lumbar spine surgery: incidence and risk factors. Spine. 2009;34(1):87–90.
52. Carragee EJ, Mitsunaga KA, Hurwitz EL, Scuderi GJ. Retrograde ejaculation after anterior lumbar interbody fusion using rhBMP-2: a cohort controlled study. Spine J. 2011;11(6):511–6.
53. Lindley EM, McBeth ZL, Henry SE, Cooley R, Burger EL, Cain CMJ, et al. Retrograde ejaculation after anterior lumbar spine surgery. Spine. 2012; 37(20):1785–9.
54. Tepper G, Rabbani R, Yousefzadeh M, Prince D. Quantitative assessment of retrograde ejaculation using semen analysis, comparison with a standardized qualitative questionnaire, and investigating the impact of rhBMP-2. Spine. 2013;38(10):841–5.
55. Shaffrey CI, Smith JS. Editorial: recombinant human bone morphogenetic protein-2. J Neurosurg Spine. 2013;18(2):109–10. Discussion 110–111.
56. Ghanayem AJ, Santaniello J. Anterior lumbar interbody fusion with recombinant human bone morphogenetic protein-2 and retrograde ejaculation: results from a non-industry sponsored. Spine J. 2012;12(9):S4.
57. Kang B-U, Choi W-C, Lee S-H, Jeon SH, Park JD, Maeng DH, et al. An analysis of general surgery-related complications in a series of 412 minilaparotomic anterior lumbosacral procedures: clinical article. J Neurosurg Spine. 2009;10(1):60–5.
58. Pappou IP, Papadopoulos EC, Sama AA, Girardi FP, Cammisa FP. Postoperative infections in interbody fusion for degenerative spinal disease. Clin Orthop Relat Res. 2006;443:120–8.
59. Scaduto AA, Gamradt SC, Warren DY, Huang J, Delamarter RB, Wang JC. Perioperative complications of threaded cylindrical lumbar interbody fusion devices: anterior versus posterior approach. J Spinal Disord Tech. 2003;16(6):502–7.

Minimally Invasive TLIF for Adult Spondylolisthesis

15

Kshitij Chaudhary and James D. Schwender

Introduction

Minimally invasive transforaminal lumbar interbody fusion (MIS TLIF) was first described in the literature in 2003 by Foley et al. in an effort to reduce post-operative morbidity associated with traditional TLIF [1]. This technique involved using sequential dilators and specialized retractors to develop a surgical corridor by exploiting the natural planes between the erector spinae muscles directly over the intended motion segment. Many comparative studies have shown that MIS TLIF, compared to conventional open TLIF, is associated with a decrease in intra-operative blood loss, lesser post-operative pain, decreased hospital stay, and early ambulation and return to work [2, 3].

Midline subperiosteal exposure in traditional TLIF causes excessive collateral damage to the paraspinal musculature, particularly to the multifidus muscle. This muscle is one of the major stabilizing muscles of the lumbar spine. Its medial location exposes it to injury by electrocautery and self-retaining retractors [4]. Moreover, it is prone to denervation injury due to its monosegmental nerve supply [5]. While it is a well-established fact that muscle injury affects acute post-operative morbidity, there is some evidence to suggest that it may also affect long-term clinical outcome [6, 7]. Dysfunctional paraspinal muscles and injury to neighboring motion segments may contribute to adjacent segment degeneration and instability [8].

Adult spondylolisthesis is one of the ideal indications for MIS TLIF. Degenerative and isthmic spondylolisthesis are the main types of spondylolisthesis seen in the adults. The spondylolisthesis tends to be low grade in this population and is quite easily amenable to MIS procedures. These patients who present with neurological symptoms of claudication or radiculopathy are best treated with decompression and fusion. Spinal fusion using the MIS technique has the advantage of decreased morbidity in the elderly and frail [9, 10].

Contraindications

As with any minimally access procedure, MIS TLIF has a prolonged learning curve. It is important for the surgeon to be comfortable with the conventional open TLIF before attempting this approach. In addition, one should gain proficiency in simple MIS decompressive procedures before MIS TLIF is attempted. Overall the con-

K. Chaudhary, M.S., D.N.B. (Ortho.)
Spine Surgery, Sir H.N. Reliance Foundation Hospital, Raja Rammohan Roy Marg, Mumbai 400 004, Maharashtra, India
e-mail: kshitijc@icloud.com

J.D. Schwender, M.D. (✉)
Twin Cities Spine Center,
913 E 26th Street, Suite 600, Minneapolis, MN 55404, USA
e-mail: jdschwender@yahoo.com

A.L. Wollowick and V. Sarwahi (eds.), *Spondylolisthesis: Diagnosis, Non-Surgical Management, and Surgical Techniques*, DOI 10.1007/978-1-4899-7575-1_15,

traindications for conventional open TLIF, such as conjoined nerves or severe osteoporosis, also apply to MIS TLIF. In addition, there are certain anatomical features, which increase the technical difficulty of MIS procedure. These relative contraindications are enumerated below. Experienced surgeons may not consider these as contraindication for MIS TLIF.

Obesity

Technically, the MIS procedure is more difficult in the obese patient due to requirement of a longer length retractor, which restricts the degree of freedom for surgical instruments. In contrast, the conventional open midline approach tends to be very invasive in the obese patient and approach-related morbidity can be dramatically reduced with minimal access. Rosen et al. found that body mass index did not have a significant relationship with most self-reported outcome measures, operative time, length of hospitalization, and complications in MIS TLIF [11].

Revision Surgery

MIS TLIF can be challenging in revision surgery due to altered anatomy and dural scarring [12]. This is especially true for contralateral decompression techniques when dural scarring is severe.

High-Grade Listhesis (Grade 3 or 4)

There are some reports of MIS TLIF in high-grade slips (Quraishi 2013); however, this is technically challenging and may require special instrumentation and implants [13]. But fortunately, high-grade slips are unusual in adult degenerative and isthmic spondylolisthesis.

Three (or More) Level Fusions

The technique described in the chapter is ideal for one and two levels of fusion. Three or more levels of fusion require alternative MIS techniques that are beyond the scope of this chapter.

Deformity Correction

MIS TLIF is not ideally suited for correction of fixed kyphosis or coronal imbalance. Mild correction, up to 3–5° per level is possible with MIS TLIF; however, if more is required, then anterior or direct lateral interbody fusion techniques are usually preferable.

Equipment Required

The procedure is done using C-arm fluoroscopy mainly in the lateral position. Several AP images are also performed as described in the procedure below. Fixed or expandable tubular retractor systems, and specialized instrumentation are available by various manufactures. Our preferred technique involves simultaneously using two expandable retractors on either side of the patient. Illumination in the surgical field is provided by either using a headlight or a fiber optic cable. Magnification is required and we prefer loupes. Alternatively, a microscope can be used for both illumination and magnification. Bayoneted instruments may be required especially if using a microscope. Advanced navigation or electro-physiological nerve root monitoring are not mandatory in most cases. However, for a novice these adjuncts may be useful to make the procedure safer and reduce exposure to ionized radiation.

Procedure

Anesthesia and Position

Muscle relaxation with general anesthesia is important to prevent muscle creep into the retractor. The patient is then positioned prone on a Wilson-type frame on a Jackson table. The use of the Wilson frame places the patient slightly flexed and therefore improves the exposure during the TLIF procedure. It is preferable to confirm that adequate fluoroscopic views are possible before proceeding further. The surgical area is then prepped and widely draped.

Procedure

The location of the skin incisions is of utmost importance and adequate planning should be performed with fluoroscopy prior to making the skin incisions. A K-wire or spinal needle is used to locate the intended level on fluoroscopy images. In the AP view, the incisions should be slightly lateral to the lateral border of the pedicles. This is usually two-finger breadths (4–5 cm) lateral to the midline spinous process. In obese patients, the incisions need to be placed future lateral to account for the increase depth to approach the spine.

The proposed skin incision is infiltrated with bupivacaine and epinephrine if not contraindicated. Two vertical incisions are made 2.5–3 cm long whether one or two levels are to be fused. The incisions are carried down until the two fascia layers are encountered. These are incised inline with the skin incision. The lumbodorsal fascia incision is critical in holding the retractor in place. Too large of a fascial incision can cause the retractor to slip out of alignment in the sagittal plane.

A small muscle dilator is used first. This is used to palpate the facet joint and the laminar surface. The direction of this dilator is 5–10° convergent to midline, which will later aid in the TLIF procedure and pedicle screw placement. The dilator direction in the lateral view is critically important. The dilator should be co-axial to each of the discs to be fused. Due to lumbar lordosis, through the same incision, one or two levels can be addressed. Once the initial dilator is placed over the facet joint to be fused, serial dilation is carried out.

After confirming the location, direction and depth of the first dilator, the tract is dilated further using sequentially larger concentric dilators (Fig. 15.1). The assembled retractor blade system is then slid down over the final dilator. The retractor should be docked over the facet joint to be fused and co-axial with the disc space. This assembly is now secured firmly the operating table with the arm extension (Fig. 15.2).

After removing the final dilator, very little muscle tissue should be seen within the confines of the retractor blades. Expansion of the retractor blades in modular systems should be limited to prevent muscle creep. Over-expansion of the retractor blades should be avoided as it does not improve exposure and causes more muscle creep. We use limited monopolar electrocautery to clear residual muscle, being careful not to create excessive tissue necrosis. Once the facet joint is encountered, this is marked for level confirmation on lateral fluoroscopy. Once the retractor is in good position and at the correct level avoid the temptation of moving the retractor frequently as this leads to muscle creep.

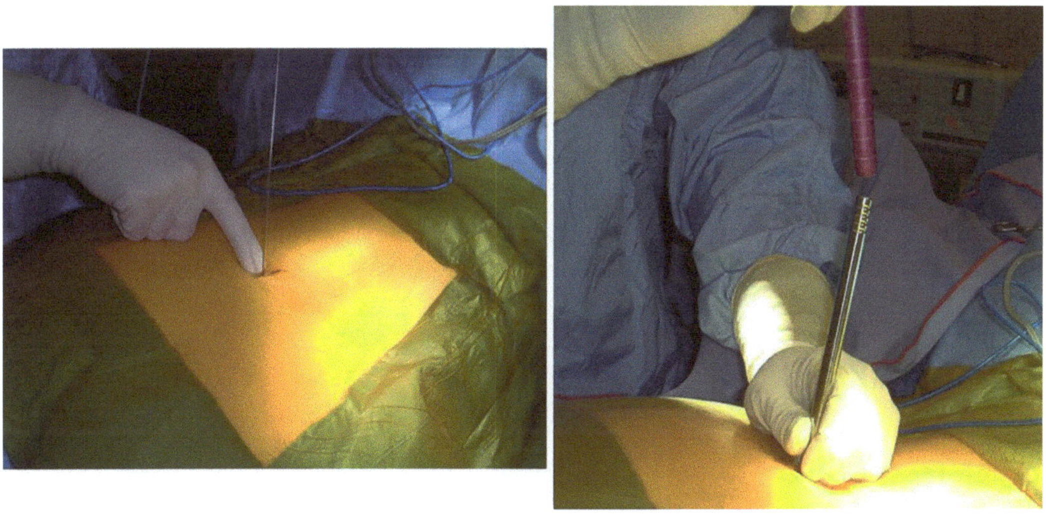

Fig. 15.1 Skin incision located with K-wire and fluoroscopy. Sequential dilation prior to retractor placement

Now that the facet joint is exposed, osteophytes are resected and the joint line is identified (Fig. 15.3). It is important to use the facet joint for orientation. This is a standard anatomical guide for the remainder of the surgical procedure including the decompression, TLIF, and pedicle screw placement. There is no need to expose the transverse process as this leads to unnecessary surgery trauma of the soft tissues and more bleeding.

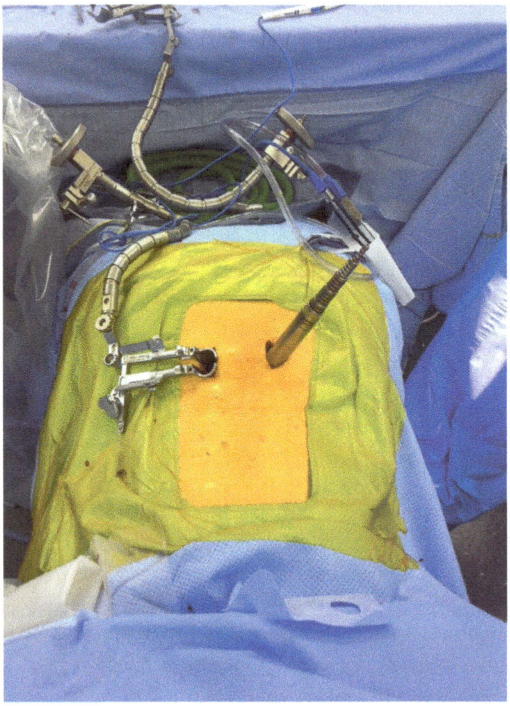

Fig. 15.2 Bilateral placement of the tubular retractor to allow for simultaneous procedure

The facetectomy side for the TLIF is chosen on the more symptomatic side. If the symptoms are bilateral, then the side of more advanced anatomical stenosis is chosen. The pars inter-articularis and lamina are identified and cleared of all soft tissue. At this point a half-inch osteotome or high-speed burr is used to complete the osteotomy of the descending articular process. The resection of the descending articular process should be such that the underlying ascending articular process should be exposed enough to visualize its medial and superior border (Fig. 15.4). The ascending articular process is then resected to expose the working TLIF portal between the exiting and traversing nerve roots. Significant epidural bleeding can be encountered while removing the ascending articular process. This can be controlled using bipolar cautery and/or collagen/thrombin paste product. The ligamentum flavum is not removed at this time and is left intact during the TLIF, as it provides protection to the underlying dura and

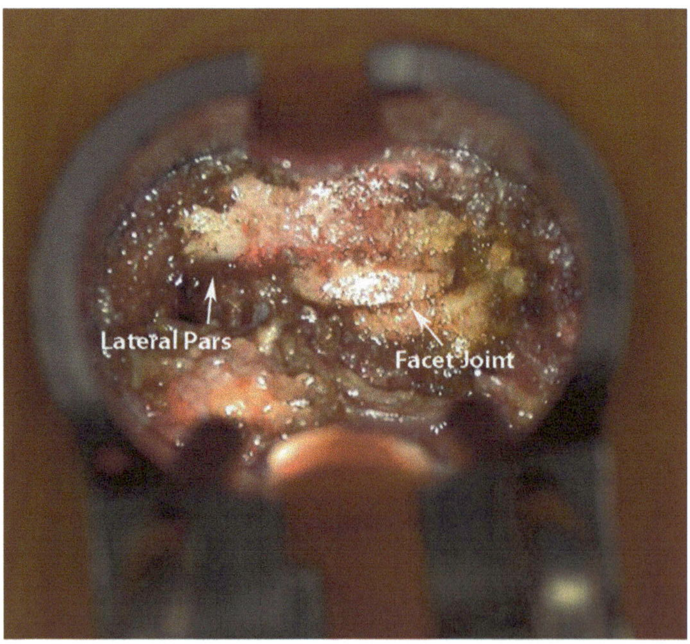

Fig. 15.3 Exposure of the motion segment. Note the minimal amount of muscle within the visual field

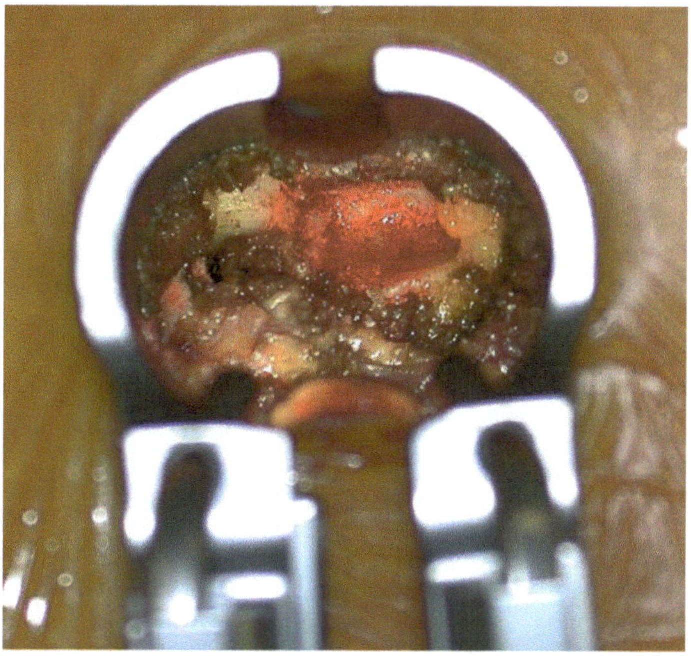

Fig. 15.4 Resection of the descending articular process prior to removal of the ascending articular process

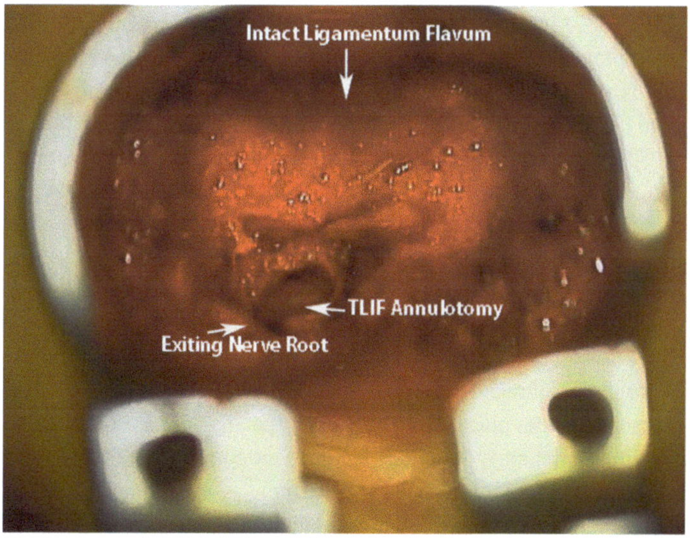

Fig. 15.5 TLIF procedure. Note the intact ligamentum flavum

traversing nerve root while the interbody work is being performed (Fig. 15.5). The exiting nerve root normally lies in the upper half of the foramen even in low-grade spondylolisthesis. This exiting nerve root need not be visualized and the overlying cranial pars inter-articularis is preserved to protect this nerve during interbody work.

A standard inter-laminar spreader or distractor cannot be used in this MIS approach as is commonly performed in the open technique. Hence, slight kyphotic positioning on a Wilson frame allows for entry into the disc space and protection of the exiting nerve root. A 15-number surgical blade is used to make a 1 cm^2 annulotomy in the

TLIF access portal. A subtotal discectomy is done in the usually fashion using a combination of curettes and paddle shavers. Adequate time should be spent preparing the disc space since this is critical in obtaining a solid interbody fusion.

In certain cases, the disc space is severely collapsed making entry into the disc space difficult. In these cases a quarter inch osteotome can be used to gain entry into the disc space followed by serial dilation. The space can be further distracted using rotating paddle shavers. Another option is to distract on the pedicle screw instrumentation on the contralateral side of the TLIF to attempt to restore disc space height while performing the TLIF.

Reduction of the spondylolisthesis is accomplished in several ways. The first is postural. Oftentimes when placing the patient in the prone position under general anesthesia with muscle relaxation partial reduction the spondylolisthesis occurs. In addition, disc height restoration most often improves the slip magnitude, as well as the slip angle. Finally, reduction instrumentation can be employed. If instrumented reduction is planned, this is done prior to placement of the interbody cage device and interbody bone grafting.

Several types of structural interbody supports are commonly used based on the surgeon's preference. Shape configurations commonly include bulleted and kidney-bean shape made of PEEK, titanium, or allograft. There are many bone graft options available. Products of decompression (local autograft) are an excellent source of bone if properly cleaned of all soft tissue. This bone is morselized and placed into the disc space and potentially the cage device. Bone graft extenders can be used in addition to the local bone.

Once the interbody work is completed, formal decompression is carried out as required on a case-by-case basis. This is done after the TLIF so that the lamina and the ligamentum flavum protect the dura and traversing nerve root from iatrogenic injury during the interbody preparation. In many cases the dura expands laterally after removal of the ligamentum flavum into the TLIF working zone. Once the ipsilateral decompression is completed the contralateral side is addressed as needed.

When contralateral decompression is required this is routinely preformed from the TLIF side. The retractor is gently redirected to the junction of the lamina and spinous process. The remaining ipsilateral lamina and the base of the spinous process are resected. The interspinous ligament is kept intact. The contralateral ligamentum flavum is now well visualized. To initiate the "over-the-top" decompression, a plane is created between the ligamentum flavum and dura. The dura and neural elements are protected and gently retracted with cottonoids as required. This is followed by using straight Kerrison ronguers for resection of any lateral recess stenosis caused by the arthritic facet joint to decompress the traversing nerve root. A formal foraminotomy can be preformed to decompress the exiting nerve root as well. Hemostasis is critical during this focused decompression and is best accomplished with judicial use of bipolar electrocautery and collagen/thrombin hemostasis products. The completed contralateral decompression is confirmed using direct visualization and a ball-tip probe (Fig. 15.6).

At this point pedicle screws are placed on the side of the TLIF and decompression (Fig. 15.7). When using a tubular retractor system, direct visualization of the anatomy for screw placement is possible. Lateral expose to the transverse processes is not generally required. The mammillary process, facet joint anatomy, and the lateral pars inter-articularis provide enough information to identify the pedicle screw starting point. Good three-dimensional orientation is a must for safe pedicle screw insertion with this technique. A standard pedicle probe is used to cannulate each of the pedicles. All pedicle sites are cannulated prior to screw placement. This allows for maximal visualization of the anatomy prior to introduction of the pedicle screws. There is no need for the use of K-wires or cannulated pedicle screws with this direct insertion technique. Lateral fluoroscopy is occasionally used during placement; however, judicial use is important. An AP is typically obtained only after all screws are placed.

Screw placement on the contralateral side can be executed in one of two ways. This can be accomplished by direct placement through the

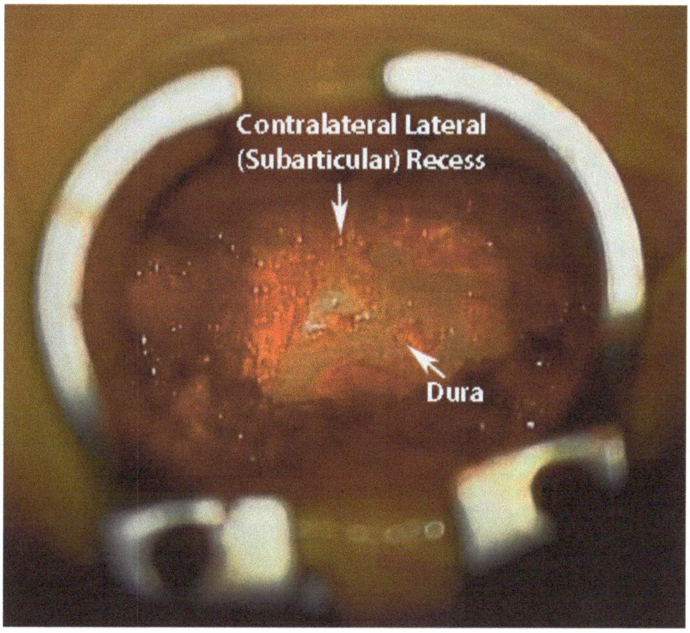

Fig. 15.6 Contralateral decompression after partial resection of the ventral spinous process and complete removal of the ligamentum flavum

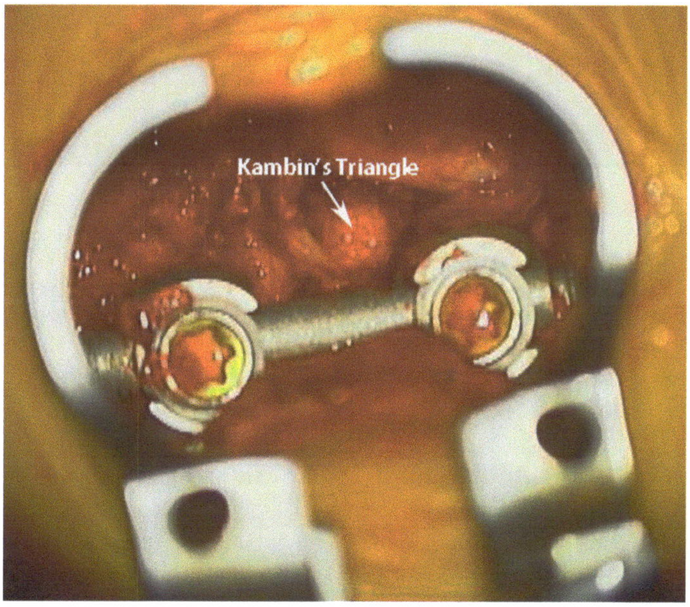

Fig. 15.7 Completed TLIF procedure with decompression and instrumentation

tubular retractor system or percutaneously. The advantages of the mini-open approach are several-fold. Radiation exposure can be reduced dramatically by avoiding multiple bi-planar views, which is required for percutaneous screw placement unless advanced imaging is available. The contralateral facet joint is exposed with the mini-open approach and fused for circumferential arthrodesis. In addition, the contralateral facet joint can be excised to provide more reduction for the spondylolisthesis correction. Finally, rods are placed either under direct visualization or percutaneously. Set screws are placed. Prior to final tightening, gentle compression is placed across the construct as needed to facilitate lordosis (Figs. 15.8, 15.9, and 15.10).

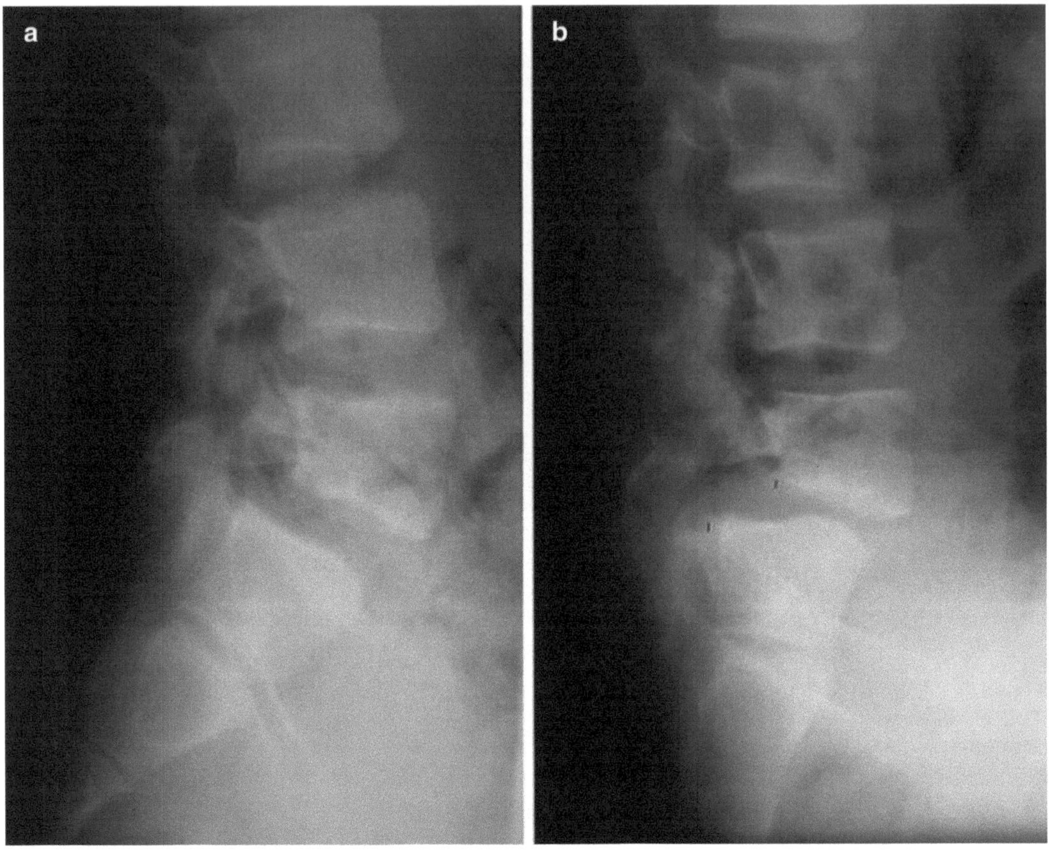

Fig. 15.8 (**a**, **b**) *Case 1: 20-year-old female with an isthmic spondylolisthesis at L5–S1 refractory to non-operative treatment. Presents with low back pain and bilateral L5 radiculopathy*. Lateral neutral and flexion radiographs showing Grade 2 slip

Special Situations

High-Grade Adult Spondylolisthesis

Reduction of high-grade spondylolisthesis (Grade 3 or 4) requires special instrumentation and surgical technique to safely perform. Fortunately, high-grade spondylolistheses are uncommon in this population. The key to safety, as with conventional approach, is to identify and decompress the exiting nerve root throughout the foramen bilaterally before reduction is attempted. This requires bilateral decompressions with facetectomies. Adequate exposure of the disc for performing the TLIF may be difficult in higher grade slips. With increasing slip magnitude the exiting nerve lies in close proximity to the disc space and this needs to be protected at all times. The annulotomy usually has to be made more medial and the lateral edge of the dura may need to be slightly retracted medially. In many cases an osteotomy of the posterior sacrum is required to gain access to the disc. Bilateral aggressive discectomy and release is required to make the motion segment is as mobile as possible.

Special reduction screws can be used to correct the translational and rotational deformity. Reduction screws are placed in the cephalad vertebra and fixed angle screws in the caudad vertebra. The rods are locked down to the caudad screws. The rods are then locked in the cephalad reduction screw so that the spondylolisthesis is slowly reduced. The procedure is best performed

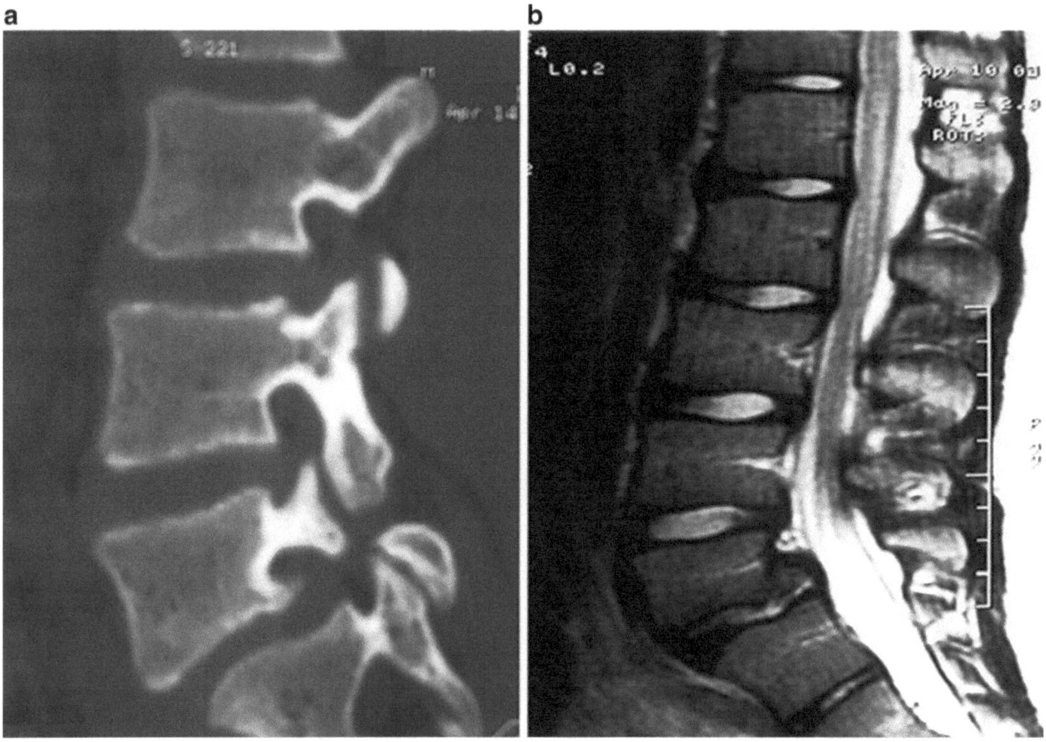

Fig. 15.9 (**a**, **b**) *Case 1*: *20-year-old female with an isthmic spondylolisthesis at L5–S1 refractory to non-operative treatment. Presents with low back pain and bilateral L5 radiculopathy*. CT and MRI revealing isthmic spondylolisthesis, disc degeneration, and a central disc herniation

under fluoroscopy and accompanying nerve root electromonitoring. Once the reduction maneuver is complete, the interbody cage and bone grafting are placed. Residual translational deformity (low grade) is acceptable and complete reduction of the spondylolisthesis should not be the goal. Adequate compression across the screws can also help improve the slip angle as well.

Two-Level Fusion

Two-level TLIF can be performed safely via this MIS approach. However, these cases are technically more difficult. Each level should be completed individually with the modular tubular retractor opened to the minimum. Only when both levels have been addressed individually in terms of the TLIF and appropriate decompress should the modular retractor be opened to accommodate for pedicle screw placement. This will reduce on the ischemia of the erector spinae musculature and reduce the creep of the muscle into the retractor.

Revision Decompression and Fusion

This is not a contraindication in performing an MIS TLIF. However, it is important to carefully review all pre-operative imaging to fully understand the current anatomy. In many cases the facetectomy for decompression and TLIF are lateral to the previous surgery, thus avoiding the epidural scarring. In addition, well-healed midline incisions are not a contraindication for the use of paramedian incisions, and in fact, are routinely performed without skin breakdown issues.

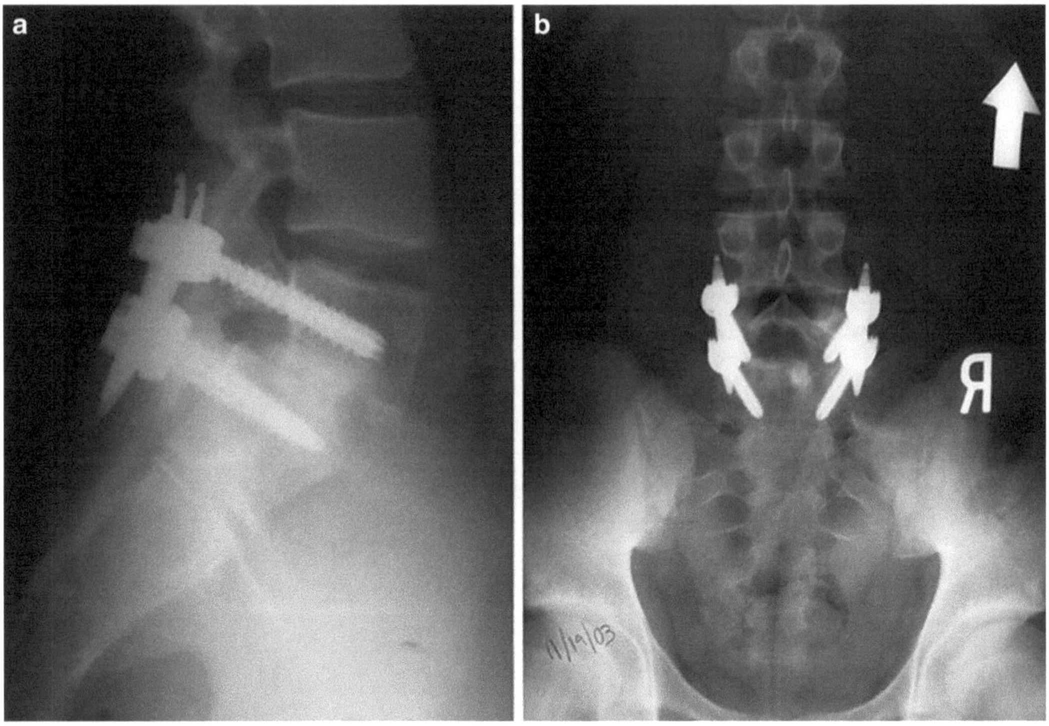

Fig. 15.10 (**a**, **b**) *Case 1*: *20-year-old female with an isthmic spondylolisthesis at L5–S1 refractory to non-operative treatment. Presents with low back pain and bilateral L5 radiculopathy*. Post-operative PA and lateral of a unilateral minimally invasive TLIF procedure. Improvement noted in slip percentage and slip angle. All pre-operative symptoms resolved

Pitfalls

Incidental Durotomy

The treatment of an incidental durotomy is the same as when encountered in a conventional midline open procedure. The aim is for a primary water-tight suture repair if possible. This is technically difficult, though not impossible, and is greatly dependent on the location and complexity of the dural tear. Supplemental dural repair patch products such as Tis-seal and Duragen can also be used. Due to the minimal dead space created in the MIS paramedian muscle approach, symptomatic pseudomeningocele formation is rare if a tight fascial closure is performed.

Poor Visualization due to Muscle Creep

Muscle creep into the tubular retractor system is often the most frustrating part of the MIS approach. To minimize this from occurring, the modular retractor system should only be opened as little as required. Remember, more exposure is not better exposure! Once the retractor is in the correct location, minimize the movement of the retractor blades. More manipulation of the blades creates a higher likelihood of inadvertent muscle entry into the confines of the retractor. Muscle can creep into the wound in spite of all precautions mentioned above. In this case it is better to entirely remove the retractor and repeat the steps of dilation to correctly replace the retractor. There is never a need to convert to an open midline exposure.

Summary

The MIS TLIF technique for the surgical treatment for adult spondylolisthesis is a popular choice amongst MIS surgeons because of its ability to address the principles of treatment for this condition. It allows for placement of a structural cage device and bone graft for fusion within the disc space. It provides access for direct decompression for both ipsilateral and contralateral stenosis. In addition, indirect decompression by disc height restoration and reduction of the spondylolisthesis are accomplished. Posterolateral facet joint fusion and pedicle screw placement are also accomplished through this technique.

References

1. Foley KT, Holly LT, Schwender JD. Minimally invasive lumbar fusion. Spine. 2003;28:S26–35.
2. Villavicencio AT, Burneikiene S, Roeca CM, et al. Minimally invasive versus open transforaminal lumbar interbody fusion. Surg Neurol Int. 2010;1:12.
3. Adogwa O, Parker SL, Bydon A, et al. Comparative effectiveness of minimally invasive versus open transforaminal lumbar interbody fusion: 2-year assessment of narcotic use, return to work, disability, and quality of life. J Spinal Disord Tech. 2011;24(8):479–84. doi:10.1097/BSD.0b013e3182055cac.
4. Kawaguchi Y, Yabuki S, Styf J, et al. Back muscle injury after posterior lumbar spine surgery. Topographic evaluation of intramuscular pressure and blood flow in the porcine back muscle during surgery. Spine. 1996;21:2683–8.
5. Macintosh JE, Bogduk N. 1987 Volvo award in basic science. The morphology of the lumbar erector spinae. Spine. 1987;12:658–68.
6. Sihvonen T, Herno A, Paljärvi L, et al. Local denervation atrophy of paraspinal muscles in postoperative failed back syndrome. Spine. 1993;18:575–81.
7. Kim D-Y, Lee S-H, Chung SK, et al. Comparison of multifidus muscle atrophy and trunk extension muscle strength: percutaneous versus open pedicle screw fixation. Spine. 2005;30:123–9.
8. Lai P-L, Chen L-H, Niu C-C, et al. Relation between laminectomy and development of adjacent segment instability after lumbar fusion with pedicle fixation. Spine. 2004;29:2527–32. discussion 2532.
9. Rouben D, Casnellie M, Ferguson M. Long-term durability of minimal invasive posterior transforaminal lumbar interbody fusion: a clinical and radiographic follow-up. J Spinal Disord Tech. 2011;24(5):288–96. doi:10.1097/BSD.0b013e3181f9a60a.
10. Karikari IO, Grossi PM, Nimjee SM, et al. Minimally invasive lumbar interbody fusion in patients over seventy years of age: analysis of peri- and post-operative complications. Neurosurgery. 2011;68(4):897–902. discussion 902.
11. Rosen DS, Ferguson SD, Ogden AT, et al. Obesity and self-reported outcome after minimally invasive lumbar spinal fusion surgery. Neurosurgery. 2008;63:956–60. discussion 960.
12. Selznick LA, Shamji MF, Isaacs RE. Minimally invasive interbody fusion for revision lumbar surgery: technical feasibility and safety. J Spinal Disord Tech. 2009;22:207–13.
13. Park P, Foley KT. Minimally invasive transforaminal lumbar interbody fusion with reduction of spondylolisthesis: technique and outcomes after a minimum of 2 years' follow-up. Neurosurg Focus. 2008;25:E16.

Surgical Technique: Lateral Interbody Fusion for Adult Spondylolisthesis

16

Luiz Pimenta, Leonardo Oliveira, and Luis Marchi

Background

Spondylolisthesis is one of the most common conditions of the spine, and its surgical treatment has been proved to be safe and effective, with marked improvement in pain and function when compared to conservative care [1, 2]. Several surgical techniques and devices have been studied to evaluate the best clinical and radiological option [3–5] but to date, no approach has been shown to be more effective than the others, with no gold standard treatment being proposed [6].

Decompression of the neural structures has been thought to be mandatory in the treatment of spondylolisthesis with irradiated pain [7] and spinal fusion with decompression had shown better clinical results and outcomes [8, 9]. However, posterior bone resection and muscle splitting, this procedure can lead to more instability and deformity of the accessed level [10].

The advent of minimal invasive spine surgery (MISS) allowed the achievement of good clinical and radiological results while minimizing collateral muscle and bone damage, with decreased risks and complications [11]. One of these techniques is the eXtreme Lateral Interbody Fusion (XLIF) that consists of an anterior interbody fusion that realigns the endplates to a horizontal position through bilateral annular release with placement of a large implant across the disc space that reaches the ring apophysis [12], maintaining intact all ligaments that play a role in ligamentotaxis, generating indirect decompression while stabilizing the motion segment [13]. Moreover, several clinical reports have emerged demonstrating the safe and effective use of the technique in comparison with other conventional surgical approaches, with the same or better clinical and radiological results [14–20], including spondylolisthesis up to grade 2 [14, 19].

This chapter describes in detail the minimally invasive transpsoas approach in the treatment of spondylolisthesis, presenting nuances in technique, surgical pitfalls, and current results already published in literature.

Surgical Procedure

Patient Selection and Indications

The XLIF approach has been utilized in the treatment of Meyerding grades I and II spondylolisthesis upper to L5 vertebral body [13, 14, 17,

L. Pimenta, M.D., Ph.D. (✉) • L. Oliveira, M.S.
L. Marchi, M.S.
Department of Minimally Invasive Spine Surgery, Instituto de Patologia da Coluna, Rua Vergueiro 1421, sala 305, São Paulo, SP 04101-000, Brazil
e-mail: luizpimenta@luizpimenta.com.br; leonardo@patologiadacoluna.com.br; marchi@patologiadacoluna.com.br

A.L. Wollowick and V. Sarwahi (eds.), *Spondylolisthesis: Diagnosis, Non-Surgical Management, and Surgical Techniques*, DOI 10.1007/978-1-4899-7575-1_16,

19, 21–23]. The L5–S1 disc space cannot be accessed due to technical limitation, as the presence of iliac crest and elevated risk of damaging the iliac vessels.

Patients must have exhausted all conservative treatments before being elective for surgery. Preoperative planning must include dynamic X-rays in order to evaluate the amount of vertebral slippage, its etiology, and the degree of instability of the targeted level [24], mandatory in the decision of performing a stand-alone construction or using posterior supplementation. When severe instability is found, percutaneous pedicle screw supplementation is indicated to enhance primary fusion, keeping slippage reduction and avoiding subsidence of the cage. Magnetic resonance imaging and/or computed tomography must be taken in order to confirm spinal stenosis and possible fractures.

Furthermore, disc level, age, gender, and bone quality are significant issues that must be analyzed preoperatively to avoid subsidence. A higher incidence of subsidence was shown to be related to osteoporotic, elderly, and female patients, while L4–L5 seems to be the most susceptible disc level to subside [25–27].

Other important factor that must be taken into account is the amount of disc height when planning for stand-alone interbody fusion. As higher is the disc, more difficult will be to generate indirect decompression by ligamentotaxis, as the ligaments are already stretched. Also, the impactation of the cage tends not to be ideal, and stabilization will be at risk of not being achieved properly.

Surgical Technique

Neuromonitoring

The first step in the operating room is placing the surface electrodes of the electromyography system (NeuroVision, NuVasive, CA, USA) to monitor lumbar plexus during transpsoas approach, which is mandatory in this kind of procedure. Four muscle groups per side must be monitored as represent bilateral spinal nerve distributions from L2–S2: vastus medialis, anterior tibialis, biceps femoris, and medial gastrocnemius (Fig. 16.1). Also, a reference electrode is placed upper to the lateral thigh, and a return electrode is placed superior to the operative site, such as on the latissimus dorsi muscle. Proper skin preparation must be performed to ensure good electrical conductivity.

Appropriate Patient Positioning

The patient is placed into a radiopaque bendable surgical table in a direct lateral decubitus position (90°), perpendicular to the table, with the trochanter directly positioned over the table break and with legs and knees slightly bent. Patient is then attached to the table by four adhesive strips: (1) torso, (2) iliac crest, (3) leg and knee, (4) knee and foot (Fig. 16.2). This configuration increases the space between iliac crest and ribs, especially relevant when accessing thoracolumbar junction or L4–L5 level.

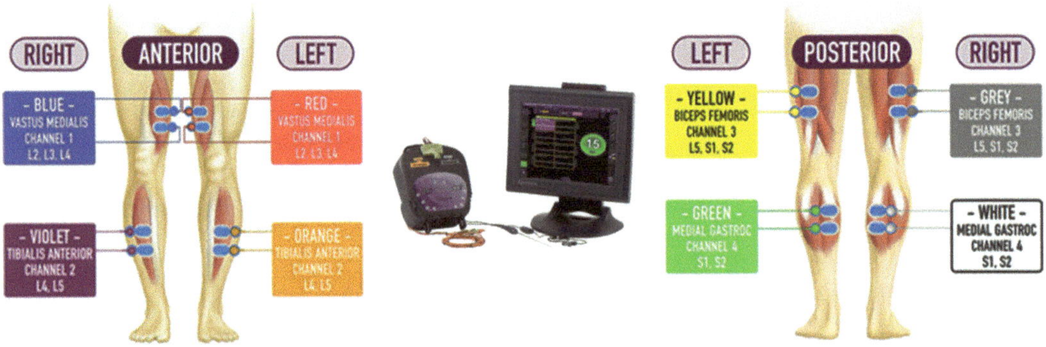

Fig. 16.1 Four muscle groups per side that represent spinal nerve distributions from L2–S2 are monitored by EMG. Each electrode is identified by a specific color and must be connected to the correspondent muscle

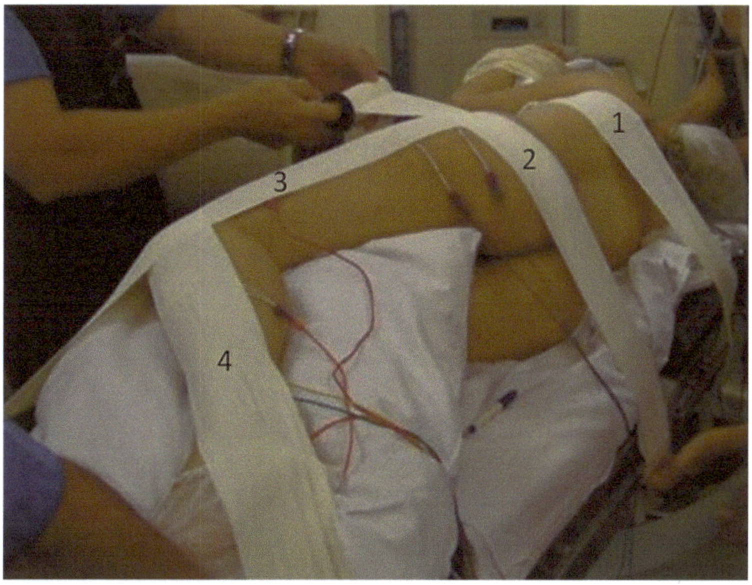

Fig. 16.2 Positioning of the patient at the surgical table for lateral access surgery. Patient is attached to the table by four adhesive strips: (*1*) torso, (*2*) iliac crest, (*3*) leg and knee, (*4*) knee and foot. Patient is in direct lateral decubitus position (90°), perpendicular to the table, with the trochanter directly positioned over the table break and with legs and knees slightly bent

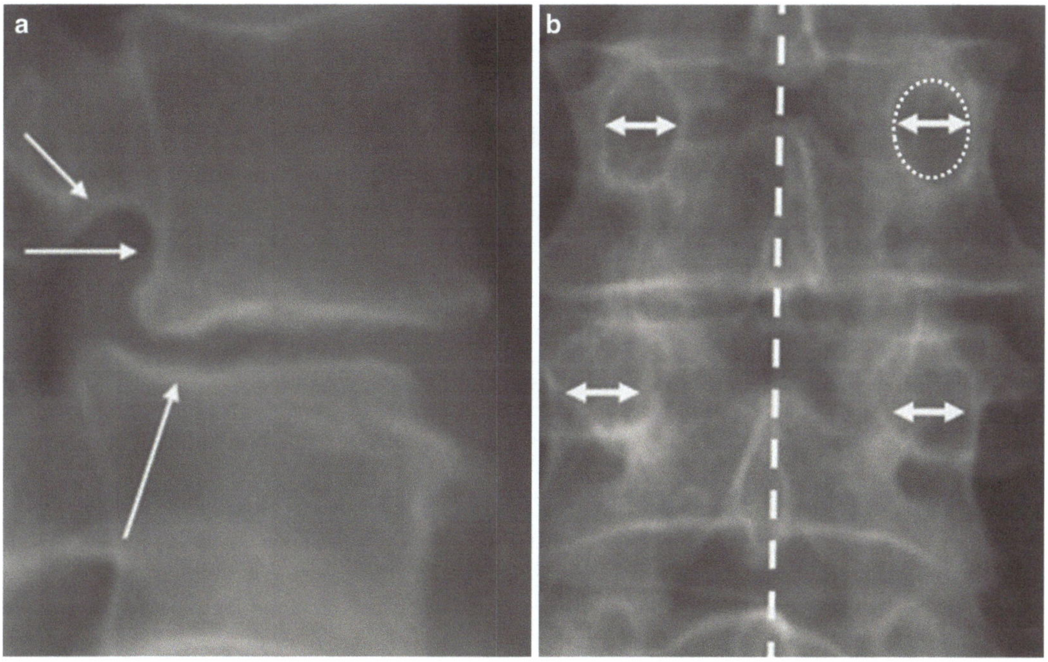

Fig. 16.3 (**a**) Lateral image shows superior pedicles and vertebral plateaus aligned, presented as a single line (*white arrows*). (**b**) AP image confirms the spinous processes in a middle position (*dotted line*), and pedicles as circumferences (*dotted circle*)

To confirm the ideal positioning, fluoroscopy is used to ensure that when at 0°, the C-arm provides a true anteroposterior (AP) image, and when at 90°, a true lateral image. It is substantial that the lateral fluoroscopic images show both vertebral plateaus and superior pedicles aligned, presented as a single line, and that the AP image reveals the spinous processes in a middle position, and pedicles as circumferences (Fig. 16.3).

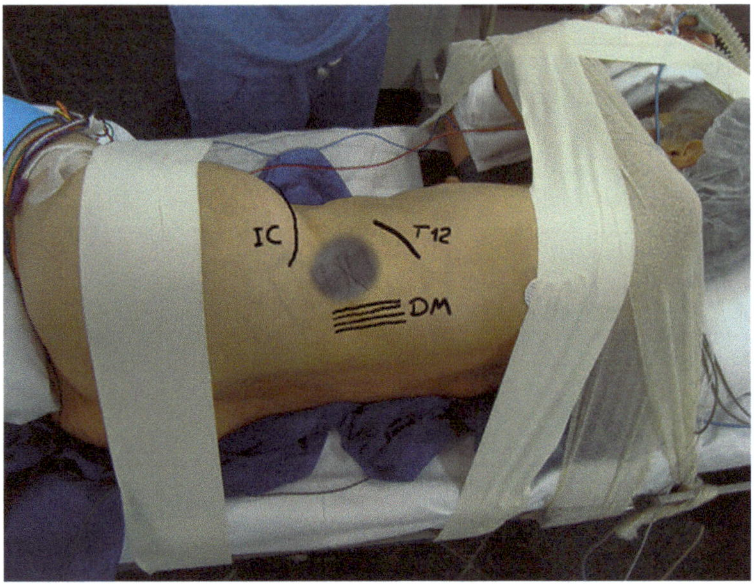

Fig. 16.4 Skin identification of the iliac crest (*IC*), twelfth rib (*T12*), and dorsal musculature (quadrates lombaris—*DM*). Using two Kirschner wires and lateral fluoroscopic image, central position of the targeted disc can be easily identified

Retroperitoneal Access

It is recommended to identify into the skin the iliac crest, the transition between the last rib and the posterior abdominal wall muscle and the quadratus lumborum muscle. After skin asepsis, the central position of the targeted disc can be identified using two Kirschner wires and lateral fluoroscopic images (Fig. 16.4). Then, a mark is made on the side of the patient, covering the center of the affected disc space. A longitudinal skin incision is made, over the intersection between the posterolateral muscles of the abdominal wall (abdominal internal oblique, abdominal external oblique, and transverse abdominus). A first fascia incision is made posteriorly to allow the surgeon to introduce the index finger into the retroperitoneal space and gently create a pathway and ensure that all attachments of the peritoneum are released, providing a safe lateral entry. Once identified the retroperitoneal space, a second fascia incision in made below the first skin mark to introduce the initial dilator. The index finger will safely escort the dilator up to the psoas muscle, protecting intra-abdominal contents (Fig. 16.5).

Psoas Traverse

The first dilator is then placed over the surface of the psoas muscle, upon the posterior third of the disc, confirmed by AP and lateral fluoroscopy. The fibers are gently separated by the initial blunt dilator until the side surface of the disc be reached, with concomitant EMG monitoring for assessing the closeness to the lumbar plexus (Fig. 16.5). The dilator can be rotated in position to determine not just proximity, but also the direction of nerves. Larger dilators are placed in sequence over the previous, always checking the EMG, until the final placement of the three blades retractor, still closed. The retractor is connected to a suspension arm in order to prevent unwanted movement. After confirming the ideal position by fluoroscopy, the working portal can be selectively adjusted to the desired diameter. A bifurcated optical fiber cable is attached to the retractor for optimal direct visualization of the exposure (Fig. 16.6).

In patients with spondylolisthesis, the meticulous realization of the procedure is essential to avoid neurological deficit, as the neural structures

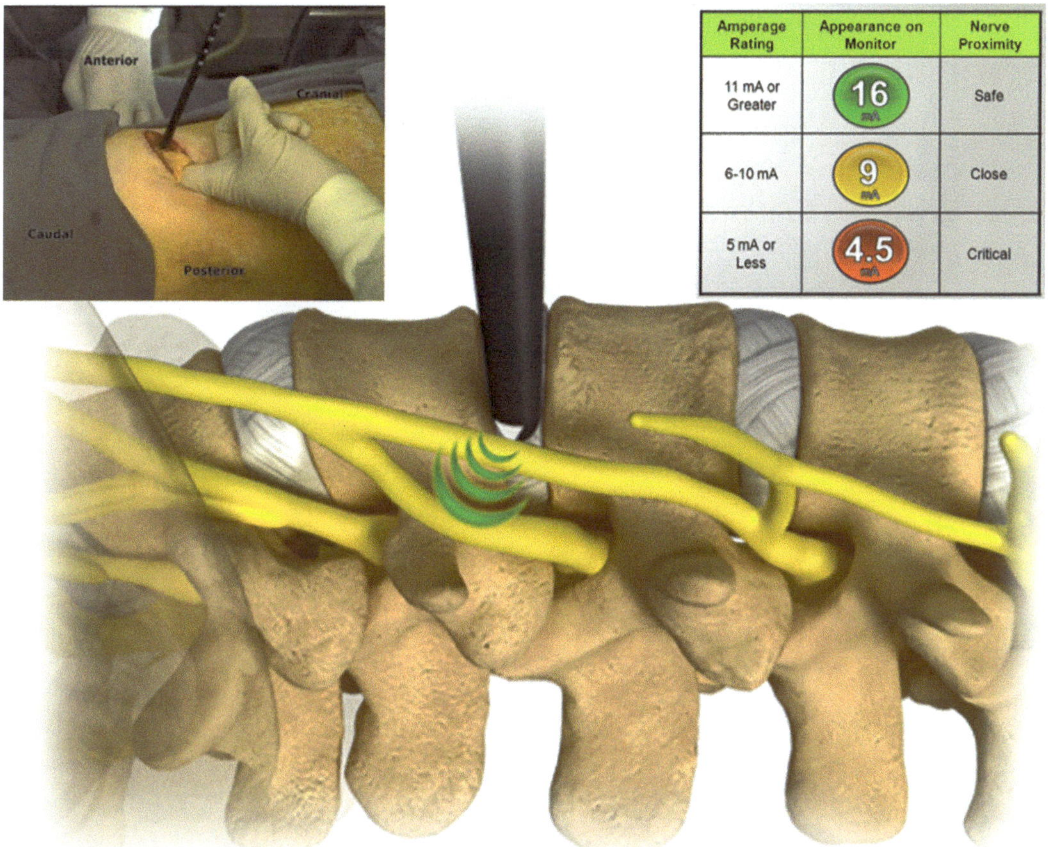

Fig. 16.5 The index finger will safely escort the dilator up to the psoas muscle, protecting intra-abdominal contents (*upper left*). EMG monitoring is mandatory for assessing the closeness and direction of the contents of lumbar plexus (*middle*). The monitoring system emits sounds, graduating by color the proximity of nerves (*upper right*)

are shifted ventrally by the L4 vertebral body slipping [19]. Moreover, the retractor opening must be minimal, with the shorter duration of muscle spreading as possible, since the lumbar plexus must be compressed during psoas traverse.

Disc Space Preparation

Under direct visualization, a wide discectomy is performed with standard instruments. The anterior and posterior portions of the disc containing the longitudinal ligaments are preserved with discectomy focused in the center of the disc, with a sufficient AP dimension to accommodate a large implant. Laterolateral disc removal and contralateral ring release with a Cobb are essential to ensure symmetrical distraction, properly bilateral decompression and avoid coronal iatrogenic changes. Furthermore, this maneuver offers the opportunity to place an implant that covers both side edges of the cortical apophyseal ring, maximizing the spinal plateau support (Fig. 16.7). The complete removal of cartilage and rasping the cortical bone layer are essential to providing blood precursor cells and bone growth factors for the successful bone ingrowth.

In spondylolisthesis, the accurate discectomy itself partially reduces the vertebral slippage. The maintenance of the anterior and posterior

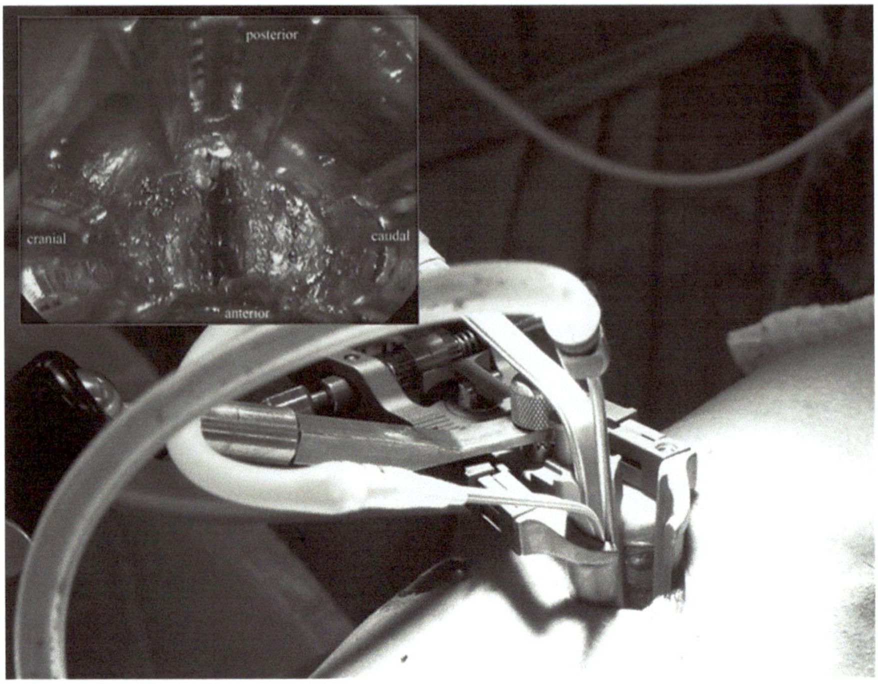

Fig. 16.6 Working portal and direct visualization of the disc space, illuminated by optical fiber cable

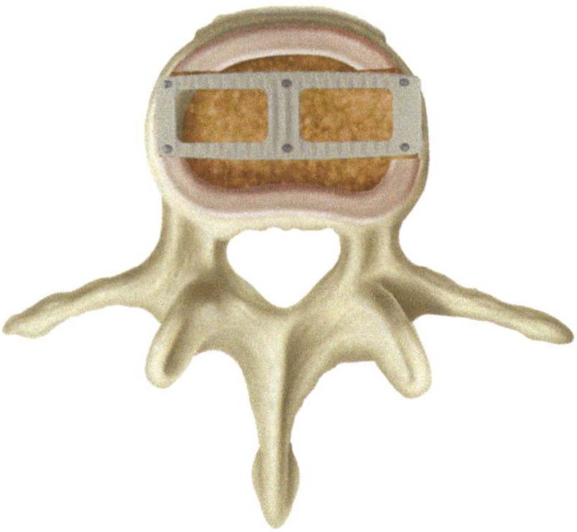

Fig. 16.7 Lateral access surgery allows the implantation of a device that covers both side edges of ring apophysis, increasing biomechanical support of the cage

portions of the disc, keeping intact the longitudinal ligaments, allows ligamentotaxis, partly responsible for slippage reduction and indirect decompression of the neural structures [13, 14, 28].

Device Insertion

To determine the correct spacer to be inserted, implant proofs of height, length, and angle should be inserted into the disc space to find the most suitable for the stipulated objectives, guiding the entire process by fluoroscopic imaging. The ideal placement of the device is centered across the disc space from an AP view, and between the anterior third and middle third of the disc space from a lateral view. The ideal implant positioning also restores focal lordosis, usually lost in this kind of deformity, especially at L4–L5 [15].

As a minimally invasive option, it is recommended to use synthetic bone grafts instead of autologous bone, avoiding major postoperative morbidity. The final position of the implant must be checked on AP and lateral fluoroscopy.

Closure

After washing the surgical site, the retractor is closed and slowly removed in order to observe the psoas muscle closure and confirm hemostasis. The incisions are closed in a standard fashion and no drain is required. The construct may be supplemented with the internal fixation system of choice, when indicated.

Postoperative Care

Patients should be encouraged to walk the same day to aid their recovery and muscle function, also avoiding deep venous thrombosis and pulmonary thromboembolism. Postoperative pain tends to be minimal, and patients may be discharged after only an overnight hospital stay. Literature shows low rate of complications in the immediate postoperative period, including hip flexion weakness (psoas weakness) or numbness ipsilateral to the surgical access (plexopaties), and less frequently quadriceps transitory weakness, the great majority resolved within 6 months [13, 15, 29, 30].

Current Results

There are several published papers regarding XLIF that include patients with spondylolisthesis in total cohort [17, 21–23]. Rodgers et al. [19] have operated 63 patients by lateral approach for the treatment of spondylolisthesis grade 2 using posterior supplementation, showing good clinical and radiological results. The hospital stay averaged 1.2 days, with no infections or persistent neurologic deficits. All patients achieved fusion at last follow-up, with improvement in self-assessment questionnaires. They have found only complications in only 3.4 % of total cohort, one patient with ileus and second having a broken pedicle screw in consequence of a car accident 14 months after surgery. Figure 16.8 shows a case example of spondylolisthesis grade 2 treated by lateral approach with posterior supplementation.

Marchi et al. [14] followed 52 patients who underwent XLIF surgery for the treatment of low

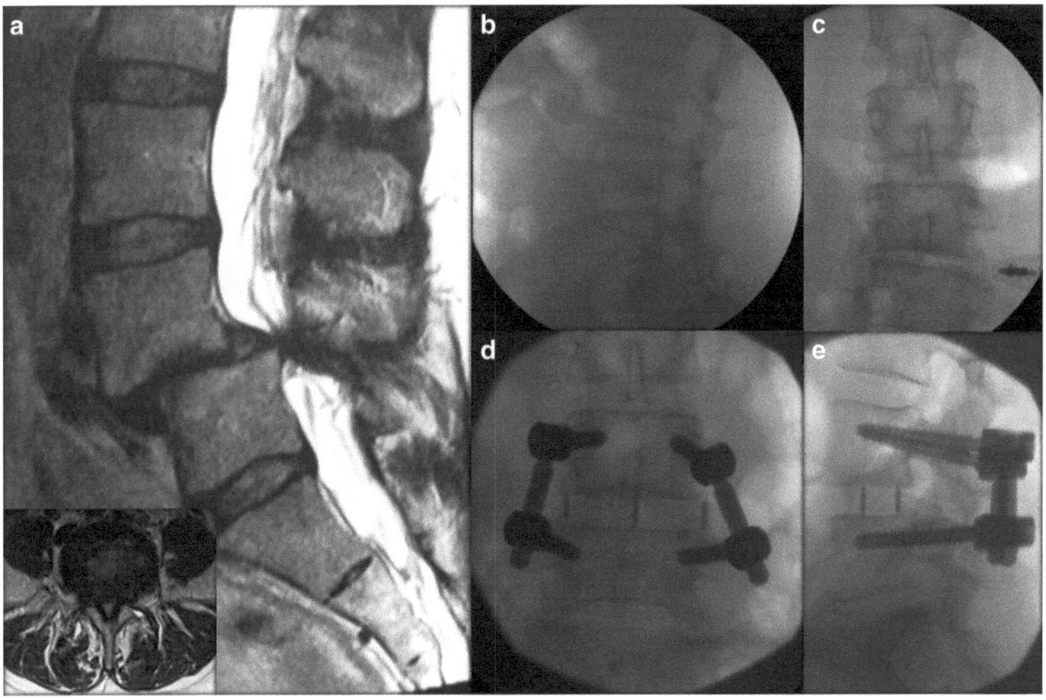

Fig. 16.8 Case example 1. Grade 2 spondylolisthesis (**a**). Ideal positioning and the accurate discectomy partially reduce the vertebral slippage (**b** and **c**). Posterior supplementation due to severe instability (**d** and **e**)

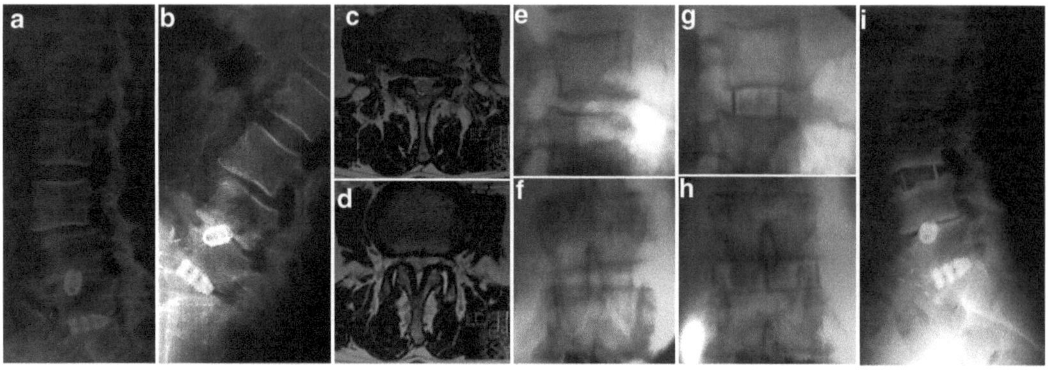

Fig. 16.9 Case example 2. Grade 1 spondylolisthesis. Dynamic X-rays show a stable deformity (**a** and **b**). Axial MRI shows stenosis (**c**) and mobile facets with liquid (**d**). Preoperative fluoroscopy (**e** and **f**). Postoperative fluoroscopy (**g** and **h**). Three-month X-ray showing good positioning of the device, increase in disc height and slippage reduction (**i**)

grade spondylolisthesis, all stand-alone constructions. They found a mean surgical duration of 73.2 ± 31.4 min (mean ± standard deviation), with less than 50 ml of blood loss and no intraoperative complications or infection. Symptoms of psoas weakness were found in 10 patients (19.2 %), while 5 patients (9.6 %) had anterior thigh numbness, both conditions resolved within 6 weeks after surgery without any special care. Clinical results of Visual Analogue Scale (VAS) and Oswestry Disability Index (ODI) were significantly improved. Radiological results have shown statistical significance in olisthesis reduction and improvement in global lordosis. Fusion was seen in 86.6 % of total cases at last follow-up, with no signals of pseudoarthrosis. Revision surgery to perform direct decompression and to place pedicle screws was necessary in seven levels (13.5 %), 5 cases in consequence of high-grade subsidence with instability/restenosis and two cases in which indirect decompression was not achieved. Other four cases of severe subsidence did not require surgical intervention. Figure 16.9 shows a case example of spondylolisthesis grade 1 treated by stand-alone lateral interbody fusion.

Conclusion

Lateral transpsoas surgery is a safe and effective treatment for spondylolisthesis up to grade 2, with remarkable clinical and radiological improvement which is maintained in long term. Strictly follow the technique step by step, using real-time neurologic monitoring, is mandatory for the success of the procedure.

References

1. Weinstein JN, Lurie JD, Tosteson TD, Zhao W, Blood EA, Tosteson ANA, et al. Surgical compared with nonoperative treatment for lumbar degenerative spondylolisthesis. Four-year results in the Spine Patient Outcomes Research Trial (SPORT) randomized and observational cohorts. J Bone Joint Surg Am. 2009; 91(6):1295–304.
2. Weinstein JN, Lurie JD, Tosteson TD, Hanscom B, Tosteson ANA, Blood EA, et al. Surgical versus nonsurgical treatment for lumbar degenerative spondylolisthesis. N Engl J Med. 2007;356(22):2257–70.
3. Kim J-S, Kang B-U, Lee S-H, Jung B, Choi Y-G, Jeon SH, et al. Mini-transforaminal lumbar interbody fusion versus anterior lumbar interbody fusion augmented by percutaneous pedicle screw fixation: a comparison of surgical outcomes in adult low-grade isthmic spondylolisthesis. J Spinal Disord Tech. 2009;22(2):114–21.
4. Lauber S, Schulte TL, Liljenqvist U, Halm H, Hackenberg L. Clinical and radiologic 2–4-year results of transforaminal lumbar interbody fusion in degenerative and isthmic spondylolisthesis grades 1 and 2. Spine. 2006;31(15):1693–8.
5. Moro T, Kikuchi S, Konno S, Yaginuma H. An anatomic study of the lumbar plexus with respect to retroperitoneal endoscopic surgery. Spine. 2003;28(5): 423–8. discussion 427–428.
6. Resnick DK, Choudhri TF, Dailey AT, Groff MW, Khoo L, Matz PG, et al. Guidelines for the performance of fusion procedures for degenerative disease

of the lumbar spine. Part 9: fusion in patients with stenosis and spondylolisthesis. J Neurosurg Spine. 2005;2(6):679–85.

7. Gill GG, Manning JG, White HL. Surgical treatment of spondylolisthesis without spine fusion; excision of the loose lamina with decompression of the nerve roots. J Bone Joint Surg Am. 1955;37-A(3):493–520.
8. Martin CR, Gruszczynski AT, Braunsfurth HA, Fallatah SM, O'Neil J, Wai EK. The surgical management of degenerative lumbar spondylolisthesis: a systematic review. Spine. 2007;32(16):1791–8.
9. Yan D, Pei F, Li J, Soo C. Comparative study of PILF and TLIF treatment in adult degenerative spondylolisthesis. Eur Spine J. 2008;17(10):1311–6.
10. Papagelopoulos PJ, Peterson HA, Ebersold MJ, Emmanuel PR, Choudhury SN, Quast LM. Spinal column deformity and instability after lumbar or thoracolumbar laminectomy for intraspinal tumors in children and young adults. Spine. 1997;22(4):442–51.
11. McAfee PC, Phillips FM, Andersson G, Buvenenadran A, Kim CW, Lauryssen C, et al. Minimally invasive spine surgery. Spine. 2010;35(Suppl):S271–3.
12. Ozgur BM, Aryan HE, Pimenta L, Taylor WR. Extreme Lateral Interbody Fusion (XLIF): a novel surgical technique for anterior lumbar interbody fusion. Spine J. 2006;6(4):435–43.
13. Oliveira L, Marchi L, Coutinho E, Pimenta L. A radiographic assessment of the ability of the extreme lateral interbody fusion procedure to indirectly decompress the neural elements. Spine. 2010; 35(Suppl):S331–7.
14. Marchi L, Abdala N, Oliveira L, Amaral R, Coutinho E, Pimenta L. Stand-alone lateral interbody fusion for the treatment of low-grade degenerative spondylolisthesis. Sci World J. 2012;2012:456346.
15. Marchi L, Oliveira L, Amaral R, Castro C, Coutinho T, Coutinho E, et al. Anterior elongation as a minimally invasive alternative for sagittal imbalance—a case series. HSS J. 2012;8(2):122–7.
16. Oliveira L, Marchi L, Coutinho E, Abdala N, Pimenta L. The use of rh-BMP2 in Standalone eXtreme Lateral Interbody Fusion (XLIF®): clinical and radiological results after 24 months follow-up. World Spinal Column J. 2010;1(1):19–25.
17. Ozgur BM, Agarwal V, Nail E, Pimenta L. Two-year clinical and radiographic success of minimally invasive lateral transpsoas approach for the treatment of degenerative lumbar conditions. SAS J. 2010;4(2): 41–6.
18. Pimenta L, Marchi L, Oliveira L, Coutinho E, Amaral R. A prospective, randomized, controlled trial comparing radiographic and clinical outcomes between stand-alone lateral interbody lumbar fusion with either silicate calcium phosphate or rh-BMP2. J Neurol Surg A Cent Eur Neurosurg. 2013;74(6): 343–50.
19. Rodgers WB, Lehmen JA, Gerber EJ, Rodgers JA. Grade 2 spondylolisthesis at L4-5 treated by XLIF: safety and midterm results in the "Worst Case Scenario". Sci World J. 2012;2012:1–7.
20. Rodgers WB, Gerber EJ, Rodgers JA. Lumbar fusion in octogenarians. Spine. 2010;35(Suppl):S355–60.
21. Khajavi K, Shen A, Lagina M, Hutchison A. Comparison of clinical outcomes following minimally invasive lateral interbody fusion stratified by preoperative diagnosis. Del Mar, California: May 10th, 2013.
22. Kepler CK, Sharma AK, Huang RC, Meredith DS, Girardi FP, Cammisa Jr FP, et al. Indirect foraminal decompression after lateral transpsoas interbody fusion. J Neurosurg Spine. 2012;16(4):329–33.
23. Youssef JA, McAfee PC, Patty CA, Raley E, Debauche S, Shucosky E, et al. Minimally invasive surgery: lateral approach interbody fusion: results and review. Spine. 2010;35(Suppl 26S):S302–11.
24. Luk KDK, Chow DHK, Holmes A. Vertical instability in spondylolisthesis: a traction radiographic assessment technique and the principle of management. Spine. 2003;28(8):819–27.
25. Park SH, Park WM, Park CW, Kang KS, Lee YK, Lim SR. Minimally invasive anterior lumbar interbody fusion followed by percutaneous translaminar facet screw fixation in elderly patients. J Neurosurg Spine. 2009;10(6):610–6.
26. Hou Y, Luo Z. A study on the structural properties of the lumbar endplate: histological structure, the effect of bone density, and spinal level. Spine. 2009;34(12):E427–33.
27. Marchi L, Abdala N, Oliveira L, Amaral R, Coutinho E, Pimenta L. Radiographic and clinical evaluation of cage subsidence after stand-alone lateral interbody fusion. J Neurosurg Spine. 2013;19(1):110–8.
28. Deukmedjian AR, Dakwar E, Ahmadian A, Smith DA, Uribe JS. Early outcomes of minimally invasive anterior longitudinal ligament release for correction of sagittal imbalance in patients with adult spinal deformity. Sci World J. 2012;2012:1–7.
29. Rodgers WB, Cox CS, Gerber EJ. Early complications of extreme lateral interbody fusion in the obese. J Spinal Disord Tech. 2010;23(6):393–7.
30. Marchi L, Oliveira L, Amaral R, Castro C, Coutinho T, Coutinho E, et al. Lateral interbody fusion for treatment of discogenic low back pain: minimally invasive surgical techniques. Adv Orthop. 2012;2012:1–7.

17 Presacral Fusion for Adult Spondylolisthesis

Gurpreet S. Gandhoke and Peter C. Gerszten

Introduction

Spine surgery is constantly making strides towards mastering the most minimally invasive route to treat the most severe pathology. Low-grade spondylolisthesis has been traditionally treated with decompressive laminectomy and posterolateral, interbody fusion, or a combination of both.

The parasagittal fibular strut, keyhole interbody rod, and vertebral body replacement devices all use the principle that the spine is an axial column with orthogonal axes defining the sagittal, bending, lateral bending, and torsional movements [1, 2]. The instantaneous axis of rotation where spinal bending and loading movements are centered is in the anterior column of the spine. An axial construct is favorably oriented to resist many of these movements, especially in combination with posterior fixation [1, 2].

The combination of an axial presacral approach combined with percutaneous pedicle screw fixation for lumbosacral discectomy and fusion offers a minimally invasive alternative procedure for the surgical management of low-grade lumbosacral spondylolisthesis. Several studies have documented the clinical success of this approach for spondylolisthesis in the setting of low-grade lumbosacral isthmic, degenerative, and post-laminectomy spondylolisthesis [3–7].

Anatomy of the Region of Interest, the Presacral Space

The midline entry point into the sacral promontory is at the level of the S1-2 interspace. At this level, the iliac vessels and the sympathetic plexus have diverged laterally. The middle sacral artery may be encountered in the midline over the sacrum but is usually small at the S1-2 level. The rectum and the sigmoid colon are separated from the sacrum by the presacral space which provides a cushion of areolar tissue and fat. This space can be easily traversed with a blunt obturator or needle. Li et al. [8] did an extensive cadaver study on the anatomy of the AxiaLIF approach. They illustrated five layers of the presacral fascial structures: Periosteum, the parietal presacral fascia, the recto-sacral fascia, autonomic nerve fascia, and the fascia propria of the rectum. They advocated that surgeons should pay attention to traverse veins and the pelvic splanchnic nerves. Injury of these structures can cause pelvic hematoma and sexual or urinary dysfunction.

G.S. Gandhoke, M.D.
P.C. Gerszten, M.D., M.P.H., F.A.C.S. (✉)
Department of Neurological Surgery, University of Pittsburgh Medical Center, UPMC Presbyterian, 200 Lothrop Street, Suite B400, Pittsburgh, PA 15213, USA
e-mail: gandhokegs@upmc.edu; gerspc@upmc.edu

A.L. Wollowick and V. Sarwahi (eds.), *Spondylolisthesis: Diagnosis, Non-Surgical Management, and Surgical Techniques*, DOI 10.1007/978-1-4899-7575-1_17,

Biomechanics of Axial fusion

Akesen et al. [9] performed the biomechanical studies of AxiaLIF in human cadavers and showed that stand-alone trans-sacral fixation significantly reduced the range of motion of segments. They demonstrated that the advantage of axial fixation is leaving the annulus intact and achieving indirect decompression with distraction. In order to obtain the optimal biomechanical properties, however, they recommended that posterior fixation, such as facet screws or pedicle screws, should be added to supplement the construct.

Ledet et al. [10] compared the biomechanical properties of the AxiaLIF with those of multiple preexisting fixation methods including cages, plates, and rod systems in bovine lumbar motion segments. Results showed a significant increase in stiffness in AxiaLIF fixation compared to the intact specimen. AxiaLIF fixation showed significantly higher stiffness than all other cage designs in terms of lateral and sagittal bending motion. In extension and axial compression, axial fixation also showed comparable stiffness to plate and rod constructs. They concluded that axial placement provides favorable biomechanical properties compared to other fixation methods. This result also was reproduced in other studies.

More recently, a biomechanical study of AxiaLIF in a long construct was performed in human cadaveric spine [11]. Fleischer and coauthors compared the S1 screw strain among four different constructs: pedicle screw alone (L2-S1), pedicle screw with an anterior interbody device, pedicle screw with axial fixation, and pedicle screw with iliac screws. The results showed that S1 screw strain was the greatest in pedicle screws alone, decreased by 38 % after anterior interbody augmentation, decreased by 75 % after using axial fixation, and decreased by 78 % after iliac screw augmentation. The study demonstrated that AxiaLIF can provide similar biomechanical properties to iliac screws.

In the subsequent sections, the technique is presented in a stepwise manner, in addition to the possible pitfalls and steps to avoid complications in treating low-grade spondylolisthesis with presacral axial interbody fusion.

Preoperative Planning and Positioning

Multiplanar imaging with MR and CT is required to determine if the patient is an appropriate surgical candidate to access the presacral space. Preoperative imaging should be thoroughly evaluated with emphasis on perirectal fat pad thickness, identification of the rectum/sacrum interface, aberrant vasculature, and anticipated trajectory. Relative contraindications for the presacral approach include insufficient presacral fat pad, previously explored presacral space, aberrant large vessels crossing the presacral space, and anatomic abnormalities that preclude placement of an axial rod through the lower lumbar segments.

After induction of general anesthesia, the patient is positioned prone on a table compatible with fluoroscopy. Bolsters are positioned under the hip in a manner such that the sacrum is raised. The operative site is excluded from the perineum with an adhesive barrier. We utilize one C-arm switching between the AP and lateral planes during the procedure.

Access

Dissection (Mini-Open Technique)

The paracoccygeal notch serves as the window of entry into the presacral space. This notch is defined medially by the coccyx and superiorly by the ligamentous arch of the caudal sacral segment. Make a 2–3 cm skin incision, 1 cm lateral to coccyx. The incision is below the ligamentous arch (Fig. 17.1)

Insert a Weitlaner retractor and mobilize the incision medially until it is positioned over the narrow bony coccyx.

The coccyx now acts as a rigid "backstop" for the dissection. Continue soft tissue dissection on the dorsal surface of coccyx. The dissection continues laterally and ventrally along the coccyx. This is the point of entry to the presacral space,

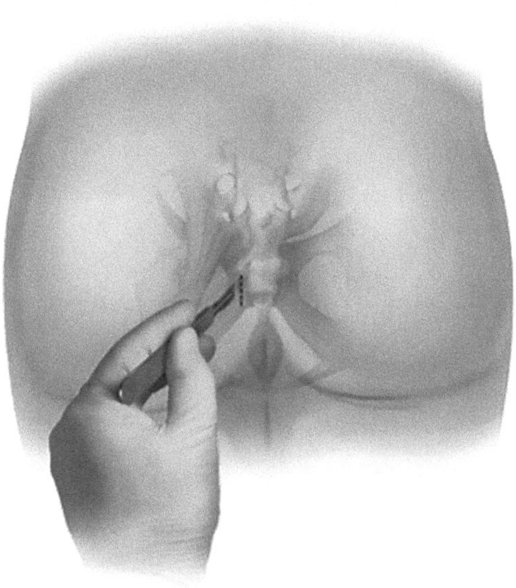

Fig. 17.1 Incision

and should be in the narrow bony part of the coccyx below the transverse process of the coccyx (Fig. 17.2).

Carefully dissect through the parietal fascia, which extends laterally from the ventral surface of the coccyx. When the fascial defect is large enough to insert a finger, begin blunt dissection of the presacral space (Fig. 17.3).

Complication Avoidance

Use of the mini-open technique will help to minimize bowel perforations at the incision site. Historically, some surgeons would create the incision lateral to the coccyx and dissect through the soft tissue. It is at this point in the procedure a bowel perforation at the incision site may happen. Dissecting against a hard back stop is the best option. Below are optional types of incisions with the applicable advantages and disadvantages of each (Table 17.1).

Presacral Access

After making the initial paracoccygeal skin incision using the mini-open techniques, use an 8″ Curved Kelly clamp turned to the anterior face of the sacrum to bluntly dissect down to the parietal fascia. Penetrating the fascia is necessary to access the retroperitoneal space and the anterior face of the sacrum. Penetrating the fascia can be accomplished using one of the following methods: (1) Finger dissection (2) blunt guide pin dissection, or (3) a combination of the two.

Finger Dissection: Dissect with your index finger to create a pathway to the sacrum while gently pushing the rectum anteriorly from the mesorectal soft tissue plane. While advancing towards the S1-S2 intersection, you can palpate the peritoneal layer of tissue (Waldeyer's fascia) that runs between the rectum and sacrum [13]. When you palpate this anatomy with your finger, you will note the retro rectal space. Use your index finger to sweep away tissue from the anterior face of the sacrum (Fig. 17.4).

Blunt Dissection: Use the Curved Dissecting Tool to penetrate the fascia immediately below the ligaments. Advance the Curved Dissecting Tool cephalad along the midline, keeping the tip engaged on the anterior cortex of the sacrum to approximately the sacral promontory. Continue to check the A/P and lateral fluoroscopic views. This maneuver is accomplished with "fingertip" control on the handle of the Dissecting Tool and should be completed using fluoroscopic guidance in both A/P and lateral planes (Fig. 17.5).

Extend the dissection bi-laterally taking care to avoid the sacral foramina. This step should be accomplished with guidance from AP fluoroscopy (Fig. 17.6).

Remove the Curved Dissector and insert the Inserter with the attached Bowel Retractor into the dissected presacral space, ensuring the tip of the Inserter/Bowel Retractor is in contact with the sacrum. Deliver the Bowel Retractor to the sacral promontory or the endpoint of the dissection (Fig. 17.7a).

Fill the 30 cc Syringe with a mixture comprised of 10 cc of contrast (intended for enteral use, i.e. Omnipaque, Gastrograffin, etc.) and 20 cc of saline (Fig. 17.7b).

Reposition inflated Bowel Retractor close to promontory (Fig. 17.7c).

Remove Inserter by pulling Inserter while slightly pushing forward at neck of Bowel Retractor (Fig. 17.7d).

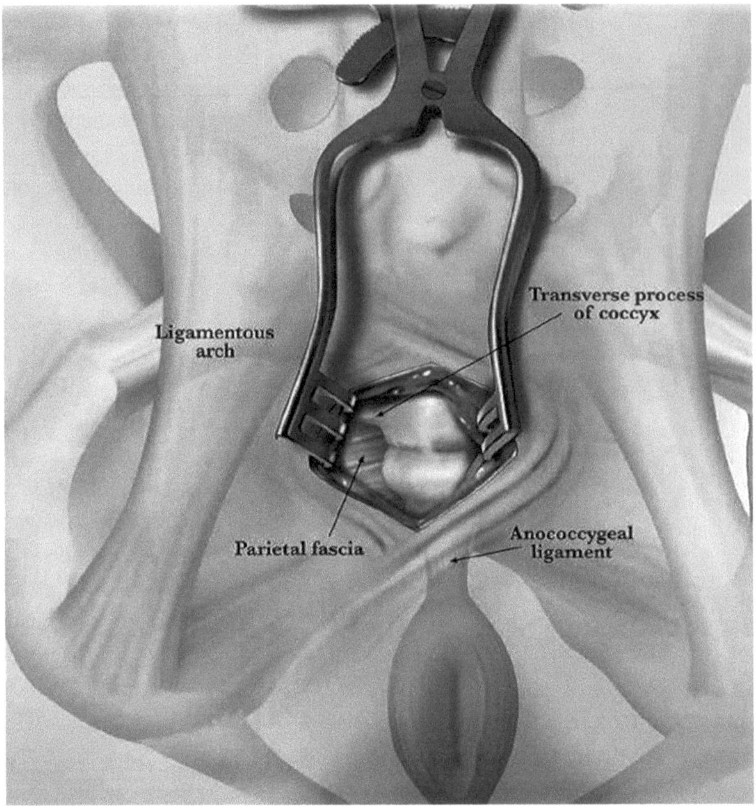

Fig. 17.2 Entry into the presacral space

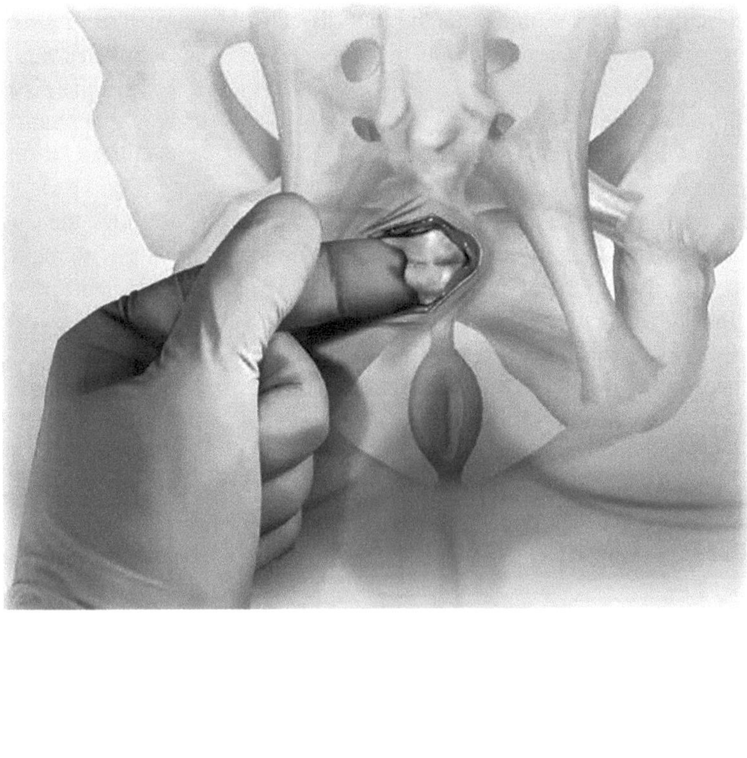

Fig. 17.3 Blunt dissection of the presacral space

Complication Avoidance

Use of the bowel retractor to mitigate the risk of bowel perforation during dissection is a maneuver which can substantially reduce the risk on an untoward injury to the rectum. The bowel retractor is a radiolucent inflatable barrier that pushes the bowel anteriorly away from the field of view and allows the instrumentation to advance while protecting the bowel.

Trajectory

Once the dissection has been completed and the bowel retractor is in place, the trajectory is then obtained. Use the dissecting tool to match the trajectory suggested by the template during the preoperative planning session. If the Dissecting Tool cannot match the trajectory suggested by the template, adjust the template to the obtainable trajectory of the Dissecting Tool and verify. Once the trajectory is established, exchange the Dissector Stylet inside the Dissecting Tool for the Beveled Guide Pin then insert the Beveled Guide Pin into the Guide Pin Handle. Insert the Guide Pin Handle through the Dissecting Tool. While maintaining the correct trajectory, the Guide Pin Handle is tapped with the Slap Hammer or a small mallet to dock the Beveled Guide Pin into the sacrum (Fig. 17.8).

Confirm trajectory with AP and lateral fluoroscopy and gently tap the Beveled Guide Pin through the sacrum and 1–2 mm into the L5 vertebral body. Using fluoroscopy, confirm the trajectory of the Beveled Guide Pin for proper placement of the implant.

Table 17.1 Advantages and disadvantages of the two different access incisions

Incision	Advantages	Disadvantages
Horizontal	May reduce wound dehiscence and less scarring due to Langer's lines [12]; can potentially allow for better lateral trajectory correction	Potentially more difficult A/P trajectory correction
Vertical	Potentially allow for better A/P trajectory correction; most common incision approach	Potentially more difficult lateral trajectory correction

Complication Avoidance

The trajectory should plan for implant placement between the pedicles. If the trajectory is too lateral, this may affect placement of pedicle screws later in the procedure or lead to breaching of the lateral wall of the vertebral body. If resulting placement of the beveled guide pin is unsatisfactory, the beveled guide pin should be removed

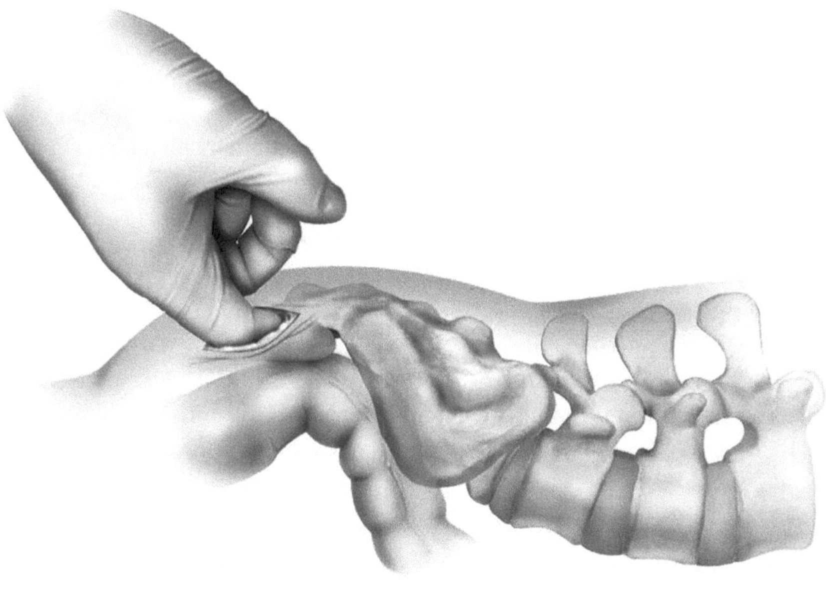

Fig. 17.4 Blunt dissection of the rectum away from the field of surgery

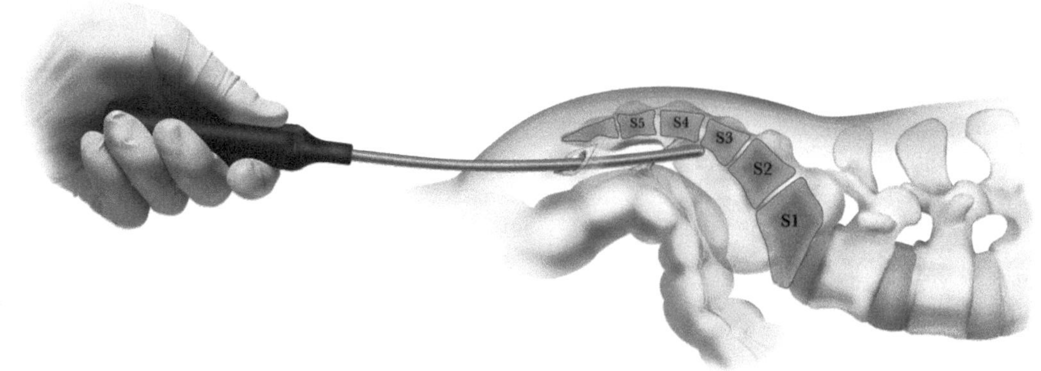

Fig. 17.5 Expansion of dissection of the rectum off the presacral space

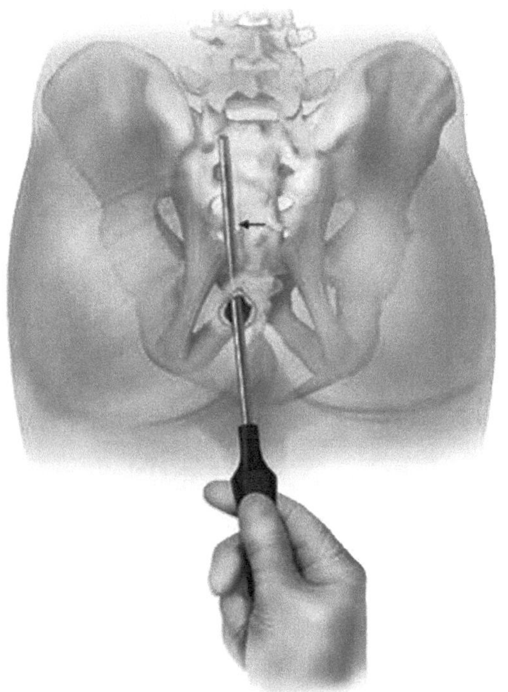

Fig. 17.6 Further expansion of dissection of the rectum off the presacral space

and reinserted until the proper trajectory is achieved.

Remove the Guide Pin Knob from the Guide Pin Handle. Remove the Guide Pin Handle and attach the Guide (Fig. 17.9).

Dilating

After the trajectory has been set and confirmed with the Beveled Guide Pin, a series of instruments are then used to sequentially dilate the soft tissue and sacral corticocancellous bone to create the working channel. Starting with the 6 mm Dilator, slide the Dilator over the Beveled Guide Pin. Use the Slap Hammer to advance the Dilator into the sacrum approximately halfway to the disc space. Remove the 6 mm Dilator, leaving the Beveled Guide Pin in place, and repeat with the 8 mm Dilator. Remove the 8 mm Dilator and repeat with the 10 mm Dilator Assembly. The 10 mm Dilator is assembled together with the 10 mm Dilator Sheath, which slides over the 10 mm Dilator body and engages with a pin and slot configuration. Advance the 10 mm Dilator far enough into the sacrum to ensure the outer diameter of the 10 mm Dilator Sheath is placed completely within the sacral cortex (Fig. 17.10).

Drilling S1: 9 mm Drill

Once the dilation of the sacrum is complete, a channel to the L5-S1 disc space is then created by inserting the 9 mm Cannulated Drill over the Beveled Guide Pin through the 10 mm sheath. Create the channel to the L5-S1 disc space by

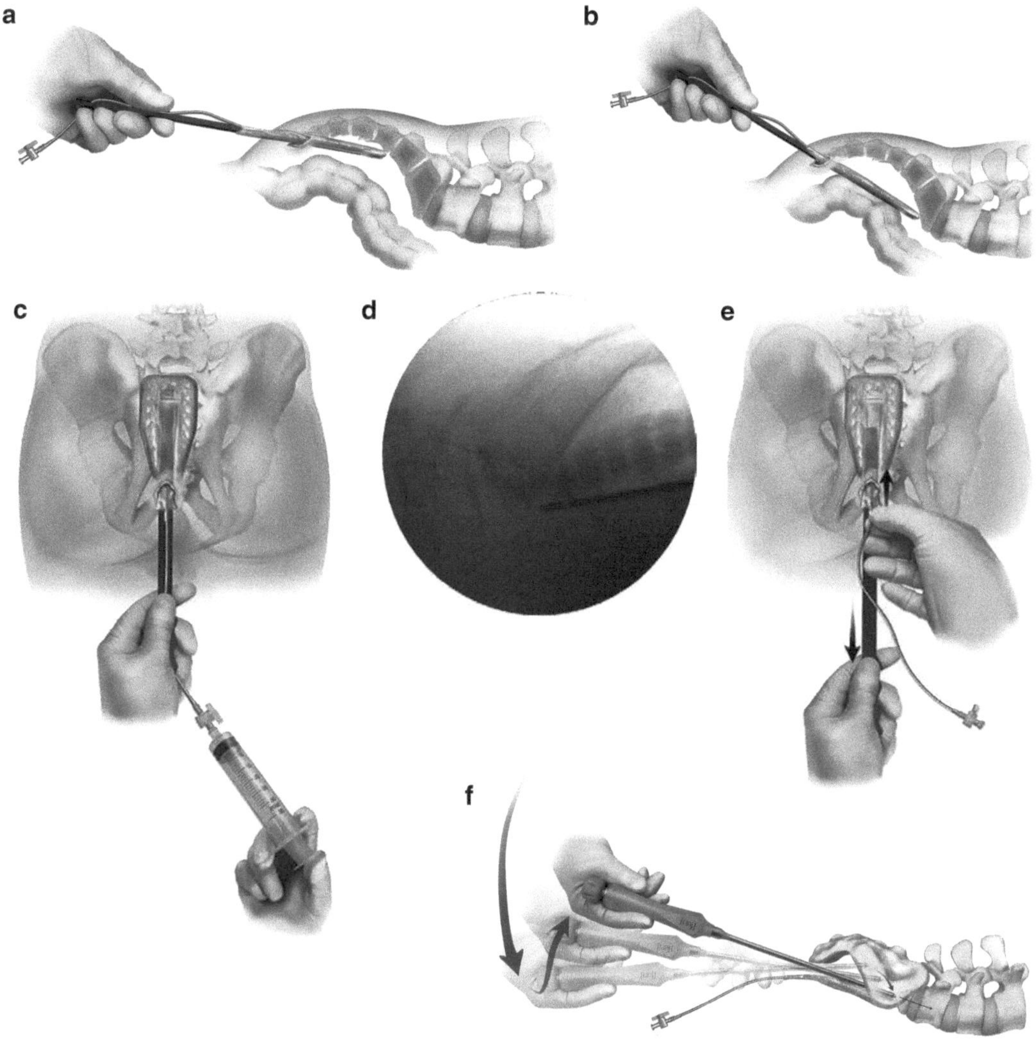

Fig. 17.7 (**a**, **b**) Role and use of the bowel retractor. (**c**) Controlled dissection in the presacral space with the bowel retractor balloon. Reposition inflated bowel retractor close to promontory. (**d**) Fluoroscopic guidance during the presacral dissection. (**e**, **f**) Pulling inserter while slightly pushing forward at neck of bowel retractor

rotating the drill in a clockwise motion. Live fluoroscopy should be used when drilling to ensure both correct trajectory and confirmation of the channel into the L5-S1 disc space. Once the channel has been confirmed, remove the 9 mm Cannulated Drill. When extracting the drill, continue rotating in a clockwise motion. This technique helps to hold pieces of bone in the flutes of the drill. These can be placed aside to be used later in the procedure as supplemental bone graft material (Fig. 17.11).

Discectomy at L5/S1

With the channel to the L5-S1 disc space confirmed, a series of Nitinol Disc Cutters, varying in length and shape, are then used to prepare the disc space. (Each cutter is designed to debulk the nucleus pulposus and lightly abrade the endplates circumferentially up to a 3 cm diameter to create a bleeding bed for fusion.)

Retract the flexible Nitinol blade of the Small Radial Cutter into the cutter sleeve, and then

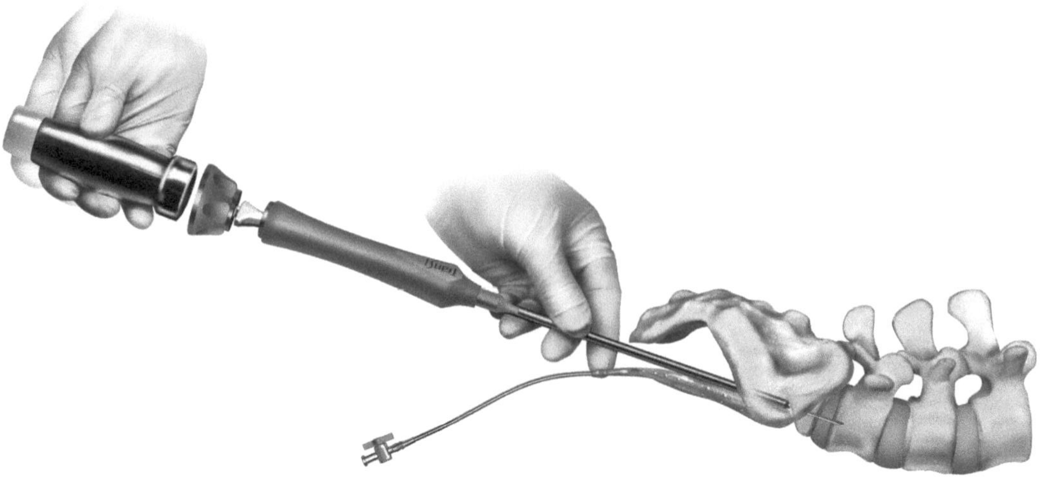

Fig. 17.8 Docking of the beveled guide pin into the sacrum

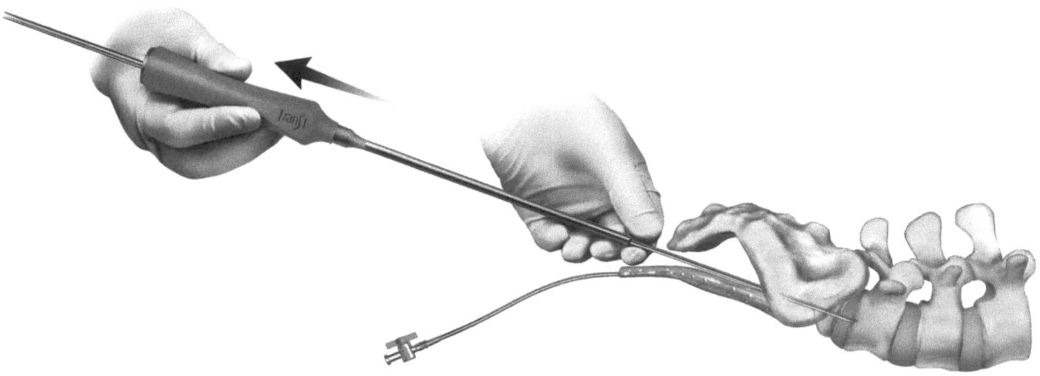

Fig. 17.9 Removal of the guide pin handle and attachment of the guide

insert the cutter through the 10 mm Dilator Sheath into the disc space. Once inside the disc space, deploy the blade in the direction that provides the most space for deployment. Typically this will be laterally or anteriorly. Using both lateral and AP fluoroscopic views, verify that the blade will not violate the annulus. Begin a series of cutting motions by rotating the handle in 90° turns to cut and remove tissue. The double-edged blade allows cutting in both directions. Repeat the process with the Large Radial Cutter, Small Radial Down cutter, and Large Radial Down cutter, in that order. (Fig. 17.12a–c)

Two series of cutters, followed by disc removal, should be performed. The first series of cutters (Small and Large Radial Cutters) are to debulk the nucleus near L5 and the second series of cutters (Small and Large Radial Down cutters) are to debulk the nucleus near S1. Tissue extractors are used to remove disc material loosened by the cutters. Tissue extractors may be used after each cutter. Retract the Tissue Extractor head into the sheath before inserting it through the 10 mm Dilator Sheath. Advance the Tissue Extractor to the L5 endplate and deploy the Tissue Extractor head. Rotate the Tissue Extractor Knob no more than six full revolutions counterclockwise and remove by pulling the entire extractor unsheathed through the dilator sheath. Discard the extractor and repeat as necessary.

The endplate rasps are then utilized to prepare the endplates. The up-cutter prepares L5 while the down-cutter prepares S1. After the endplates have been prepared, tissue extractors are once again utilized to remove the cartilaginous material (Fig. 17.13).

Complication Avoidance

This step is the most crucial in the procedure. The discectomy portion should not be rushed and should be expected to last at least 20 min. Improper disc preparation may affect the fusion process. During the disc preparation and depending on the trajectory established, the range of dissection could be affected. Always use fluoroscopy to establish where the tips of the cutters and endplate rasps are, as you do not want to compromise the annulus and increase the risk of graft extrusions due to a compromised annulus.

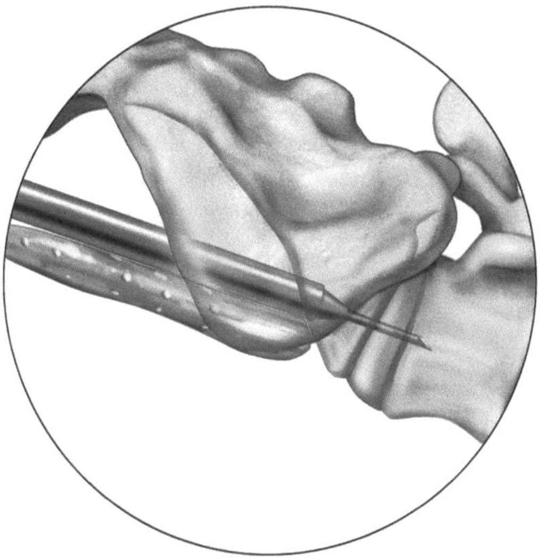

Fig. 17.10 Sequential dilation

Bone Grafting at L5/S1

Prepare the bone graft material (i.e., autogenous bone and allogenic demineralized bone matrix (DBM) mixed with autologous blood) for the L5/S1 disc space by utilizing the autologous material harvested during the drilling. Typically, a total of 7–10 cc of grafting material will be required to fill the disc space. Therefore, insert 2–3 cc of bone graft per tube. Use the Bone Graft Inserter to place the bone graft material into the L5/S1 disc space. Take care not to advance the beveled edge of the Bone Graft Inserter Cannula into L5. Push the material into the disc space and pack it by pushing the Bone Graft Inserter Plunger through the cannula. Repeat the loading process until the disc space is full, rotating the beveled tip to deliver the material into the disc space in quadrants. Check trajectory with A/P and lateral fluoroscopic views (Fig. 17.14a, b).

Complication Avoidance

To minimize the prospect of non-fusion due to the grafting material, it is recommended to use the following materials for AxiaLIF procedures:

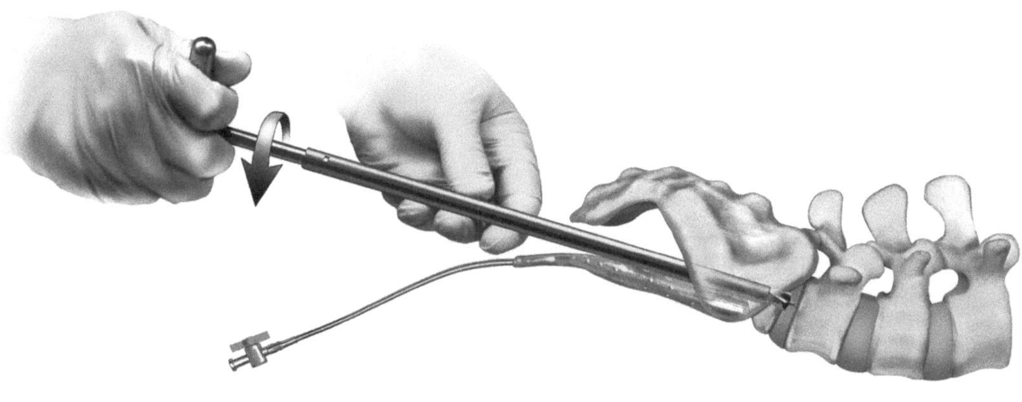

Fig. 17.11 Sacral dilation

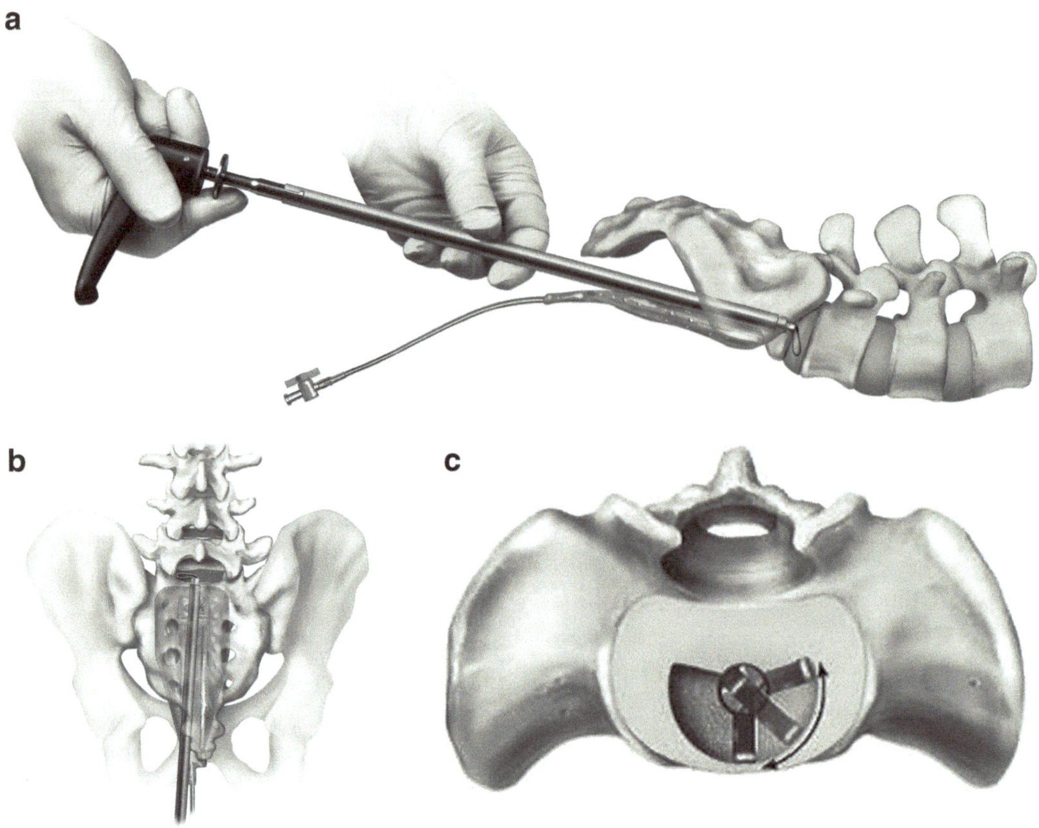

Fig. 17.12 (**a–c**) Discectomy at L5-S1

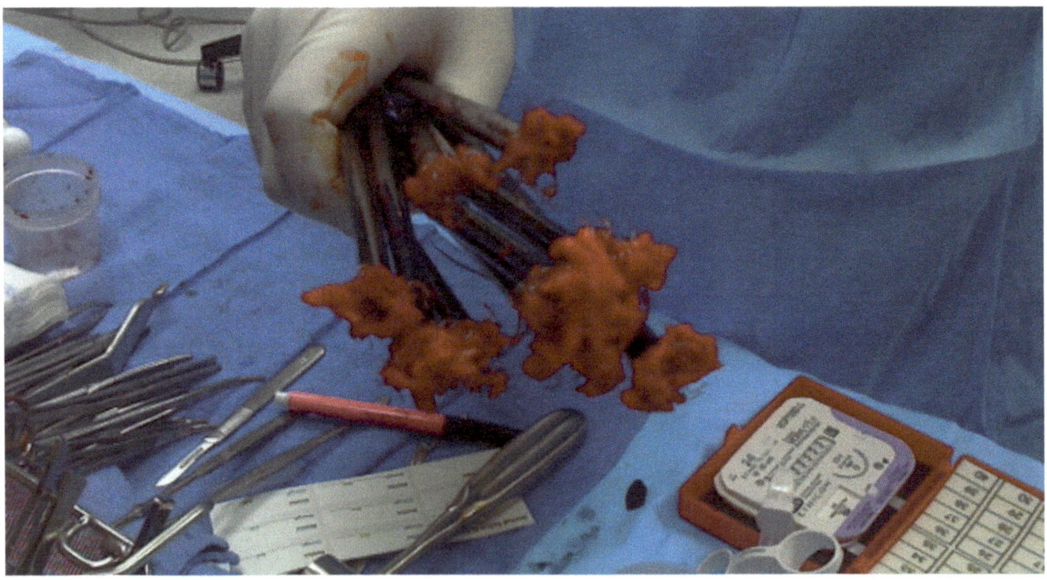

Fig. 17.13 Discectomy and preparation of the end plates

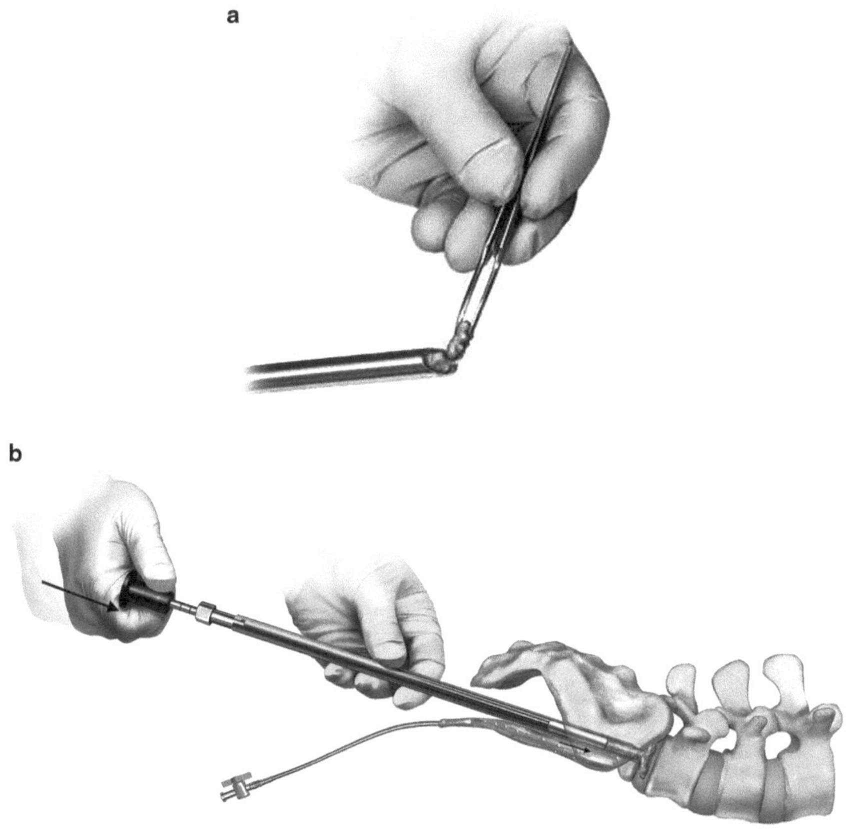

Fig. 17.14 (**a**, **b**) Bone grafting

- Autograft
  - 5–8 cc per fused level
  - Autograft may be combined with appropriately cleared osteoinductive agents and/or osteoconductive matrices, such as bone graft extenders for use with autograft bone in spinal fusion applications
- Bone Marrow Aspirate
  - Harvested from iliac crest or vertebral body (pedicle approach)
  - The aspirate should then be combined with an appropriately cleared matrix, ceramic or allograft chips

Dilating: 12 mm Dilator

Insert the Beveled Guide wire and remove the 10 mm sheath. Utilizing the 8 mm dilator insert the 12 mm Dilator with Sheath Assembly over the Beveled Guide Pin. Use the Slap Hammer to dock the Dilator with Sheath in the sacrum. Advance the 12 mm Dilator far enough into the sacrum to ensure the outer diameter of the sheath is placed completely within the sacral cortex (Fig. 17.15).

Disengage the 12 mm Dilator from the 12 mm Dilator Sheath and remove the 12 mm Dilator. The Dilator Sheath should remain anchored to the sacrum to serve as a protected working channel for subsequent instrumentation.

Drilling S1: 10.5 mm Drill

Working through the 12 mm dilator, insert the 10.5 mm Drill through the Dilator Sheath and rotate the handle clockwise, drilling until just through the sacrum or past the S1 endplate. Fluoroscopy is used to verify how far to drill into the sacrum and disc.

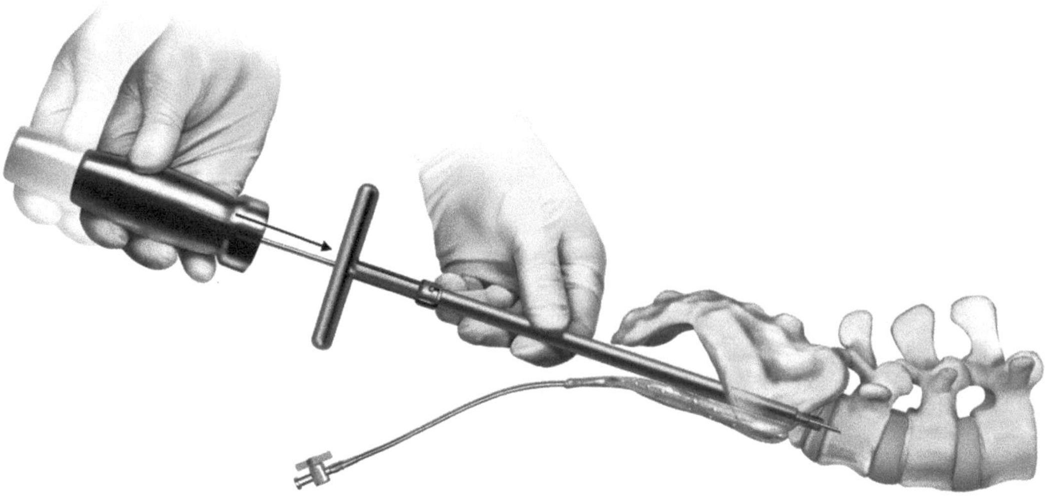

Fig. 17.15 Twelve millimeter dilation

When extracting the Drill, twist in a counterclockwise motion. This technique ensures bone graft will be left in the disc space (Fig. 17.16).

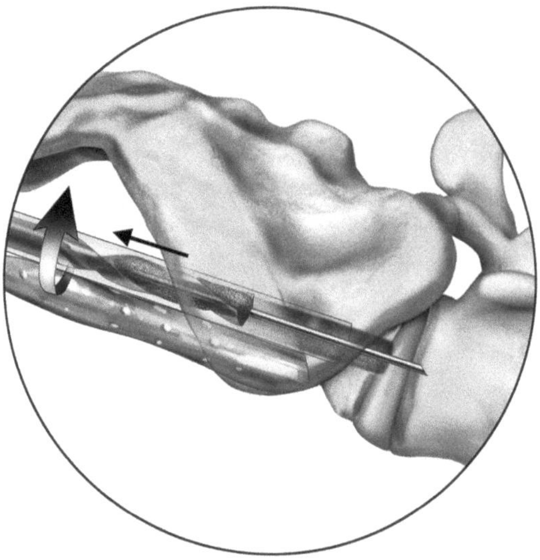

Fig. 17.16 Use of the 10.5 mm drill

Advance 12 mm Sheath

Reinsert the beveled guide pin and tap into the L5 endplate. Using the 12 mm Dilator Tamp, advance the 12 mm Dilator Tamp and Sheath with the Slap Hammer up to the L5 vertebral body so that the tip of the sheath is flush against the inferior endplate of the L5 vertebral body. Once the 12 mm Dilator Sheath is flush against the inferior endplate of the L5 vertebral body, remove the Dilator body from the Sheath (Fig. 17.17).

Drilling L5 Endplate: 10.5 mm Drill

Through the 12 mm dilator sheath, insert the 10.5 mm drill over the beveled guide wire and drill 10–15 mm (or 1/3 to 1/2) into the L5 vertebral body. This enables the L5 Dilator Trial to be inserted into L5. Fluoroscopy is used to verify drill depth into the L5 vertebral body. Remove the beveled guide pin after drilling (Fig. 17.18).

Complication Avoidance

In situations where soft bone has been identified, and to minimize the complication of subsidence, more dilation or smaller drill channel creation should be incorporated. Either use the 9 mm Drill to create the drill channel of 3 mm into L5, use of the Dilator Trial to create a channel in L5 or a combination of both.

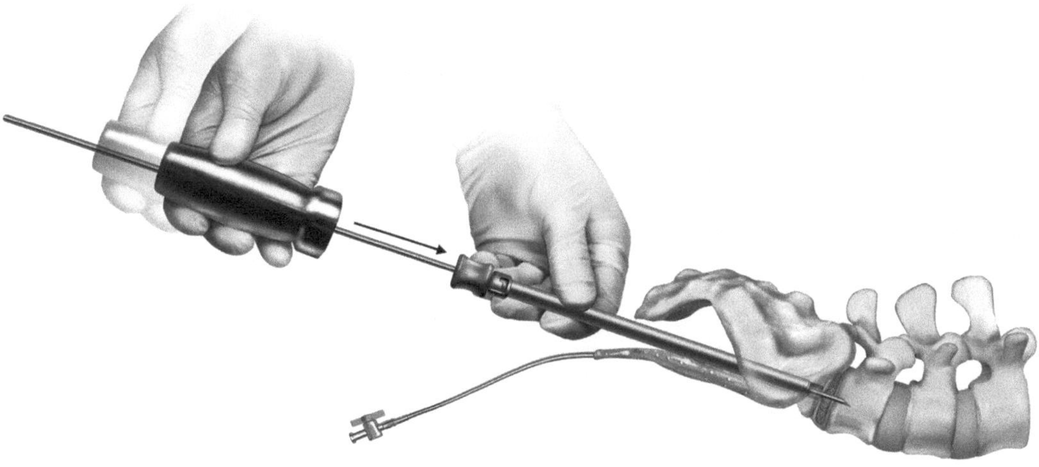

Fig. 17.17 Advance 12 mm sheath

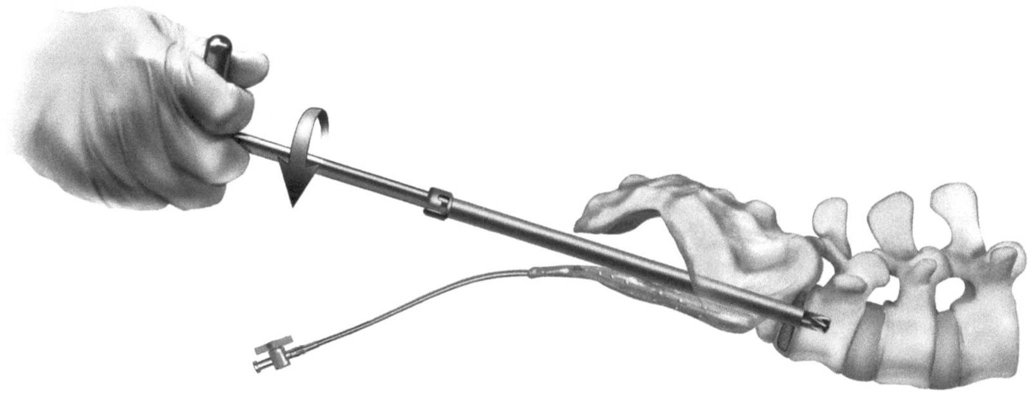

Fig. 17.18 Drilling the L5 Endplate

Dilator Trial Insertion and Implant Size Selection

Insert the 20 mm L5 Dilator Trial through the 12 mm sheath until the shoulder is in line with the inferior L5 endplate. If the dilator trial tip is 2/3 to 3/4 of the way into the L5 vertebral body, then take measurements using the 20 mm L5 Dilator Trial. If the dilator trial tip can go deeper, then remove the 20 mm trial and insert the 22.5 mm trial until the shoulder is in line with the inferior L5 endplate (Fig. 17.19).

If the L5 tip of the Dilator Trial is 2/3rds to 3/4ths depth in L5, then look at the lateral cross holes in the Dilator Trial shaft to determine the S1 Anchor size. The hole that is closest to the sacral face will represent which S1 Anchor size to select. The hole closest to the L5 tip represents the 25 mm S1 Anchor and each of the adjacent holes is 5 mm apart.

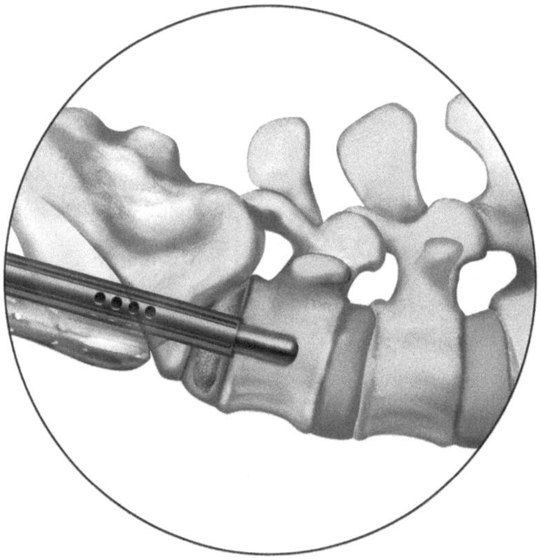

Fig. 17.19 Dilator trial insertion and implant size selection

Exchange System

Evaluate the sacral face in the lateral view to choose which Exchange System (30°, 45° or 60°) best matches the contact angle. Insert the Single Piece Guide Wire and remove the Dilator Sheath using the 12 mm Dilator while leaving the Single Piece Guide Wire in place. Place the selected Exchange Bushing over the Single Piece Guide Wire, advancing it with the long laser mark facing dorsal until it contacts the sacral face. Verify correct placement using fluoroscopy. Simultaneously rotate the Bushing 180° and continue advancing the bushing until the angled surface of the bushing meets the sacral face (exposing the short laser mark on the dorsal side). Advance the conformable tip tubular retractor (CTTR) over the bushing with the arrow pointing dorsal until the angled, flexible tip the contacts sacral face. Again, verify correct placement with fluoroscopy. The CTTR has two channels for Fixation Wires, which are used to secure the Retractor to the sacrum. Insert a Fixation Wire by hand through one of the two small lumens at the handle end of the Retractor until the tip contacts the sacrum. Advance the Fixation Wire 1–2 cm into the sacrum using a wire driver. Bend the Wire out of the way and insert the second Fixation Wire in a similar fashion (Fig. 17.20).

Complication Avoidance

Use of the CTTR will help to minimize bowel perforations at the sacral face due to the flexible tip. The CTTR is designed to keep the bowel out of the area of the sacral face during implant insertion.

Implant Delivery

Assemble the selected L5 Anchor, S1 Anchor and Distraction Rod onto the large hexalobe of the Dual Driver. Secure all implant components using the Retention Tube (Fig. 17.21).

Insert the assembled implant construct into the Tubular Retractor and over the Single Piece Guide Wire and carefully advance the Dual Driver until the superior end of the implant is engaged with the sacrum. While maintaining the position of the Tubular Retractor, advance the construct by rotating the Dual Driver clockwise. Axial pressure may be required to initially engage the rod threads into bone. Continue implant insertion until the L5 Anchor is fully engaged in the L5 vertebral body. The waist section between the S1 and L5 Anchors must be in the L5/S1 disc space to allow for distraction. The inferior portion of the S1 Anchor should be proud on the face of the sacrum by one or two threads. Remove the Retention Tube by unthreading it in a counterclockwise direction. To remove the Dual Driver, put the ratcheting handle in the fixed or neutral position and pull back while lightly rocking back and forth (Fig. 17.22).

S1 Distraction

To obtain distraction of the L5-S1 disc space, insert the Counter Torque Tube over the Single Piece Guide Wire and through the Tubular Retractor and rotate slightly until engaged in the back of the S1 Anchor. Remove the Single Piece Guide Wire and insert the Distraction Driver through the Counter Torque Tube and press forward while initially rotating to engage it in the Distraction Rod. Use the Distraction Driver to distract the L5-S1 disc space by slowly rotating the handle clockwise while at the same time

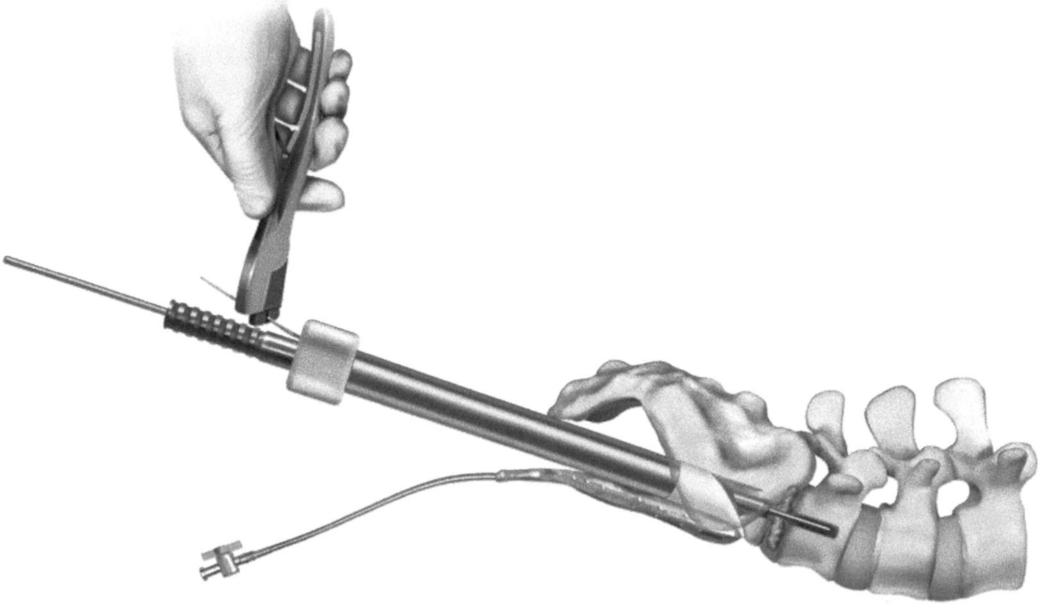

Fig. 17.20 Role and use of the exchange system

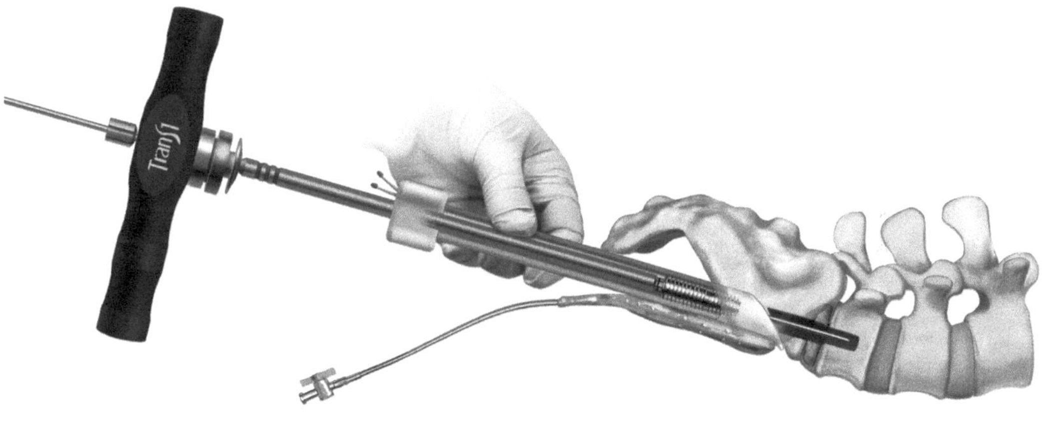

Fig. 17.21 Implant delivery-1

maintaining the rotational position of the Counter Torque Tube. One full rotation of the handle will produce approximately 1.25 mm of distraction.

Complication Avoidance

Typical distraction in normal bone can be as great as 5 mm. For patients with soft bones it is possible to achieve a 12 mm maximum distraction. However, this is not recommended due to potential risk of implant strippage/migration due to poor bone quality. The use of fluoroscopy during distraction will help mitigate this complication (Fig. 17.23).

Fixation Rod Insertion

Once distraction has been attained, the implant fixation rod must be inserted. To accomplish this, connect the ratcheting torque limiting

(RTL) handle to the quick connect portion of the Fixation Rod Driver (either end). Assemble the Fixation Rod onto the small hex of the Fixation Rod Driver. Next thread the Retention Tube into the back of the RTL Handle and Fixation Rod Driver and turn it clockwise until it is fully tightened into the Fixation Rod. Insert the Fixation Rod through the Tubular Retractor and engage it in the internal threads of the L5 Anchor portion of the AxiaLIF Plus 1-Level construct by turning clockwise. Continue turning using a light touch until the Fixation Rod is fully seated as indicated by an initial positive stop on the driver as well as visual fluoroscopy confirmation. This must be performed while closely monitoring under fluoroscopy to ensure the L5 Anchor does not advance. Remove the Retention Tube by rotating counterclockwise and then remove the Fixation Rod Driver (Fig. 17.24).

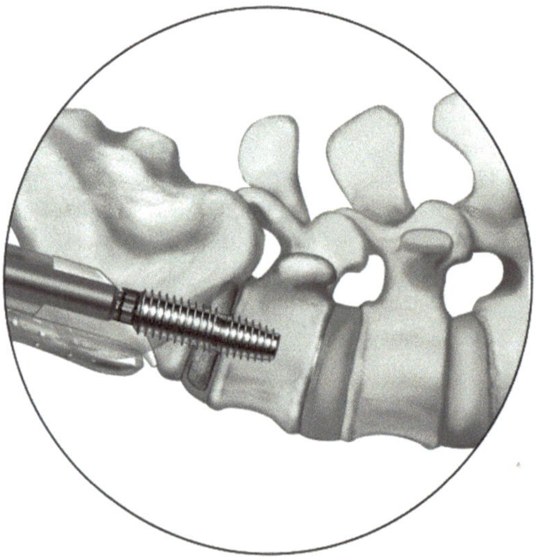

Fig. 17.22 Implant delivery-2

Complication Avoidance

If the L5 Anchor starts advancing during this step, STOP and remove the Retention Tube and driver. In situations of soft bone, it is critical that fixation rod implantation is closely watched. Soft bone will not cause the driver to reach the torque measurement; thus, it is very possible to continue to advance the implant further than anticipated.

Finish and Close

To complete the implantation of the AxiaLIF system, flush and aspirate the presacral corridor as needed with an antibiotic. Remove the Fixation Wires and then remove the Tubular Retractor. Close the skin in routine fashion and apply a dressing to the access site. Complete the L5/S1 anterior construct with percutaneous posterior instrumentation [5] (Fig. 17.25a–c).

Complication Avoidance

To minimize the occurrence of presacral hematomas, before removing the Tubular Retractor, insert an anti-coagulant product such as Flo-Seal, down the retractor and into the presacral space near the site of implant insertion. Careful attention should also be given to the wound closure. Utilize deep dermal skin approximation. In our

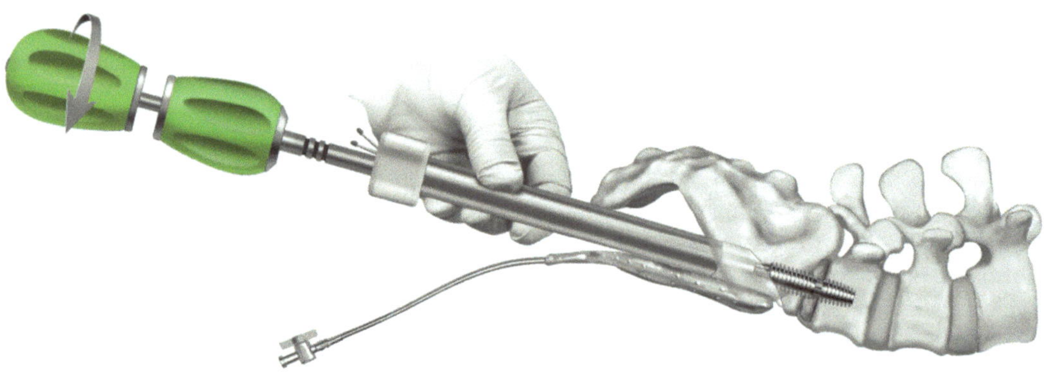

Fig. 17.23 S1 distraction

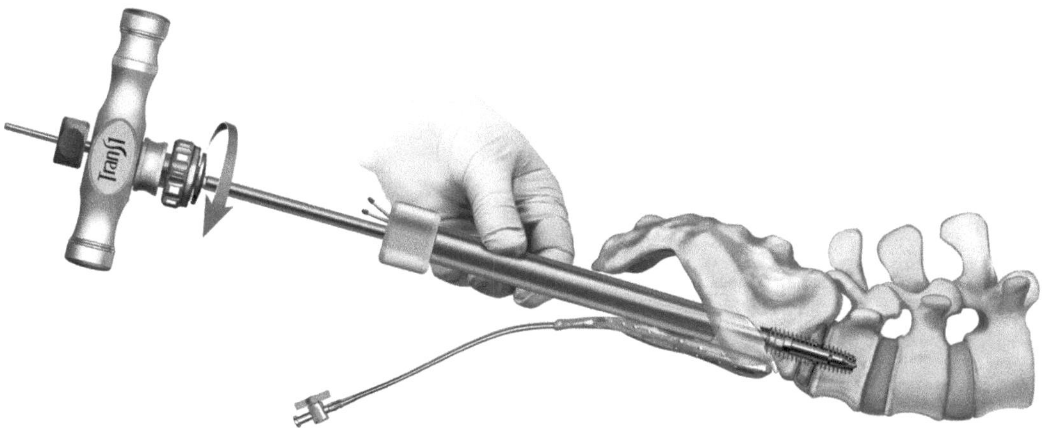

Fig. 17.24 Fixation rod insertion

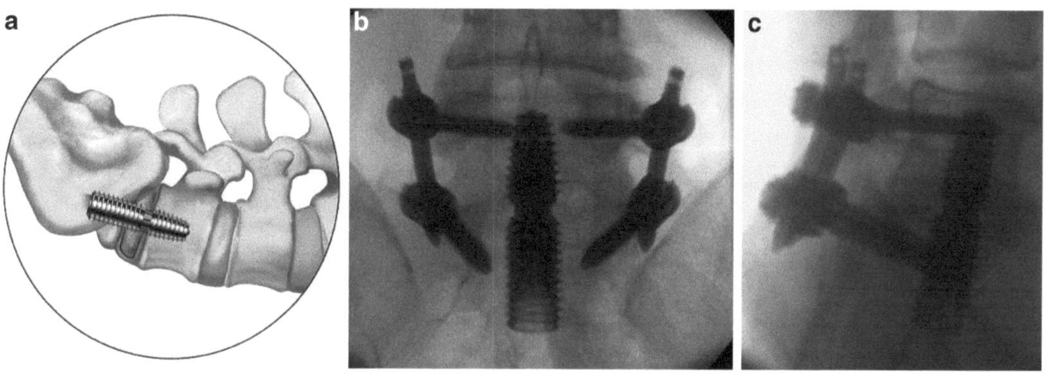

Fig. 17.25 (a–c) Final result

experience the procedure is associated with minimal blood loss and postoperative pain. Patients are usually discharged home on the first postoperative day.

Conclusion

The AxiaLIF System is not intended to treat severe spondylolisthesis (grade 3 or 4). Overall, the minimally invasive ALIF through a presacral approach combined with percutaneous posterior fixation is a technically feasible treatment for symptomatic spondylolisthesis that is associated with high fusion rates, significant improvements in pain, and low complication rates.

References

1. Meyers AM, Noonan KJ, Mih AD, Idler R. Salvage reconstruction with vascularized fibular strut graft fusion using posterior approach in the treatment of severe spondylolisthesis. Spine. 2001;26(16):1820–4. PMID: 11493859.
2. MacMillan M, Fessler RG, Gillespy M, Montgomery WJ. Percutaneous lumbosacral fixation and fusion: anatomic study and two-year experience with a new method. Neurosurg Clin N Am. 1996;7(1):99–106. PubMed PMID: 8835150.
3. Aryan HE, Newman CB, Gold JJ, Acosta Jr FL, Coover C, Ames CP. Percutaneous axial lumbar interbody fusion (AxiaLIF) of the L5-S1 segment: initial clinical and radiographic experience. Minim Invasive Neurosurg. 2008;51(4):225–30. PMID: 18683115.
4. Cragg A, Carl A, Casteneda F, Dickman C, Guterman L, Oliveira C. New percutaneous access method for

minimally invasive anterior lumbosacral surgery. J Spinal Disord Tech. 2004;17(1):21–8. PMID: 14734972.
5. Gersztcn PC, Tobler W, Raley TJ, Miller LE, Block JE, Nasca RJ. Axial presacral lumbar interbody fusion and percutaneous posterior fixation for stabilization of lumbosacral isthmic spondylolisthesis. J Spinal Disord Tech. 2012;25(2):E36–40. PMID: 21964453.
6. Tender GC, Miller LE, Block JE. Percutaneous pedicle screw reduction and axial presacral lumbar interbody fusion for treatment of lumbosacral spondylolisthesis: a case series. J Med Case Rep. 2011;5:454. PMID: 21910878. PMCID: 3179763.
7. Tobler WD, Gerszten PC, Bradley WD, Raley TJ, Nasca RJ, Block JE. Minimally invasive axial presacral L5-S1 interbody fusion: two-year clinical and radiographic outcomes. Spine. 2011;36(20):E1296–301. PMID: 21494201.
8. Li X, Zhang Y, Hou Z, Wu T, Ding Z. The relevant anatomy of the approach for axial lumbar interbody fusion. Spine. 2012;37(4):266–71. PMID: 21494190.
9. Akesen B, Wu C, Mehbod AA, Transfeldt EE. Biomechanical evaluation of paracoccygeal transsacral fixation. J Spinal Disord Tech. 2008;21(1): 39–44. PMID: 18418135.
10. Ledet EH, Tymeson MP, Salerno S, Carl AL, Cragg A. Biomechanical evaluation of a novel lumbosacral axial fixation device. J Biomech Eng. 2005;127(6): 929–33. PMID: 16438229.
11. Fleischer GD, Kim YJ, Ferrara LA, Freeman AL, Boachie-Adjei O. Biomechanical analysis of sacral screw strain and range of motion in long posterior spinal fixation constructs: effects of lumbosacral fixation strategies in reducing sacral screw strains. Spine. 2012;37(3):E163–9. PMID: 21857409.
12. Gibson T. Karl Langer (1819–1887) and his lines. Br J Plast Surg. 1978;31(1):1–2. PMID: 342024.
13. Crapp AR, Cuthbertson AM. William Waldeyer and the rectosacral fascia. Surg Gynecol Obstet. 1974; 138(2):252–6. PMID: 4589911.

Surgical Techniques: Management of High-Grade Spondylolisthesis Including Reduction Techniques

18

Scott C. Wagner, Harry L. Shufflebarger, and Ronald A. Lehman

Introduction

Surgical management of high-grade spondylolisthesis is an area of controversy. Multiple techniques for reduction and fixation have been described, and before beginning a discussion regarding these techniques, an understanding of the current classification schemes and pathomechanics of high-grade spondylolisthesis is required.

Pathomechanics of High-Grade Spondylolisthesis

Significant anatomic changes are common in patients with high-grade spondylolisthesis, including primarily dysplastic posterior elements of the lumbosacral junction. The changes occur typically secondary to deficiency in the pars interarticularis, and include facet and laminar dysplasia, or spina bifida occulta of the sacrum [1–3]. Elongation of the pars or stress fracture is the primary deficiency that leads to development of spondylolisthesis, with resultant instability of the lumbosacral junction that allows for anterior translation of L5. Wedging of the vertebral body of L5, kyphosis, and doming of the sacrum are all secondary changes that progressively develop. Subsequently, changes in the alignment of the spine in relation to the pelvis occur, with alteration in the sagittal orientation of the sacrum and pelvis that significantly changes the vector of shear forces at the lumbosacral junction [1]. Normally, these forces are resisted by the pars interarticularis posteriorly, and the intervertebral disc anteriorly; when deficient, progressive deformity occurs [3]. These changes in spinopelvic alignment are the basis for a new classification of high-grade spondylolisthesis [1, 2].

Classification of Spondylolisthesis

The original Meyerding classification of spondylolisthesis is based on the percentage of lumbar vertebral slip in relation to the sacrum. Grades I and II represent 0–25 % and 26–50 % vertebral translation, respectively, and are typically referred to a "low-grade slips." High-grade spondylolisthesis is composed of grades III and IV, which are defined as 51–75 % and 76–100 % translation, respectively. Grade V, which represents greater than 100 % translation, is termed spondyloptosis.

S.C. Wagner, M.D. (✉) • R.A. Lehman, M.D.
Department of Orthopaedic Surgery, Walter Reed National Military Medical Center, 8901 Wisconsin Avenue, Bethesda, MD 20889, USA
e-mail: scott.cameron.wagner@gmail.com; armyspine@yahoo.com

H.L. Shufflebarger, M.D.
Department of Orthopaedic Surgery, Miami Children's Hospital, 3100 SW 62 Avenue, Miami, FL 33155, USA
e-mail: hthook@aol.com

A.L. Wollowick and V. Sarwahi (eds.), *Spondylolisthesis: Diagnosis, Non-Surgical Management, and Surgical Techniques*, DOI 10.1007/978-1-4899-7575-1_18,

Recently, the Spinal Deformity Study Group (SDSG) proposed a modified classification system based on each patient's pelvic incidence, sacro-pelvic balance, and spinal balance as measured radiographically [4]. This classification identifies specific lumbosacral morphology associated with high-grade slips, and allows these deformities to be subsequently categorized into two generalized subgroups: balanced deformities, in which the pelvic incidence and sacral slope are similar, and unbalanced deformities, in which the pelvic tilt is high but the sacral slope is low [5]. Almost all patients with high-grade slips have pelvic incidence values greater than 60° [6]. Furthermore, patients with a retroverted pelvic posture had significantly higher rate of positive sagittal imbalance [2, 4]. Figure 18.1 shows the lateral lumbar radiographs of patients with high-grade slips but variations in their pelvic anatomy, suggestive of balanced and unbalanced deformities [6]. The surgical management of high-grade spondylolisthesis remains an area of significant controversy, though 90 % of these patients are typically symptomatic and, untreated, their slips are often progressive [7]. The most common presenting complaints in patients with high-grade spondylolisthesis include low back pain and sciatica, though some may have impaired sphincter control manifesting as stress incontinence of urine [7]. Motor or sensory loss is relatively rare.

Treatment Algorithm: High-Grade Spondylolisthesis

Patients with high-grade slips are usually symptomatic, and their deformities are well established; therefore, surgical management is generally the preferred method of treatment for high-grade slips. The primary endpoints of treatment in these patients are

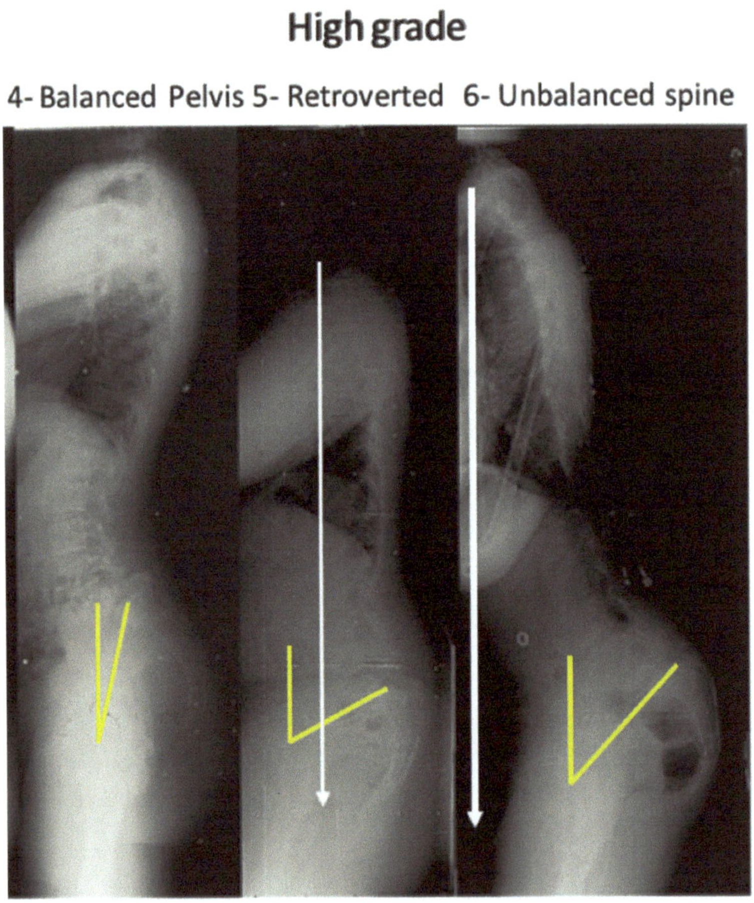

Fig. 18.1 Classification of high-grade spondylolisthesis as proposed by SDSG for spino-pelvic posture in high-grade spondylolisthesis. [Reprinted from Labelle H, Mac-Thiong JM, Roussouly P. Spino-pelvic sagittal balance of spondylolisthesis: a review and classification. Eur Spine J. 2011;20 Suppl 5:641-646. With permission from Wolters Kluwer Health]

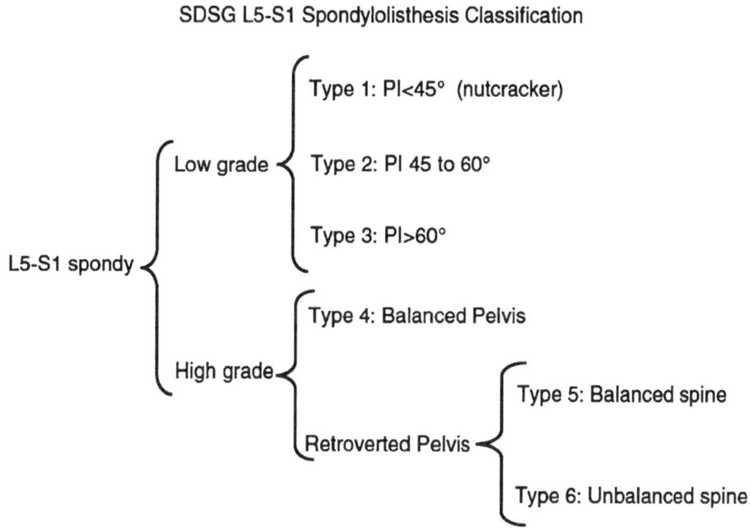

Fig. 18.2 Classification algorithm of spondylolisthesis based on spino-pelvic posture. [Reprinted from Labelle H, Mac-Thiong JM, Roussouly P. Spino-pelvic sagittal balance of spondylolisthesis: a review and classification. Eur Spine J. 2011;20 Suppl 5:641-646. With permission from Wolters Kluwer Health]

satisfactory reduction of the slip and fusion of the lumbosacral junction to prevent any further slippage, with the overall goals of surgery being to restore lumbosacral lordosis while minimizing neurological complications and improving neurologic function for those patients who have deficits [7]. Restoration of the ability to withstand shear forces at the lumbosacral junction is crucial to successful surgical management, and it is only accomplished with establishment of the posterior tension band (normally provided by the pars interarticularis) and the anterior column support [3]. Standing lateral radiographs of the lumbar spine and pelvis are requirements for appropriate classification, as patients with unbalanced deformities may necessitate reduction of sagittal misalignment [6, 8]. Figure 18.2 is the proposed SDSG classification algorithm, with suggestion that reduction may be indicated for some type 5 deformities, and mandatory for all type 6 deformities [6]. In addition, inclusion of full length lateral 36″ scoliosis radiographs are imperative to further classify overall sagittal balance. However, while many techniques for reduction and fusion have been described, the ideal treatment remains an area of ongoing debate [9].

Controversies

Significant controversy exists regarding the necessity of reduction of the slip, as well as the timing and most effective means of achieving reduction. Even maintaining the reduction while the fusion mass heals is an area of contention. While low-grade spondylolistheses treated with in situ fusion have shown relatively good outcomes, high-grade slips treated without reduction were thought to be prone to high rates of nonunion or slip progression [10–13]. A 6 % incidence of cauda equina syndrome has also been reported with in situ fusion without reduction [14], and pseudarthrosis, progression of the deformity and persistent symptoms have all be described without reduction [15, 16]. One study comparing in situ fusion with reduction and arthrodesis found better functional results at 15-year follow-up for the in situ group, but reductions were not anatomic, and the patient population was relatively small [17]. It has been theorized that when fusion is performed without reduction, the graft remains in tension, which is not conducive to formation of a fusion mass [18]. However, some recent studies have suggested that only patients with an unbalanced pelvis require reduction, while patients with high-grade slips but balanced deformities may benefit from in situ fusion without reduction [8]. A separate controversy exists regarding open versus minimally invasive surgical techniques for reduction and fusion, though the literature has recently shown favorable outcomes—lower estimated blood loss, shorter surgical time, and shorter hospital stay—utilizing minimally invasive techniques [19–21].

Described Surgical Techniques

The literature is replete with various techniques for the surgical management of high-grade spondylolisthesis, including open, minimally invasive, and "mini-open" procedures, as well as various techniques for reduction of the slip. These principles apply primarily to high-grade isthmic spondylolisthesis at the L5-S1 junction. As previously mentioned, the primary goal of surgical treatment is the restoration of both the posterior tension band and anterior structural support, which prevents the conversion of axial load to shear forces through the lumbosacral junction [3].

Open Procedure

Positioning and Approach

Positioning of the patient is one of the most important steps in the surgical procedure. A modified Jackson table is ideal. The patient is placed prone with the hips in maximal extension, which allows for partial reduction of pelvic retroversion in patients with a mobile L5-S1 segment, and may require elevation of the patient's lower extremities above the table [22].

The open procedure utilizes a standard midline exposure, elevating the paraspinal muscles from the spinous processes of the involved segments, with exposure of the transverse processes to allow visualization of the involved nerve roots [22–24].

Open Reduction

Reduction of the slip, in patients with an appropriate indication, is technically demanding with a relatively high rate of neurologic injury. Various open techniques have been described, including casting [25], Harrington rod distraction [26], staged reduction and fixation using an external fixator [27], and translation through posterior instrumentation [28].

It is essential that the involved nerve roots are decompressed bilaterally, while it is often beneficial to maintain the upper section of the L5 lamina to preserve the attachment of the ligamentum flavum when performing a reduction [23]. Removing the posterior elements and far lateral exposure allow for direct visualization of the nerve roots, and it is important to completely decompress these nerve roots before reduction is attempted to minimize these risks [14, 23].

Subsequent preparation of the involved disc space and/or removal of the dome of the sacrum is advisable to facilitate reduction. Poly-axial screws (or reduction screws which are preferable) are then placed in the pedicles of the upper and lower vertebrae, though use of Schanz pins in L5 has been reported instead of pedicle screws [22]; the pedicle screw insertion points for the sacrum are superior and lateral to the superior articular process. The insertion points for L5 are often unreliable and deformed in these patients, but the screws can be placed under direct visualization after removal of the posterior elements [24].

Distraction is then performed at the involved level using any flat instrument such as a Cobb elevator as a lever to open the intervertebral space; Harrington rods have been described for use in reduction as well [24]. Many techniques have been described including using either a rod or plate, which has been contoured to appropriate lumbar lordosis, or by utilization of a reduction tool. The sacral screw is first used as an anchor; by reducing the L5 screws to the rod or plate, a posteriorly directed force is generated that pulls the vertebral body back into alignment [23, 24].

Minimally Invasive Procedure

Positioning and Approach

The minimally invasive technique has been previously described [29, 30], though is primarily reserved for surgical patients with grade III (or lower) spondylolisthesis [31]. Positioning also involves a hyperextended, prone positioning on a radiolucent table. Three-centimeter paramedian incisions are made approximately 4–5 cm from the midline over the affected level, and blunt dissection is performed to the appropriate facets with fluoroscopic confirmation [31]. MIS retractors are placed, and either loupes with fiberoptic lights or a surgical microscope may be utilized for visualization. Standard MIS facetectomies and transforaminal lumbar interbody fusion

(TLIF) are performed bilaterally, with sequential distraction of the interbody space to allow passage of the implant; concomitant discectomy is performed to open the space completely [31].

Reduction

After the MIS approach has been completed and there is adequate exposure, spondylolisthesis reduction screws are placed under fluoroscopic guidance in the cephalad vertebral pedicles, and standard poly-axial pedicle screws in the caudad vertebra [31]. The paramedian approach allows improved access to the L5 pedicles with improved trajectory as compared to the open, midline approach. Reduction of the slipped vertebral element is performed with a rod clamped to the reduction screws, with the reduction blades facilitating posterior translation of the superior vertebra in relation to the fixed, inferior vertebral body [31].

Interbody Fusion

After adequate reduction has been achieved, whether open or MIS, it is mandatory to supplement the reduction with an adequate supporting implant and bone grafting. Without an interbody implant and appropriate grafting, the slip will be prone to loss of correction, nonunion, and long-term failure [32–34]. Interbody fusion may be achieved with either an anterior or posterior lumbar interbody fusion (PLIF) technique [12, 35, 36]. Structural interbody cages are placed bilaterally in the disc space. The pedicle screws are compressed to restore lordosis, and if the L5 nerve roots are noted to be in tension, an anterior lumbar interbody fusion (ALIF) may also be performed. Posterior fusion is completed with grafting of the transverse processes and sacrum [22].

Authors' Preferred Management

Preoperative Planning

Adequate preoperative planning is essential in the management of patients with high-grade spondylolistheses. We prefer the sagittal balance classification of Labelle et al. [4, 6] in assessing overall global sagittal alignment. If the patient is a Type 5 with compensated sagittal balance, then a reduction maneuver is not necessary. The proposed operation needs to take into account the patient's preoperative symptoms: if the patient presents with radiculopathy, a thorough nerve root decompression is warranted even if no reduction of the spondylolisthesis is to be performed.

Surgical Technique

It is the opinion of the authors that in order to best facilitate restoration of the biomechanics of the lumbosacral junction, anatomic reduction of the deformity is recommended [3, 36, 37]. Doing so reestablishes normal biomechanics and neutralizes shear forces. Restoring sagittal spino-pelvic alignment favors union and does, in theory, decrease the risk for adjacent level degeneration. Given the potential tension this maneuver will place on the L5 nerve roots, therefore, monitoring of the L5 nerve roots throughout the procedure is recommended [3].

The patient is positioned prone on a radiolucent surgical table such as a Jackson table (OSI, Union City, CA). L4 through the caudal edge of the sacrum is exposed via a low lumbar skin incision. Exposure is carried out laterally enough to expose the transverse processes of the lumbar vertebrae as well as the sacral alae. It is important to note that because there is frequent anatomic aberration in this region, care must be taken to avoid iatrogenic durotomy. For all reductions of Meyerding Grade III spondylolistheses, our preferred method is to perform a Gill laminectomy to allow access to the cauda equina and nerve roots [37]. Additionally, it allows for the use of this bone for bone graft in preparation for the fusion bed. Following Gill laminectomy, we thoroughly perform wide and extensile decompression of the L5 nerve roots. When the deformity is Grade IV or V, the nerve root often is dysmorphic in its appearance. In these settings we use free running EMGs to stimulate the nerve to ensure we are adequately identifying it.

Once this is adequately decompressed, we then turn our attention to performing a PLIF approach bilaterally. Exposure of the lumbosacral disc space is accomplished by medial retraction of the S1 nerve root. Multiple small epidural veins are encountered at the base of the S1 pedicle, and we recommend bipolar electrocautery to control them. Once the lumbosacral disc and posterior cephalad portion of the sacrum have been exposed, the posterior longitudinal ligament is incised and excised. The disc material is removed with complete exposure of the sacral dome. If a sacral dome osteotomy needs to be performed, we do this under direct and fluoroscopic visualization with an osteotome while protecting the dura and exiting nerve roots. This step is, essentially, equivalent to pedicle subtraction osteotomy in the more proximal segments of the spine [3]. The cut is directed towards the anterior cortex of the sacrum, and cephalad to the tips of the sacral screws. Extension of the osteotomy bilaterally under the dural sac and laterally into the alae also facilitates reduction [3]. Following thorough and complete discectomy, we place a Cobb elevator to the level of the anterior annulus and obtain a lateral fluoroscopic image to ensure that the segment is mobile. If it is not, we reassess and perform additional release of the disc and annulus.

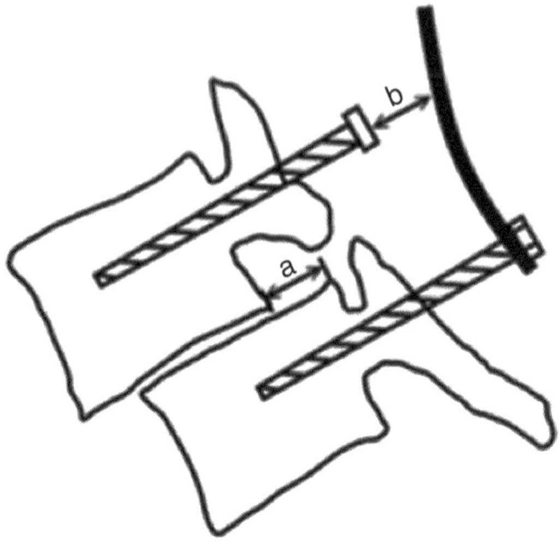

Fig. 18.3 Illustration showing the placement of screws with the posterior rod contoured in approximation of lumbar lordosis, prior to reduction. [Adapted from Lian XF, Hou TS, Xu JG, et al. Single segment of posterior lumbar interbody fusion for adult isthmic spondylolisthesis: reduction or fusion in situ. Eur Spine J. 2014; 23(1):172-179. With permission from Springer-Verlag]

Next, we place interbody cages bilaterally. Instrumentation can be done before or after the decompression, but in general we prefer to instrument first. Larger sacral screws, usually 7.5 mm diameter, are placed "tricortically" in the sacrum [38]. Then we place large reduction screws into L5, which are typically 6.5–7.5 mm, but this varies depending on the anatomy and size of the patient. The rods are contoured to approximate lumbar lordosis prior to insertion. For larger grade III, IV, and V slips, L4 is instrumented with reduction type screws as well. Figure 18.3 demonstrates the placement of screws with the posterior rod contoured in approximation of lumbar lordosis, prior to reduction [9]. With the interbody grafts in place, distraction is performed across this segment with the use of a lamina spreader and the L5 screw is gently pulled back to the level of the L4 and S1 screws heads. Intermittent distraction is a key component to this maneuver to allow for successful reduction of the slip. Figure 18.4 illustrates the distraction maneuver utilized during reduction [9]. Also, it is imperative that the L5 nerve roots be continually palpated and rechecked to ensure they are not being trapped during the reduction maneuver. If any deterioration in function is detected, exploration

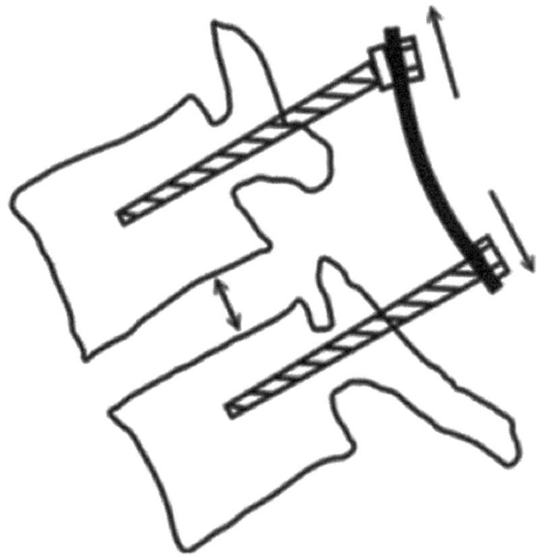

Fig. 18.4 Illustration demonstrating the interbody distraction utilized during the reduction maneuver. [Adapted from Lian XF, Hou TS, Xu JG, et al. Single segment of posterior lumbar interbody fusion for adult isthmic spondylolisthesis: reduction or fusion in situ. Eur Spine J. 2014; 23(1):172-179. With permission from Springer-Verlag]

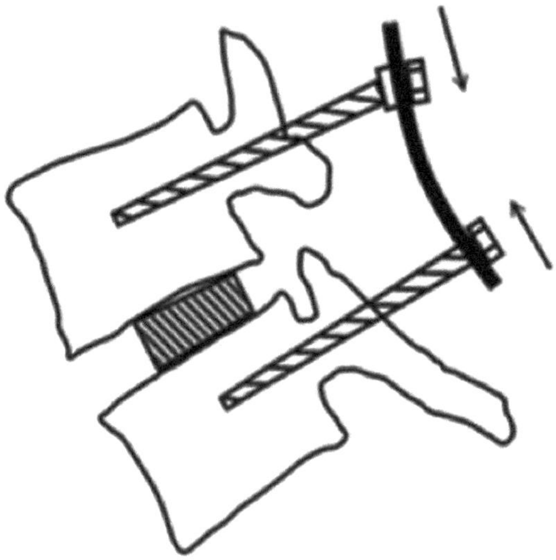

Fig. 18.5 Illustration demonstrating the final lateral view with compression across intervertebral space. [Adapted from Lian XF, Hou TS, Xu JG, et al. Single segment of posterior lumbar interbody fusion for adult isthmic spondylolisthesis: reduction or fusion in situ. Eur Spine J. 2014; 23(1):172-179. With permission from Springer-Verlag]

of the nerve root with further decompression should be performed. If there is no compression, consideration must be given to reducing tension on the nerve root. If EMG deterioration remains despite these techniques, the sacrum can be further shortened, or staging of the procedure may also be considered [3]. If the L5 screws loosen during distraction, which is not infrequent, these should be replaced with larger diameter screws and reassessment of soft tissue and osseous releases. Lateral fluoroscopy should be checked intermittently during reduction as well. Final reduction is confirmed under C-arm, and modifications to the rod contour can be made if further lumbosacral lordosis is required [3]. We also check the position of our pedicle screws to ensure there none has loosened. Figure 18.5 demonstrates the final lateral view with compression across intervertebral space [9]. We then perform posterolateral fusion to supplement the interbody grafts. It is our routine practice to place a collagen material over the dura to decrease adherence of the scar tissue that will be formed to the dura. Closure is typically performed over a subcutaneous drain [3].

Post-operatively, the patients are kept in either a TLSO or a simple elastic lumbosacral corset. Ambulation begins on post-operative day one, but most other activities are restricted until at least 3 months after surgery [3].

Complications

Intraoperative hemorrhage, while not a complication per se, can lead to significant problems during surgery if not appropriately controlled. As noted, ligation or bipolar cauterization of epidural veins early in the case is advised before they are torn. Thrombin gelfoam is also useful for hemostasis.

The most common neurologic complication encountered by the authors after spondylolisthesis reduction is radiculopathy, primarily of the L5 nerve roots. In our experience, as well as Dr. Harms', the occurrence of temporary or permanent radiculopathy is relatively low [39, 40]. With anatomic reduction, occurrence of pseudarthrosis is also low.

Conclusions

There exists significant controversy in the literature regarding the surgical treatment of high-grade spondylolisthesis: in situ fusion versus reduction, the timing of surgery, and the techniques for achieving fixation are extremely varied. The classification of spondylolisthesis and management modalities continue to evolve, but in the authors' experience, anatomic reduction with posterior-instrumented arthrodesis has yielded highly encouraging results.

References

1. Mac-Thiong JM, Labelle H. A proposal for a surgical classification of pediatric lumbosacral spondylolisthesis based on current literature. Eur Spine J. 2006; 15(10):1425–35.
2. Mac-Thiong JM, Wang Z, de Guise JA, Labelle H. Postural model of sagittal spino-pelvic alignment and its relevance for lumbosacral developmental

spondylolisthesis. Spine (Phila Pa 1976). 2008; 33(21):2316–25.
3. Shufflebarger HL. High dysplastic spondylolisthesis: anatomic reduction. The Harms/Shufflebarger technique. In: DeWald RL, Bridwell KH, editors. The textbook of spinal surgery. 3rd ed. Philadelphia, PA: Lippincott Williams & Wilkins; 2011. p. 660–7.
4. Labelle HRP, Berthonnaud E, Mac-Thiong JM, Hresko T, Dimar, J, Parent S, Weidenbaum M, Brown C, Hu S. Spondylolisthesis classification based on spino-pelvic alignment. Podium presentation at the 2009 Scoliosis Research Society Annual Meeting. San Antonio, USA; 2009.
5. Hresko MT, Labelle H, Roussouly P, Berthonnaud E. Classification of high-grade spondylolistheses based on pelvic version and spine balance: possible rationale for reduction. Spine (Phila Pa 1976). 2007;32(20):2208–13.
6. Labelle H, Mac-Thiong JM, Roussouly P. Spino-pelvic sagittal balance of spondylolisthesis: a review and classification. Eur Spine J. 2011;20 Suppl 5: 641–6.
7. Vialle R, Benoist M. High-grade lumbosacral spondylolisthesis in children and adolescents: pathogenesis, morphological analysis, and therapeutic strategy. Joint Bone Spine. 2007;74(5):414–7.
8. Martiniani MLC, Specchia N. "In situ" fusion or reduction in high-grade dysplastic developmental spondylolisthesis. Eur Spine J. 2012;21 Suppl 1:S134–40.
9. Lian XF, Hou TS, Xu JG, et al. Single segment of posterior lumbar interbody fusion for adult isthmic spondylolisthesis: reduction or fusion in situ. Eur Spine J. 2014;23(1):172–9.
10. DeWald RL, Faut MM, Taddonio RF, Neuwirth MG. Severe lumbosacral spondylolisthesis in adolescents and children. Reduction and staged circumferential fusion. J Bone Joint Surg Am. 1981;63(4): 619–26.
11. Johnson JR, Kirwan EO. The long-term results of fusion in situ for severe spondylolisthesis. J Bone Joint Surg Br. 1983;65(1):43–6.
12. Poussa M, Schlenzka D, Seitsalo S, Ylikoski M, Hurri H, Osterman K. Surgical treatment of severe isthmic spondylolisthesis in adolescents. Reduction or fusion in situ. Spine (Phila Pa 1976). 1993;18(7):894–901.
13. Akamaru T, Kawahara N, Tim Yoon S, et al. Adjacent segment motion after a simulated lumbar fusion in different sagittal alignments: a biomechanical analysis. Spine (Phila Pa 1976). 2003;28(14):1560–6.
14. Schoenecker PL, Cole HO, Herring JA, Capelli AM, Bradford DS. Cauda equina syndrome after in situ arthrodesis for severe spondylolisthesis at the lumbosacral junction. J Bone Joint Surg Am. 1990;72(3): 369–77.
15. Grzegorzewski A, Kumar SJ. In situ posterolateral spine arthrodesis for grades III, IV, and V spondylolisthesis in children and adolescents. J Pediatr Orthop. 2000;20(4):506–11.
16. Molinari RW, Bridwell KH, Lenke LG, Ungacta FF, Riew KD. Complications in the surgical treatment of pediatric high-grade, isthmic dysplastic spondylolisthesis. A comparison of three surgical approaches. Spine (Phila Pa 1976). 1999;24(16):1701–11.
17. Poussa M, Remes V, Lamberg T, et al. Treatment of severe spondylolisthesis in adolescence with reduction or fusion in situ: long-term clinical, radiologic, and functional outcome. Spine (Phila Pa 1976). 2006;31(5):583–90. discussion 591–582.
18. Hanley Jr EN, Levy JA. Surgical treatment of isthmic lumbosacral spondylolisthesis. Analysis of variables influencing results. Spine (Phila Pa 1976). 1989; 14(1):48–50.
19. Dhall SS, Wang MY, Mummaneni PV. Clinical and radiographic comparison of mini-open transforaminal lumbar interbody fusion with open transforaminal lumbar interbody fusion in 42 patients with long-term follow-up. J Neurosurg Spine. 2008;9(6):560–5.
20. Holly LT, Schwender JD, Rouben DP, Foley KT. Minimally invasive transforaminal lumbar interbody fusion: indications, technique, and complications. Neurosurg Focus. 2006;20(3):E6.
21. Logroscino CA, Proietti L, Pola E, Scaramuzzo L, Tamburrelli FC. A minimally invasive posterior lumbar interbody fusion for degenerative lumbar spine instabilities. Eur Spine J. 2011;20 Suppl 1:S41–5.
22. Lamartina C, Zavatsky JM, Petruzzi M, Specchia N. Novel concepts in the evaluation and treatment of high-dysplastic spondylolisthesis. Eur Spine J. 2009;18 Suppl 1:133–42.
23. Chung JY, Parthasarathy S, Avadhani A, Rajasekaran S. Reduction of high grade listhesis. Eur Spine J. 2010;19(2):353–4.
24. Rengachary SS, Balabhandra R. Reduction of spondylolisthesis. Neurosurg Focus. 2002;13(1):E2.
25. Ds B. Treatment of severe spondylolisthesis: a combined approach for reduction and stabilization. Spine (Phila Pa 1976). 1979;4(5):423–9.
26. Harrington PR, Tullos HS. Spondylolisthesis in children. Observations and surgical treatment. Clin Orthop Relat Res. 1971;79:75–84.
27. Karampalis CGM, Shafafy M, Webb J. High-grade spondylolisthesis: gradual reduction using Magerl's external fixator followed by circumferential fusion technique and long-term results. Eur Spine J. 2012;21 Suppl 2:S200–6.
28. Curcin A, Edwards CC. Reduction and fusion of spondyloptosis: long-term follow-up. Presented at the Scoliosis Research Society Annual Meeting; September 21–24. Portland; 1994.
29. Schwender JD, Holly LT, Rouben DP, Foley KT. Minimally invasive transforaminal lumbar interbody fusion (TLIF): technical feasibility and initial results. J Spinal Disord Tech. 2005;18(Suppl):S1–6.
30. Rampersaud YR, Gurgo RD. Mini-open posterior lumbar interbody fusion for deformity. In: Mummaneni PV, Lenke L, Haid R, editors. Spinal deformity: a guide to surgical planning and management. St. Louis: Quality Medical Publishing; 2008. p. 721–48.
31. Quraishi NA, Rampersaud YR. Minimal access bilateral transforaminal lumbar interbody fusion for high-grade isthmic spondylolisthesis. Eur Spine J. 2013;22(8):1707–13.

32. Boos N, Marchesi D, Zuber K, Aebi M. Treatment of severe spondylolisthesis by reduction and pedicular fixation. A 4-6-year follow-up study. Spine (Phila Pa 1976). 1993;18(12):1655–61.
33. Edwards CE. Reduction of spondylolisthesis. In: DeWald RL, Bridwell KH, editors. The textbook of spinal surgery. 3rd ed. Philadelphia, PA: Lippincott Williams & Wilkins; 1991. p. 605–34.
34. Suk SI, Lee CK, Kim WJ, Lee JH, Cho KJ, Kim HG. Adding posterior lumbar interbody fusion to pedicle screw fixation and posterolateral fusion after decompression in spondylolytic spondylolisthesis. Spine (Phila Pa 1976). 1997;22(2):210–9. discussion 219–220.
35. Spruit M, Pavlov PW, Leitao J, De Kleuver M, Anderson PG, Den Boer F. Posterior reduction and anterior lumbar interbody fusion in symptomatic low-grade adult isthmic spondylolisthesis: short-term radiological and functional outcome. Eur Spine J. 2002;11(5):428–33.
36. Suk KS, Jeon CH, Park MS, Moon SH, Kim NH, Lee HM. Comparison between posterolateral fusion with pedicle screw fixation and anterior interbody fusion with pedicle screw fixation in adult spondylolytic spondylolisthesis. Yonsei Med J. 2001;42(3): 316–23.
37. Gill G. Long-term follow-up evaluation of a few patients with spondylolisthesis treated by excision of the loose lamina with decompression of the nerve roots without spinal fusion. Clin Orthop Relat Res. 1984;182:215–9.
38. Lehman Jr RA, Kuklo TR, Belmont Jr PJ, Andersen RC, Polly Jr DW. Advantage of pedicle screw fixation directed into the apex of the sacral promontory over bicortical fixation: a biomechanical analysis. Spine (Phila Pa 1976). 2002;27(8):806–11.
39. Harms J, Jeszenszky D, Stoltze D, et al. True spondylolisthesis reduction and monosegmental fusion in spondylolisthesis. In: Bridwell KH, Dewald RL, editors. The textbook of spine surgery. 2nd ed. Philadelphia, PA: Lippincott-Raven; 1997. p. 1337–47.
40. Shufflebarger HL, Geck MJ. High-grade isthmic dysplastic spondylolisthesis: monosegmental surgical treatment. Spine (Phila Pa 1976). 2005;30 Suppl 6: S42–8.

19 Management of Spondyloptosis

Ali M. Maziad and Oheneba Boachie-Adjei

Introduction

Spondylolysis and spondylolisthesis at the L5 vertebra has an incidence of 4.4 % in 6-year-old children and increases to 5.8 % in adulthood. Spondyloptosis is an advanced form of spondylolisthesis characterized by 100 % or more forward slip of one vertebra over the vertebra below which denotes a grade V slip based on Meyerding's grading system. It has been shown that isthmic spondylolysis with or without spondylolisthesis does not exist at birth but rather develops in the months or years following birth. While there is a higher incidence of spondylolysis in males, by a ratio of up to 2:1, females have a higher risk of progression to higher grades including spondyloptosis.

Meyerding's grading [1] is a classification that divides the vertebral body into four quadrants:
Grade 0: No slippage
1–25 %: Grade I
26–50 %: Grade II
51–75 %: Grade III,
76–100 %: Grade IV;
>100 % is Grade V in which situation, there is complete slippage past the anterior border of the vertebra below which is the sacrum as it is most commonly seen at the L5/S1 level.

Additional classification of Spondylolisthesis by Wiltse Classification [2] identifies the etiology of spondylolisthesis.

1. Dysplastic: Congenital malformation of the sacrum or neural arch of L5.
2. Isthmic: Stress fracture, elongation, or acute fracture of the pars.
3. Degenerative: Long-standing arthritic process of the zygapophyseal joints.
4. Traumatic: Neural arch fracture excluding the pars region.
5. Pathologic: Bone disease—Paget's, Metastatic disease, or Osteopetrosis.
6. Iatrogenic: Following lumbar spine surgery.

Taillard [3] suggested that two anatomical factors play an important role in the development of a slip: the shape of the fifth lumbar vertebra and the shape of the dome of the sacrum. However, it is now believed that the trapezoidal shape of the slipped vertebral body may be secondary remodeling due to the slip and not the cause of the progression of slip. Also it was noted that those remodeling changes are more common among males compared to females.

Various forms of posterior element malformations have been noticed to correlate with advanced grades of spondylolisthesis that may progress to spondyloptosis. Spina bifida occulta, facet aplasia,

A.M. Maziad, M.D., M.Sc. (✉)
O. Boachie-Adjei, M.D.
Department of Orthopedic Surgery – Scoliosis Service, Hospital for Special Surgery, 535 East 70th Street, New York, NY 10021, USA
e-mail: ali.maziad@gmail.com; oboachie@gmail.com

A.L. Wollowick and V. Sarwahi (eds.), *Spondylolisthesis: Diagnosis, Non-Surgical Management, and Surgical Techniques*, DOI 10.1007/978-1-4899-7575-1_19,

or laminar aplasia can cause decreased mechanical resistance to shear forces at the lumbosacral junction which in turn cause further progression of deformity. Curylo et al. found that the incidence of dysplasia of posterior elements in patients with spondyloptosis is 62 % [4]. There have been various reports regarding the association of spondylolisthesis with spina bifida oculta ranging from 22 to 92 %. It is generally agreed that inheritance plays a major role in the development of the pars interarticularis defect.

Additionally, patients with high pelvic incidence may have further progression of spondylolisthesis as compared to patients with low pelvic incidence. This is due to the increased pelvic tilt and lumbar lordosis associated with high pelvic incidence. Boisaubert et al. [5] have also shown that PI has a very high ($P<0.001$) statistical positive correlation with the degree of slippage in spondylolisthesis. In a study by Curylo et al., noted an increased PI in 53 patients with spondyloptosis with a mean pelvic incidence of 76°. Also patients with spondyloptosis have a decreased thoracic kyphosis as a compensation to maintain sagittal balance [6].

Traumatic spondyloptosis has also been described in the literature secondary to fracture dislocation of the thoracic or lumbar spine. The condition is often devastating and associated with high energy trauma and severe neurologic deficits which requires emergent surgical decompression and stabilization of the spine.

Nonoperative treatment is the first step in management of nonprogressive slips less than 50 % in patients who are asymptomatic. However surgical intervention maybe necessary in slips greater than 50 % or in patients with progressive neurological symptoms or back pain not responding to conservative treatment and interfering with daily activities [7–10].

The surgical management for high-grade slips including spondyloptosis is controversial. Posterior decompression and fusion in situ is the most common surgical intervention for spondyloptosis. However, it is associated with high rate of pseudoarthrosis due to the decompression associated with the procedure as well as tensile forces on the fusion mass which in turn may lead to progression of deformity along with persistent sagittal imbalance due to lack of correction of the deformity. Early results for isolated posterolateral fusion showed high rate of pseudoarthrosis up to 40 % [11].

Bradford and Boachie-Adjei recommended the combined anterior and posterior approaches with complete posterior decompression when the slippage is >75 % to decrease the risk of pseudarthrosis [12]. To avoid nonunion, interbody fusion either through anterior or posterior approaches provides additional surface for fusion as well as biomechanical advantage against tensile forces on the posterior fusion. Furthermore, interbody fusion allows for wider posterior decompression of neural elements with less concern about nonunion. Also it allows for better sagittal alignment and reduction of deformity along with a better cosmetic outcome [13–15].

Gaines has popularized a technique involving excision of the L5 vertebral body through an anterior approach followed by a posterior approach to excise the posterior elements and neural decompression with reduction of L4 onto S1 to achieve correction of deformity. This reduction is maintained by posterolateral fusion with transpedicular instrumentation from L4 to S1 [15]. Other authors described a modified technique for Gaines procedure involving partial excision of the L5 vertebral body through an anterior approach followed by posterior reduction of the slip and fixation. The advantages of this technique include preservation of the L5 pedicles of which can be used for the reduction screws, and increase the lever arm for the reduction. The procedure prevents excessive crowding of the nerve roots of L4 and L5 in one foramen which occurs with complete removal of the vertebral body of L5, additionally, less shortening of the thecal sac is expected with this procedure compared to complete resection [16].

Clinical Presentation

Patients present with low back pain that may be associated with radicular symptoms along with motor and sensory deficits in the lower extremities as the nerve roots are highly compressed. Symptoms of spinal canal stenosis similar to intermittent claudication or a cauda equina syndrome may be present along with bladder or bowel symptoms. Sagittal and coronal imbalance can be a presentation in patients with advanced degrees of spondylolisthesis and spondyloptosis secondary to lumbosacral kyphosis or associated scoliosis.

Clinical symptoms can be aggravated by increased activity and standing and maybe partially relieved by rest and recumbent position. Physical examination may show a step off during palpation of the back of patients at the slipped level. Also shortening of the trunk, flattening of the buttocks (heart shaped sacrum), and tightness of hamstrings maybe observed along with sagittal imbalance, altered gait, and loss of trunk height. Associated scoliosis may also be present. Depending on the etiology of spondylolisthesis, it has been suggested by some authors that a child with spondylolysis or spondylolisthesis can be permitted to enjoy a normal childhood and adolescence without restriction of activities and without fear of progression; however, in cases with progressive slip and spondyloptosis, surgical intervention is often required to relieve symptoms.

Diagnostic Imaging

Standing 36″ scoliosis AP and lateral X-rays are usually the first imaging modality needed to assess a patient with spondyloptosis. It is important to assess and measure spinal parameters in different regions of the spine not just lumbar in order to evaluate the overall magnitude of the deformity and spinal balance and make an accurate assessment of the magnitude of surgical correction in case surgical intervention is warranted.

Roentgenograms show severe kyphosis of the dislocated lumbosacral joint (100 % slip) and a slip angle of the fifth lumbar vertebra of more than 50°. Spondyloptosis is easy to identify on standing AP and lateral X-rays of the lumbar spine as L5 vertebra falls below the S1 upper endplate. Spina bifida can also be documented on the plain radiographs.

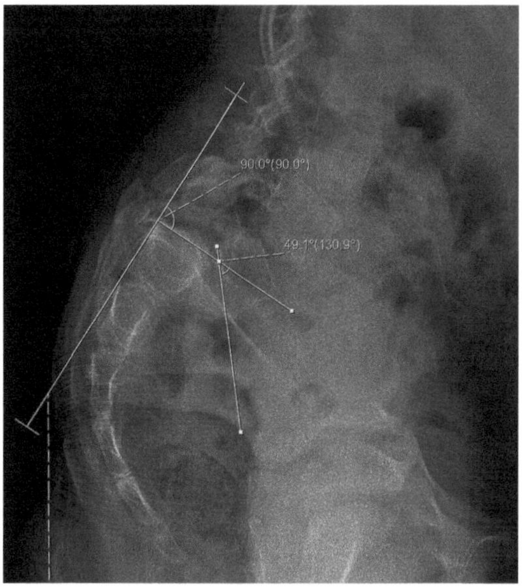

Fig. 19.1 *Slip angle* is a value that determines the severity of spondylolisthesis and is higher than 50° in spondyloptosis. It is measured between the perpendicular to a line along the posterior surface of the sacrum and a line along the inferior border of L5 (normal value is 0 to −10°

Radiographic parameters that should be considered include slip grade (Myerding classification), slip angle, lumbosacral kyphosis, sacral inclination, sacral rotation, and sagittal balance, Spinopelvic parameters; pelvic incidence, sacral slope, pelvic tilt, lumbar lordosis, and thoracic kyphosis (Figs. 19.1, 19.2, 19.3, 19.4, 19.5, 19.6, and 19.7). The three parameters form a fixed geometric relation—Pelvic Incidence = Pelvic Tilt + Sacral Slope. Lumbosacral angle is normally lordotic; however, in advanced slips, the angle becomes kyphotic which further compromises the overall sagittal balance and it is important to be corrected to near normal values during surgery to ensure a good balance and a favorable environment for fusion to occur. For the lumbar spine to be in proper sagittal balance, it needs to be aligned within 10° of the pelvic incidence. Thus, the higher the pelvic incidence, the more the lordosis that needs to be provided for the patient during surgery in order to keep them in proper sagittal alignment after surgery with minimal straining of the back and pelvic muscles.

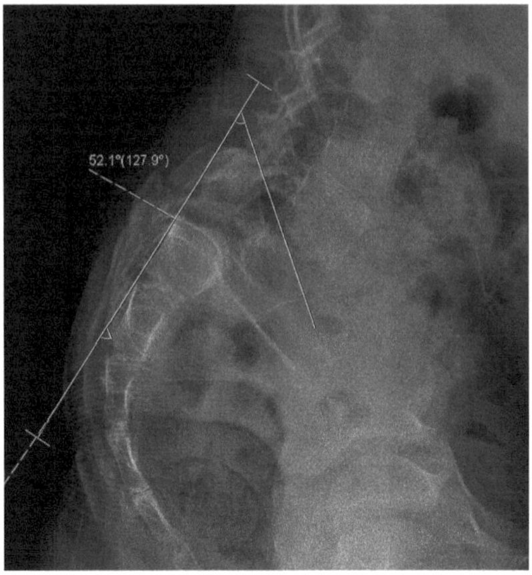

Fig. 19.2 *Lumbosacral angle* is the angle measured between the superior end plate of L5 and the posterior border of the sacrum. A lumbosacral angle of less than 100° is associated with a vertical sacrum and a sign of progressive spondylolisthesis

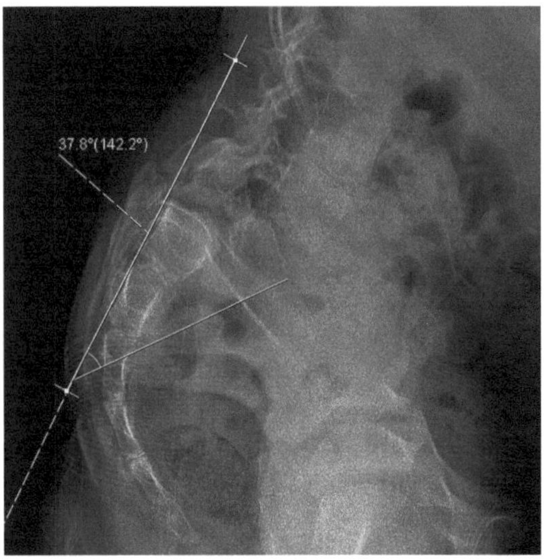

Fig. 19.3 *Sagittal rotation* which is the angle between a tangent to the posterior surface of the sacrum and the tangent to the anterior surface of L5

A sacral inclination of less than 30° signifies a vertical sacrum which compensates for high degrees of slips. It is measured between the vertical line and a line along the posterior surface of the sacrum.

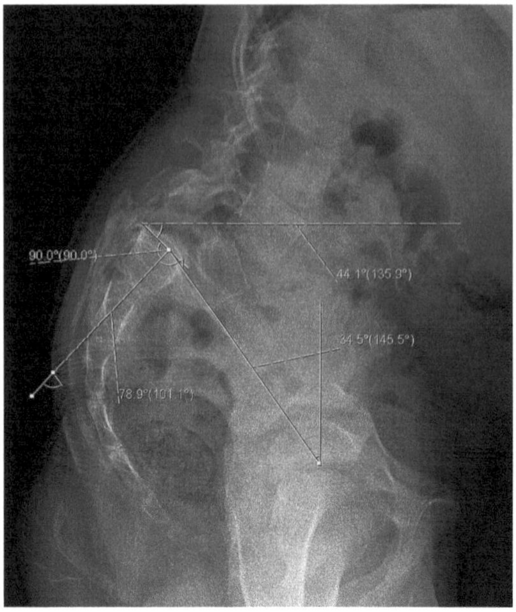

Fig. 19.4 *Spinopelvic parameters* define the relation between the pelvis and spine and are important to measure in order to evaluate the sagittal profile of the patient and determine the amount of surgical correction needed in order to achieve a balanced spinopelvic profile with the least muscle strain. This includes pelvic incidence, pelvic tilt, and sacral slope

CT scan is helpful in delineating the bony anatomy, any posterior element defects, pedicle sizes, length and orientation of vertebral bodies, presence of autofusion, disc space height, all of which can be helpful in surgical planning of instrumentation levels, interbody fusion, osteotomies, screw length, and diameter.

Posterior element defects or dysplasia can be seen on computed tomography (CT) scans and the surgeon should be mindful of any spinal anomalies to avoid inadvertently slipping into the open spinal canal and injuring the thecal sac. In cases where spontaneous fusion occurs between L5 and S1 levels, CT scan can demonstrate and confirm the boney mass which if solid can guide the surgical procedure and may obviate the need for osteotomy at the L5/S1 level which can be regarded as an extra sacral segment with surgical intervention occurring at the levels above.

Magnetic resonance imaging (MRI) is very helpful to see the neural structures, spinal and foraminal stenosis, and nerve root compressions

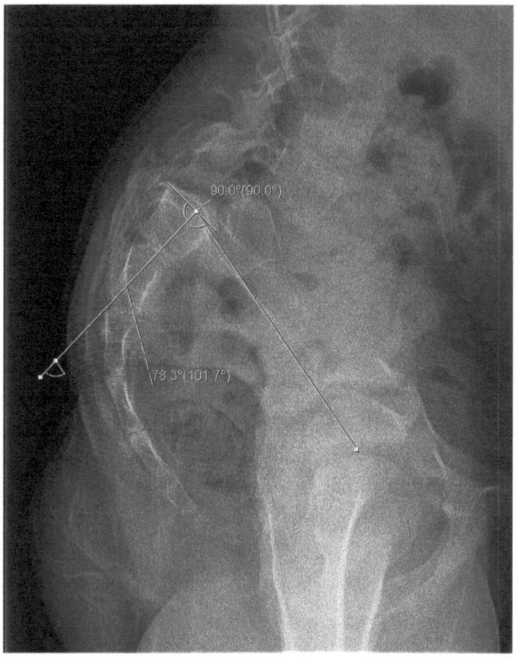

Fig. 19.5 *Pelvic incidence* (*PI*) is defined as the angle between the perpendicular to the sacral plate at its midpoint and the line connecting this point to the femoral heads axis. Higher pelvic incidence is associated with higher degrees of slips [17]

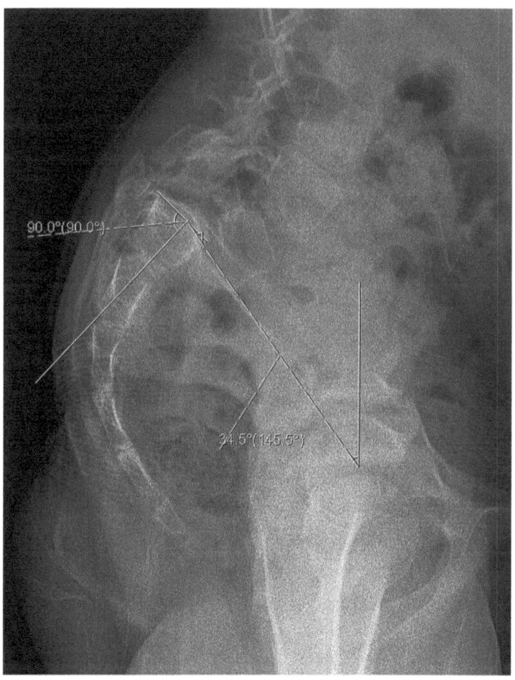

Fig. 19.6 *Pelvic Tilt* (*PT*) is defined by the angle between the vertical and the line through the midpoint of the sacral plate to femoral heads axis

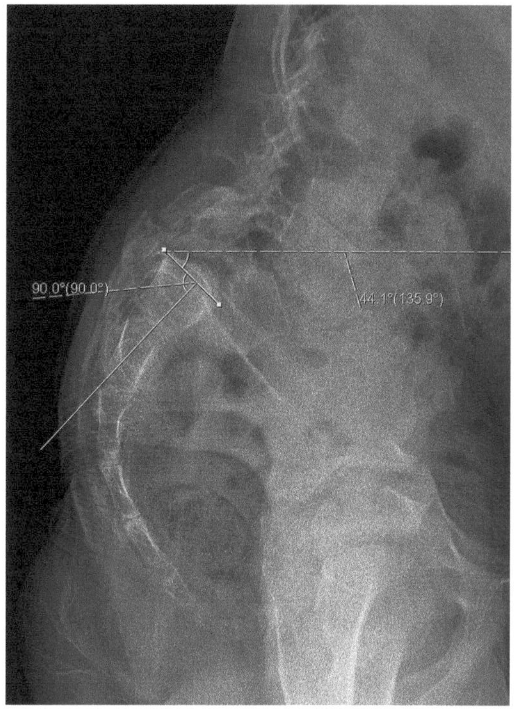

Fig. 19.7 *Sacral Slope* (*SS*) is defined as the angle between the horizontal and the sacral plate

which usually occurs due to encroaching of the L5 posterior elements on the dural sac or disc bulge at the L5/S1 level or above as well as other malformations such as tethered cord, posterior element defects which can along with the patient symptoms alert the surgeon to the need for neural decompression of stenosed segments. MRI can also detect facet joint effusion secondary to spondylolisthesis.

Although more invasive, in patients where MRI is contraindicated or previous hardware is placed, CT/myelography maybe an alternative to MRI to see neural structures.

Treatment Non-operative

While there is no study in the literature specific to the natural history of spondyloptosis, Di Martino et al. reported a case of spondyloptosis at L5/S1 diagnosed at the age of 9 with occasional low back pain treated conservatively. Spontaneous fusion was noted at the age of 36 and confirmed with CT scan. They concluded that conservative treatment may be a viable option in treatment for patients with mild symptoms, also it supports in situ fusion as a viable option for treatment of spondyloptosis [18].

Operative Management

Instrumentation is highly advised in posterior fusion of spondyloptosis, to stabilize the spine as it provides higher fusion rates and can maintain reduction in case correction of deformity is attempted. Particularly if laminectomy and destabilization of the spine is done to decompress neural elements which is often needed given the neurological symptoms associated with the deformity. In high-grade spondylolisthesis and spondyloptosis, there is no role for decompressive surgery alone unless spontaneous and complete autofusion has been confirmed by CT scan and the patient complains only of neurological symptoms without back pain.

Although excellent results from in situ fusion for high-grade slips have been reported by some authors, the outcomes are not very predictable. High rates of pseudarthrosis and bending of the fusion mass have also been reported. Fusion rates are higher with addition of anterior column support. Reduction may help restoring the overall sagittal balance of the spine and indirect decompression of spinal and foraminal stenosis. However it is associated with higher complication rates secondary to stretching of nerve roots if more than 50 % correction is attempted [19]. If there is sufficient disc height, interbody fusion is advised as it provides better spinal alignment, fusion surface, and indirect foraminal decompression as well as anterior biomechanical support, thus relieving the stress on posterior implants.

Anterior surgery poses certain risks related to the approach, major vessel manipulation or injury, retrograde ejaculation in males along with increased operative time, bowel complications, deep venous thrombosis, pulmonary complications, and hospitalization. Posterior partial reduction correcting the lumbosacral kyphosis may avoid the complications of full reduction as well as a second anterior approach. It also helps in correction of the sagittal balance. The sacral dome can cause significant anterior impingement of the dural sac in which case, partial sacral dome resection can be performed to further decompress the neural elements through a posterior approach.

Bohman et al. described placement of fibular graft through a posterior approach from S1 body across the disc space into the L5 body. This technique obviates the need for an anterior approach but involves manipulation of the thecal sac. As described by Bohlman during surgery the surgeon can protect the neural elements under fluoroscopic control with guidewire advancement through the body of S1, across the L5-S1 disc space, and up to the anterior cortex of L5. Over reaming of the guidewire can be performed under fluoroscopic guidance, beginning at 6 mm, increasing by 2 mm increments, up to 12 mm. Thereafter, a single fibula allograft can be impacted into position. A modification of the above technique can include addition of pedicle screw fixation in L4 and trans-sacral pedicle screws capturing L5 to supplement the trans-sacral fibula fixation [20].

The mainstay of operative treatment of spondylolisthesis is posterior in situ lumbosacral arthrodesis, with extension to the fourth lumbar vertebra if the slippage is more than 50 %. With this approach, symptomatic relief has been reported in 75 % or more of patients. However, it has been reported that additional slippage may occur after a posterolateral or posterior arthrodesis even if the patient is kept supine, and that progression is even more likely in patients who have had decompression combined with a posterior lateral arthrodesis. Boxall et al. reported that 46 % of their patients who had a slippage of more than 50 % and a solid posterior fusion had progression of the deformity. In these patients, the average lumbosacral kyphosis preoperatively was 50°. Continued progression also has been noted by Newman, Bosworth et al., and Laurent and Osterman and has ranged from 10 to 37 % [21, 22].

Bradford et al. reported on 22 consecutive who had severe spondylolisthesis (Grade IV and V) who were treated by a first-stage posterior decompression (Gill procedure) and a posterolateral arthrodesis, followed by halo-skeletal traction (femoral or pelvic) for 7–10 days, and then by a second-stage anterior interbody arthrodesis, followed by immobilization in a cast. They reported an average follow-up of 5 years. The slip angle averaged 71° preoperatively, was corrected to an average of 31° by reduction, and averaged 28° at follow-up. The average preoperative percentage of slippage (98 %) did not change substantially. Radicular pain improved in all 12 patients who had the complaint preoperatively. Ten patients had postoperative neurological deficits that completely resolved in all but one at follow-up. They also reported 21 % (four patients) pseudoarthrosis [12–14].

The operative treatment of severe, symptomatic spondylolisthesis (more than 50 % slippage) continues to pose a therapeutic challenge. Options for patients who have this deformity include posterior arthrodesis in situ, with or without decompression, posterior interbody arthrodes, anterior arthrodesis in situ, and reduction of the spondylolisthesis, with associated arthrodesis.

In major lumbosacral kyphosis, the fusion mass is subjected to abnormal bending forces. Progression of the deformity is less likely to occur if the kyphosis can be partially corrected and the fusion mass can be placed under compression, or less tension thus allowing a better biomechanical environment for fusion to occur.

Lumbosacral kyphosis leads to loss of sagittal balance. Thus for the patient to look forward, they have to compensate by hyperextending the upper lumbar levels, tilt the pelvis forward and flex the hips and knees with possible associated hypokyphosis of the thoracic spine. This posture places much more stresses on all the muscles and joints leading to easy fatigability.

While in situ fusion has been a mainstay in treatment of high-grade slips, reduction can aid in the outcomes of surgery as it allows decompression of the neural elements which are usually impinged by the posterior elements. It allows correction of the lumbosacral kyphosis, which results in less hyperlordosis at the upper lumbar and thoracic spine as well as less hamstring tightness or hip and knee flexion, thus giving the patient a more balanced posture with less muscular fatigue. Reduction can also restore the paraspinal and abdominal muscles to more physiologic alignment with a normal length-tension relationship, thus providing a more efficient function of those muscles with less fatigability.

Various techniques for reduction of high-grade spondylolisthesis have been described by including corrective casts by Scaglietti, which required extensive periods of bed rest, Harrington rods, wires attached to an external corrective system by Snijder, and through a two-stage procedure utilizing posterior decompression and posterolateral fusion followed by anterior reduction with fusion by Bradford [20–26].

Gaines described a technique of anterior excision of the vertebral body of L5 and the L4-5 and LS-S I discs were resected at the first stage, through a low midline transverse abdominal incision and a retroperitoneal approach. Major vessels need to be mobilized to allow access to the spine. Once exposed, the L4-5 disc is removed followed by resection of the L5 body all the way to the base of the pedicles. At this point the L5-S1 disc can be visualized and removed down to bone. All bone and intervening disc between lower endplate of L4 and upper endplate of S1 were removed with complete exposure of the dura. No correction was attempted at this stage. They waited 2 weeks until the second stage was done. During the second stage, a posterior exposure was done to excise the remaining posterior elements of L5 and compress L4 over S1 with posterolateral bone grafting [15].

Controversy still remains about the surgical treatment of high-grade spondylolisthesis. Some authors advocate that posterior decompression may not be necessary as a routine in patients with no neurological deficits and a wide spinal canal and neuroforamina and that partial reduction and fusion is sufficient to achieve good results. Decompression may destabilize the spine leading to further progression of slip as well as provide less surface area for a fusion mass if posterior only approach is to be used. Sailhan et al. reported on 44 patients with high-grade spondylolisthesis with a mean age of 20.4 years who underwent posterior fusion without decompression. There were 28 grade 3, 13 grade 4, and 3 grade 5 deformities. Twenty-one of the patients (47.7 %) underwent supplemental anterior interbody fusion of the L5-S1 disc space. No patient underwent decompression of the neurologic elements. They reported an average reduction in the percentage slip of the spondylolisthesis from 64 to 38 % displacement of L5 on S1 was achieved as well as an average reduction of the L5 incidence of 15.4° was also achieved. Both these changes were statistically significant ($P<0.05$). They reported five patients with pseudoarthrosis (four patients who had combined anterior/posterior fusion and one patient with posterior only fusion). They reported six patients who continued to have hamstring tightness and due to similarity between pain attributed to hamstring stiffness and radicular pain caused by neurogenic claudication, it was undetermined what the percentage of these patients who may have had radiculopathy secondary to spinal stenosis caused by the reduction of the spondylolisthesis. Six patients had poor results requiring revision surgery two of which had final fair results with an overall of good to fair results of 90.9 % in this series [27].

Surgical treatment of high-grade spondylolisthesis is technically demanding. Multiple studies have reported on the results obtained with posterior in situ fusion, instrumented posterior fusion with or without reduction, combined anterior and posterior procedures, spondylectomy with reduction of L4 to the sacrum (for spondyloptosis), and posterior interbody fusion with trans-sacral fixation. Regardless of the technique used, there is a significant risk of postoperative complications.

Non-instrumented in situ fusion is associated with a high rate of postoperative progression of the deformity and a failure of fusion in up to 44 % of cases. Instrumented reduction of spondyloptosis increases neurologic compromise due to excessive tension on nerve roots or direct pressure on the nerve roots by bone or and disc material extruded into the canal [20–26].

The tension on the L5 nerve root is directly proportional to the percentage of reduction, with the majority of tension (71 %) created by reducing the final 50 % of the deformity [21]. Additionally, increasing the amount of lordosis of the L5 vertebral body slightly relaxed the L5 nerve root in high-grade slips. The incidence of postoperative neurologic injuries after reduction is difficult to determine precisely as it is highly variable with published reports of deficits ranging from 0 to 75 %, since transient neurologic deficits are usually more common than reported by authors since most often only serious deficits are reported [28].

The authors believe that supplementation of fusion with bone morphogenic protein can provide higher rates of fusion with posterior only surgery and can obviate the need for supplementary anterior fusion and grafting.

Case Presentation

Surgical Technique

An immediate preoperative evaluation is advised for all patients particularly those with complex deformities. We prefer to go over the symptoms with the patient again before surgery and identify the magnitude of back pain versus leg pain, any new symptoms that may have started since patient was last seen. Neurological assessment is advised to have an immediate preoperative baseline in case any deficits are noticed postoperatively.

A walkthrough of the surgical procedures, expected OR time, and possible complications makes the patient and family aware of the magnitude of surgery (Figs. 19.8 and 19.9).

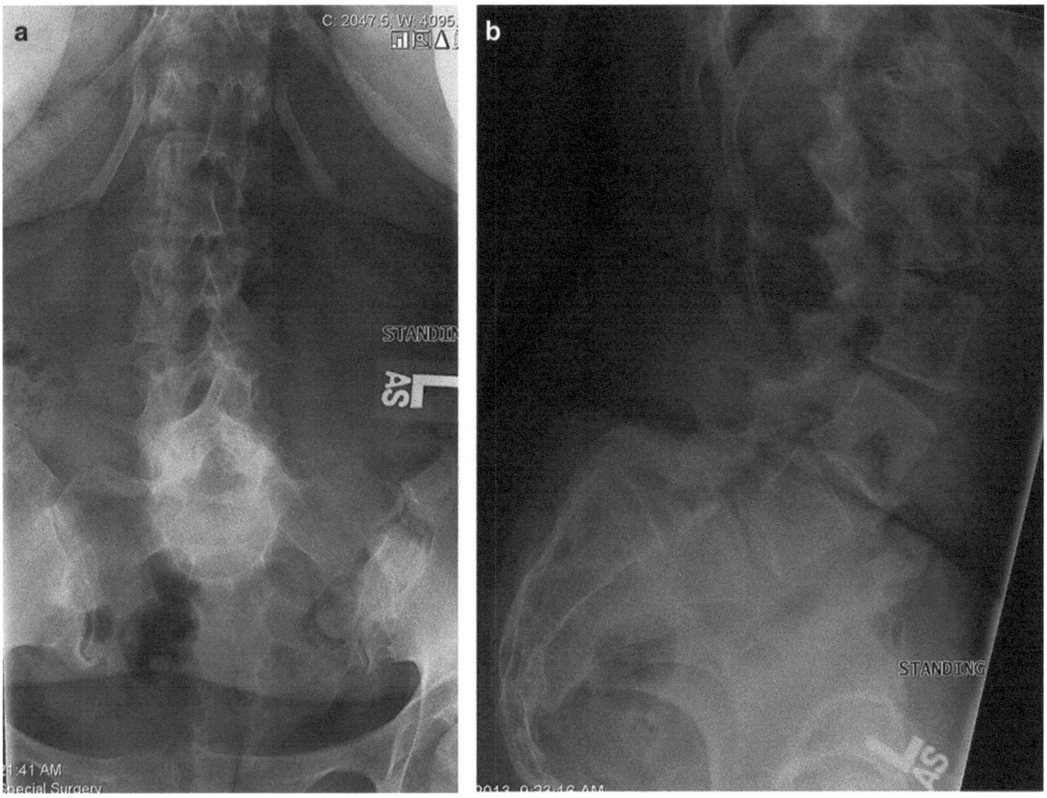

Fig. 19.8 (**a**, **b**) Case 1: AP and lateral X-ray views in a patient with advanced spondyloptosis

Patient Positioning

The patient is placed on a Jackson frame. Proper padding of boney prominences is crucial to avoid any pressure sores. It is also important to communicate the plan with the anesthesia team in order to be prepared for expected blood loss and surgical time. Additionally, the surgical team of attending, residents, and fellows should go over the images one last time before the procedure and develop an understanding of the surgical steps, implants, and expectations of the procedure. Images should be readily available in the OR either printed or in PACS and should be easily seen by all personnel in the OR. In complex cases, measurement of pedicle sizes, scrutinizing the boney anatomy, and estimation of implant sizes can guide the surgeon and save operative time during the procedure.

Isolation of the surgical site with 1,000 drapes and preoperative cleaning should precede prepping of the skin (Fig. 19.10).

Patients with spondyloptosis have exaggerated lordosis which could make dissection challenging. Staying strictly on bone can decrease bleeding and provide a good exposure.

Identification of the level with image intensifier is helpful in short fusions to avoid unnecessary dissection of higher levels to planned surgery. This can be done using a ball tip probe under the lamina or a Kocher around the lamina or transverse process.

Once the level is identified, further dissection to the proper level is done bilaterally all the way to the transverse processes.

Proper sized screws are inserted preferably with large diameters to allow good boney purchase which will aid in reduction. Osteotomies of

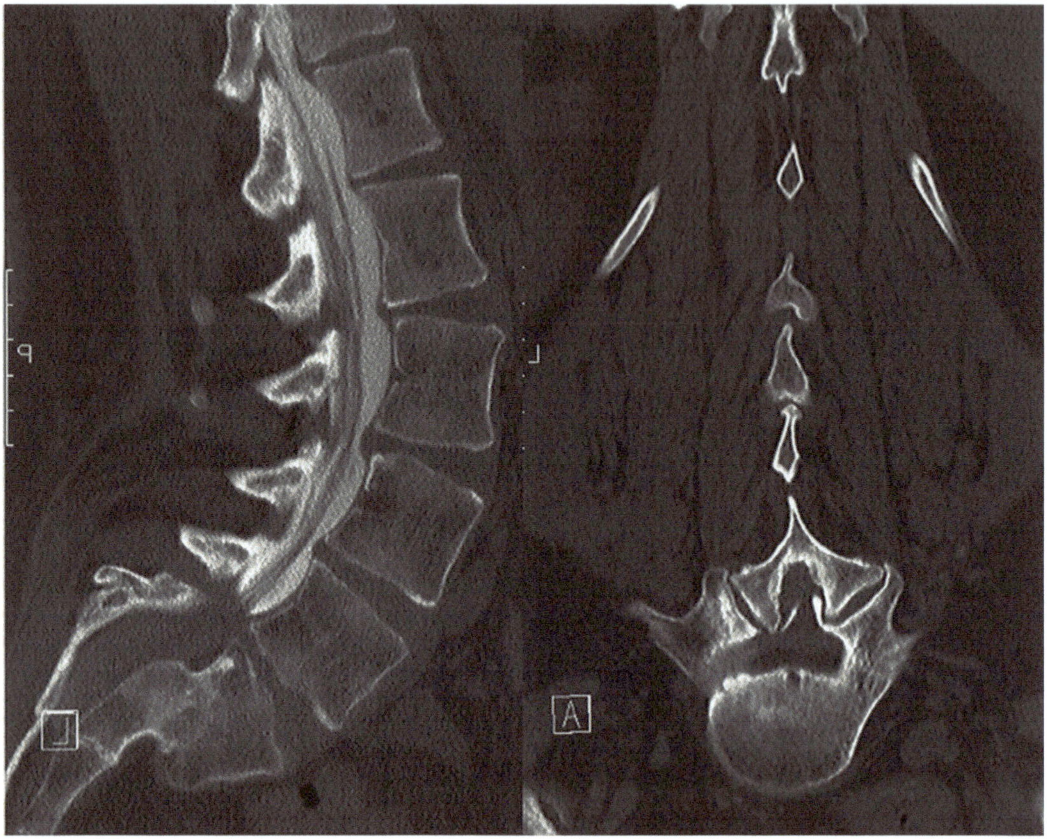

Fig. 19.9 *CT scan*: showing advanced spondyloptosis with autofusion at the L5/S1 level

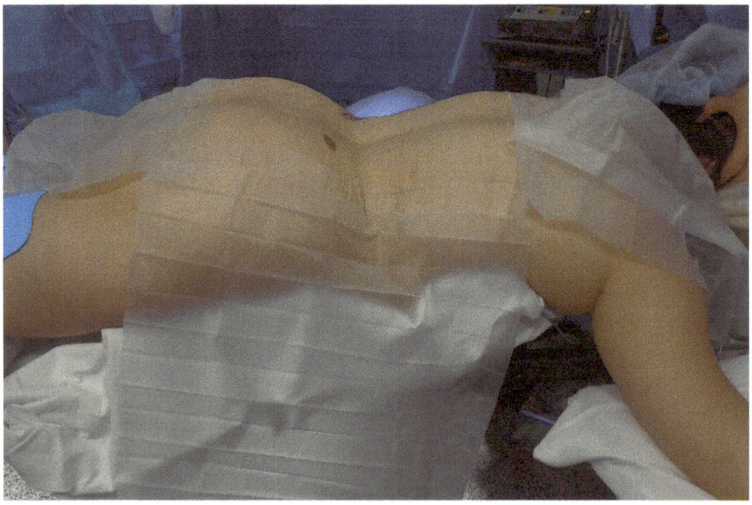

Fig. 19.10 Patient positioning on Jackson frame

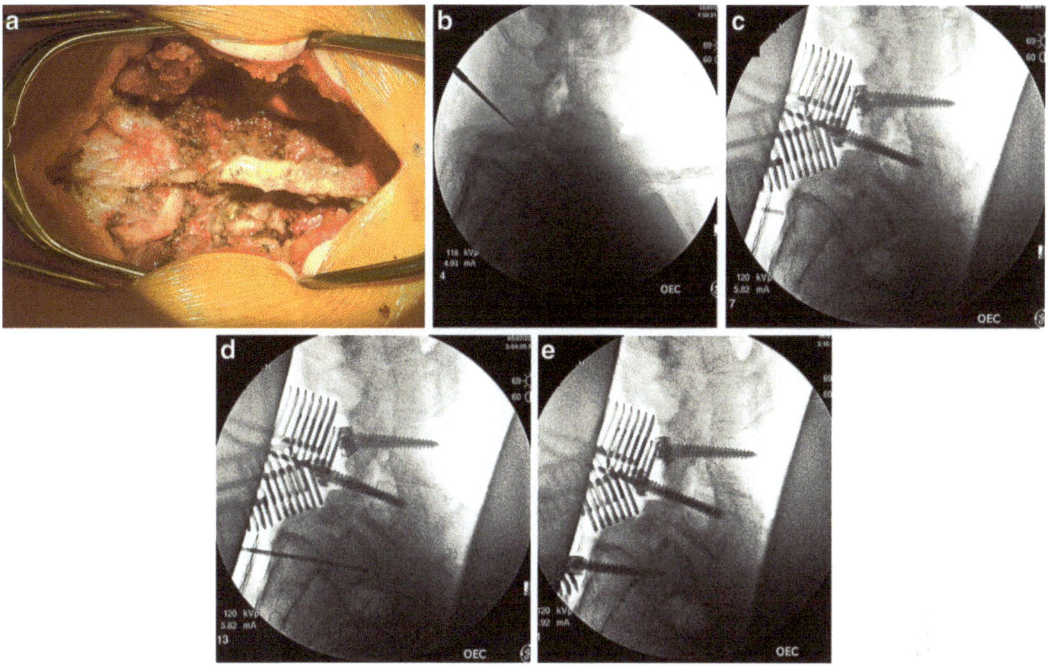

Fig. 19.11 (**a**–**e**) Exposure, identifying the level and pedicle screw placement under fluoroscopy

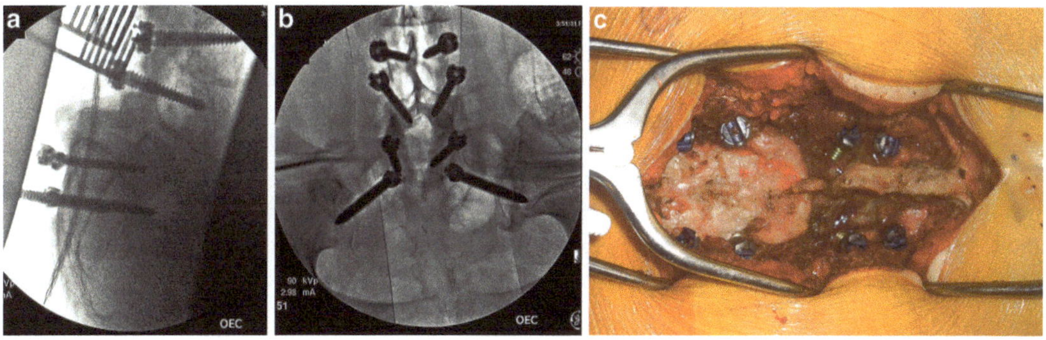

Fig. 19.12 (**a**–**c**) Pedicle screws placed

the facet joints can be done before or after screw placement. Screws were placed at the L3 and L4 levels. Transfixing screws from S1 to L5 vertebral body were placed under image intensifier to ensure proper length is used. We found that S2 screws are helpful as an additional point of fixation aiding in reduction of the slip (Figs. 19.11 and 19.12).

K2M Mesa® Rail system was used in this case which provides additional rod stiffness in the sagittal plane given its beam like design compared to cylindrical Co.Cr. rods of the same

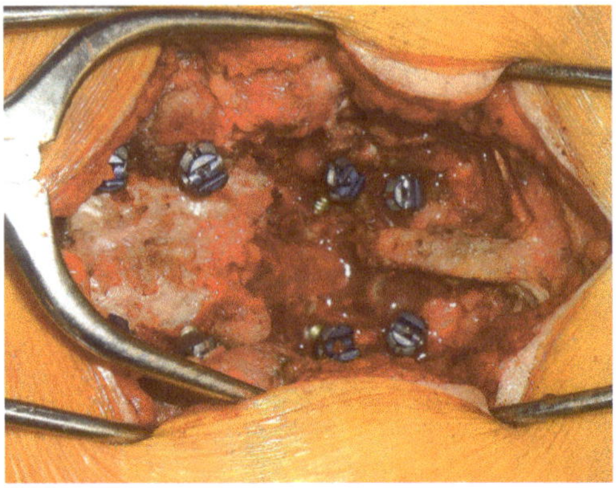

Fig. 19.13 Following wide posterior decompression

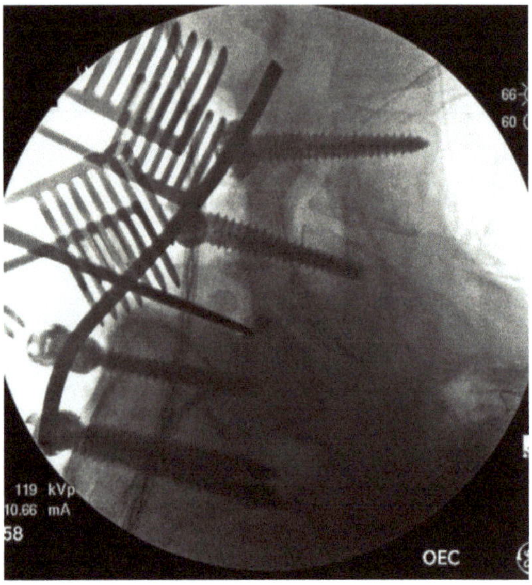

Fig. 19.14 Partial corpectomy of L5 under fluoroscopy

diameter. Following screw placement, decompression of the spinal canal at the stenosed levels as well as foraminal stenosis using rongeurs, kerrisons, and pituitaries was done (Fig. 19.13).

If in situ fusion is planned, contouring the rods to the spine and locking screws is done.

Partial reduction was attempted, so further decompression of the nerve roots all the way laterally to the transverse process was done since further tension on the roots is expected with reduction. Also discectomy of the L4-5 and partial corpectomy of the L5 vertebral body was done to aid in reduction. Corpectomy of the posterior ridge of the L5 body under image intensifier followed in order to create a flat surface for the L4 vertebral body to lie on top of the L5/S1 complex (Fig. 19.14).

Following locking of the distal screws S1 and S2, gradual simultaneous tightening of the L4 and L3 screws bilaterally was done to reduce the L4 vertebra to the contoured rod meanwhile, assessment of the L4 and L5 nerve roots was done to estimate the amount of tension on the nerve roots. Continuous neuromonitoring is essential to detect any changes. Additionally, direct EMG stimulation of nerve roots may detect latency in conduction if excessive stretch is present (Fig. 19.15).

Additional posterior compression of screws puts the vertebral bodies under compressive forces and adds lordosis to the lumbar spine. Boney contact between L4 and L5 vertebrae was confirmed by fluoroscopy. Final tightening of instrumentation was done followed by burring of the boney surfaces to facilitate fusion. Care must be taken to avoid injury to the exposed dura and nerve roots. Local bone graft along with allograft is used. If BMP is to be used, we advise using a dural sealant before its application to avoid irritation of the nerve roots. We prefer to wash using pulse lavage prior to bone grafting. Deep drain was used followed by application of 1 g of Vancomycin powder locally for better infection control (Figs. 19.16, 19.17, and 19.18).

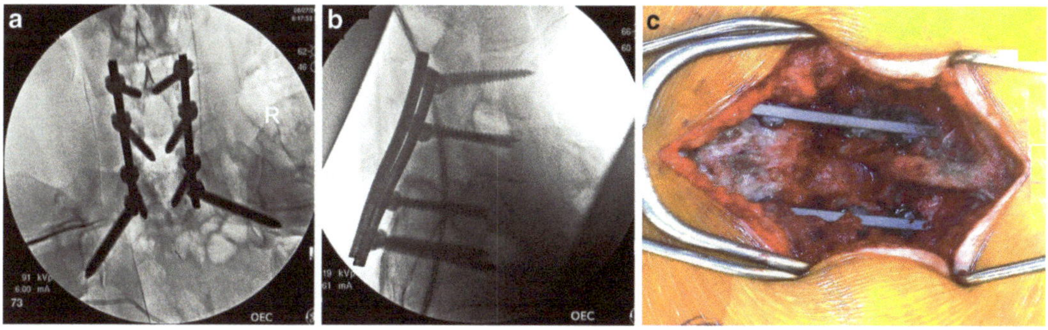

Fig. 19.15 (**a**–**c**) Following insertion of rail rods

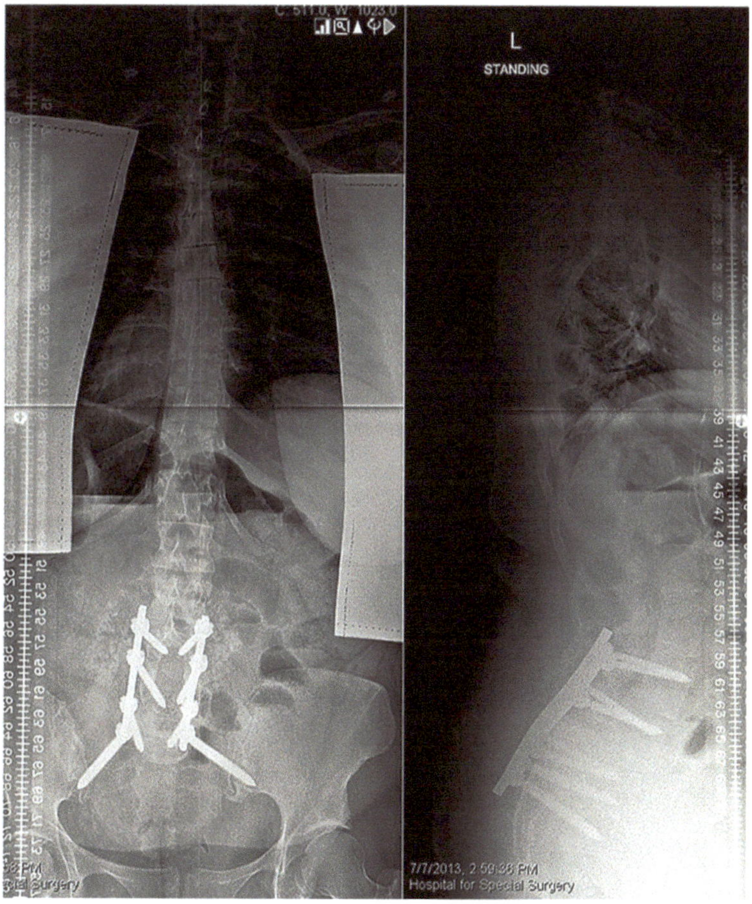

Fig. 19.16 Case 1: postoperative AP/lateral X-rays

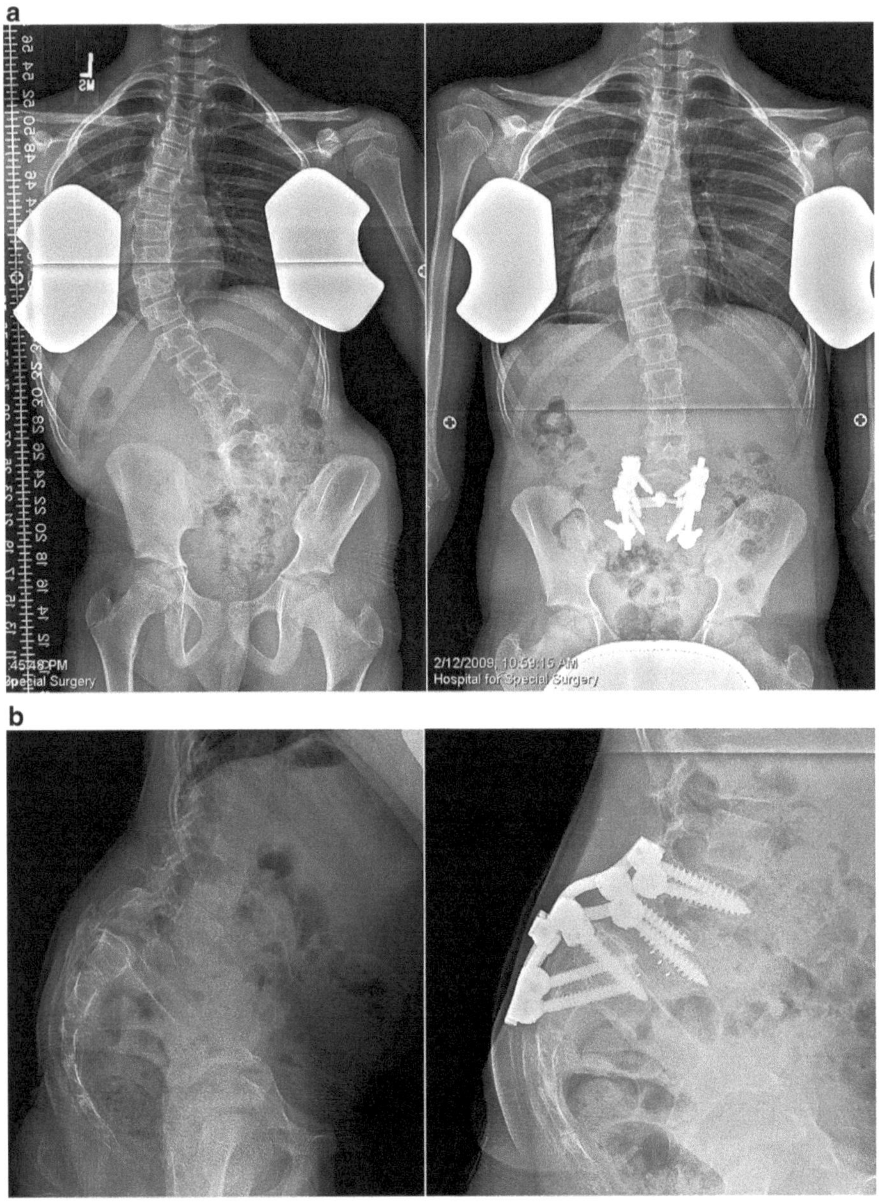

Fig. 19.17 (**a**, **b**) Case 2: AP/lateral view pre- and post-operative

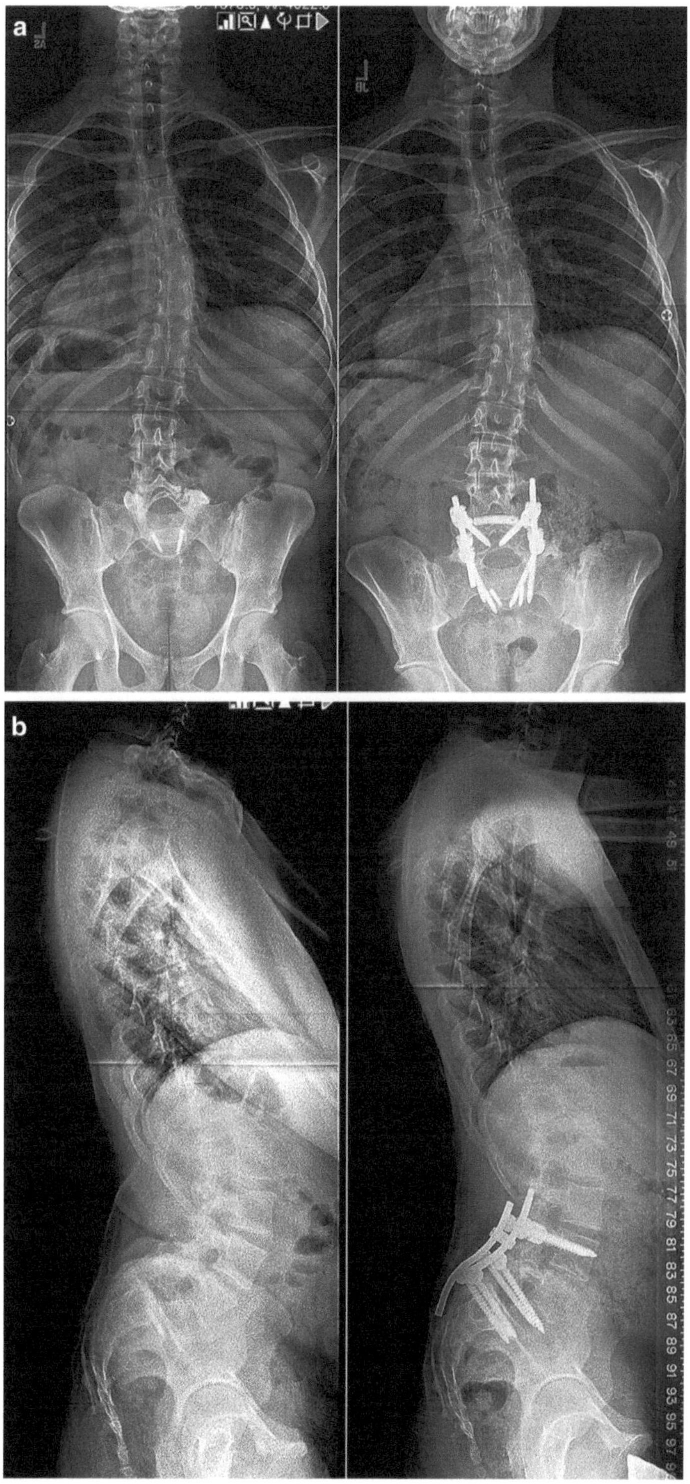

Fig. 19.18 (**a**, **b**) Case 3: AP/Lat view pre- and post-operative

References

1. Meyerding HW. Low backache and sciatic pain associated with spondylolisthesis and protruded intervertebral disc: incidence, significance and treatment. J Bone Joint Surg. 1941;23:461–70.
2. Wiltse L, Newman PH, Macnab I. Classification of spondylolysis and spondylolisthesis. Clin Orthop. 1976;117:23.
3. Curylo LJ, Edwards C, Dewald RW. Radiographic markers in spondyloptosis implications for spondylolisthesis progression. Spine. 2002;27(18):2021–5.
4. Taillard W. Les Spondylolisthesis chez l'enfant et l'adolescent. Acta Orthop Scand. 1955;24:115.
5. Boisaubert B, Montigny JP, Duval-Beaupere G, et al. Incidence, sacrum, spondylolisthesis. Rachis. 1997; 9:187–92.
6. Labelle H, Roussouly P, Berthonnaud E, et al. The importance of spino-pelvic balance in L5-s1 developmental spondylolisthesis: a review of pertinent radiologic measurements. Spine. 2005;30:S27–34.
7. Matsunaga S, Ijiri K, Hayashi K. Nonsurgically managed patients with degenerative spondylolisthesis: a 10- to 18-year follow-up study. J Neurosurg. 2000;93: 194–8.
8. Seitsalo S. Operative and conservative treatment of moderate spondylolisthesis in young patients. J Bone Joint Surg Br. 1990;72:908–13.
9. Fredrickson BE, Baker D, McHolick WJ, et al. The natural history of spondylolysis and spondylolisthesis. J Bone Joint Surg Am. 1984;66:699–707.
10. Floman Y. Progression of lumbosacral ishtmic spondylolisthesis in adults. Spine. 2000;25:342.
11. Smith JA, Deviren V, Berven S, et al. Clinical outcome of trans-sacral interbody fusion after partial reduction for high-grade l5-s1 spondylolisthesis. Spine. 2001;26:2227–34.
12. Bradford DS, Boachie-Adjei O. Treatment of severe spondylolisthesis by anterior and posterior reduction and stabilization. A long-term follow-up study. J Bone Joint Surg Am. 1990;72:1060–6.
13. Bradford D. Treatment of severe spondylolisthesis: a combined approach for reduction and stabilization. Spine. 1979;4:423–9.
14. Bradford D, Gotfried Y. Staged salvage reconstruction of grade IV and V spondylolisthesis. J Bone Joint Surg Am. 1987;69:191–202.
15. Gaines RW, Nichols WK. Treatment of spondyloptosis by two stage L5 vertebrectomy and reduction of L4 onto S1. Spine. 1985;10:680–6.
16. Kalra K, et al. A modified Gaines procedure for spondyloptosis. J Bone Joint Surg Br. 2010;92:1589–91.
17. Vaz G, Roussouly P, Berthonnaud E, et al. Sagittal morphology and equilibrium of pelvis and spine. Eur Spine J. 2002;11:80–7.
18. Di Martino A, et al. Spontaneous fusion of L5 spondyloptosis: should we learn from nature? Spine J. 2012;12(6):529.
19. Kawahara N, Tomita K, Kobayashi T, et al. Influence of acute shortening on the spinal cord: an experimental study. Spine. 2005;30:613–20.
20. Bohlman HH, Cook SS. One-stage decompression and posterolateral and interbody fusion for lumbosacral spondyloptosis through a posterior approach. Report of two cases. J Bone Joint Surg Am. 1982; 64:415–8.
21. Laursen M, Thomsen K, Eiskjaer SP, et al. Functional outcome after partial reduction and 360 degree fusion in grade III-V spondylolisthesis in adolescent and adult patients. J Spinal Disord. 1999;12:300–6.
22. Molinari RW, Bridwell KH, Lenke LG, et al. Anterior column support in surgery for high-grade, isthmic spondylolisthesis. Clin Orthop Relat Res. 2002;394:109–20.
23. Boxall D, Bradford DS, Winter RB, Moe JH. Management of severe spondylolisthesis in children and adolescents. J Bone Joint Surg. 1979;61A:479–95.
24. Ishikawa S, Kumar SJ, Torres BC. Surgical treatment of dysplastic spondylolisthesis. Results after in situ fusion. Spine. 1994;19:1691–6.
25. Hanson DS, Bridwell KH, Rhee JM, et al. Dowel fibular strut grafts for high-grade dysplastic isthmic spondylolisthesis. Spine. 2002;27:1982–8.
26. Schoenecker PL, Cole HO, Herring JA, et al. Cauda equina syndrome after in situ arthrodesis for severe spondylolisthesis at the lumbosacral junction. J Bone Joint Surg Am. 1990;72:369–77.
27. Sailhan F, Gollogly S, Roussouly P. The radiographic results and neurologic complications of instrumented reduction and fusion of high-grade spondylolisthesis without decompression of the neural elements: a retrospective review of 44 patients. Spine. 2006;31(2):161–9.
28. Petraco DM, Spivak JM, Cappadona JG, et al. An anatomic evaluation of L5 nerve stretch in spondylolisthesis reduction. Spine. 1996;21:1133.

Management of Traumatic Spondylolisthesis: Cervical and Lumbar

20

Kelley Banagan and Steven C. Ludwig

Introduction

Spondylolisthesis refers to the anterior translation of one vertebral body in relation to another. It occurs most commonly in the lumbar spine but is also seen clinically in the cervical spine. It can be further classified with the commonly applied Wiltse classification based on etiology with dysplastic, isthmic, degenerative, pathological, and traumatic as the recognized subdivisions. Most commonly, spondylolisthesis is of the degenerative variety in the lumbar spine. Acute traumatic spondylolisthesis is rare and must be distinguished from acute isthmic spondylolisthesis occurring secondary to preexisting spondylolysis [1]. The most commonly recognized traumatic spondylolisthesis is that of the axis, or the so-called *hangman's fracture*. However, a variety of case reports in the literature describe traumatic slips within the subaxial cervical spine and the lumbar spine. It is generally recognized that mechanism of injury and anatomy play crucial roles in the development of traumatic fracture patterns, including the development of instability and spondylolisthesis. Furthermore, the nature of the injury and the degree of instability and/or degree of the slip dictate and guide appropriate management.

K. Banagan, M.D. • S.C. Ludwig, M.D. (✉)
Department of Orthopaedics, University of Maryland Medical System, 110 S. Paca St., Floor 6, Suite 300, Baltimore, MD 21201, USA
e-mail: kbanagan@umoa.umm.edu; sludwig@umoa.umm.edu

Cervical Spine: Anatomic Considerations in Injury Patterns

The highest incidence of traumatic cervical injury occurs at the upper segments of the cervical spine. The specific injury pattern that results is directly related to the force applied and the anatomy of the region. In the craniocervical spine, the direction of the skull contact forces in part dictates the injury incurred, whereas in the subaxial spine, the pattern of injury relates to the forces applied directly to the vertebra, or a lever arm applied to several adjacent segments. The orientation of the facet joints in the cervical spine also predisposes the area to specific injury patterns. The coronal nature of the joints accounts for the higher occurrence of facet dislocations in this region of the spine [1, 2]. Bauze and Ardran [3], in 1978, reported their experience with experimental dislocation of the cervical spine in cadaveric specimens. The experiment attempted to simulate a naturally occurring event, and the authors concluded that the forward displacement of one vertebra on another seemed to be related to maximal force in combination with rupture of the posterior ligaments and stripping of the anterior longitudinal ligament (ALL) [3].

A.L. Wollowick and V. Sarwahi (eds.), *Spondylolisthesis: Diagnosis, Non-Surgical Management, and Surgical Techniques*, DOI 10.1007/978-1-4899-7575-1_20,

The axis also has unique anatomic considerations that can specifically predispose it to injury. It is a transitional vertebra, articulating superiorly with the atlas and inferiorly with a normal cervical vertebra. Synovial joints on the upper surface are relatively unyielding. Inferiorly, the intervertebral disc and coronally oriented facets share the weight and load bearing. Separating the two areas is a narrow isthmus of bone, which the foramen transversarium traverses and weakens. Furthermore, the axis is essentially a double vertebra and, from a mechanical standpoint, the dens increases the lever arm that can be applied to the body, thereby increasing the potential for fracture.

Traumatic Spondylolisthesis of the Axis

Traumatic spondylolisthesis of the axis (TSA; hangman's fracture) was first described in 1913 in an article titled "The Ideal Lesion in Judicial Hanging" [4]. The fracture produced as a result of the submental knot is created by distraction and extension [5]. However, distinctions exist between the classically described hangman's fracture and the commonly occurring TSA. Presently, the most common causes of TSA are motor vehicle collisions and falls. The commonly proposed mechanism is flexion or hyperextension with axial loading. Associated with TSA are high incidences of injuries to the head (16 %–46 %), other portions of the cervical spine (13 %), and thorax (43 %). Also associated with TSA are generally low incidences of neurological injury and nonunion [6].

TSA usually involves bilateral fractures through the neural arch of the axis and can result in anterior displacement of C2 on C3 [6]. Various classifications of TSA have been developed. Francis et al. [7] defined two categories based on the limits of stability proposed by Johnson et al.: [8] 3.5 mm of translation and 11° of angulation. Pepin and Hawkins [9] and Effendi et al. [10] classified the hangman's fracture based on radiographic displacement of the fracture [6, 11]. Effendi et al. [10] described the cervicocranial concept with which the cephalad element consists of the skull, atlas, dens, and body of the axis and the caudal element consists of the arch of the atlas, the third cervical vertebra, and the remaining cervical spine. They classified hangman's fractures based on appearance. Type I fractures are isolated hairline fractures of the ring of the atlas with minimal displacement of the body of C2. The mechanism is axial loading and hyperextension. Type II fractures are characterized by displacement of the anterior fragment with disruption of the disc and are caused by hyperextension and rebound flexion. Type III is fixed displacement and angulation of the anterior segment with locked facets caused by a flexion rotation moment. Levine and Edwards [12] further modified this classification scheme to include the Type IIa hangman's fracture, incorporating a flexion-distraction injury [11].

Management of TSA

In 1968, Cornish [5] presented his experience in the management of 14 cases of TSA. He asserted that treatment should be based on recognition of the deforming force and the extent of injury. Primary treatment of unstable lesions was recommended to allow for early stabilization and mobilization. Skull traction was discouraged because it runs parallel to the mechanism of injury and can further propagate the fracture [5]. The treatment algorithms proposed by Cornish rest on the premise that the fracture is inherently unstable. However, debate exists regarding the inherent stability of the injury.

Müller et al. [6] examined 39 patients who sustained hangman's fractures and were treated at one institution. The fractures were classified according to the Effendi classification, and the group proposed a stability scale for the different Type II fractures and a corresponding treatment rationale. Type I fractures were considered stable, and application of a rigid cervical orthosis remains the treatment method of choice. With Type II flexion injuries, or the Levine and Edwards Type IIa, the axis body fragment hinges around the intact ALL. Radiographic evaluation of these fractures usually reveals moderate to severe angulation of the body fragment with little to no anterior displacement. Treatment with rigid external immobilization is appropriate for the majority of the injuries. With Type II extension injuries, the axis fragment hinges around an intact posterior longitudinal ligament (PLL), and the ALL and anterior disc are ruptured. The group also found these lesions to be stable, with non-rigid immobilization advocated as the treatment of choice.

However, Type IIa spondylolisthesis injuries need to be carefully differentiated. These lesions are highly unstable secondary to rupture of the C2–C3 disc, in addition to the ALL and PLL. Nonoperative management of these fractures has been associated with a substantial rate of failure of stabilization (33 %) and nonunion (11 %) in a series of 39 patients [6]. In that series, solid fusion was achieved in all fractures treated with internal stabilization. Coric et al. [13] stated that as much as 6 mm of anterior displacement was tolerated in this group as long as the fragments were in stable position, but Müller et al. [6] maintained that internal stabilization is necessary. Images of a 23-year-old man with a Type II hangman's fracture are presented (Fig. 20.1).

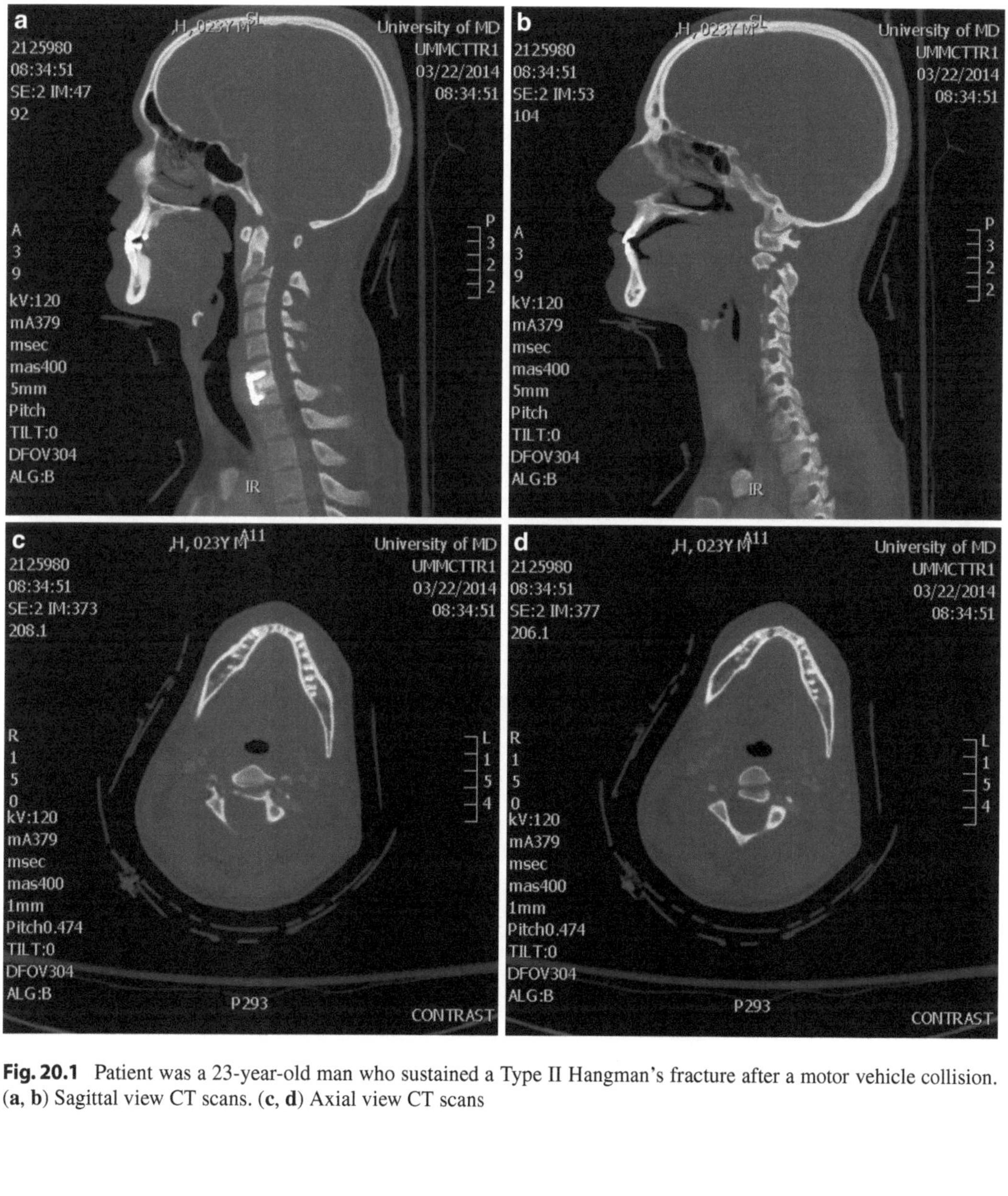

Fig. 20.1 Patient was a 23-year-old man who sustained a Type II Hangman's fracture after a motor vehicle collision. (**a**, **b**) Sagittal view CT scans. (**c**, **d**) Axial view CT scans

The patient was treated nonoperatively with a rigid cervical orthosis (Fig. 20.2).

Several biomechanical studies have been conducted to assess which method of stabilization is most appropriate for fracture fixation. Surgical options include anterior fusion, posterior fusion, or a combined anterior and posterior approach (more specifically, C2–C3 anterior cervical discectomy and fusion or C1–C3 versus C2–C4 posterior spinal fusion and instrumentation). Chittiboina et al. [11] examined anterior versus posterior fixation in human cadaveric specimens in which TSA was created. They found that posterior constructs had increased stiffness in all parameters tested in the biomechanics laboratory: rotation, flexion, extension, and lateral bending. However, posterior fixation that spans C1–C2 by default results in a clinically significantly decreased range of motion across the segment and increased dorsal pain. Furthermore, posterior fixation in this region can be technically challenging, with a narrow margin of error for screw placement. As such, the high stiffness afforded by posterior fixation might not warrant the associated risk, especially considering that anterior fixation constructs were adequate in restoring stiffness and clinically can yield identical fusion rates [11].

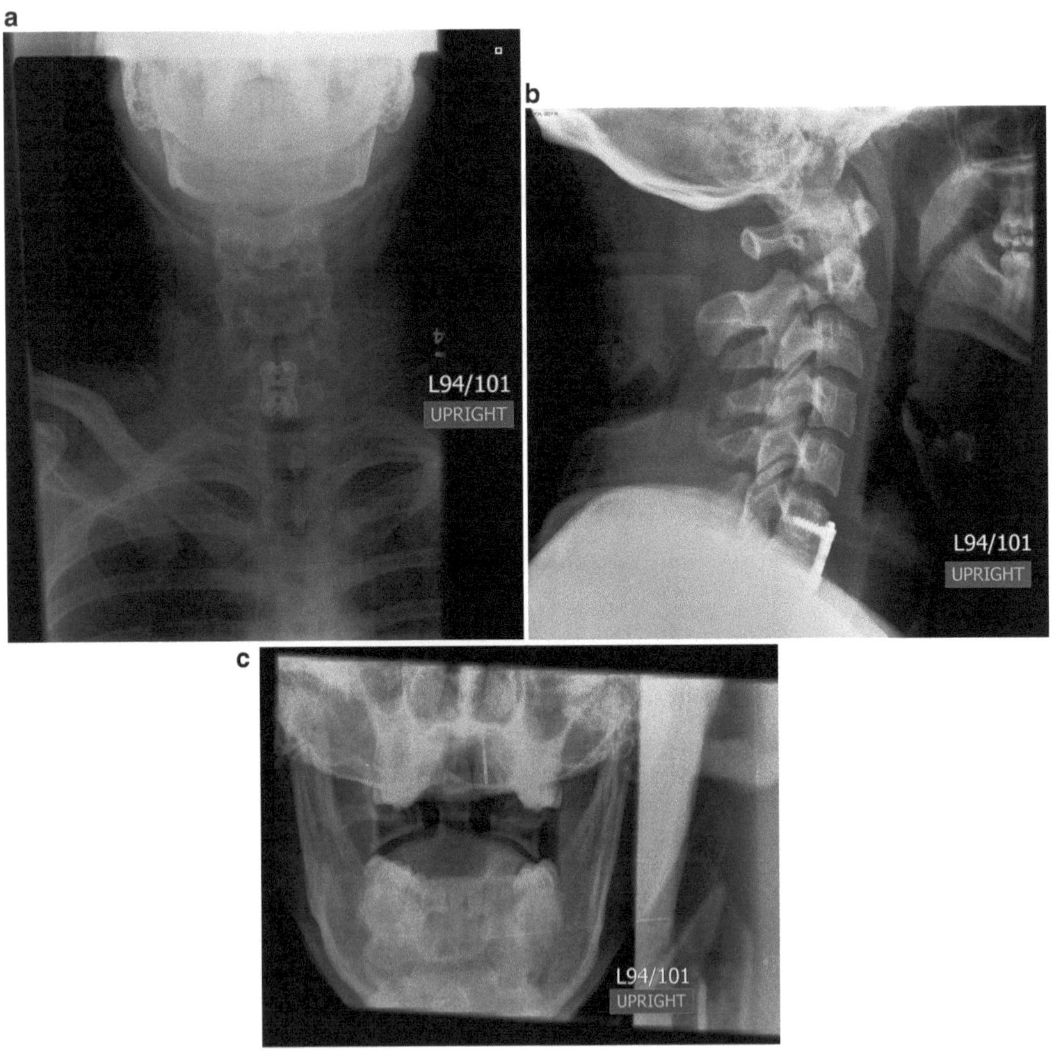

Fig. 20.2 Same patient shown in Fig. 20.1, with the collar applied. (**a**) Anteroposterior upright view. (**b**) Lateral upright view. (**c**) Open mouth upright view

Arand et al. [14] conducted a similar biomechanical study in which a clinically relevant instability model of traumatic spondylolisthesis of C2 was created such that various stabilizing constructs could be tested. The group found clinically relevant signs of destabilization across C2–C3 with only low-grade lesions of the anterior discoligamentous structures. They therefore concluded that from a biomechanical standpoint, the most accurate and stable method of stabilization was anterior plate fixation. Only in isthmus fractures of C2 without discoligamentous lesions was posterior fixation more suitable [14].

Traumatic Spondylolisthesis of the Subaxial Cervical Spine

Traumatic spondylolisthesis of the subaxial cervical spine is a rare occurrence, and few cases have been reported. Ido et al. [15] reported that the condition was first described by Perlman and Hawes in 1951. Patients usually present with a complete, or rarely a partial, neurological deficit with radicular symptoms. Historically, a combined anterior and posterior fusion procedure is advocated for these unstable injuries [16]. The vast majority of literature regarding traumatic spondylolisthesis of the lower portion of the cervical spine is in the form of case reports.

Srivastava et al. [16] presented their management of a C3–C4 spondyloptosis in a 35-year-old man who suffered a fall of approximately 20 feet and landed on his forehead. He had complete spondyloptosis of C3 on C4 with bilateral pedicle fractures at C3, fracture of the C1 arch, and bilateral C2 pedicle fractures secondary to severe hyperextension force with associated axial load. The patient was neurologically intact. Computed tomographic (CT) scanning and magnetic resonance imaging (MRI) were performed and revealed no lamina or facet fractures and no spinal cord compression or signal abnormality. MRI is essential in this patient population to rule out the presence of disc fragments within the spinal canal. The group elected to treat the patient first with a reduction maneuver. An awake, nasotracheal fiberoptic intubation was performed, and, with the patient awake, gradual weight was added to Gardner-Wells tongs and traction was applied. Fluoroscopic guidance was used to assess reduction. The neck was kept in neutral flexion-extension during the reduction maneuver. Once acceptable alignment was achieved and the patient remained neurologically intact, anterior cervical discectomy and fusion were performed at C3–C4. The group opted for anterior stabilization only, as opposed to a multi-stage anterior and posterior procedure, in an effort to avoid the destabilizing effects that can result from a posterior procedure. However, the requirement for anterior-only stabilization is anatomic reduction of the posterior elements with acceptable alignment and appropriate postoperative immobilization to allow for fracture healing. Furthermore, in cases in which neurological deficit is present, a posterior procedure might be necessary such that decompression can be performed [16].

Similarly, Shah and Rajshekhar [17] and Ido et al. [15] described, in their respective case reports, management of a C7–T1 spondyloptosis and C6–C7 traumatic spondylolisthesis, respectively. Again, both patients suffered a fall from height with associated hyperextension injuries and axial load. In each instance, a reduction maneuver was performed with careful assessment of neurological function. Anterior cervical discectomy and fusion were then performed. In each case, an anterior-only construct was thought to afford adequate stability and the patient was spared the morbidity of a combined approach [15, 17].

Lumbar Spine: Anatomic Considerations and Traumatic Spondylolisthesis

Traumatic spondylolisthesis of the lumbar spine is a rare entity, with only 100 reported cases since Watson-Jones [18] described the condition in 1940. The majority of reported cases are traumatic lumbosacral dislocations, with dislocation at the L5–S1 level. In the lumbar spine, the facets are able to slide past each other in extension. This minimizes the chance of facet fracture occurring secondary to hyperextension in the lumbar spine, as is often seen in the cervical spine. The facet joints in the lumbar spine are oriented in a sagittal plane, making them able to resist rotation but not flexion or translation. They do not support an axial load unless an extension posture is assumed. Furthermore, the angle of the sacrum in relation to the L5 body at the lumbosacral junction will impact the development of a pathological process in this region (i.e., the greater the lumbosacral joint angle is, the greater the applied translation force will be). The coronal nature of the facet joints at L5–S1 also explains why traumatic spondylolisthesis occurs most frequently at this level [1].

A variety of mechanisms have been proposed as the mechanism of injury in traumatic spondylolisthesis of the lumbar spine. Watson-Jones [18] suggested hyperextension stress, and Roaf [19] suggested hyperflexion, axial rotation, and compression forces. According to Deniz et al. [1], many cite hyperflexion and compression as the main deforming force for anterior or anterolateral lumbosacral dislocation, although some case reports of direct force tangential to the apophyseal joint and hyperextension with compression have been presented. The injury is characterized by disruption of the supra- and intraspinous ligaments and the joint capsules. The ALL, PLL, and disc might remain intact [20].

Vialle et al. [21] published a series of 11 patients who had suffered lumbosacral dislocation. The purpose of the study was to investigate the mechanism of injury, the nature of the injury, and the preferred treatment method. The group proposed a novel anatomic classification based on the injury patterns observed in the treatment group. Type I fractures represent pure dislocation of the articular facets in the absence of fracture. Type IA is unilateral rotatory dislocation, Type IB is bilateral facet dislocation with lateral displacement secondary to hyperflexion and lateral translation, and Type IC is bilateral facet dislocation with anterior slippage of the L5 vertebra secondary to flexion and distraction forces. Type II fractures are characterized by a unilateral articular process fracture dislocation. Type III is bilateral facet fracture dislocation with disc injury. Type IIIA fractures are caused by flexion-distraction forces, and Type IIIB fractures have rotational deformities [21].

Regardless of the mechanism of injury, Vialle et al. [21] found that traumatic spondylolisthesis of the lumbar and lumbosacral spine is produced by high-energy trauma. As such, the injury is rarely isolated and patients frequently suffer from associated pulmonary, abdominal, vascular, and brain injuries. The presence of transverse process fractures in the lumbosacral spine on initial imaging can serve as a "sentinel" sign and raise the suspicion for lumbosacral injury. CT scanning and MRI are essential to further define the injury and identify the potential presence of a disc herniation and compromise of the L5 neural foramen [21]. Operative intervention is the preferred management of choice for this injury, and all 11 patients in the group presented by Vialle et al. [21] were treated with posterior spinal fusion and instrumentation. Images of a 23-year-old woman with bilateral L5–S1 facet fractures, an S1 superior endplate fracture, and resultant traumatic L5–S1 spondylolisthesis are presented (Fig. 20.3). The patient was treated operatively with posterior spinal fusion and instrumentation. Interbody fusion was deferred secondary to the endplate fracture of S1 (Fig. 20.4).

Fabris et al. [20] presented their experience with the management of three patients with traumatic spondylolisthesis of L5–S1. All three patients were treated operatively with posterior stabilization. Open procedures with L5 laminectomy were advocated because they allow for direct visualization and control of the neural structures, which are essential if a reduction maneuver becomes necessary, in the setting of neurological compromise, or if fragments of disc require removal. Both groups [20, 21] advocate performing an interbody fusion if considerable disruption of the disc is shown by preoperative MRI. Interbody fusion allows for a higher degree of stability and a higher fusion rate, with the anterior support reducing the risk of implant failure. Interbody fusion can be performed from an anterior or posterior approach [1].

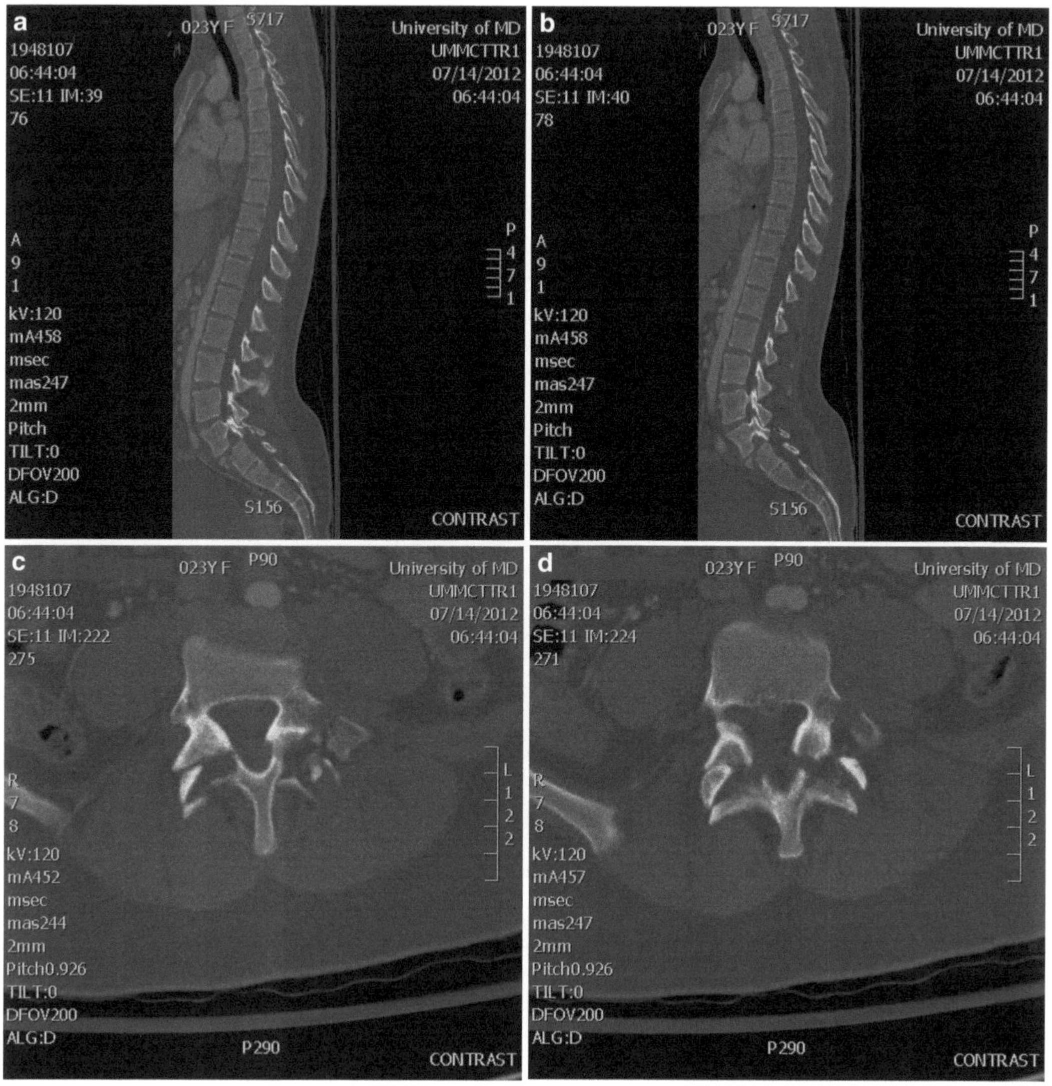

Fig. 20.3 Patient was a 23-year-old woman who sustained traumatic spondylolisthesis at L5–S1 after a motor vehicle collision. (**a**, **b**) Sagittal view CT scans, two different views. (**c**, **d**) Axial view CT scans obtained at L5–S1 reveal traumatic spondylolisthesis

Conclusion

Traumatic spondylolisthesis is a rare condition, usually the result of a high-energy mechanism. TSA, or a hangman's fracture, is the most commonly recognized traumatic spondylolisthesis. It is important to recognize the pattern of injury because it will guide the decision regarding operative versus nonoperative treatment. Traumatic spondylolisthesis of the subaxial cervical spine and the lumbar spine is less common, often associated with facet fractures and usually requiring operative intervention.

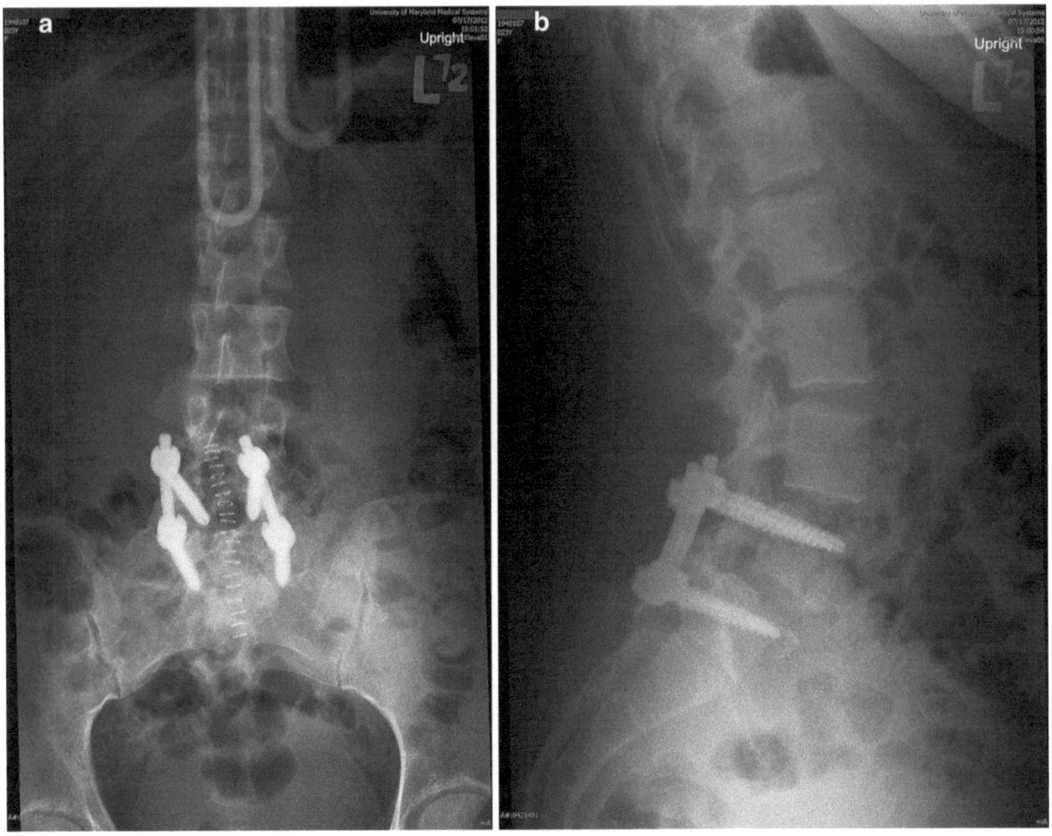

Fig. 20.4 Postoperative upright radiographs of same patient shown in Fig. 20.3. (**a**) Anteroposterior view. (**b**) Lateral view

Acknowledgment The authors thank Dori Kelly, MA, senior editor and writer, for editing the manuscript and formatting the figures.

References

1. Deniz FE, Zileli M, Cagli S, Kanyilmaz H. Traumatic L4–L5 spondylolisthesis: case report. Eur Spine J. 2008;17 suppl 2:S232–5.
2. Cusick JF. Yoganandan. Biomechanics of the cervical spine 4: major injuries. Clin Biomech (Bristol, Avon). 2002;17:1–20.
3. Bauze RJ, Ardran GM. Experimental production of forward dislocation in the human cervical spine. J Bone Joint Surg Br. 1978;60:239–45.
4. Wood-Jones F. The ideal lesion in judicial hanging. Lancet. 1913;181:53.
5. Cornish BL. Traumatic spondylolisthesis of the axis. J Bone Joint Surg Br. 1968;50:31–43.
6. Müller EJ, Wick M, Muhr G. Traumatic spondylolisthesis of the axis: treatment rationale based on the stability of the different fracture Types. Eur Spine J. 2000;9:123–8.
7. Francis WR, Fielding JW, Hawkins RJ, Pepin J, Hensinger R. Traumatic spondylolisthesis of the axis. J Bone Joint Surg Br. 1981;63:313–8.
8. Johnson RM, Crelin ES, White III AA, Panjabi MM, Southwick WO. Some new observations on the functional anatomy of the lower cervical spine. Clin Orthop Relat Res. 1975;111:192–200.
9. Pepin JW, Hawkins RJ. Traumatic spondylolisthesis of the axis: Hangman's fracture. Clin Orthop Relat Res. 1981;157:133–8.
10. Effendi B, Roy D, Cornish B, Dussault RG, Laurin CA. Fractures of the ring of the axis: a classification based on the analysis of 131 cases. J Bone Joint Surg Br. 1981;63:319–27.
11. Chittiboina P, Wylen E, Ogden A, Mukherjee DP, Vannemreddy P, Nanda A. J Neurosurg Spine. 2009; 11:379–87.

12. Levine AM, Edwards CC. The management of traumatic spondylolisthesis of the axis. J Bone Joint Surg Am. 1985;67:217–26.
13. Coric D, Wilson JA, Kelly Jr DL. Treatment of traumatic spondylolisthesis of the axis with nonrigid immobilization: a review of 64 cases. J Neurosurg. 1996;85:550–4.
14. Arand M, Neller S, Kinzl L, Claes L, Wilke HJ. The traumatic spondylolisthesis of the axis: a biomechanical in vitro evaluation of an instability model and clinical relevant constructs for stabilization. Clin Biomech (Bristol, Avon). 2002;17:432–8.
15. Ido K, Murakami H, Kawaguchi H, Urushidani H. An unusual reduction technique prior to surgical treatment for traumatic spondylolisthesis in the lower cervical spine. J Clin Neurosci. 2002;9:664–6.
16. Srivastava SK, Agrawal KM, Sharma AK, Agrawal MD, Bhosale SK, Renganathan SR. C3–C4 spondyloptosis without neurological deficit: a case report. Spine J. 2010;10:e16–20.
17. Shah KC, Rajshekhar V. Successful management of posttraumatic C7–T1 spondyloptosis with uninstrumented ventral surgery. Surg Neurol. 2004;62:431–4.
18. Watson-Jones R. Fractures and other bone and joint injuries. Br J Surg. 1940;27:616–7.
19. Roaf R. Spinal injuries. Burma Med J. 1960;8:139–43.
20. Fabris D, Costantini S, Nena U, Lo Scalzo V. Traumatic L5–S1 spondylolisthesis: report of three cases and a review of the literature. Eur Spine J. 1999;8:290–5.
21. Vialle R, Charosky S, Rillardon L, Levassor N, Court C. Traumatic dislocation of the lumbosacral junction diagnosis, anatomical classification and surgical strategy. Injury. 2007;38:169–81.

Spondylolisthesis Associated with Scoliosis

21

Cara L. Sedney and John C. France

Abbreviation

AP Anteroposterior

Scoliosis: Definition and Classification

Scoliosis is defined as a lateral curvature of the spine, and may either be idiopathic (most common, and actually related to complex genetic and familial factors), or result from a variety of congenital, neuromuscular, pathologic, or degenerative processes. Scoliosis is most generally grouped in terms of its cause and age of onset, with pediatric and adolescent forms of scoliosis being considered as different from degenerative adult scoliosis. Adolescent idiopathic scoliosis is most commonly classified by the Lenke classification, which takes into account curve location, structurality, kyphosis, and lumbar apical vertebra [1]. Adult classification schemes are not as commonly accepted, with several proposed schemes currently in use.

C.L. Sedney, M.D.
Department of Neurosurgery, West Virginia University, HSC PO Box 9183, Morgantown, WV 26505, USA
e-mail: csedney@hsc.wvu.edu

J.C. France, M.D. (✉)
Department of Orthopaedics, West Virginia University, HSC PO Box 9196, Morgantown, WV 26505, USA
e-mail: jfrance@hsc.wvu.edu

Causation and Association of Scoliosis and Spondylolisthesis

An association of scoliosis and spondylolisthesis has long been recognized; however, the relationship of these two entities is a subject of debate. The incidence of scoliosis found in patients with spondylolisthesis ranges from 15 to 43 % [2]. Conversely, the incidence of spondylolisthesis in patients with scoliosis is only 6 %, similar to that found in the general population (6.2 %) [2]. Scoliosis is more commonly associated with spondylolisthesis if the spondylolisthesis is present at L4-5, is dysplastic in nature, or is of higher Meyerding grade [3]. The reasons for this are association in children are thought to be partly genetic, with subtle connective tissue disorders such as Ehlers-Danlos variants implicated by some [4]. The association of these two entities is stronger in an elderly population with degenerative spondylolisthesis and scoliosis, due to the similar pathologic processes at work.

Spondylolisthesis Presenting with Scoliosis

In general, spondylolisthesis in association with scoliosis may present either co-existent with scoliosis, or after scoliosis or other fusion surgery. Spondylolisthesis seen co-existent with scoliosis may be a cause of the scoliosis, or be an unrelated

A.L. Wollowick and V. Sarwahi (eds.), *Spondylolisthesis: Diagnosis, Non-Surgical Management, and Surgical Techniques*, DOI 10.1007/978-1-4899-7575-1_21,

finding. Spondylolisthesis is felt to contribute to scoliosis through two possible mechanisms. In children it is theorized that sciatic irritation and muscle spasm from spondylolisthesis can result in a "sciatic scoliosis" which is generally a mild lumbar or thoracolumbar scoliotic curve, but curves of up to 50° have been reported [5]. A negative family history of scoliosis supports this diagnosis according to Peterson [6]. Rotation is minimal or absent. A second mechanism is through asymmetric rotation and torsion at the level of the spondylolisthesis, termed "torsional scoliosis." These cases generally have significant rotation and translation in both coronal and sagittal planes, with the apex of the scoliotic curve also being the level of the spondylolisthesis.

Scoliosis which follows normal adolescent idiopathic patterns and involves the thoracic spine is more often unrelated to spondylolisthesis (which is generally isthmic in nature) and is felt to represent a separate entity. However, although there are no known causative relationship, the spondylolisthesis does require consideration when planning surgical intervention for the scoliosis, which will be described below.

In adults with degenerative scoliosis, spondylolisthesis is a common co-existent finding and both findings likely contribute to further asymmetric degenerative changes, which will be discussed elsewhere.

Spondylolisthesis Developing After Scoliosis

In contrast, spondylolisthesis seen after a scoliosis surgery, or other spinal fusion, may be related to post-surgical stresses or simply a manifestation of degenerative processes. Again, the causation is debatable with a paucity of literature on the subject. Some experts argue that the increased biomechanical stress on inferior spinal levels may play a role [7], while others feel that spondylolisthesis reflects normal spinal degeneration [8]. Although in clinical practice such cases are seen, only a single case report describes a degenerative spondylolisthesis after previous fusion for scoliosis: Winter and Silverman present the case of a 32-year-old female who presented with a spondylolisthesis at L4-5 after a fusion of T1 to T12 at 11 years of age [9]. Because her intervening discs were healthy, the authors postulate no relationship between her scoliosis surgery and her subsequent development of spondylolisthesis [9]. Koptan and colleagues reported ten pediatric patients who developed a painful spondylolysis 2–7 years after a scoliosis fusion, with three of these having a grade I spondylolisthesis [10]. Danielsson and Nachemson conducted a 22-year follow-up study on patients undergoing posterior fusion for adolescent idiopathic scoliosis and found similar lumbar degenerative disease in these patients compared to patients who had bracing of scoliosis, but increased disc degeneration when compared to control subjects [11]. They did not, however, comment specifically on spondylolisthesis. In 1963, Harris and Wiley reported a series of six patients who suffered subsequent spondylolysis after a spinal fusion done for non-scoliosis diagnoses [12].

A final form of spondylolisthesis includes a slip of the vertebral body above a previous fusion, a form of adjacent segment disease. Although literature describing this phenomenon is sparse as compared to kyphotic changes, this form of spondylolisthesis generally relates to sagittal imbalance or hypermobility above a fusion because of increased biomechanical stresses at this level.

Diagnosis and Symptoms

While the diagnoses of spondylolisthesis and scoliosis are largely radiographic, teasing out whether one finding or both are responsible for symptoms is a more complex issue. Spondylolisthesis may be an asymptomatic finding present on imaging studies such as scoliosis films, or may present with such symptoms as back pain and/or bilateral radiculopathy. Lower grade spondylolisthesis is more likely to be asymptomatic than higher grade cases, where up to 90 % may be symptomatic. Spondylolisthesis associated with cephalad adjacent segment disease may be associated with upper lumbar or thoracic back pain, or a "pitched forward" position. Scoliosis in children is not considered to be a painful condition, although some children and adolescents will complain of pain. Both conditions may contribute to axial back pain.

Surgical Techniques and Considerations

The major treatment dilemma surrounding scoliosis and spondylolisthesis which present simultaneously is whether to treat only one condition, or both. This decision-making process often centers on whether one condition is felt to cause the other. Arlet and colleagues advocate treating each condition separately, but note that in nine of their 82 patients, the scoliosis seemed directly related to the spondylolisthesis and improved after reduction and arthrodesis of the spondylolisthesis [13]. Seitsalo has reported resolution of sciatic scoliosis in 25 out of 39 patients who underwent lumbosacral fusion for spondylolisthesis, while 19 of 28 cases of torsional type scoliosis had good result from lumbosacral fusion only [14]. They therefore recommend consideration for correction of the scoliosis if a significant rotational component is present, while correction of the spondylolisthesis alone may resolve non-rotational curves [14]. However, they do advocate surgical correction of the spondylolisthesis prior to the scoliotic curve becoming structural, after which time it may also require treatment regardless of its original etiology [14]. Furthermore, the curves in question were lumbar curves; thoracic and thoracolumbar curves were treated as separate entities in this study [14]. Zhou and colleagues also report a single case of resolution of a scoliotic curve with reduction and fusion of a Meyerding grade IV spondylolisthesis, supporting the assertions of previous literature regarding torsional scoliosis being caused by spondylolisthesis [5]. Their patient had a lumbar curve with compensatory thoracic curve, both of which corrected on bending films [5]. In cases where a significant scoliotic curve was present, both Arlet and Seitsalo reported a strategy of staging the reduction and fusion of a high-grade spondylolisthesis, followed by scoliosis correction surgery several months later, but similarly advocate acting before the curve becomes structural [13, 14]. Crostelli and Mazza emphasize the fact that treatment must be based upon the characteristics of each entity considered separately, regardless of the association of the two [4]. They further postulate that a lumbar curve of greater than 15° is unlikely to resolve with treatment of the spondylolisthesis alone [4]. In general, it seems to be supported by most authors that a thoracic or thoracolumbar scoliosis is unrelated to a spondylolisthesis and the symptomatic pathology should be treated. For lumbar curves, in particular mild ones not associated with a rotational component, sciatic scoliosis may be suspected and the spondylolisthesis would be treated. Torsional lumbar scoliosis, that associated with a rotational component, is more controversial; however, attempting to correct the spondylolisthesis initially may be prudent. The scoliotic curve may be followed and corrected in a staged manner if it progresses, fails to resolve, and/or is symptomatic (Fig. 21.1). Alternatively, both may be corrected as a single surgery, in particular if the scoliotic curve appears structural on bending films.

In contrast, spondylolisthesis presenting after a spinal fusion for scoliosis, trauma, or other diagnoses may require special consideration because of the altered biomechanical forces at work on the spine, rather than because of causation. Koptan and colleagues have presented ten pediatric patients with spondylolysis and low-grade spondylolisthesis after a posterior fusion for scoliosis and recommended direct repair of the spondylolysis in these cases to preserve motion segments in these patients with already decreased spinal motion [10]. However, this strategy is only feasible for young patients without degenerative disease and with very minimal spondylolisthesis. For other patients, fusion is generally required if surgical treatment is to be pursued.

When fusion below a long construct is considered, a number of factors must be taken into account: whether to connect to the previous fusion, caudal extent, anterior support, and overall sagittal balance. Connection to the previous fusion should be considered if the spondylolisthesis is adjacent to the previous fusion or within one or two spinal levels of it; if there is additional degenerative changes between the previous fusion and the new spondylolisthesis; or if there

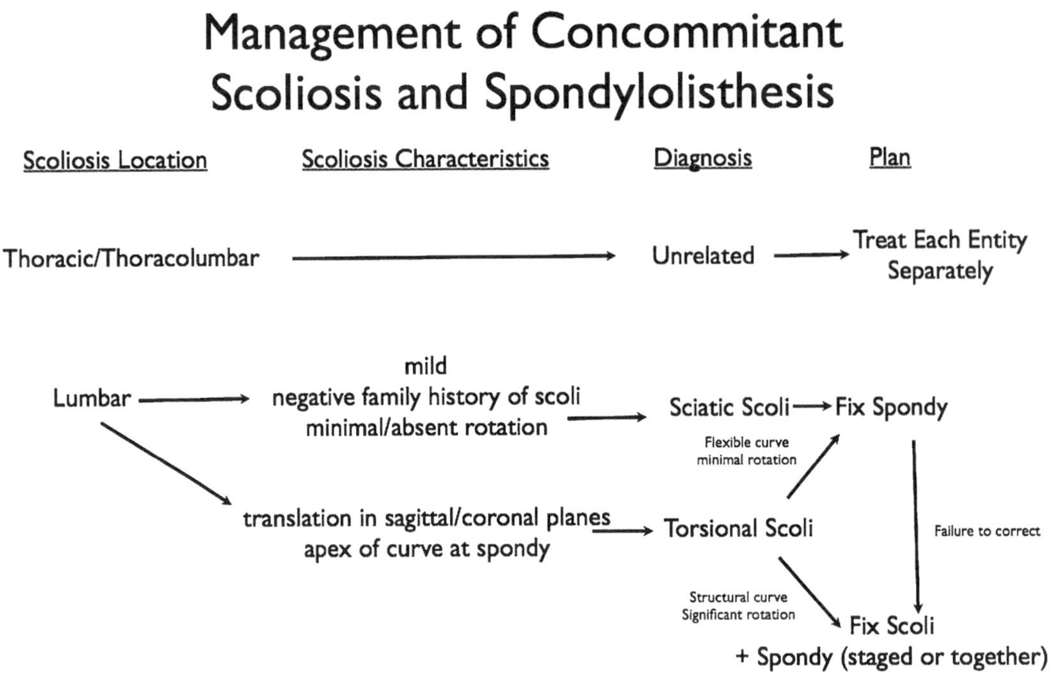

Fig. 21.1 Flowchart demonstrating management of concommitant scoliosis and spondylolisthesis

is curve progression inferior to the previous construct. If connection to the previous construct is elected, an assessment of the bony fusion should be made so that the decision to remove or replace hardware or explore the existing fusion can be acted upon at the same surgery. If the fusion is found to be solid, fewer points of fixation within the fusion levels will be required. If a non-union is detected, this area should be repaired and included among the instrumented levels.

The caudal extent of the fusion may be a straightforward-decision if the spondylolisthesis levels are not being connected to the previous fusion. However, if a long construct is planned, consideration should be given to pelvic fixation. Additionally, interbody support at L5-S1 might be required for purposes of encouraging fusion at this critical point of the construct. An anterior approach for lumbar interbody fusion works well both for this purpose and also for spondylolisthesis reduction and lordosis preservation and is the approach of choice for the senior author. The overall sagittal balance should be assessed because of the importance of preserving lordosis and preventing "flat back syndrome" which may necessitate extensive osteotomy correction in the future if this critical component is neglected, especially when long constructs are planned.

Clinical Cases

36-Year-Old Female

A 36-year-old female presented to the clinic with a 5-year history of axial back pain. She had undergone a posterior scoliosis fusion at the age of 12 from the upper thoracic spine to L1. At the time of presentation her back pain was significantly impacting her ability to function and was resistant to conservative treatment including anti-inflammatory medications, physical therapy, chiropractic care, and a series of facet blocks. Her symptoms improved with sitting. Her neurologic examination was normal. Standing scoliosis radiographs (Fig. 21.2) demonstrated a Meyerding grade I spondylolisthesis of L5-S1, approximately 75° of lumbar lordosis, progressive lumbar scoliotic curve with degenerative change at L1-L2, and good sagittal balance.

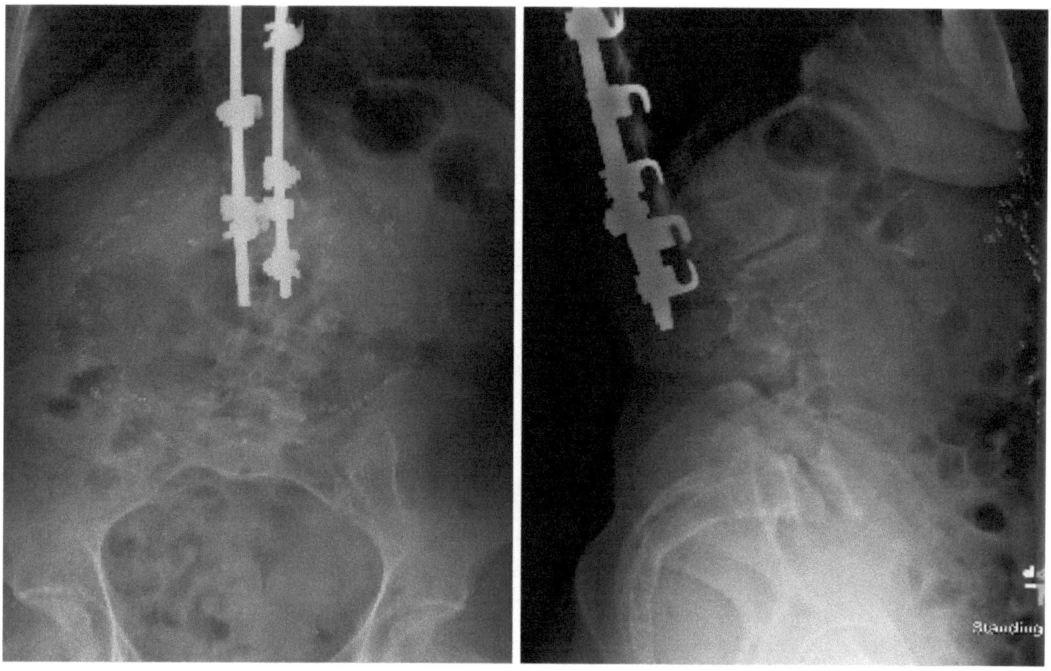

Fig. 21.2 Anteroposterior (AP) and lateral standing radiographs demonstrating spondylolisthesis of L5 on S1 with long fusion segment above

Surgery was offered to her based upon her refractory symptoms. Because she had both an L5-S1 spondylolisthesis as well as adjacent segment degeneration at L1-2, it was felt necessary to address both of these issues. An L5-S1 anterior lumbar interbody fusion was performed for reduction of her spondylolisthesis and to aid in fusion, and a posterior approach for removal of hardware with exploration of her previous fusion was performed. Finding no evidence of nonunion, pedicle screw instrumentation was placed from T9 to the pelvis, with facetectomies performed to aid in reduction of the lumbar scoliosis and to preserve lordosis. Post operative radiographs demonstrated good reduction of the deformity as well as the spondylolisthesis (Fig. 21.3).

45-Year-Old Male

A 45-year-old male presented to the clinic with progressive back and bilateral lower extremity weakness and pain, with a history of a previous fusion from T3 to L3 for scoliosis done in childhood. His current symptoms were consistent with lumbar stenosis, and lumbar myelogram confirmed stenosis as well as spondylolisthesis at L3-4, L4-5, and L5-S1 (Fig. 21.4). His neurologic exam was normal. These symptoms were resistant to conservative therapy and the patient was requesting surgical intervention. He underwent a decompression for his stenosis, as well as a fusion from L3 to the iliac wings bilaterally, connecting to his old hardware. Iliac screws were included due to the long construct. An L5-S1 anterior interbody graft was placed to aid in fusion (Fig. 21.5).

12-Year-Old Female

A 12-year-old female was followed since age 8 with spondylolisthesis of L5-S1 as well as a thoracolumbar scoliotic curve which progressed despite bracing from a Cobb angle of 13 to a Cobb angle of 70 in a period of 4 years. Syrinx and tumor were ruled out on MRI and the patient underwent a T6 to L4 fusion. The spondylolisthesis had been stable and was not addressed in the index procedure.

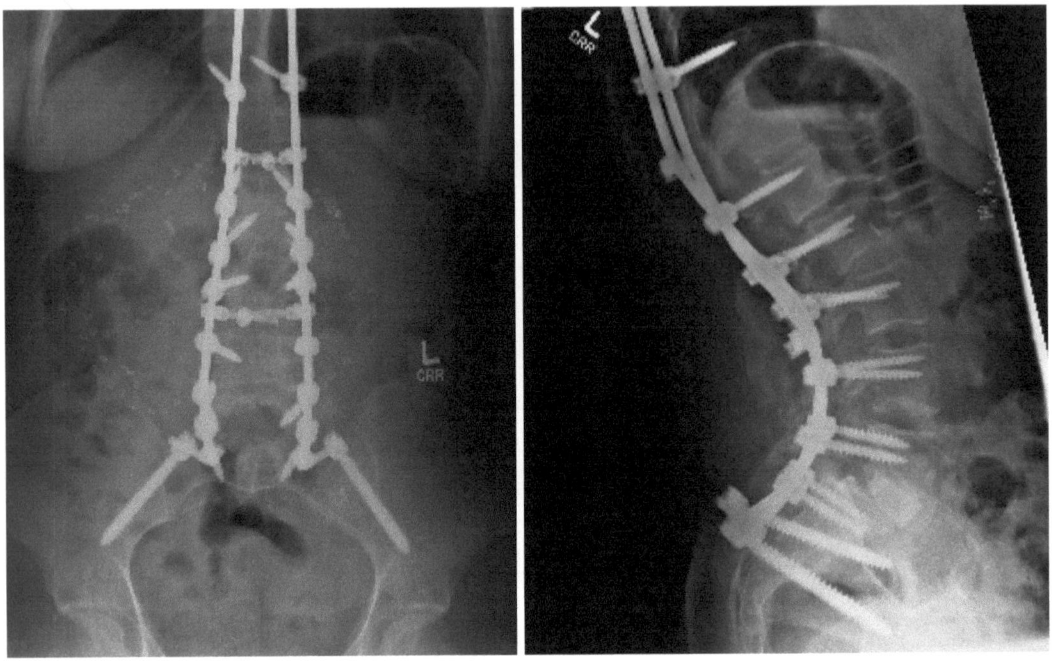

Fig. 21.3 AP and lateral lumbar radiographs demonstrating post operative correction of spondylolisthesis and extension of fusion to pelvis

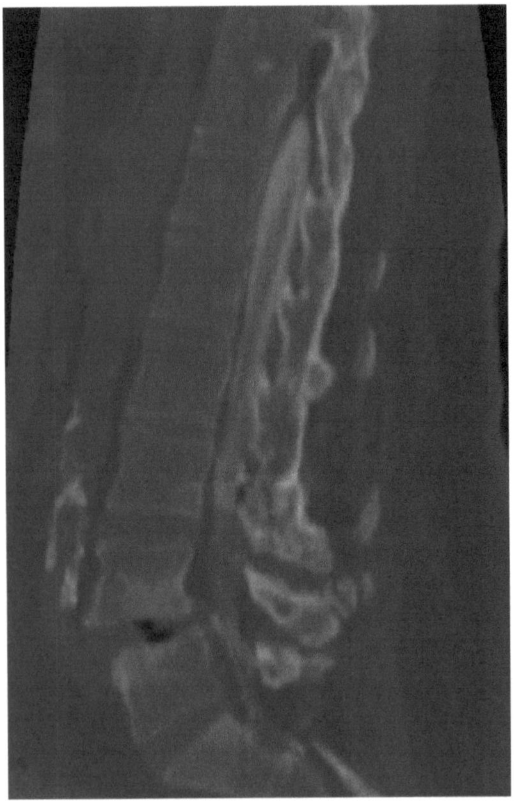

Fig. 21.4 Preoperative computed tomography sagittal view demonstrating spondylolisthesis at L4-5 below long fusion construct with spinal stenosis

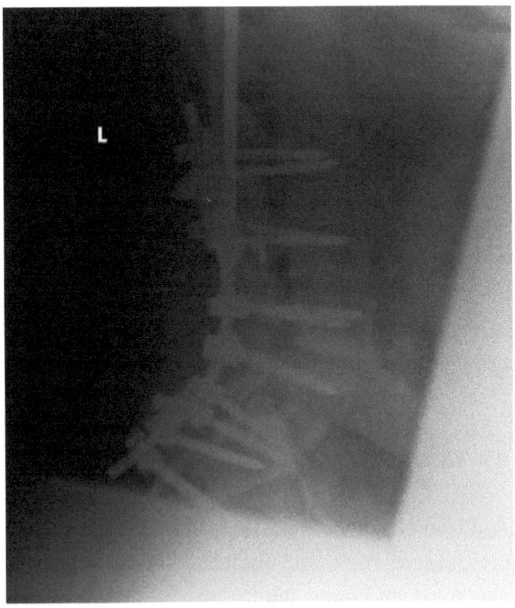

Fig. 21.5 Upright lateral radiographs after extension of fusion to pelvis with L5-S1 ALIF placement to aid in fusion

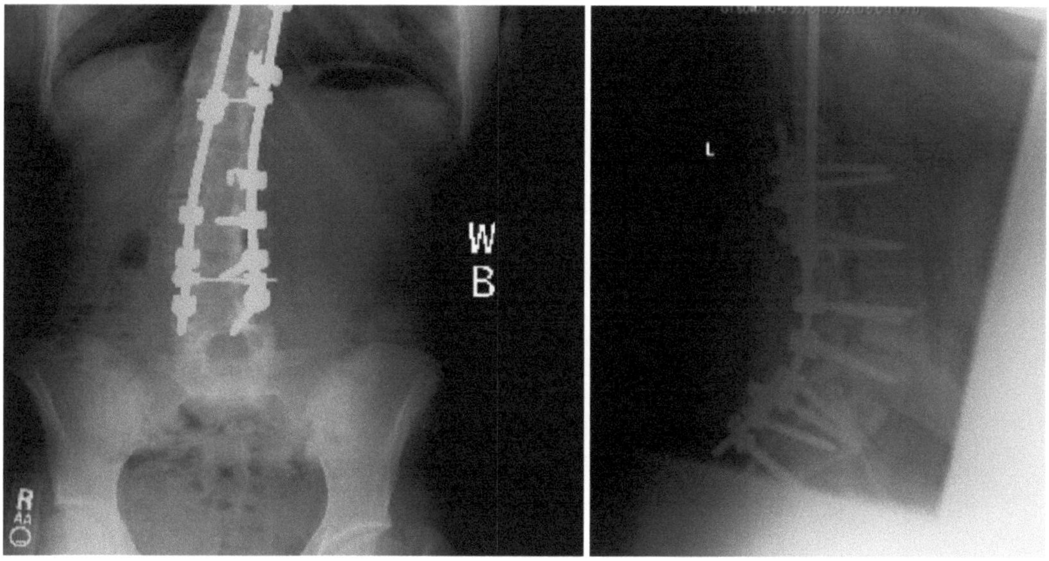

Fig. 21.6 AP and lateral standing lumbar radiographs demonstrating high-grade spondylolisthesis and previous fusion for scoliosis

By 4 years after her index procedure, she had persisting back pain and the spondylolisthesis progressed, and her fusion was extended down to the sacrum via a posterior-only approach (Fig. 21.6).

References

1. Lenke LG, Betz RR, Harms J, Bridwell KH, Clements DH, Lowe TG, et al. Adolescent idiopathic scoliosis: a new classification to determine extent of spinal arthrodesis. J Bone Joint Surg Am. 2001;83-A(8):1169–81.
2. Pneumaticos SG, Esses SI. Scoliosis associated with lumbar spondylolisthesis: a case presentation and review of the literature. Spine J. 2003;3(4):321–4.
3. McPhee IB, O'brien JP. Scoliosis in symptomatic spondylolisthesis. J Bone Joint Surg Br. 1980; 62-B(2):155–7.
4. Crostelli M, Mazza O. AIS and spondylolisthesis. Eur Spine J. 2013;22 Suppl 2:S172–84.
5. Zhou Z, Song Y, Cai Q, Kong Q. Spontaneous resolution of scoliosis associated with lumbar spondylolisthesis. Spine J. 2013;13(5):e7–10.
6. Peterson JB, Wenger DR. Asymmetric spondylolisthesis as the cause of childhood lumbar scoliosis—can new imaging modalities help clarify the relationship? Iowa Orthop J. 2008;28:65–72.
7. Nachemson A, Cochran T. Late structural and functional effects in the spine of surgically fused patients with idiopathic scoliosis followed up in adulthood. Orthop Abstracts. 1981;3:444.
8. Dickson JH, Erwin WD, Rossi D. Harrington instrumentation and arthrodesis for idiopathic scoliosis. A twenty-one-year follow-up. J Bone Joint Surg Am. 1990;72:687–83.
9. Winter RB, Silverman BJ. Degenerative spondylolisthesis at the L4-L5 in a 32-year-old female with previous fusion for idiopathic scoliosis: a case report. J Orthop Surg (Hong Kong). 2003;11(2): 202–6.
10. Koptan WM, ElMiligui YH, ElSharkawi MM. Direct repair of spondylolysis presenting after correction of adolescent idiopathic scoliosis. Spine J. 2011; 11(2):133–8.
11. Danielsson AJ, Nachemson AL. Radiologic findings and curve progression 22 years after treatment for adolescent idiopathic scoliosis: comparison of brace and surgical treatment with matching control group of straight individuals. Spine. 2001;26(5):516–25.
12. Harris RI, Wiley JJ. Acquired spondylolysis as a sequel to spine fusion. J Bone Joint Surg Am. 1963; 45:1159–70.
13. Arlet V, Rigault P, Padovani JP, Touzet P, Finidori G, Guyonvarch G. Scoliosis, spondylolysis, and lumbosacral spondylolisthesis. A study of their association appropos of 82 cases in children and adolescents. Rev Chir Orthop Reparatrice Appar Mot. 1990;76(2): 118–27.
14. Seitsalo S, Osterman K, Poussa M. Scoliosis associated with lumbar spondylolisthesis: a clinical survey of 190 young patients. Spine. 1988;13(8):899–904.

Part III

Results of Treatment and Complications

22 Results of Surgical Treatment of Adult Degenerative Spondylolisthesis

Theodore D. Koreckij and Jeffrey S. Fischgrund

Very few studies have provided evidence of the natural history of degenerative spondylolisthesis and, as will be shown in the coming text, few high quality studies (randomized and prospective in nature) exist that demonstrate clinical improvement with surgical intervention over conservative therapy. The Maine Lumbar Spine Study was a nonrandomized observational study of a mixed cohort of patients treated by community-based orthopedic spine surgeons and neurosurgeons for symptoms related to spinal stenosis from degenerative conditions, with and without spondylolisthesis. This study initially enrolled 148 patients that were treated with either conservative therapy or surgery. Surgery in these patients ($n=72$) typically consisted of a decompressive laminectomy (88 %, with only three receiving a noninstrumented fusion). One, 4, and 10-year results of this study have been published [1, 2]. At 1 year, 77 % of surgically treated patients reported improvement in their predominant symptoms (leg or back pain) compared to 44 % of patients treated conservatively. The 4 years (70 % and 52 %, respectively) and 10 years (54 % and 42 %, respectively) indicate a deterioration of the effects of surgical intervention but remained improved over conservative therapy. It should be noted that there were baseline differences in the patients amongst treatment arms and there was a significant loss to follow-up (97 patients) at 10 years. Despite its limitations, this study represents much of the best evidence available regarding long-term results of surgery compared to non-operative treatment.

Recently, the results of the Spine Patients Outcomes Research Trial (SPORT) have come to the forefront of discussions. The SPORT trial is a large prospective multicenter study involving surgical candidates from 13 centers in 11 states. At its outset, it focused on the treatment of disc herniation, spinal stenosis, and degenerative spondylolisthesis. Its study design consisted of both a randomized cohort and an observational cohort of patients that declined randomization. The surgical treatments for degenerative spondylolisthesis cohort included decompression with or without fusion and with or without instrumentation. Non-operative interventions included today's standard therapies (i.e., NSAIDS, physical therapy, epidural injections). It also used validated outcome measures, setting it apart from most of the other studies discussed in this chapter.

T.D. Koreckij, M.D.
Department of Orthopaedic Surgery, University of Missouri-Kansas City School of Medicine, St. Luke's Hospital of Kansas City, Dickson-Diveley Midwest Orthopaedic Clinic, Kansas City Orthopaedic Institute, 3651 College Blvd, Leawood, KS 66211, USA
e-mail: tkoreckij@gmail.com

J.S. Fischgrund, M.D. (✉)
Department of Orthopaedics, William Beaumont Hospital, Royal Oak, Michigan Orthopaedic Institute, PC, 26025 Lahser Road, 2nd Floor, Southfield, MI 48033, USA
e-mail: jsfischgrund@comcast.net

A.L. Wollowick and V. Sarwahi (eds.), *Spondylolisthesis: Diagnosis, Non-Surgical Management, and Surgical Techniques*, DOI 10.1007/978-1-4899-7575-1_22,

The degenerative spondylolisthesis study enrolled 607 patients; 304 in the randomized cohort and 303 in the observation cohort. The 2 and 4 years results have been published [3, 4]. Analysis of as-treated results (due to significant cross-over in the randomized group) revealed significant improvements in all primary and secondary outcomes measures in the surgically treated groups. This treatment effect was seen as early as 6 weeks after surgery and was maintained throughout the 4-year follow-up time period. However, it should be noted that non-surgical treatment resulted in modest improvement in most patients. This study represents our best mid-term data regarding surgical treatment of degenerative spondylolisthesis. However, long-term data will not be available for many years.

Surgical Options

Decompression Without Fusion

Decompression without fusion for spinal stenosis, as with much spine literature, is limited in terms of the quality of studies available. Further complicating the issue, comparisons between studies is also difficult due to different scoring methodologies used to determine outcomes. Nonetheless, there are published studies available arguing both for and against decompression without fusion.

Katz et al. demonstrated unsatisfactory results with decompression without fusion in a retrospective study published on 88 patients with degenerative spondylolisthesis with an average follow-up of 4.6 years. This data demonstrated poor outcomes in 47 % of patients at final follow-up which had deteriorated from 11 % at 1 year follow-up. Additionally, at final follow-up, 18 % of patients required repeat surgery for instability or recurrent stenosis [5]. Postacchini et al. analyzed outcomes in 64 patients over a mean of 8 years follow-up. Only 67 % of patients reported clinically satisfactory outcomes with 20 % of patients reporting worsening of symptoms over time [6]. This same author demonstrated bone regrowth of the posterior elements after laminectomy in 88 % of patients (n=40, 16 with degenerative spondylolisthesis) 8.6 years after index surgery. Increased amounts of bone regrowth were noted in patients with worse outcomes which may account for deterioration in clinical outcomes over time [7]. The results of these studies are in line with a meta-analysis of 216 patients which demonstrated that 69 % of patients reported satisfactory results with decompression alone. In this meta-analysis a slip progression was noted at an incidence of 31 % [8]. However, of the ten studies in this review documenting slip progression, only the study mentioned below by Bridwell et al. [9] found a correlation between slip progression and clinical outcomes.

Other studies offer a different experience of decompression without fusion. Herno et al. examined 108 patients that underwent decompression without fusion at a 7- and 13-year follow-up. The data demonstrated that results remained stable over time with 65–67 % of patients reporting positive outcomes at final follow-up. However, they also highlight that 9 % of patients did require repeat surgery for additional stenosis [10]. Another study in support of decompression without fusion reviewed 290 patients with one or two-level spondylolisthesis. This data showed that 82 % of patients had excellent or good results with surgery at 10-year follow-up. In this study, only 3 % of patients required repeat surgery for recurrent stenosis or instability [11].

There have been two randomized studies utilizing decompression without fusion as one of their treatment arms for degenerative spondylolisthesis. In a landmark study, Herkowitz and Kurz randomized 50 patients to either a decompressive laminectomy or a decompressive laminectomy with posterolateral fusion for one-level degenerative spondylolisthesis. In the fusion group, 24 patients (96 %) reported excellent/good results at mean of 3 years follow-up compared to 11 patients (44 %) reporting excellent/good results without fusion [12]. They reported a 36 % pseudoarthrosis rate in this study (with no effect on clinical outcome), the significance of which will be discussed later. In another randomized prospective study, patients undergoing decompression without fusion reported significantly worse outcomes and increased olisthesis progression compared to patients receiving a posterolateral fusion with or without instrumentation. Interpretation of these results should be done with caution as only ten patients that underwent isolated decompression were available at final follow-up (2 years) with small numbers included in study as whole ($n=43$ divided into three groups) [9]. Additionally, this study is one of the few studies that correlate a link between slip progression and worse clinical outcomes following surgical treatment of degenerative spondylolisthesis.

A more recent article published by Amundsen et al. reported on the 10-year outcomes on 100 patients treated for spinal stenosis. Patient allocation was not randomized except for a smaller subset of the patient cohort ($n=29$ with 18 undergoing decompression without fusion and 11 undergoing conservative treatment). In the randomized cohort, treatment with surgery afforded better clinical outcomes compared to conservative therapy (92 % and 47 %, respectively) at 4 years and was maintained throughout the follow-up period. These results were similar to those seen in the nonrandomized portion of this study. However, the authors also wished to emphasize that delays in surgery (3–27 months) in lieu of more conservative management did not appear to affect surgical outcomes in those patients that later crossed-over to surgery. Slip progression was not associated with worse clinical outcomes in this study [13].

The method used for decompression may also be important in determining outcomes. A prospective study of 67 patients was reviewed in which patients were to receive either a laminectomy or multiple level laminotomy with a mean of 3.7 years follow-up. Although confounding factors are present in the study with patient crossover to laminectomy treatment arms, they found similar clinical results with excellent/good results observed in 78–81 % of patients regardless of treatment. However, patients undergoing laminotomy had significantly better improvement in back pain compared to laminectomy patients whereas laminectomy patients found significantly greater improvement in radicular symptoms. There were three patients treated with laminectomy that develop post-operative instability requiring fusion and none with the laminotomy group. Ultimately, those authors concluded that multiple level laminotomy is preferred in patients with mild disease whereas laminectomy is indicated for more severe stenosis provided the diseased segment is stable [14].

Decompression with Fusion Without Instrumentation

There are several earlier studies that have shown improved outcomes with posterolateral fusion (Fig. 22.1) over non-fusion patients. In 1985, Lombardi et al. retrospectively reviewed the outcomes of 47 patients with degenerative spondylolisthesis treated utilizing 3 surgical techniques. Group 1 ($n=6$) received a wide laminectomy with facet joint removal, group 2 ($n=20$) received bilateral laminectomies with facet joint preservation and Group 3 ($n=21$) had a similar decompression to Group 2 with the addition of a posterolateral fusion using autogenous iliac crest bone graft. Only 33 % of patients in Group 1 reported good/excellent results whereas 80 % of patients did so in Group 2. Those patients in Group 3 reported 90 % good/excellent results. Most patients demonstrated progression of slip but this did not correlate with clinical outcome until slip progressed beyond 50 %. Two patients developed a pseudoarthrosis determined by bending X-rays. One patient, who was asymptomatic for 2 years after index operation, subsequently developed pain and was found to have a pseudoarthrosis and underwent revision with an excellent result and the other refused surgery and had a poor result [15].

A prospective nonrandomized trial utilizing decompression with posterolateral fusion versus two different types of posterior instrumentation in 147 patients was reviewed. Results of this study are difficult to extrapolate secondary to array of diagnoses (degenerative scoliosis, isthmic spondylolisthesis, and degenerative disc disease) included without a clear breakdown on the results of each. Nonetheless, the data demonstrated that 71 % of patients reported good/excellent results with a 65 % fusion rate in noninstrumented fusion patients. However this study is also limited secondary to short follow-up of 2 years [16].

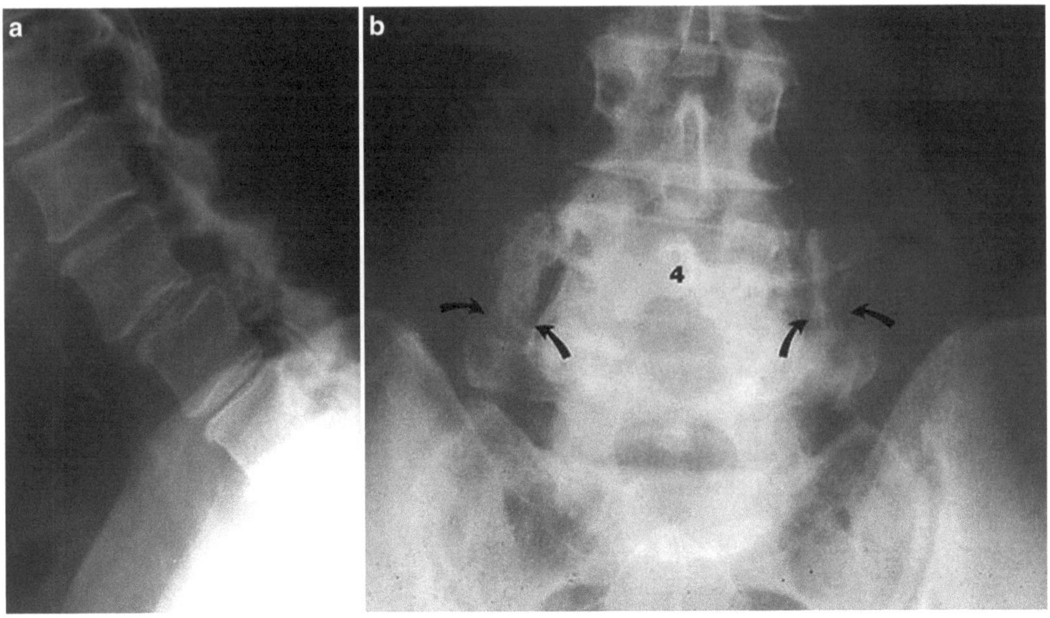

Fig. 22.1 (**a**) Representative lateral radiograph of degenerative spondylolisthesis; (**b**) AP radiograph of a noninstrumented posterolateral fusion. *Arrows* demonstrate a cleft in the intertransverse process fusion mass, indicative of a pseudoarthrosis

As mentioned early, the Herkowitz and Kurz study was the first prospective, randomized trial comparing decompression with and without posterolateral in situ fusion [12]. The initial results of study were reported at 3 years. Satisfactory outcomes in the fusion group were 96 % compared to 44 % for the non-fusion group with a significantly higher percentage of patients reporting excellent results in the fusion group. Scores for back and leg symptoms were also significantly better in those patients having underwent a fusion. This study reported a pseudoarthrosis rate of 36 % but stated that in these patients, a pseudoarthrosis did not appear to have a deleterious effect on outcome with all patients reported good/results. Seven of 25 patients demonstrated slip progression despite attempted arthrodesis. All seven of those patients went on to excellent or good results. In the non-fusion patients, 24 of 25 patients developed slip progression with only 11 of those 24 reporting excellent or good results and 13 reporting a fair or poor result. The authors concluded that a fibrous union may add enough stability to provide for improved clinical outcomes but literature of longer follow-up discussed subsequently disputes this finding.

A meta-analysis of published results between 1970 and 1993 demonstrated improved outcomes with noninstrumented fusion over decompression alone. In this review, six papers with a total of 71 patients of short to mid-term follow-up revealed 90 % satisfactory results with fusion compared to 67 % of patients with decompression alone. This review highlights a large discrepancy in published solid fusion rates ranging 30–100 % [8]. More recent literature has continued to defend that patients undergoing a posterolateral fusion have improved outcomes over decompression alone. In 2004, Ghogawala et al. published a prospective nonrandomized multi-institutional study comparing decompression alone ($n=14$) to decompression with instrumented fusion ($n=20$). Although both groups reported improved Oswestry Disability Index and Short-Form 36 scores, fusion patients reported significantly greater improvement in both over decompression alone. Although a strength of this study is its using of a validated outcome measures to determine clinical success, a major weakness is its 1-year follow-up data [17].

The importance of long-term follow-up is highlighted in several key studies. One such study was a follow-up of that original study by Herkowitz and Kurz. Kornblum et al. reviewed 47 patients that developed a pseudoarthrosis after noninstrumented posterolateral fusion of a one-level degenerative spondylolisthesis. Follow-up in this study averaged 8 years after index surgery. Eighty-six percent of patients that attained a solid fusion reported good/excellent outcomes in regard to pain and activity level versus 56 % of patients that developed a pseudoarthrosis [18]. Tsutsumimoto et al. further highlight the importance of long-term follow-up in a review of 47 patients that underwent a posterolateral fusion without instrumentation at a mean follow-up of 9.5 years. Using a validated outcome measure and VAS scores for back and leg pain, the data demonstrated improved clinical outcomes in patients that achieved solid fusion. Important to note, no differences were seen at the 1 year follow-up and it was not until 5 years did significant differences in outcomes become evident [19].

Posterolateral Fusion with Instrumentation

Although the literature regarding decompression with and without fusion is fairly supportive on the side of fusion, the use of instrumentation to augment fusion is less concrete. The driving force behind the use of instrumentation is an attempt to create a more rigid environment affording a greater potential for fusion.

Zdeblick et al. compared noninstrumented posterolateral fusion and two different types of instrumentation. These results revealed that the use of semi-rigid instrumentation afforded a fusion rate of 77 %, significantly greater than the 65 % fusion rate seen with noninstrumented fusions. Rigid fixation improved fusion rates to 95 %. Clinical outcomes demonstrated 89 and 95 % good or excellent results for semi-rigid and rigid instrumentation although no statistical analyses were performed on these results. However, a limitation of this study is its relatively short follow-up of 1 year [16].

One of the largest retrospective reviews to date was accomplished through the pooled data of more than 314 spine surgeons performing fusion surgery over a 1 year period from January 1991 through December of that year. The results of 2,684 patients demonstrated improved fusion rates with instrumentation over noninstrumented fusion, 89 % vs. 71 %, respectively. However, due to its retrospective nature, numerous baseline differences among treatment groups existed (i.e., age at time of surgery, previous operations, workers compensation status) which make inferences on clinical outcomes difficult [20]. In the meta-analysis by Mardetko et al., 239 patients across nine studies were reviewed which received various methods of instrumentation. Posterolateral fusion with instrumentation yielded between 93 and 95 % fusion rates. This did not significantly increase the rate of satisfactory outcomes compared to noninstrumented fusions [8].

A prospective randomized study of 68 patients with degenerative spondylolisthesis by Fischgrund et al. analyzed outcomes comparing decompression and noninstrumented posterolateral fusion with decompression and an instrumented fusion at 2-year follow-up [21]. Fusion rates were significantly higher in instrumented patients compared to noninstrumented fusions, 83 % vs. 45 %, respectively. Clinical outcomes in terms of pain relief and activity level were not significantly different between the two groups (76 % vs. 85 % excellent/good results).

A more recent meta-analysis was reviewed which analyzed randomized control trials and comparative observation studies between 1966 and 2005. Six studies were included in the review, including three observational and three randomized studies. Data from these studies revealed a significantly improved relative risk (RR) of achieving a solid fusion using instrumentation over noninstrumented fusions. The randomized studies demonstrated a greater RR of achieving solid fusion than did the observational studies (1.96 vs. 1.20) highlighting the importance of randomized control studies. The authors went on to conclude that although clear evidence exists

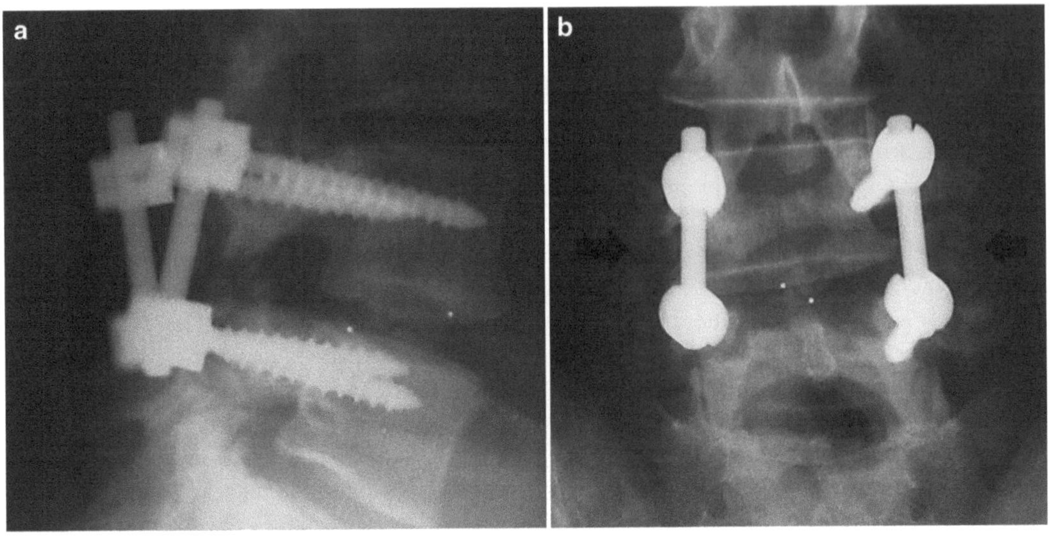

Fig. 22.2 (**a**) Lateral radiograph of an instrumented posterolateral fusion. Radiolucent markers demonstrate the borders of the interbody device; (**b**) AP radiograph. *Arrows* point to posterolateral fusion mass

that fusion rates are improved by the addition of instrumentation, however, current literature has been unable to show a definitive clinical improvement using an instrumented fusion over a noninstrumented fusion [22].

As mentioned previously, the SPORT trial's surgical intervention arm in the treatment of degenerative spondylolisthesis was decompression with or without fusion, with or without instrumentation, and with or with anterior column support. A 4-year analysis of those treatments was reviewed [23]. Clinical outcomes demonstrated significant improvements in pain with an instrumented fusion over noninstrumented fusion at short-term follow-up (1 and 2 year) but this difference was no longer evident at 3- and 4-year follow-up. Physical function scores were not significantly different at 3 and 4 years follow-up but some small differences in favor of instrumentation with anterior support were seen at 2 years. Fusion rates (assessed mostly with X-ray) demonstrated at 67 % rate for noninstrumented fusion, 85 % for a posterolateral instrumented fusion, and 87 % for an instrumented fusion with anterior support. However, the follow-up in Fischgrund et al. and the SPORT trial is 2 and 4 years, respectively. Longer term follow-up may be the deciding factor in a determination of whether an instrumented solid fusion will offer improved clinical outcomes over a noninstrumented solid fusion.

Anterior Column Support

The use of anterior interbody support (Fig. 22.2) is rooted in several theoretical advantages: additional surface area for fusion, biomechanical stability, improved sagittal alignment, and indirect reduction of neuroforaminal and central stenosis by restoration of disc height. There are a number of techniques utilized to obtain anterior support including: anterior lumbar interbody fusion (ALIF), posterior lumbar interbody fusion (PLIF), transforaminal lumbar interbody fusion (TLIF), and the direct lateral or transpsoas interbody fusion (DLIF). Each technique is associated with its own set of challenges and morbidity which is beyond the scope of this chapter. Most studies to date comparing the utilization of anterior support versus instrumented posterolateral fusion are retrospective case series of a mixed cohort of patients making interpretations to its effectiveness difficult. No high quality randomized controlled trials in the setting of degenerative spondylolisthesis have been done to assess whether the additional of anterior support improves clinical outcomes over those seen with a solid posterolateral fusion.

Biomechanical studies have shown improved stability with the use of anterior support. A study on calf specimens that underwent nondestructive flexion-extension testing was reviewed. In order to examine the effects of different types of reconstruction on adjacent levels, the L5-S1 level received pedicle screw fixation with and without anterior support. The contours of the rods were bent in order to duplicate restoration of sagittal alignment providing the theoretical advantage of anterior support. This was compared to kyphotically placed rods with and without anterior support. Restoration of sagittal balance with a lordotic PLIF/posterior instrumentation construct decreased motion across the operative segment but also yielded the highest strain at the adjacent level disc space. Compared with a kyphotic posterolateral fusion, PLIF may lead to even higher load at the superior adjacent level because of the increased stiffness of the fixed segments even if local kyphosis is corrected by PLIF [24]. This increased strain at adjacent levels will be discussed later in this chapter during the discussion of dynamic stabilization devices.

Yashiro et al. retrospectively reviewed 58 patients with degenerative spine disease (31 with degenerative spondylolisthesis) treated with instrumented posterolateral fusion or a PLIF. They reported a 60 % union rate in instrumented posterolateral fusion versus 91 % union rate in PLIF group. This lower union rate in the posterolateral fusion group is lower than other reported series for instrumented posterolateral fusion and was not explained in the article. The authors did report improved sagittal alignment and maintenance of disc height in the PLIF group. No clinical outcomes, however, were reported in this study [19].

A retrospective review of 85 patients with degenerative lumbar spine disease, not isolated degenerative spondylolisthesis, and radiologic evidence of instability was reviewed. Fifty-five patients were treated with an instrumented posterolateral fusion alone and 30 received PLIF/posterolateral fusion. The patients were followed for a mean period of 32 months. Of these patients, 86 % improved with respect to their pain symptoms, but only 46 % had a good to excellent overall result. Patients treated with a posterolateral fusion plus PLIF did not demonstrate superior clinical outcomes compared to those with a posterolateral fusion alone [25]. A study of 35 isthmic spondylolisthesis patients receiving either a posterior lumbar fusion ($n = 18$) or a posterior lumbar fusion and PLIF ($n = 17$) demonstrated correction of subluxation, disc height, and foraminal area in the group in which a PLIF procedure was performed, but not in the posterolateral fusion-only group. Again, no statistical differences were demonstrated in terms of neurological or functional improvement or in terms of fusion rate; follow-up was only 2 years [26].

Lauber et al. performed a prospective study on a mixed cohort of patients suffering from degenerative ($n = 19$), isthmic ($n = 19$), and dysplastic ($n = 1$) spondylolisthesis. Follow-up at 2- and 4-year intervals was presented. Overall fusion rate was 94.8 % and this study did not separate out the different pathologies. The functional outcomes and pain scores showed rapid deterioration to baseline pre-operative levels at 4 years. However, in subset analysis, those patients with an isthmic spondylolisthesis had significantly better clinical improvement, highlighting the importance of well-designed studies, as not all types of spondylolisthesis are similar [27].

A prospective randomized trial investigating instrumented posterolateral fusion, PLIF, and posterolateral fusion/PLIF was performed on mixed cohort of degenerative spine patients (42 with degenerative spondylolisthesis). No differences in union rates were found amongst the groups at 2 years (92 %, 95 %, and 96 %, respectively). Again, although the groups undergoing a PLIF demonstrated improved sagittal alignment and disc height, this did *not* result in improved clinical outcomes [28].

With the lack of randomized, prospective studies comparing anterior support to posterolateral fusion in degenerative spondylolisthesis, its undertaking should be done with caution. Although posterolateral fusion compared to decompression alone has been associated with increased morbidity [29–31], the addition of anterior support further adds to this risk. Reported rates of complications with addition of anterior support have ranged between 8 and 80 % [32]. Although many of the same complications exist with decompression and instrumented posterolateral fusion (i.e., dural tear, hardware breakage, etc.), the increased technical demands associated with the addition of anterior support lend itself to an increased risk of these complications. Again, an examination of the risks associated with these procedures is difficult to account for due to low quality evidence available and differences in reporting major and minor complications.

In the current health care setting, increasing attention is being placed on cost utility of additional procedures, devices, and technologies. In a 10-year study, Kim et al. demonstrated that fusion with instrumentation significantly increases cost per quality adjusted life year (QALY). Compared with decompression alone, decompression plus instrumented fusion was associated with an improvement in quality of life at a cost of $185,878 per QALY [33]. In a health care system with limited resources, this additive cost may be prohibitive especially in the setting of limited clinical improvement afforded by these additional devices.

Role of Biologics

Historically, spinal fusions were augmented with autogenous bone graft, either local bone from the decompression or from the iliac crest. However, for longer spinal fusions or in revision situations, autogenous grafting can be inadequate. Additionally, harvest site morbidity has always been a source of debate. Although various bone graft substitutes and extenders exist, none has made more of an impact than the use of bone morphogenetic proteins (BMP). Recombinant human derivatives of BMP 2 and 7 (rhBMP 2 and rhBMP7) have both received limited FDA approval for the use in spinal fusion, of which rhBMP2 is most widely used. Controversy exists regarding the complications that exist, which may have been under-reported in the original studies [34, 35].

There have been several well-designed studies that highlight the success of BMP2 in achieving posterolateral fusion in the setting of degenerative spondylolisthesis. In the study by Boden et al., groups were compared utilizing rhBMP2 with and without posterior pedicle instrumentation as well as a group receiving autograft and instrumentation. Although a small study of only 25 patients, it demonstrated improved rates of fusion with the use of BMP as well as quicker improvements in clinical outcomes. The group undergoing posterolateral fusion without instrumentation showed the quickest improvement in clinical outcomes. Interestingly, this group also had a 100 % fusion rate while affording the shortest operative time by avoiding the instrumentation [36]. In 2009, a study of 463 patients with degenerative spondylolisthesis was reported in which one group received instrumented posterolateral fusion with rhBMP2 ($n=239$) and another group received an instrumented posterolateral fusion with iliac crest bone graft ($n=224$). At 2-year follow-up, the rhBMP2 group had a 96 % fusion rate compared to 89 % for the iliac crest group, which was statistically significant; however, clinical outcomes did not show superiority for either group. Both operative time and blood loss were lower in the rhBMP groups and in this study, 60 % of patients reported continued pain at the donor site at final follow-up. The authors concluded that given the improved fusion rates and equivalent clinical outcomes, the use of rhBMP2 is advantageous by avoiding the donor site morbidity of iliac crest bone graft [37].

The use of rhBMP7 has also been shown advantageous in augmenting a posterolateral fusion. In a prospective, randomized, multicenter study, Vaccaro et al. compared the use of rhBMP7 to autogenous iliac crest bone grafting in 36 patients undergoing posterolateral fusion without instrumentation. At 2-year follow-up, 55 % of patients receiving rhBMP7 achieved a solid fusion compared to 40 % of autograft patients. Improvements in clinical outcome measures were found to be similar between groups [38]. In a 4-year follow-up of the same patients, fusion rates in the rhBMP7 and autograft groups improved to 68 % and 50 % respectively, with similar improvements observed in clinical outcomes. Unfortunately, small numbers of patients available at final follow-up precluded the formation of statistically significant results [39].

The original studies leading to FDA approval of both rhBMP 2 and 7 reported almost no adverse events steaming from the use of BMP during surgeries involving either anterior support [40–42] or posterolateral fusion [37, 43, 44]. Although these studies were of high quality design (randomized, prospective), they were biased by their industry sponsorship. Since these original studies, there have been numerous complications reported with the use of BMP. A recent review was performed which highlights some of the major adverse events associated with the use of rhBMP2 [34]. The authors reviewed the original peer-reviewed literature as well as publicly available FDA databases and summaries associated with rhBMP2. In those studies involving posterolateral fusion, there appeared to be increased morbidity with the use of BMP in the early post-operative period relating to increased pain scores, functional outcomes, and wound complications compared to those patients undergoing iliac crest bone graft harvest. This result is counterintuitive in that the treatment effect of not performing the additional surgery associated with iliac crest bone harvest should be highest in the early post-operative period in favor of those patients receiving rhBMP. Published FDA documents also show higher rates of adverse events related to back and leg pain in rhBMP2 patients compared to controls (16 % vs. 4.8 %, respectively) which was not discussed in any of the peer-reviewed articles. Other reported adverse events include end-plate osteolysis and graft subsidence with anterior support devices, radiculitis, bone overgrowth, and increased rates of delayed infection.

Dynamic Stabilization

Despite its popularity for the treatment of a wide range of spine disorders, lumbar fusion is not without its pitfalls. Biomechanical studies have demonstrated that spinal fusion increases intradiscal pressures in levels above and below the fusion and that the pressure increases with the number of levels fused [24, 45]. This additional strain brings the added concern for development "adjacent segment degeneration" (Fig. 22.3). However, clinical trials to date have not definitively determined

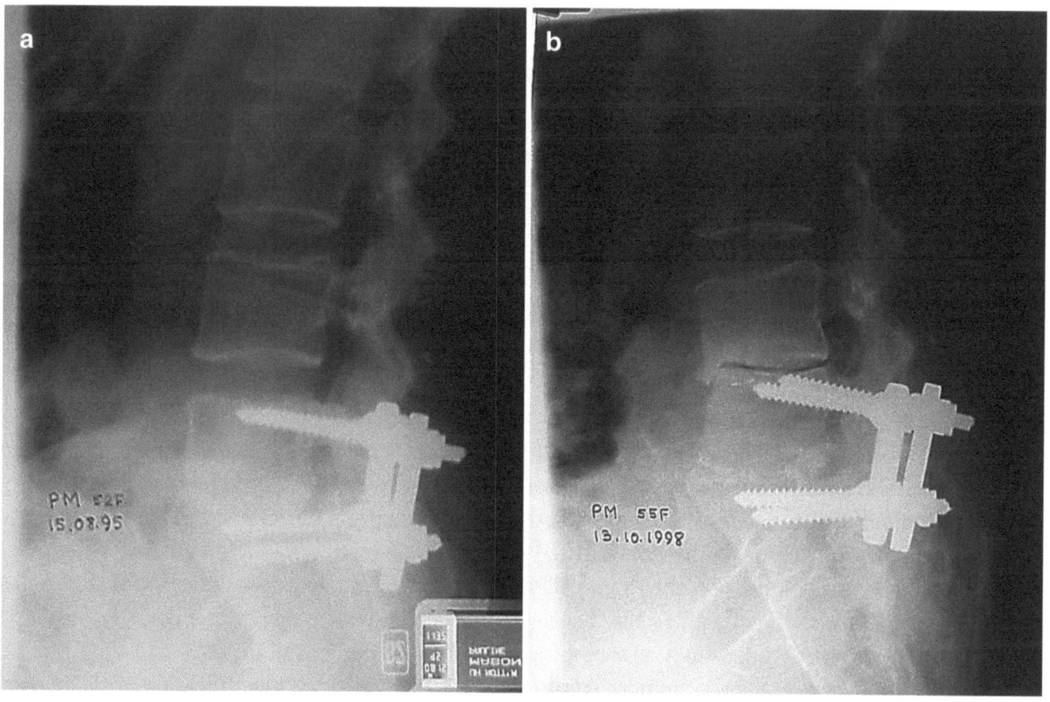

Fig. 22.3 (**a**) Lateral radiograph of an instrumented fusion; (**b**) 3 years after fusion demonstrate adjacent segment degeneration of the level above the instrumented fusion

whether this adjacent segment degeneration is a result of the fusion [46, 47] or if it represents the natural history of degenerative disease [48]. There is also added concern that should revision surgery be necessary for adjacent segment disease, a previous fusion may lead to higher rates of pseudoarthrosis [49]. These concerns have led to development of motion preserving technologies in hopes of controlling motion, as opposed to a fusion which attempts to completely inhibit motion, thereby theoretically decreasing the incidence of adjacent segment disease.

There are several reports on the use of the Dynesys system (Zimmer Spine, Minneapolis, MN). One the first series to report results with this technology was by Stoll et al. In a series of 73 patients of mixed degenerative pathologies (39 with degenerative spondylolisthesis) with a 38-month follow-up, they reported significant improvement in pain and function. However, seven patients required further surgery for adjacent segment disease [50]. A 2-year follow-up study on 26 patients with degenerative spondylolisthesis utilizing dynamic stabilization resulted in significant reductions in pain scores and walking distance. In this study, no radiographic evidence of slip progression was noted, but six patients did have evidence of degeneration in levels above or below the fusion [51]. In a 4-year follow-up of these patients, Scharaen et al. reported maintenance of clinical improvement. However, adjacent disc disease was now present in 47 % of patients [52].

The Graf dynamic stabilization system (SEM, CO, Mountrouge, France) is another motion preserving technology that has been studied. The 3-year results of prospective study investigating outcomes of decompression alone ($n=42$) and with Graf stabilization ($n=46$) were published by Konno and Kikuchi [53]. The authors report equivalent "good/excellent" results (60 % and 61 %, respectively) with both cohorts experiencing significant reductions in both back and leg pain, although these results worsened from the 1- to 3-year follow-up time points. No results were reported regarding adjacent segment disease in this study as it was not a comparison to fused patients but the authors conclude that the Graf system was not able to reduce the clinical deterioration seen after decompressive surgery. Long-term results of the Graf dynamic stabilization system were published on 56 patients. Of those 56 participants, 23 carried the diagnosis of degenerative spondylolisthesis. Although the study reported significant improvements in pain and function and that patients with degenerative spondylolisthesis faired best, no analysis of those results was provided. Radiographic results demonstrated maintenance of lordosis in 90 % of patients and retained segmental motion in 70 %. Three patients required surgery for adjacent segment disease [54].

Additional devices are currently under investigation. The use of tension band system (Ligament Vertebral de Renfort, Cousin Biotech, Wervicq-Sud, France) that acts as an interspinous ligamentoplasty to limit flexion was recently reported on with mid-term results [55]. Compared to a control group consisting of bilateral laminotomy alone, the tension band system plus laminotomy reported less symptomatic instability (4.3 % vs. 27.8 %, respectively) and a greater improvement in pain and functional scores. Both groups demonstrated decreases in disc height but the tension band system significantly improved lordosis and control of translational movement.

In contrast to the flexion limiting devices, a number of interspinous devices aimed at placing the diseased segment into extension are under investigation. Placing a vertebral segment into extension has shown both in vitro and clinical to increase central and neuroforaminal area and thus reducing symptoms related to neurogenic claudication [56, 57]. One such device, the X STOP (Kyphon Inc., Sunnyvale, CA, USA) has been evaluated in several prospective, randomized studies of patients with mixed etiologies for spinal stenosis [58–60]. Those studies demonstrated 37 % improvement in symptoms at 2 years compared to controls (non-operative care), and 75 % of patients were ultimately satisfied with treatment. However, analysis of this device in patients specifically with degenerative spondylolisthesis has yielded higher failure rates and there are no long-term studies on the utilization of this device for this diagnosis [61].

Another interspinous device, Coflex (Paradigm Spine, GmbH, Wurmlingen, Germany), is designed to stabilize the diseased segment after direct surgical decompression without concomitant fusion rather than place the diseased segment into extension, setting it apart from other interspinous devices. In a multicenter, randomized trial comparing Coflex ($n=215$) with laminectomy and posterolateral instrumented fusion ($n=107$) at 2-year follow-up, Coflex demonstrated equivalent improvements in VAS back and leg pain scores, with greater improvements in SF-12 Physical Health outcomes as well as all components of the Zurich Claudication Questionnaire compared to fusion. Utilizing an FDA composite for overall success, it demonstrated non-inferiority compared to fusion [62]. Although these results are encouraging for the use of this device in the treatment of degenerative spondylolisthesis, long-term studies will be necessary to determine the durability of these outcomes.

Conclusions

The optimal treatment of degenerative spondylolisthesis remains elusive. However, as with any surgical specialty, patient specific treatments held in discussion with medical comorbidities is paramount to a successful outcome. Spine surgery is not without its complications and a large decompression with an instrumented fusion may not be the most preferred treatment in the elderly infirm patient. This population may continue to be better served with isolated decompression (laminectomy or laminotomy) without fusion. While this may not afford complete resolution of symptoms, literature does demonstrate clinical improvement with these procedures. As always, discussions between physician and patient are necessary to properly establish treatment goals and mitigate risk.

In the young, healthy patient treatment should be aimed at relief of symptoms. It is not infrequent that a patient will present with an isolated radiculopathy but has imaging consistent with multi-level disease. Clearly, not all diseased elements need to be addressed and isolated decompression in the form of laminotomy/foramenotomy or unilateral laminectomy is all that is warranted.

In the often encountered setting of bilateral radiculopathy or symptoms related to central stenosis and back pain in a young, active patient, a bilateral laminectomy, while an option, does carry the risk of increased instability particularly in the setting of spondylolisthesis. In this population decompression with fusion appears to offer better and more sustained clinical improvement over decompression alone. It also appears that achieving a solid arthrodesis is critical to ascertaining long-term clinical success. The addition of posterior instrumentation does appear to improve fusion rates but no studies have demonstrated that fusion with posterior instrumentation results in a better clinical outcome than a solid fusion achieved without instrumentation.

The use of anterior support, although backed by sound theoretical advantages, has not been shown to provide any improvement in clinical outcomes over posterolateral fusion. Although some studies have reported increased fusion rates with the use of anterior support, little is known regarding the long-term effects of those improved rates. This improvement in fusion rates afforded by the addition of anterior support should be tempered against the added morbidity associated with these procedures. Additionally, in the current health care setting, cost of additional procedures and devices needs be considered.

The utility of dynamic stabilization technologies have yet to be compared in well-designed head-to-head studies with posterolateral fusion. Although these devices do allow for controlled motion of instrumented segments, their ability to reduce adjacent segment disease remains to be seen. Clearly, further studies with these technologies are warranted prior to widespread implementation. The same sentiment can be used regarding the role of biologics, namely rhBMP2. The use of BMP does appear to come with its own set of complications. Further, non-industry sponsored studies will be necessary for accurate reporting of the risks involved and to determine whether their risk profile is any better than iliac crest bone graft.

Clearly, the medical community has made some significant strides in our understanding of the treatment of degenerative spondylolisthesis. Although we have demonstrated improved clinical outcomes with surgery, further high quality studies with long-term follow-up are necessary to arrive at the preferred treatment.

References

1. Atlas SJ, Deyo RA, Keller RB, Chapin AM, Patrick DL, Long JM, et al. The Maine Lumbar Spine Study, part III. 1-year outcomes of surgical and nonsurgical management of lumbar spinal stenosis. Spine. 1996;21(15):1787–94. Discussion 1794–5.
2. Atlas SJ, Keller RB, Robson D, Deyo RA, Singer DE. Surgical and nonsurgical management of lumbar spinal stenosis: four-year outcomes from the Maine lumbar spine study. Spine. 2000;25(5):556–62.
3. Weinstein JN, Lurie JD, Tosteson TD, Hanscom B, Tosteson ANA, Blood EA, et al. Surgical versus nonsurgical treatment for lumbar degenerative spondylolisthesis. N Engl J Med. 2007;356(22):2257–70.
4. Weinstein JN, Lurie JD, Tosteson TD, Zhao W, Blood EA, Tosteson ANA, et al. Surgical compared with nonoperative treatment for lumbar degenerative spondylolisthesis. Four-year results in the spine patient outcomes research trial (SPORT) randomized and observational cohorts. J Bone Joint Surg Am. 2009;91(6):1295–304.
5. Katz JN, Lipson SJ, Larson MG, McInnes JM, Fossel AH, Liang MH. The outcome of decompressive laminectomy for degenerative lumbar stenosis. J Bone Joint Surg Am. 1991;73(6):809–16.
6. Postacchini F, Cinotti G, Gumina S, Perugia D. Long-term results of surgery in lumbar stenosis. 8-year review of 64 patients. Acta Orthop Scand Suppl. 1993;251:78–80.
7. Postacchini F, Cinotti G. Bone regrowth after surgical decompression for lumbar spinal stenosis. J Bone Joint Surg. 1992;74(6):862–9.
8. Mardjetko SM, Connolly PJ, Shott S. Degenerative lumbar spondylolisthesis. A meta-analysis of literature 1970–1993. Spine. 1994;19(20 Suppl):2256–65S.
9. Bridwell KH, Sedgewick TA, O'Brien MF, Lenke LG, Baldus C. The role of fusion and instrumentation in the treatment of degenerative spondylolisthesis with spinal stenosis. J Spinal Disord. 1993;6(6):461–72.
10. Herno A, Airaksinen O, Saari T. Long-term results of surgical treatment of lumbar spinal stenosis. Spine. 1993;18(11):1471–4.
11. Epstein NE. Decompression in the surgical management of degenerative spondylolisthesis: advantages of a conservative approach in 290 patients. J Spinal Disord. 1998;11(2):116–22. Discussion 123.
12. Herkowitz HN, Kurz LT. Degenerative lumbar spondylolisthesis with spinal stenosis. A prospective study comparing decompression with decompression and intertransverse process arthrodesis. J Bone Joint Surg Am. 1991;73(6):802–8.
13. Amundsen T, Weber H, Nordal HJ, Magnaes B, Abdelnoor M, Lilleâs F. Lumbar spinal stenosis: conservative or surgical management?: A prospective 10-year study. Spine. 2000;25(11):1424–35. Discussion 1435–6.
14. Postacchini F, Cinotti G, Perugia D, Gumina S. The surgical treatment of central lumbar stenosis. Multiple laminotomy compared with total laminectomy. J Bone Joint Surg. 1993;75(3):386–92.
15. Lombardi JS, Wiltse LL, Reynolds J, Widell EH, Spencer C. Treatment of degenerative spondylolisthesis. Spine. 1985;10(9):821–7.
16. Zdeblick TA. A prospective, randomized study of lumbar fusion. Preliminary results. Spine. 1993; 18(8):983–91.
17. Ghogawala Z, Benzel EC, Amin-Hanjani S, Barker FG, Harrington JF, Magge SN, et al. Prospective outcomes evaluation after decompression with or without instrumented fusion for lumbar stenosis and degenerative grade I spondylolisthesis. J Neurosurg Spine. 2004;1(3):267–72.
18. Kornblum MB, Fischgrund JS, Herkowitz HN, Abraham DA, Berkower DL, Ditkoff JS. Degenerative lumbar spondylolisthesis with spinal stenosis: a prospective long-term study comparing fusion and pseudarthrosis. Spine. 2004;29(7):726–33. Discussion 733–4.
19. Tsutsumimoto T, Shimogata M, Yoshimura Y, Misawa H. Union versus nonunion after posterolateral lumbar fusion: a comparison of long-term surgical outcomes in patients with degenerative lumbar spondylolisthesis. Eur Spine J. 2008;17(8):1107–12.
20. Yuan HA, Garfin SR, Dickman CA, Mardjetko SM. A historical cohort study of pedicle screw fixation in thoracic, lumbar, and sacral spinal fusions. Spine. 1994;19(20 Suppl):2279–96S.
21. Fischgrund JS, Mackay M, Herkowitz HN, Brower R, Montgomery DM, Kurz LT. 1997 Volvo award winner in clinical studies. Degenerative lumbar spondylolisthesis with spinal stenosis: a prospective, randomized study comparing decompressive laminectomy and arthrodesis with and without spinal instrumentation. Spine. 1997;22(24):2807–12.
22. Martin CR, Gruszczynski AT, Braunsfurth HA, Fallatah SM, O'Neil J, Wai EK. The surgical management of degenerative lumbar spondylolisthesis: a systematic review. Spine. 2007;32(16):1791–8.
23. Abdu WA, Lurie JD, Spratt KF, Tosteson ANA, Zhao W, Tosteson TD, et al. Degenerative spondylolisthesis: does fusion method influence outcome? Four-year results of the spine patient outcomes research trial. Spine. 2009;34(21):2351–60.
24. Sudo H, Oda I, Abumi K, Ito M, Kotani Y, Hojo Y, et al. In vitro biomechanical effects of reconstruction on adjacent motion segment: comparison of aligned/kyphotic posterolateral fusion with aligned posterior lumbar interbody fusion/posterolateral fusion. J Neurosurg. 2003;99(2 Suppl):221–8.

25. Rompe JD, Eysel P, Hopf C. Clinical efficacy of pedicle instrumentation and posterolateral fusion in the symptomatic degenerative lumbar spine. Eur Spine J. 1995;4(4):231–7.
26. La Rosa G, Conti A, Cacciola F, Cardali S, La Torre D, Gambadauro NM, et al. Pedicle screw fixation for isthmic spondylolisthesis: does posterior lumbar interbody fusion improve outcome over posterolateral fusion? J Neurosurg. 2003;99(2 Suppl):143–50.
27. Lauber S, Schulte TL, Liljenqvist U, Halm H, Hackenberg L. Clinical and radiologic 2-4-year results of transforaminal lumbar interbody fusion in degenerative and isthmic spondylolisthesis grades 1 and 2. Spine. 2006;31(15):1693–8.
28. Kim K-T, Lee S-H, Lee Y-H, Bae S-C, Suk K-S. Clinical outcomes of 3 fusion methods through the posterior approach in the lumbar spine. Spine. 2006;31(12):1351–7. Discussion 1358.
29. Turner JA, Ersek M, Herron L, Haselkorn J, Kent D, Ciol MA, et al. Patient outcomes after lumbar spinal fusions. JAMA. 1992;268(7):907–11.
30. Deyo RA, Cherkin DC, Loeser JD, Bigos SJ, Ciol MA. Morbidity and mortality in association with operations on the lumbar spine. The influence of age, diagnosis, and procedure. J Bone Joint Surg Am. 1992;74(4):536–43.
31. Gibson JN, Waddel G. Surgery for degenerative lumbar spondylosis: updated Cochrane review. Spine (Phila Pa 1976). 2005;30(20):2312–20.
32. Chrastil J, Patel AA. Complications associated with posterior and transforaminal lumbar interbody fusion. J Am Acad Orthop Surg. 2012;20(5):283–91.
33. Kim S, Mortaz Hedjri S, Coyte PC, Rampersaud YR. Cost-utility of lumbar decompression with or without fusion for patients with symptomatic degenerative lumbar spondylolisthesis. Spine J. 2012;12(1):44–54.
34. Carragee EJ, Hurwitz EL, Weiner BK. A critical review of recombinant human bone morphogenetic protein-2 trials in spinal surgery: emerging safety concerns and lessons learned. Spine J. 2011;11(6):471–91.
35. Simmonds MC, Brown JVE, Heirs MK, Higgins JPT, Mannion RJ, Rodgers MA, et al. Safety and effectiveness of recombinant human bone morphogenetic protein-2 for spinal fusion: a meta-analysis of individual-participant data. Ann Intern Med. 2013;158(12):877–89.
36. Boden SD, Kang J, Sandhu H, Heller JG. Use of recombinant human bone morphogenetic protein-2 to achieve posterolateral lumbar spine fusion in humans: a prospective, randomized clinical pilot trial: 2002 Volvo award in clinical studies. Spine. 2002; 27(23):2662–73.
37. Dimar JR, Glassman SD, Burkus JK, Pryor PW, Hardacker JW, Carreon LY. Clinical and radiographic analysis of an optimized rhBMP-2 formulation as an autograft replacement in posterolateral lumbar spine arthrodesis. J Bone Joint Surg Am. 2009;91(6): 1377–86.
38. Vaccaro AR, Anderson DG, Patel T, Fischgrund J, Truumees E, Herkowitz HN, et al. Comparison of OP-1 Putty (rhBMP-7) to iliac crest autograft for posterolateral lumbar arthrodesis: a minimum 2-year follow-up pilot study. Spine. 2005;30(24):2709–16.
39. Vaccaro AR, Whang PG, Patel T, Phillips FM, Anderson DG, Albert TJ, et al. The safety and efficacy of OP-1 (rhBMP-7) as a replacement for iliac crest autograft for posterolateral lumbar arthrodesis: minimum 4-year follow-up of a pilot study. Spine J. 2008;8(3):457–65.
40. Burkus JK, Heim SE, Gornet MF, Zdeblick TA. Is INFUSE bone graft superior to autograft bone? An integrated analysis of clinical trials using the LT-CAGE lumbar tapered fusion device. J Spinal Disord Tech. 2003;16(2):113–22.
41. Burkus JK, Gornet MF, Dickman CA, Zdeblick TA. Anterior lumbar interbody fusion using rhBMP-2 with tapered interbody cages. J Spinal Disord Tech. 2002;15(5):337–49.
42. Burkus JK, Transfeldt EE, Kitchel SH, Watkins RG, Balderston RA. Clinical and radiographic outcomes of anterior lumbar interbody fusion using recombinant human bone morphogenetic protein-2. Spine. 2002;27(21):2396–408.
43. Glassman SD, Dimar JR, Burkus K, Hardacker JW, Pryor PW, Boden SD, et al. The efficacy of rhBMP-2 for posterolateral lumbar fusion in smokers. Spine. 2007;32(15):1693–8.
44. Dimar JR, Glassman SD, Burkus KJ, Carreon LY. Clinical outcomes and fusion success at 2 years of single-level instrumented posterolateral fusions with recombinant human bone morphogenetic protein-2/compression resistant matrix versus iliac crest bone graft. Spine. 2006;31(22):2534–9. Discussion 2540.
45. Weinhoffer SL, Guyer RD, Herbert M, Griffith SL. Intradiscal pressure measurements above an instrumented fusion. A cadaveric study. Spine. 1995;20(5):526–31.
46. Lehmann TR, Spratt KF, Tozzi JE, Weinstein JN, Reinarz SJ, el-Khoury GY, et al. Long-term follow-up of lower lumbar fusion patients. Spine. 1987; 12(2):97–104.
47. Luk KD, Lee FB, Leong JC, Hsu LC. The effect on the lumbosacral spine of long spinal fusion for idiopathic scoliosis. A minimum 10-year follow-up. Spine. 1987;12(10):996–1000.
48. Penta M, Sandhu A, Fraser RD. Magnetic resonance imaging assessment of disc degeneration 10 years after anterior lumbar interbody fusion. Spine. 1995; 20(6):743–7.
49. Whitecloud TS, Davis JM, Olive PM. Operative treatment of the degenerated segment adjacent to a lumbar fusion. Spine. 1994;19(5):531–6.
50. Stoll TM, Dubois G, Schwarzenbach O. The dynamic neutralization system for the spine: a multi-center study of a novel non-fusion system. Eur Spine J. 2002;11 Suppl 2:S170–8.
51. Schnake KJ, Schaeren S, Jeanneret B. Dynamic stabilization in addition to decompression for lumbar spinal stenosis with degenerative spondylolisthesis. Spine. 2006;31(4):442–9.
52. Schaeren S, Broger I, Jeanneret B. Minimum four-year follow-up of spinal stenosis with degenerative

spondylolisthesis treated with decompression and dynamic stabilization. Spine. 2008;33(18):E636–42.
53. Konno S, Kikuchi S. Prospective study of surgical treatment of degenerative spondylolisthesis: comparison between decompression alone and decompression with graf system stabilization. Spine. 2000;25(12):1533–7.
54. Kanayama M, Hashimoto T, Shigenobu K, Togawa D, Oha F. A minimum 10-year follow-up of posterior dynamic stabilization using Graf artificial ligament. Spine. 2007;32(18):1992–6. Discussion 1997.
55. Hong S-W, Lee H-Y, Kim KH, Lee S-H. Interspinous ligamentoplasty in the treatment of degenerative spondylolisthesis: midterm clinical results. J Neurosurg Spine. 2010;13(1):27–35.
56. Sobottke R, Schlüter-Brust K, Kaulhausen T, Röllinghoff M, Joswig B, Stützer H, et al. Interspinous implants (X Stop, Wallis, Diam) for the treatment of LSS: is there a correlation between radiological parameters and clinical outcome? Eur Spine J. 2009;18(10):1494–503.
57. Siddiqui M, Karadimas E, Nicol M, Smith FW, Wardlaw D. Influence of X Stop on neural foramina and spinal canal area in spinal stenosis. Spine. 2006;31(25):2958–62.
58. Zucherman JF, Hsu KY, Hartjen CA, Mehalic TF, Implicito DA, Martin MJ, et al. A multicenter, prospective, randomized trial evaluating the X STOP interspinous process decompression system for the treatment of neurogenic intermittent claudication: two-year follow-up results. Spine. 2005;30(12):1351–8.
59. Zucherman JF, Hsu KY, Hartjen CA, Mehalic TF, Implicito DA, Martin MJ, et al. A prospective randomized multi-center study for the treatment of lumbar spinal stenosis with the X STOP interspinous implant: 1-year results. Eur Spine J. 2004;13(1):22–31.
60. Kuchta J, Sobottke R, Eysel P, Simons P. Two-year results of interspinous spacer (X-Stop) implantation in 175 patients with neurologic intermittent claudication due to lumbar spinal stenosis. Eur Spine J. 2009;18(6):823–9.
61. Verhoof OJ, Bron JL, Wapstra FH, Van Royen BJ. High failure rate of the interspinous distraction device (X-Stop) for the treatment of lumbar spinal stenosis caused by degenerative spondylolisthesis. Eur Spine J. 2008;17(2):188–92.
62. Davis RJ, Errico TJ, Bae H, Auerbach JD. Decompression and Coflex® interlaminar stabilization compared to decompression and instrumented spinal fusion for spinal stenosis and low-grade degenerative spondylolisthesis: two-year results from the prospective, randomized, multicenter food and drug ad. Spine. 2013;38(18):1529–39.

Results of Surgical Treatment of Low-Grade Adult Isthmic Spondylolisthesis

23

Christina L. Goldstein and Stephen J. Lewis

Introduction

The purpose of this chapter is to examine the literature pertaining to the results of surgical treatment of adult lumbar spondylolysis and adult isthmic spondylolisthesis with the goal of maximizing clinical outcomes.

Pars Repair

Patients with symptomatic spondylolysis can usually be managed non-operatively and rarely require surgical intervention after adolescence in the absence of spondylolisthesis and disc degeneration. However, patients presenting with spondylolysis and extension-based low back pain unresponsive to 3–6 months or more of standard conservative treatment may occasionally be considered for direct pars repair (Fig. 23.1). The best indication for repair include the following four criteria:

1. Extension-based lumbo-sacral back pain unresponsive to non-surgical care
2. Normal disc [1]
3. No slip [1]
4. Excellent relief of pain with a direct pars injection with lidocaine and steroid [2].

Though no specific age cutoff for performance of direct pars repair exists, less favorable clinical and radiologic results have consistently been reported in patients older than 20–30 years of age [3–6].

Kimura was the first to report on direct pars bone grafting without supplemental internal fixation in 1968 [7]. That same year Scott developed a cerclage-wiring fixation technique to provide compression across and augment stability of the pars defect, though these results were not reported until 1986 [8]. In 1970 Buck described the use of a single lag screw for pars osteosynthesis [9] with multiple descriptions of surgical outcomes using this technique being reported. Subsequently, Morscher [10] developed a modular hook-screw construct in which a custom screw inserted across the pars defect could attach to a hook inserted under the lamina which, when tightened via a lock nut, would provide additional compression across the defect. Finally, with the introduction of Cotrel-Dubosset instrumentation, intrasegmental spondylolysis fixation using a pedicle screw-hook or pedicle screw-rod construct was developed, with the first

C.L. Goldstein, M.D., F.R.C.S.C.
Department of Orthopaedic Surgery, University of Missouri, Missouri Orthopaedic Institute, 1100 Virginia Ave, MO 65212, Columbia
e-mail: goldsteincl@health.missouri.edu

S.J. Lewis, M.D., M.Sc., F.R.C.S.C. (✉)
Department of Orthopaedics, Toronto Western Hospital, 399 Bathurst St., Toronto, ON, Canada, M5T 2S8
e-mail: Stephen.Lewis@UHN.CA

A.L. Wollowick and V. Sarwahi (eds.), *Spondylolisthesis: Diagnosis, Non-Surgical Management, and Surgical Techniques*, DOI 10.1007/978-1-4899-7575-1_23,

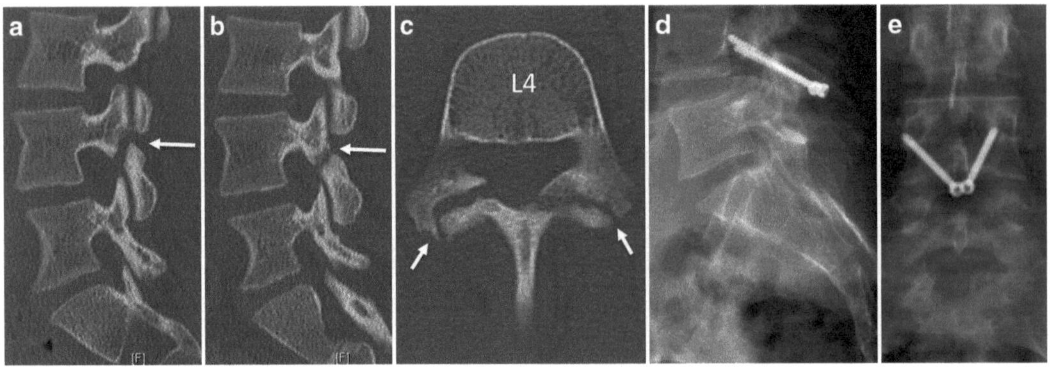

Fig. 23.1 Radiographs of a 16-year-old female with a 2-year history of chronic low back pain worse in extension. Right (**a**) and left (**b**) CT sagittal reconstruction and axial (**c**) of L4 demonstrate bilateral L4 pars defects (*arrows*). Postoperative lateral (**e**) and AP (**f**) following 4.5 mm titanium laminar screws placed across the pars defects after decompressing the defects and placement of structural grafts harvested from the iliac crest through the same incision

report appearing in 1991 [2]. This contemporary construct for direct pars repair has continued to evolve with each generation of spinal implants with favorable outcomes being reported.

In 2011 Drazin and colleagues [11] presented a comprehensive overview of direct surgical repair of spondylolysis in athletes, including a systematic review of 60 years of the English-language literature pertaining to the clinical and radiologic outcomes of pars defect repair in patients aged 24 years or younger. A total of 18 articles using a variety of surgical techniques were identified, with half of them reporting specifically on outcomes of pars repair in athletes. Clinical and radiologic outcome data were summarized and the modified Henderson criteria [12] were applied to subjectively assess patients' postoperative pain and ability to return to preoperative activity level. None of the included studies were level I randomized controlled trials with the majority being retrospective case series. The predominant level of involvement was L5 in both athletes and non-athletes (96 % and 92 % respectively) with patient age ranging from 12 to 60 years between the 18 studies.

The most commonly used surgical technique identified by Drazin et al. [11] was Buck's single lag screw fixation with six of the studies reporting on this method. Excellent results were consistently identified by study authors with >90 % of athletes returning to their preoperative level of physical activity [13–17]. Buck reported somewhat lower success rates in his original series of non-athletes with 81 % of patients reporting no or minimal symptoms postoperatively [9]. The less rigid Scott wiring technique has been shown to provide less satisfactory clinical results with 0–75 % of patients reporting good or excellent outcomes [5, 15, 18, 19]. Modifications of the Scott, or Songer [20] technique using pedicle screws and a cerclage wire have provided 73–100 % good or excellent results [3, 21]. The earliest report of pars repair by pedicle screw-hook fixation [22] identified 81 % good or excellent outcomes, though the mean age of this cohort was 32.4 years. More recent studies examining outcomes of contemporary screw-hook constructs have observed excellent results, with 100 % of patients <30 years of age achieving good or excellent postoperative function [6, 23].

Since the publication of this systematic review, ongoing investigations into the outcome of pars repair have been performed. At an average follow-up of 9 years Giudici et al. [24] observed good or excellent results according to Odom's criteria in 43 %, 63 %, and 84 % in 52 patients age 25 years or less undergoing surgery using Buck's, Scott's, or modified Scott's technique respectively. In general, patients experiencing a poor outcome had bone graft resorption and progression of slippage. Clegg et al. [25] who reported on 49 patients (mean age 17.4 years) undergoing pars also used a modified Scott. At an average of 21.7 months following surgery, 96 % of patients reported no or mild to moderate symptoms on the ODI or SF-36. Kim et al. [26] performed a Buck's fusion in 25 patients aged 15–29 with spondylolysis and reported 88 % good or excellent results according to Kirkaldy–Willis criteria [27].

In a cohort of patients with symptomatic lumbar spondylolysis who responded to direct pars injection and negative discography treated by Shin et al. [28] pars repair using either a pedicle screw-hook construct ($n=23$) or direct pars screw ($n=17$) was performed. Clinical outcomes rated by the oswestry disability index (ODI) and VAS scores were better in the pars screw patients than in those treated with a screw-hook construct with patients demonstrating successful union having better postoperative results. Hioki et al. [29] reported a similar phenomenon in 44 athletes with a mean age of 24.2 years treated with cerclage wiring of their pars defect, with patients obtaining bilateral bony union (67.4 %) achieving higher postoperative JOA score improvements than those with unilateral union (13 %) or nonunion (19.6 %).

Minimally invasive approaches to pars repair have also recently been reported with satisfactory clinical results. Amoretti et al. [30] performed percutaneous CT-guided cannulated screw fixation of bilateral L5 spondylolysis defects in ten consecutive patients with an average age of 57 years. Patients tolerated the outpatient procedure well with minimal blood loss and no cases of screw malposition. Significant decreases in VAS measurements (7.8 ± 0.9 preop to 1.5 ± 1.1 at 2 years, $p<0.001$) and ODI scores (62.3 ± 17.2 preop to 15.1 ± 6.0 at 2 years, $p<0.001$) were observed with no cases of slip progression or instrumentation failure. More recently, Widi et al. [31] employed a similar approach of cannulated screw placement across the pars under fluoroscopic guidance through tubular retractors in three patients with a mean age of 21.7 years. All three patients demonstrated satisfactory bone healing at 6 months postoperatively and had returned or were planning to return to their preoperative sporting activities.

Decompression and Fusion for Low-Grade Isthmic Spondylolisthesis

While low-grade spondylolisthesis is present from early childhood, symptoms in adults generally present once the disc at L5-S1 degenerates, leading to foraminal compression of the L5 nerve roots (Fig. 23.2). Adult patients with isthmic spondylolysis who do not meet the criteria for pars repair and who fail traditional methods of conservative management are candidates for surgical decompression and stabilization. Though controversy exists regarding the optimal surgical technique for management of low-grade adult isthmic spondylolisthesis, three surgical interventions should rarely, if ever, be used in this patient population and are worth mentioning.

1. Dynamic stabilization techniques should not be used in patients with isthmic spondylolisthesis given that motion across the spondylolysis contributes to patient symptomatology and solid stabilization is required for symptom relief [32].
2. Indirect decompression via interspinous process spacer placement is also not indicated given that these devices require intact posterior elements to create distraction and therefore will not function as intended in the presence of a pars defect.
3. Decompression alone has extremely poor results in patients with lytic spondylolisthesis. While decompression alone can be an option in some cases of degenerative spondylolisthesis, decompression and instrumented fusion is the gold standard in treating symptomatic low-grade adult isthmic spondylolisthesis [33].

A variety of anterior, posterior, and combined (360°) surgical approaches exist for the surgical management of low-grade adult isthmic spondylolisthesis, each with their own proposed advantages and disadvantages. Posterior lumbar decompression and instrumented fusion is the most commonly employed technique for surgical management of adult low-grade isthmic spondylolisthesis. It can be performed through bilateral paramedian (i.e., Wiltse) approaches or the widely

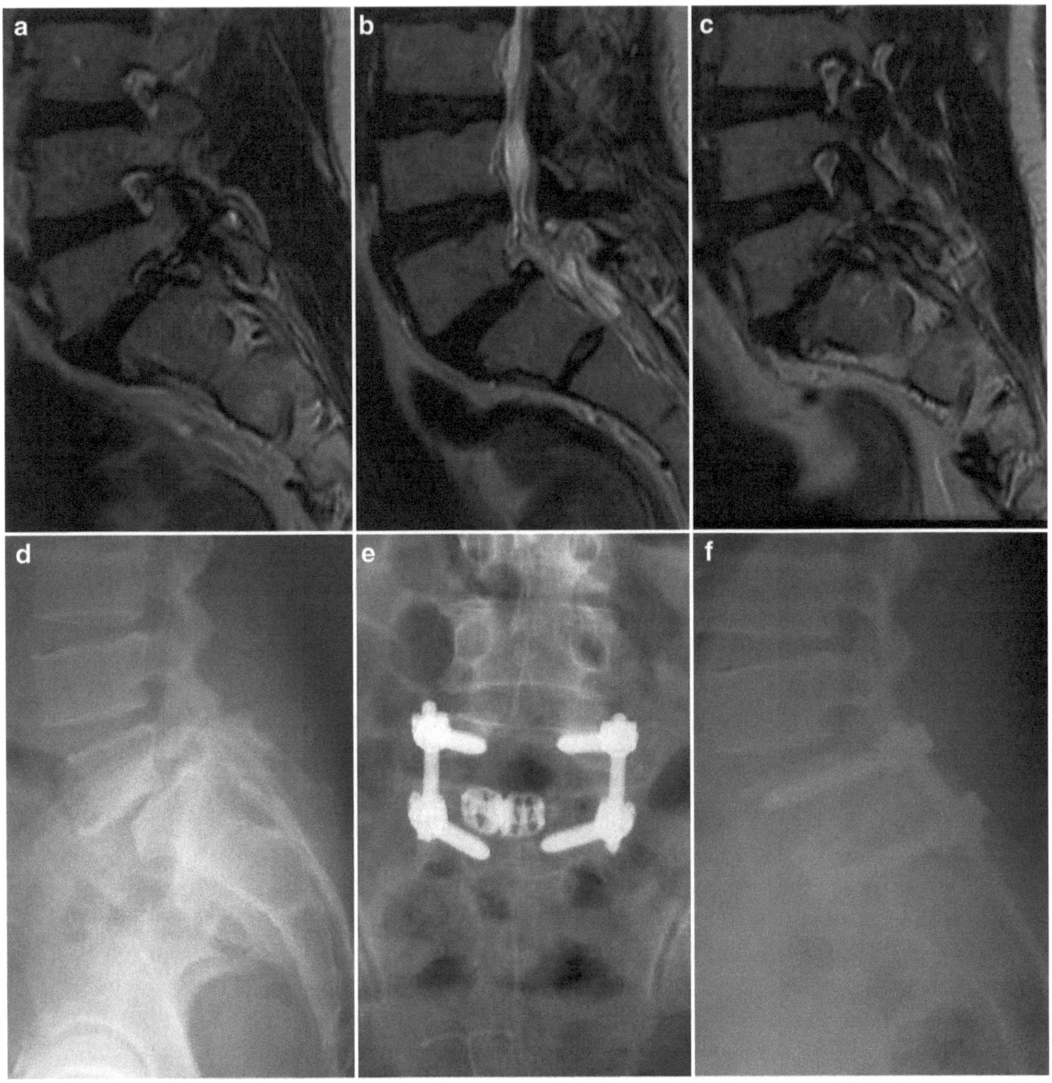

Fig. 23.2 Preoperative and postoperative images of a 51-year-old woman with bilateral L5 radiculopathy. Preoperative right (**a**), mid, and left (**c**) sagittal T2 (**b**) demonstrate a grade 1 isthmic spondylolisthesis with bilateral L5 foraminal compression secondary to disc. Preoperative (**d**) and postoperative PA (**e**) and lateral (**f**) radiographs following posterior decompression with Gill laminectomy and bilateral disc excision. Reconstruction is performed with bilateral pedicle screws and a posterior lumbar interbody cage

familiar midline posterior incision and has the advantage of allowing for direct decompression of the neural elements. If concerns regarding the ability to obtain a posterolateral fusion (PLF) exist, or one wishes to attempt to restore lumbar lordosis across the degenerated disc or release the annulus to facilitate slip reduction, interbody fusion through either a posterior (PLIF) or transforaminal (TLIF) approach can be added to obtain a 360° or circumferential fusion. While interbody fusion can be associated with higher rates of neural injury, adequate release of perineural adhesions and avoidance of overzealous nerve retraction can help minimize these complications. Distraction of the posterior elements during the decompression, either through the pedicle screws or the bone, helps provide more room around the nerve to gain safer access to the disc space.

Stand-alone anterior lumbar interbody fusion (ALIF) has been used for many years to treat spondylolisthesis and has the advantages of a large surface area for fusion with low postoperative pain and rapid surgical recovery. However, removal of the last remaining restraints to anterior translation, the anterior longitudinal ligament, and annulus fibrosus, in the setting of compromised posterior elements can exacerbate instability and may result in graft extrusion and/or slip progression, resulting in recommendations for the performance of supplemental posterior instrumented fusion [34]. Further, this technique relies solely on indirect decompression of the neural elements and may be associated with significant approach-related complications including retrograde ejaculation [35] and vascular injury [36]. In light of these disadvantages and the development of techniques to reconstruct and fuse the anterior column from a posterior approach, stand-alone ALIF is rarely performed in this patient population.

Two previous systematic reviews have examined the evidence pertaining to surgical management of adult low-grade isthmic spondylolisthesis in an attempt to identify the optimal method of treatment. In 2005 Kwon et al. summarized English-language studies examining surgical management of adult low-grade isthmic spondylolisthesis in at least five patients and reporting on fusion rate and/or clinical outcome. Their primary objective was to determine which surgical technique, posterior alone, anterior alone, or a 360° procedure, led to superior radiographic fusion and clinical outcome. A total of 34 studies reporting on more than 1,000 patients were included, four of which were prospective randomized controlled trials. The remaining 30 were retrospective studies with only six describing a comparison of two surgical techniques.

With respect to radiographic outcome, patients undergoing a combined anterior (ALIF, PLIF, or TLIF) and posterior procedure demonstrated a significantly higher fusion rate (98.2 %, 167/170) compared to patients undergoing isolated posterior (83.3 %, 741/890) or anterior (74.0 %, 57/77) surgery ($p<0.0001$). Clinical success, as defined by the authors of each individual study, was significantly higher in both the stand-alone anterior (89.6 %, 60/67) and combined groups (86.4 %, 108/125) compared to the posterior-only group (74.8 %, 609/814, $p=0.005$), though no difference between the anterior and combined groups was observed ($p=0.65$). Subgroup analysis demonstrated significantly improved radiographic fusion rates (90.2 % vs. 77.4 %, $p<0.0001$) and rates of clinical success (84.9 % vs. 64.4 %, $p<0.0001$) in patients in whom internal fixation had been placed. Success rates were also substantially lower in smokers and patients involved in workers compensation or litigation. After identifying the limitations and weakness of the current literature, the authors conclude that the highest rates of radiographic and clinical success were observed in patients undergoing combined anterior and posterior approaches with the placement of posterior instrumentation.

Subsequently, Jacobs et al. [37] performed a similar review of studies in which a minimum of ten patients were treated with surgery for low-grade isthmic spondylolisthesis in which at least one radiographic, functional, or clinical outcome was reported. A total of 29 studies, including eight prospective RCTs, were identified for study inclusion. In attempting to determine the best method of surgical treatment, instrumented versus uninstrumented PLF was examined in four of the RCTs with no significant benefit of supplemental instrumentation being observed in any of these studies [38–41]. Results from the remaining RCTs also failed to demonstrate a clinical benefit of the addition of ALIF [42], supplemental direct decompression [43], or bone graft substitute [44] to PLF.

In the remaining 21 case series, 24 surgical treatment groups were reported. Good or excellent clinical outcomes were observed in 60–98 % of patients undergoing PLF (15 groups) with fusion rates ranging from 81 % to 100 %. ALIF was employed in five groups with fusion occurring in 47–90 % of patients and 85–94 % experiencing a good or excellent clinical outcome. Only two groups reported on the use of posterior interbody fusion, with 80 and 95 % of patients obtaining radiographic fusion, but only 45 % of patients having a good or excellent clinical outcome (one group). Based on these results, the authors conclude that, though PLF is the most common treatment method employed and therefore appears to be the accepted gold standard, scientific evidence to support this consensus does not exist. They also state that further RCTs examining the role of instrumentation in posterior lumbar fusion and comparing surgical approaches (anterior vs. posterior vs. circumferential) in the treatment of low-grade adult isthmic spondylolisthesis are required.

Since publication of these systematic reviews investigators continue to work towards identifying the optimal treatment strategy for adult low-grade isthmic spondylolisthesis, with three English-language RCTs comparing alternative surgical techniques having been published [45–47]. In 2011 Audat et al. examined surgical fixation with or without reduction and PLIF for the treatment of symptomatic low-grade isthmic spondylolisthesis in a prospective, randomized, double-blinded study. No significant difference was observed between the groups with regard to operative time or LOS. Complication rates were also similar between the two groups during the hospital stay. At final follow-up, only one patient in the in situ fusion group ($n = 21$) experienced a pseudarthrosis requiring reoperation, while all patients in the reduction and PLIF group ($n = 20$) obtained a solid fusion. While both groups demonstrated improvements in quality of life following surgery, improvements on the ODI were significantly better in the reduction and PLIF group compared to the in situ PLF group at 3 years (0.04 vs. 0.15, $p < 0.005$).

A similar investigation involving randomization of 50 adult patients with symptomatic low-grade isthmic spondylolisthesis was performed that same year [46]. All patients underwent a posterior decompressive laminectomy, medial facetectomy, and foraminotomy, with those in the PLIF group undergoing complete bilateral facetectomies, discectomy, and placement of two interbody titanium cages packed with local autologous bone graft. Operative times were similar in the two groups, though patients undergoing PLIF lost significantly less blood than those in the PLF group (830±215 vs. 1,100±280 mL, $p < 0.05$). No significant difference in intraoperative or short-term postoperative complications, including incidental durotomy, nerve injury, or deep infection, was observed between the groups. At 2 years the postoperative fusion rates were 84 % in the PLF group compared to 100 % in the PLIF group. At a mean follow-up of 3.3 years, patients who had undergone PLIF had less postoperative back pain (VAS score 1.20±0.57 vs. 1.80±0.57, $p = 0.001$) and better scores on the Short-Form 36 (85.9±5.6 vs. 81.5±6.8, $p = 0.015$), though no significant difference in ODI scores was observed between the groups at final follow-up (PLF = 14.1 ± 2.4 vs. PLIF = 13.4 ± 1.9).

The role of the addition of PLIF to instrumented PLF was also the topic of investigation in an RCT involving 80 patients by Farrokhi et al. [47]. All patients underwent direct decompression and placement of pedicle screw fixation with half undergoing intertransverse fusion and half having a PLIF (though the method of anterior column reconstruction was not reported). Trends towards increased operative times and blood loss were observed in the PLIF cohort while those undergoing PLF alone experienced less back pain and received less narcotic medication in the immediate postoperative period ($p = 0.016$). At 1-year follow-up patients in the PLIF group complained more frequently of neurogenic claudication (33.3 % vs. 7.3 %, $p = 0.004$) and demonstrated lower improvements in quality of life on the Oswestry low back pain disability scale (17.1±13.0 vs. 25.0±9.36, $p = 0.004$) despite lower rates of "good" fusion (66.7 % vs. 89.1 %, $p = 0.012$).

In addition to ongoing investigations of traditional surgical techniques for treatment of adult isthmic spondylolisthesis, minimally invasive methods are increasingly being applied to this patient population. While no prospective randomized studies comparing traditional open versus minimally invasive instrumented lumbar interbody fusion for the management of low-grade adult isthmic spondylolisthesis exist, five cohort studies have examined these techniques in 339 adult patients with either degenerative or isthmic spondylolisthesis [48–52]. Surgical time was similar between the open and MIS cohorts in all five studies though patients experienced significantly less blood loss [48, 50–52] and lower rates of transfusion [48–51] following MIS fusion. A significantly shorter length of hospital stay (LOS) was observed following MIS fusion in three of the four studies reporting on this outcome [48–50].

No significant difference in union rates was observed between the open and MIS cohorts with 100 % ($n=80$) and 97.6 % ($n=85$) of patients achieving successful union in the open and MIS cohorts of the two studies reporting radiographic outcome [50, 52]. Clinical outcome was assessed using the ODI in three of the five studies, with Wang et al. [50] reporting no significant difference at a mean follow-up of 26.3 months, while significantly better ODI scores following MIS fusion were reported at 12 and 24 months postoperatively by Rampersaud et al. [51] and Kotani et al. [52] respectively. Finally, four of the studies reported on absolute complication rates with two showing no significant difference between the cohorts [50, 52] and two favoring MIS fusion [48, 51], though the definitions of complications and methods of diagnosis varied among the studies. In light of this level III evidence, it would appear that MIS lumbar fusion may be considered an optional technique for treating low-grade adult isthmic spondylolisthesis and has the potential to provide radiographic and clinical outcomes at least equivalent to traditional open decompression and instrumented fusion.

Conclusions

Though the number of adult patients who will be candidates for direct pars repair is small, multiple case series have reported favorable outcomes with direct pars repair, with more rigid fixation using pedicle screw-hook or direct pars screw constructs demonstrating improved postoperative clinical outcomes using a variety of measurement tools. These fixation strategies also appear to result in higher rates of bony union that appears to lead to improved clinical outcomes. Thus, in the appropriately selected patient, spondylolysis repair using pedicle screw-hook constructs or screw osteosynthesis through a traditional midline surgical approach is a viable surgical treatment option. While minimally invasive approaches to spondylolysis repair have been described, the long-term results of these new techniques remain undetermined.

In those patients who are not candidates for direct pars repair, posterior lumbar decompression and instrumented fusion does appear to be the optimal surgical strategy for management of low-grade adult isthmic spondylolisthesis. While definitive evidence in favor of one fusion technique over another is lacking, it is clear that posterior decompression and instrumented fusion can produce high rates of good to excellent radiographic and clinical results with low complication rates. 360° fusion may produce improved radiographic and clinical results outcomes. An all-posterior approach with performance of a PLIF or TLIF provides results that are similar to ALIF and supplemental posterior fixation while avoiding the morbidity of dual anterior and posterior approaches. Finally, though the evidence regarding MIS instrumented TLIF for low-grade adult isthmic spondylolisthesis is limited, it may be considered an option, and at the very least seems to provide equivalent radiographic and clinical results compared to open decompression and instrumented fusion.

References

1. Gillet P, Petit M. Direct repair of spondylolysis without spondylolisthesis, using a rod-screw construct and bone grafting of the pars defect. Spine. 1999;24:1252–6.
2. Gupta P, Gupta MC. Pars repair. In: Bridwell KH, Dewald RI, editors. The textbook of spinal surgery. 3rd ed. Philadelphia: Lippincott Williams & Wilkins; 2011. p. 581–9.
3. Johnson GV, Thompson AG. The Scott wiring technique for direct repair of lumbar spondylolysis. J Bone Joint Surg. 1992;74:426–30.
4. Ivanic GM, Pink TP, Achatz W, Ward JC, Homann NC, May M. Direct stabilization of lumbar spondylolysis with a hook screw: mean 11-year follow-up period for 113 patients. Spine. 2003;28:255–9.
5. Nozawa S, Shimizu K, Miyamoto K, Tanaka M. Repair of pars interarticularis defect by segmental wire fixation in young athletes with spondylolysis. Am J Sports Med. 2003;31:359–64.
6. Debusscher F, Troussel S. Direct repair of defects in lumbar spondylolysis with a new pedicle screw hook fixation: clinical, functional and CT-assessed study. Eur Spine J. 2007;16:1650–8.
7. Kumura M. My method of filling the lesion with spongy bone in spondylolysis and spondylolisthesis. Seikei Geka. 1968;19:285–96.

8. Nicol RO, Scott JH. Lytic spondylolysis. Repair by wiring. Spine. 1986;11:1027–30.
9. Buck JE. Direct repair of the defect in spondylolisthesis. Preliminary report. J Bone Joint Surg. 1970;52:432–7.
10. Morscher E, Gerber B, Fasel J. Surgical treatment of spondylolisthesis by bone grafting and direct stabilization of spondylolysis by means of a hook screw. Arch Orthop Trauma Surg. 1984;103:175–8.
11. Drazin D, Shirzadi A, Jeswani S, Ching H, Rosner J, Rasouli A, Kim T, Pashman R, Johnson JP. Direct surgical repair of spondylolysis in athletes: indications, techniques, and outcomes. Neurosurg Focus. 2011;31(5):E9–20.
12. Henderson ED. Results of the surgical treatment of spondylolisthesis. J Bone Joint Surg Am. 1966; 48:619–42.
13. Hardcastle P, Annear P, Foster DH, Chakera TM, McCormick C, Khangure M, et al. Spinal abnormalities in young fast bowlers. J Bone Joint Surg. 1992;74:421–5.
14. Reitman CA, Esses SI. Direct repair of spondylolytic defects in young competitive athletes. Spine J. 2002; 2:142–4.
15. Debnath UK, Freeman BJ, Gregory P, de la Harpe D, Kerslake RW, Webb JK. Clinical outcome and return to sport after the surgical treatment of spondylolysis in young athletes. J Bone Joint Surg. 2003;85:244–9.
16. Ranawat VS, Dowell JK, Heywood-Waddington MB. Stress fractures of the lumbar pars interarticularis in athletes: a review based on long-term results of 18 professional cricketers. Injury. 2003;34:915–9.
17. Brennan RP, Smucker PY, Horn EM. Minimally invasive image-guided direct repair of bilateral L-5 pars interarticularis defects. Neurosurg Focus. 2008;25(2):E13.
18. Askar Z, Wardlaw D, Koti M. Scott wiring for direct repair of lumbar spondylolysis. Spine. 2003;28:354–7.
19. Schlenzka D, Remes V, Helenius I, Lambert T, Tervahartiala P, Yrjönen T, et al. Direct repair for treatment of symptomatic spondylolysis and low-grade isthmic spondylolisthesis in young patients: no benefit in comparison to segmental fusion after a mean follow-up of 14.8 years. Eur Spine J. 2006; 15:1437–47.
20. Songer MN, Rovin R. Repair of the pars interarticularis defect with a cable-screw construct. A preliminary report. Spine. 1998;21:2041–5.
21. Bozarth GR, Fogel GR, Toohey JS, Neidre A. Repair of pars interarticularis defect with a modified cable-screw construct. J Surg Orthop Adv. 2007;16:79–83.
22. Kakiuchi M. Repair of the defect in spondylolysis. Durable fixation with pedicle screws and laminar hooks. J Bone Joint Surg Am. 1997;79(6):818–25.
23. Noggle JC, Sciubba DM, Samdani AF, Anderson DG, Betz RR, Asghar J. Minimally invasive direct repair of lumbar spondylolysis with a pedicle screw and hook construct. Neurosurg Focus. 2008;25(2):E15.
24. Giudici F, Minoia L, Archetti M, Corriero AS, Zagra A. Long-term results of the direct repair of spondylolisthesis. Eur Spine J. 2011;20 Suppl 1:S115–20.
25. Clegg T, Carreon L, Mutchnick I, Puno R. Clinical outcomes following repair of the pars interarticularis. Am J Orthop. 2013;42(2):72–6.
26. Kim YT, Lee H, Lee CS, Lee DH, Hwang CJ, Ahn TS. Direct repair of the pars interarticularis defect in spondylolysis. J Spinal Disord Tech. 2012 [August 29; ePub ahead of print].
27. Kirkaldy-Willis WH, Paine KW, Cauchoix J, McIvor G. Lumbar spinal stenosis. Clin Orthop Relat Res. 1974;99:30–50.
28. Shin M, Ryu K, Rathi NK, Park C. Direct pars repair surgery using two different surgical methods: pedicle screw with universal hook system and direct pars screw fixation in symptomatic lumbar spondylosis patients. J Korean Neurosurg Soc. 2012;51:14–9.
29. Hioki A, Miyamoto K, Sadamasu A, Nozawa S, Ogawa H, Fushimi K, Hosoe H, Shimizu K. Repair of pars defects by segmental transverse wiring for athletes with symptomatic spondylolysis. Relationship between bony union and postoperative symptoms. Spine. 2012;37(9):802–7.
30. Amoretti N, Huwart L, Hauger O, Browaeys P, Marcy P, Nouri Y, Ibba C, Boileau P. Computed tomography- and fluoroscopy-guided percutaneous screw fixation of low-grade isthmic spondylolisthesis in adults: a new technique. Eur Radiol. 2012;22:2841–7.
31. Widi GA, Williams SK, Levi AD. Minimally invasive direct repair of bilateral lumbar spine pars defects in athletes. Case Rep Med. 2013; 5 pp. Article ID 659078 [ePub ahead of print].
32. Kwon BK, Hilibrand AS, Malloy K, Savas PE, Silva MT, Albert TJ, et al. A critical analysis of the literature regarding surgical approach and outcome for adult low-grade isthmic spondylolisthesis. J Spinal Disord Tech. 2005;18 Suppl 1:S30–40.
33. Mardjetko S, Albert T, Andersson G, Bridwell K, DeWald C, Gaines R, Geck M, Hammerberg K, Herkowitz H, Kwon B, Labelle H, Lubicky J, McAfee P, Ogilvie J, Shufflebarger H, Whitesides T. Spine/SRS spondylolisthesis summary statement. Spine. 2005;30(6S):S3.
34. Agabegi SS, Fischgrund JS. Contemporary management of isthmic spondylolisthesis: pediatric and adult. Spine J. 2010;10:530–43.
35. Lindley EM, McBeth ZL, Henry SE, Cooley R, Burger EL, Cain CMJ, Patel VV. Retrograde ejaculation after anterior lumbar spine surgery. Spine. 2012;37(20):1785–9.
36. Quraishi NA, Konig M, Booker SJ, Shafafy M, Boszczyk BM, Grevitt MP, Mehdian H, Webb JK. Access related complications in anterior lumbar surgery performed by spinal surgeons. Eur Spine J. 2013;22 Suppl 1:S16–20.
37. Jacobs WCH, Vreeling A, De Kleuver M. Fusion for low-grade adult isthmic spondylolisthesis: a systematic

review of the literature. Eur Spine J. 2006;15:391–402.
38. McGuire RA, Amundson GM. The use of primary internal fixation in spondylolisthesis. Spine. 1993;18(12):1662–72.
39. Thomsen K, Christensen FB, Eiskjaer SP, Hansen ES, Fruensgaard S, Bunger CE. 1997 Volvo award winner in clinical studes. The effect of pedicle screw instrumentation on functional outcome and fusion rates in posterolateral lumbar spinal fusion: a prospective, randomized clinical study. Spine. 1997;22(24):2813–22.
40. France JC, Yaszemski MJ, Lauerman W, et al. A randomized prospective study of posterolateral lumbar fusion outcomes with and without pedicle screw instrumentation. Spine. 1999;24(6):553–60.
41. Moller H, Hedlund R. Instrumented and noninstrumented posterolateral fusion in adult spondylolisthesis – a prospective randomized study: part 2. Spine. 2000;25(1):1716–21.
42. Christensen FB, Hansen ES, Eiskjaer SP, et al. Circumferential lumbar spinal fusion with Brantigan cage versus posterolateral fusion with titanium Cotrel-Dubousset instrumentation: a prospective, randomized clinical study of 146 patients. Spine. 2002;27(23):2674–83.
43. Carragee EJ. Single-level posterolateral arthrodesis, with or without posterior decompression, for the treatment of isthmic spondylolisthesis in adults. A prospective, randomized study. J Bone Joint Surg Am. 1997;79(8):1175–80.
44. Johnsson R, Stromqvist B, Aspenberg P. Randomized radiostereometric study comparing osteogenic protein-1 (BMP-7) and autograft bone in human noninstrumented posterolateral lumbar fusion: 2002 Volvo award in clinical studies. Spine. 2002;27(23):2654–61.
45. Audat ZM, Darwish FT, Al Barbarawi MM, Obaidat MM, Haddad WH, Bashaireh KM, Al-Aboosy IA. Surgical management of low grade isthmid spondylolisthesis; a randomized controlled study of the surgical fixation with and without reduction. Scoliosis. 2011;6:14–9.
46. Musluman AM, Yilmaz A, Cansever T, et al. Posterior lumbar interbody fusion versus posterolateral fusion with instrumentation in the treatment of low-grade isthmic spondylolisthesis: midterm clinical outcomes. J Neurosurg Spine. 2011;14:488–96.
47. Farrokhi MR, Rahmanian A, Masoudi MS. Posterolateral versus posterior interbody fusion in isthmic spondylolisthesis. J Neurotrauma. 2012;29:1567–73.
48. Isaacs RE, Podichetty VK, Santiago P, Sandhu FA, Spears J, Kelly K, Rice L, Fessler RG. Minimally invasive microendoscopy-assisted transforaminal lumbar interbody fusion with instrumentation. J Neurosurg Spine. 2005;3:98–105.
49. Gahreman A, Ferch RD, Rao PJ, Bogduk N. Minimal access versus open posterior lumbar interbody fusion in the treatment of spondylolisthesis. Neurosurgery. 2010;66(2):296–304.
50. Wang J, Zhou Y, Zhang ZF, Li CQ, Zheng WJ, Liu J. Comparison of one-level minimally invasive and open transforaminal lumbar interbody fusion in degenerative and isthmic spondylolisthesis grades 1 and 2. Eur Spine J. 2010;19:1780–4.
51. Rampersaud YR, Gray R, Lewis SJ, Massicotte EM, Fehlings MG. Cost-utility analysis of posterior minimally invasive fusion compared with conventional open fusion for lumbar spondylolisthesis. SAS J. 2011;5:29–35.
52. Kotani Y, Abumi K, Ito M, Sudo H, Abe Y, Minami A. Mid-term clinical results of minimally invasive decompression and posterolateral fusion with percutaneous pedicle screws versus conventional approach for degenerative spondylolisthesis with spinal stenosis. Eur Spine J. 2012;21:1171–7.

Results of Surgical Treatment of Pediatric Spondylolysis and Spondylolisthesis

24

Adam C. Shaner and Paul D. Sponseller

As discussed in previous chapters, the recommendations for surgical treatment of pediatric spondylolysis and spondylolisthesis are based primarily upon the work originally performed by Wiltse et al. In evaluation of the pediatric patient with spondylolysis and/or listhesis, it is important to characterize the nature of the defect (congenital vs. other etiology) as well as its severity and the presence of symptoms including pain, radiculopathy, or myelopathy. Taken together, these factors dictate the indications for operative management [1].

Patients requiring surgery fall into the categories presented in Table 24.1. The grading system of Meyerding is based upon the percentage of anterior slip of the vertebral body on the adjacent segment which is divided into quarters [2].

The focus of this chapter will be to discuss the results of those patients who have undergone surgery for management of their deformity. We will first focus on symptomatic low grade spondylolysis that has failed conservative management before transitioning to management of high grade spondylolisthesis.

A.C. Shaner, M.D.
Department of Orthopaedic Surgery, Johns Hopkins Hospital, Baltimore, MD 21287-0882, USA
e-mail: ashaner1@jhmi.edu

P.D. Sponseller, M.D., M.B.A. (✉)
Department of Orthopaedic Surgery, John Hopkins Bloomberg Children's Hospital, Baltimore, MD 21287, USA
e-mail: psponse@jhmi.edu

Results of Management of Low Grade Pediatric Spondylolysis and Spondylolisthesis

The indications for treatment of spondylolysis with grade I or II slip are defined by the presence of symptoms. For the majority of patients, the chief complaint is pain. Failure of nonsurgical management including activity modification, physical therapy, NSAIDs, and occasionally bedrest are indications for operative intervention.

In situ bilateral lateral fusion performed at the site of the pars defect is the mainstay of surgical treatment, which may be accomplished via several methods.

Kimura and Buck originally described the technique of direct repair consisting of a posterior approach to the pars interarticularis and arthrodesis using laminar screws with autograft [3, 4]. Buck later rewrote on the technical difficulty of proper screw placement for this procedure [5]. Follow-up for this was examined by for 18 patients undergoing this technique, with 15 patients having satisfactory results based on the Henderson criteria (Table 24.2). For the remaining three patients who had a poor outcome, repeat imaging showed a pseudarthrosis at the site of the defect of the pars interarticularis [6].

A similar approach has also been described by Nicol and Scott using 18-gauge stainless steel wire around the transverse process bilaterally and

A.L. Wollowick and V. Sarwahi (eds.), *Spondylolisthesis: Diagnosis, Non-Surgical Management, and Surgical Techniques*, DOI 10.1007/978-1-4899-7575-1_24,

Table 24.1 Treatment recommendations based on myerding classification and symptoms

Grade slip	Symptoms present	Treatment
I/II	No	Radiographic follow-up
I/II	Yes	Activity modification, bracing; surgery for failed conservative management
III/IV	No	Fusion
III/IV	Yes	Fusion

Table 24.2 Subjective assessment guidelines

Excellent: No pain, return to normal occupation and normal sport
Good: Occasional pain after strenuous activity, return to normal occupation and less strenuous sport
Poor: Pain persists, unable to return to occupation and to partake in sport

Table 24.3 Macnab outcome criteria

Excellent: No pain; no restriction of activity
Good: Occasional pain of sufficient severity to interfere with the patient's ability to do his/her normal work or his capacity to enjoy leisure hours
Fair: Improved functional capacity, but handicapped by intermittent pain of sufficient severity to curtail or modify work or leisure activities
Poor: No improvement or insufficient improvement to enable increase in activities; further operative intervention required

then tightening the wires to each other inferiorly to the posterior spinal process. Multiple modifications of this procedure have been described with similar results [7, 8]. Larger patient series using this technique in patients with Grade I spondylolysis yielded satisfactory results in 20 of 22 patients, with 16 excellent and 4 good outcomes. Radiographically, the 17 patients whose defects healed had excellent (14) or good (3) results [9, 10]. A series performed by Askar et al. in patients younger than 25 years undergoing Scott wiring for symptomatic spondylolysis also further reinforced this, yielding "good" or "excellent" results in 12 of 14 patients with a mean follow-up period of 10.9 years [11].

Long-term follow-up results on 62 patients for isthmic repair performed with Buck, Scott, or a modified Scott technique showed an excellent result observed in 83.3 % of patients operated with the modified Scott technique. This was in comparison with patients operated with the Scott (62.5 %) and the Buck technique (28.5 %). Of those patients with clinical and radiological failure, 57 % of patients with the Buck technique received a subsequent posterior fusion compared to 12.5 % with the Scott technique and 2.7 % with the Scott modified technique. The most common reason for revision was symptomatic pseudarthrosis and progression of spondylolisthesis [10].

This approach was further modified with the advent of pedicle screws as an anchor for fixation. Rovin and Songer described a combination of the Scott technique and the Morscher technique, using a hook screw in place of cables. The combined technique, the modified pedicle screw-cable construct was performed in 1998 and involved placing a special pedicle cable-screw into the pedicle of the involved vertebra. Seven patients underwent this procedure with five rating outcomes as excellent and in two as good, according to the Prolo score [12]. Further retrospective analysis of this technique showed excellent results clinically and on radiographic examination [13].

Similarly good outcomes have been described using this technique and the similar pedicle screw-laminar hook method by several authors [14–17]. Shah et al. performed a similar retrospective analysis comparing direct laminar screw fixation to that of pedicle screw-rod-hook technique. Using the Macnab criteria (Table 24.3) for pain assessment, results showed excellent or good outcome in eight of nine patients in the direct laminar screw group and six of seven patients in the pedicle screw-rod-hook group. However, there was a significant increase in surgical time and estimated blood loss among the pedicle screw group, as it required greater surgical exposure [18]. This was confirmed by a larger study examining 47 consecutively enrolled patients who underwent pedicle screw with universal hook system or direct pars screw fixation. Successful bone fusion rate was 78.3 % in the pedicle screw group, and 93.3 % in the direct pars screw group, with decreased operation time, amount of blood loss, hospital stay, as well as better clinical outcome in the latter cohort [19].

To combat this trend, minimally invasive methods have been devised to attempt to lower

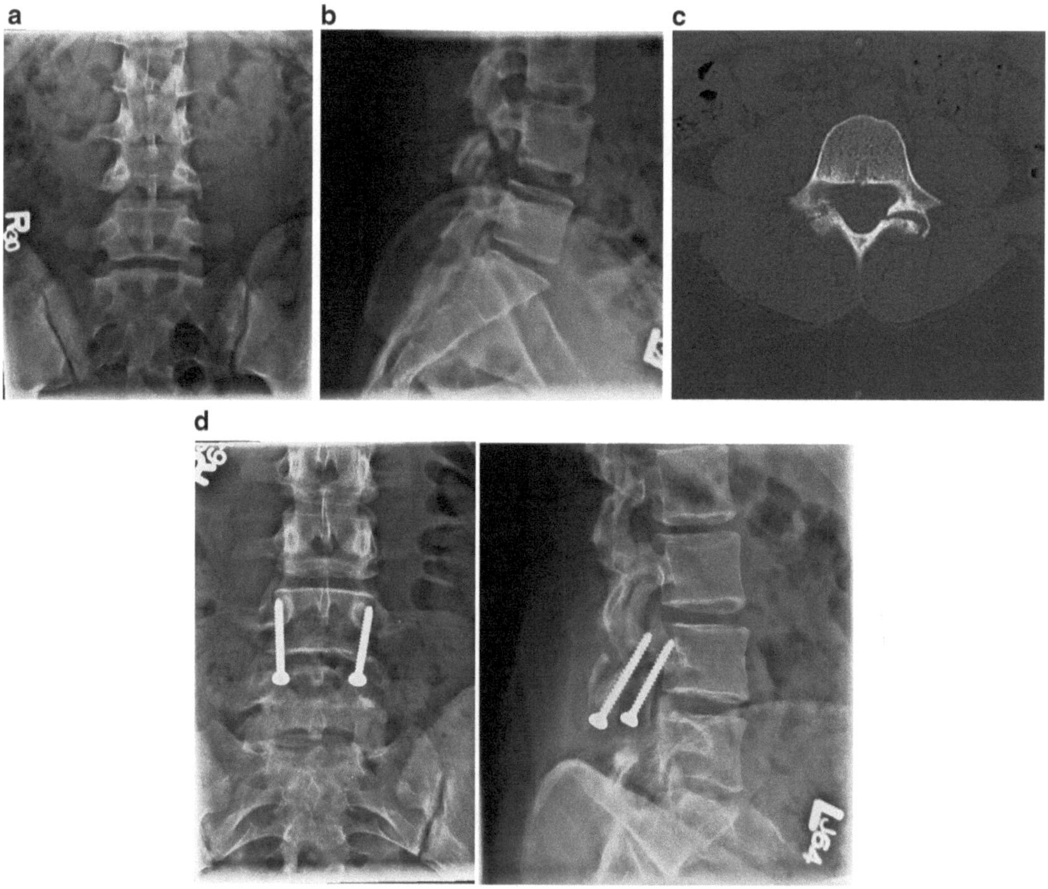

Fig. 24.1 (**a–c**) Preoperative imaging showing pars defect in a pediatric patient. (**c, d**) Postoperative imaging after direct pars interarticularis repair using compression screw technique with bone graft

blood loss and decrease hospital stay time. The neurosurgery group at John Hopkins reported on a series of consecutive pediatric patients with bilateral L5 spondylolysis treated utilizing a minimally invasive direct repair using a pedicle screw and cable construct with direct repair of the pars defect. Early follow-up in the first 8 months yielded excellent result with resolution of symptoms in all patients [20].

The orthopedic surgery group at Johns Hopkins retrospectively analyzed 31 patients undergoing intralaminar screw fixation for spondylolisthesis with a minimum follow-up time of 2 years. Preoperative pain was reduced by VAS scores and of the 25 athletes who underwent the procedure, 19 returned to competitive sports with a mean postoperative VAS score of 1 point at a mean of 6 months after surgery. One patient required revision posterior fusion and two patients sustained unilateral intralaminar screw fractures. Also of note, MRI findings, age, and degree of disc degeneration had no effect on outcome which goes against the current practice standard of mandatory MRI evaluation of the involved discs at the level of the defect to assess degeneration which have been hypothesized to prevent a positive outcome [21] (Fig. 24.1).

Alternatives to Direct Repair

In addition to excellent results in the majority of patients undergoing direct pars interarticularis repair, definitive posterior fusion can achieve similar positive results. In those patients failing or not candidates for direct repair, a single level posterior spinal fusion has been advocated and has been described both with and without the use of postoperative immobilization in either brace or cast [19, 22–24]. Retrospective analyses of patients treated with uninstrumented posterolateral fusion for grade I and grade II disease demonstrated fusion rates greater than 83 % and relief of symptoms in more than 75 % [22, 25].

To compare results of posterolateral fusion to direct repair, long-term follow-up in 23 patients treated by Scott's repair was contrasted with 25 patients treated by posterolateral segmental fusion without instrumentation. At mean follow-up time of 54 months, 87 % of the Scott's group and 96 % of the fusion group had occasional pain which did not interfere with daily activities or no pain at all. There was no statistical difference in the subjective, clinical, or functional outcome between the two operation groups [26]. At long-term follow-up of 15 years, the previously improved ODI slowly decreased for the direct repair group compared to the segmental fusion which was statistically significant, but only moderately apparent in terms of difference in clinical exam [15]. As such, patients with direct repair may not do as well as those with single level fusion long term, possibly due to the fact that direct repair does not protect the disc of the lytic/olisthetic segment from further degeneration. In comparing posterior vs. posterolateral fusion at 20-year long-term follow-up, nonunion was present in 34 % of patients after posterior fusion and in 13 % after posterolateral fusion, with 14 % of patients reporting back pain often or very often at rest [27].

Comparison of posterior lumbar interbody fusion versus posterolateral fusion with instrumentation in the treatment of low grade isthmic spondylolisthesis showed good or excellent results in 22 (88 %) cases in the PLIF group and 19 (76 %) cases in the PLF group. Fusion rates were 100 % in the PLIF group and 84 % in the PLF group with no difference in the complication rates for each group at 3.3 year mean follow-up [28]. Overall, satisfactory long-term results and patient satisfaction can be anticipated with direct repair as well as posterior/posterolateral fusion techniques for low grade spondylolisthesis.

Results of Management of High Grade Pediatric Spondylolisthesis

Surgical management of spondylolisthesis should be reserved for the subset of patients who have failed conservative management who have persistent pain or a limitation to their physical activities. Again using the original treatment guidelines set by Wiltse, skeletally immature patients with slip greater than 50 % are recommended for surgical fusion regardless of the presence or absence of symptoms. For higher grade spondylolisthesis (III and greater), the algorithm of treatment becomes more unclear and has numerous possibilities in terms of fixation type, levels of fusion, and reduction vs. in situ fusion. These cases often present the greatest challenges to the pediatric spine surgeon and are associated with increased risk of complication and morbidity [29, 30]. Here, we will compare results of these interventions including rates of pseudarthrosis, outcomes, and neurologic risk.

Obtaining a thorough history and documentation of physical exam findings, particularly those of nerve root compression (e.g., radiculopathy, weakness, and sensory deficit). In these cases, decompression of the nerve root alone or with fusion (instrumented vs. non-instrumented) is advised. Historically, decompression was performed without concurrent fusion and often resulted in slip progression and pseudarthrosis. This procedure, first described by Gill in 1955 involved removal of the loose posterior element showed good outcomes in early results, but increased slip in 14 % of patients, in long-term follow-up [31]. However, this was difficult to repeat as subsequent studies have shown poorer long-term results with or without slip progression [32, 33]. As such, current recommendations advocate for the use of spinal fusion with instrumentation as an adjunct to any decompression of the posterior elements. In doing so, the surgeon weighs the risk of increased instability against wider decompression of the neural elements. By utilizing instrumentation with fusion of the affected vertebral levels, both stability and adequate release of the involved nerve roots can be obtained. The fusion itself can be performed with or without reduction of the slip with anterior or posterior procedures including posterolateral or interbody fusion.

Masoudi et al. compared outcomes of posterolateral fusion against lumbar interbody fusion using instrumentation using Oswestry low back pain disability scale and the visual analog scale and showed that posterolateral fusion had better clinical results and decreased back pain, but a lower rate of fusion compared to PLIF [34].

In Situ Fusion

In situ fusion of the spine is advocated by many as it serves to prevent further slip and decrease overall pain, but to stabilize the spine for decompression. In situ fusion has shown good results with or without postoperative cast immobilization [35–38]. Long-term follow-up for patients with high grade (<60 %) slip undergoing in situ uninstrumented fusion via anterior, posterior, or circumferential technique was analyzed by Poussa et al. and revealed slightly improved clinical outcomes measured by the ODI in circumferential fusion group, with and associated decrease in lumbar range of motion. Despite the high grade slip and radiologic evidence of nerve root compression, clinical findings of nerve weakness were not usually present [15, 30, 39–41]. Likewise, other groups have advocated for circumferential fusion with addition of a fibular allograft or autograft strut through the S1–L5 vertebral bodies or trans-sacral hollow modular anchorage screws to provide the best opportunity to limit symptomatic pseudarthrosis while obtaining good functional outcomes and limiting slip progression [29, 42–45]. However, even in situ fusion without reduction carries a risk of development of acute cauda equina. In these instances, immediate decompression that includes resection of the posterosuperior rim of the dome of the sacrum and the adjacent intervertebral disc is recommended [46, 47].

For those patients with unsatisfactory results including cauda equina or symptomatic pseudarthrosis, the majority who undergo reoperation achieve good results [37]. Overall, patient satisfaction of greater than 80 % can be expected for those with high grade spondylolisthesis undergoing in situ fusion [48] (Fig. 24.2).

Reduction of Slip

Reduction of high grade spondylolisthesis offers several advantages compared to in situ fusion at the risk of increased surgical time, higher technical demand, and risk of L5 nerve radiculopathy (most common complication) [49]. Several techniques for reduction of high grade slip have been described, and are reserved primarily for patients with severe sagittal imbalance, high mobility of the slip on lateral flexion–extension radiographs, and preoperative radiculopathy requiring wide decompression.

Numerous reduction techniques have been described including single and multiple stage procedures with use of traction, anterior, posterior, combined fusion, as well as interbody fusion. Bradford and Boachie-Adjei described a two-stage procedure with posterior decompression and posterolateral fusion followed by temporary halo-skeletal traction. The second stage then utilized ALIF followed by cast immobilization, resulting in correction of sagittal alignment, solid fusion, and only one incident of persistent back pain with radiculopathy [50]. Similarly good outcomes were obtained using Harrington distraction rods to obtain reduction with concurrent posterolateral fusion followed by anterior lumbosacral fusion using two bicortical wedge-shaped iliac grafts, or pedicular fixation using posterolateral fusion combined with PLIF [42, 51].

A long-term comparison of patients who had undergone in situ fusion vs. in situ with reduction and postoperative cast immobilization showed a decreased rate of progression of slip and lumbosacral kyphosis, but overall similar clinical and functional outcomes. The authors advocated that reduction should only be performed if it results in an improvement in the rate of fusion, functional outcome, or cosmesis [52]. Partial reduction of high grade spondylolisthesis combined with wide decompression of the posterior elements has also

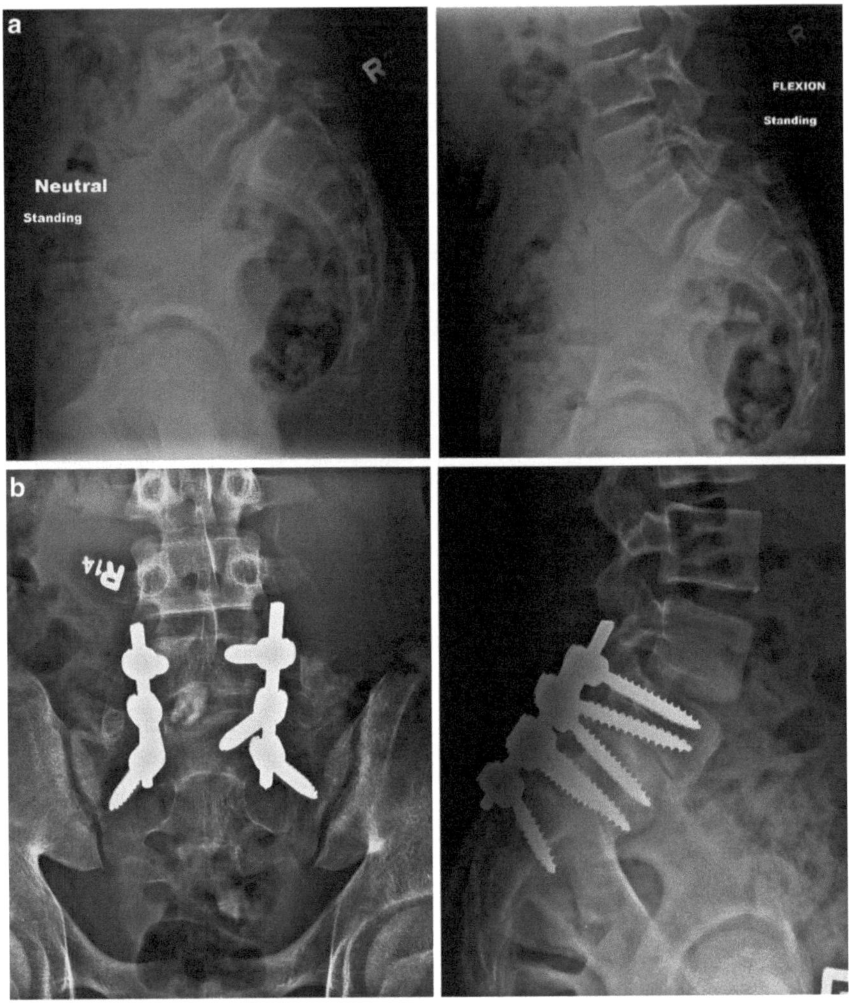

Fig. 24.2 (**a**) Preoperative neutral and forward flexion films showing Grade I/II L5–S1 slip. (**b**) Postoperative radiographs after reduction and posterolateral fusion

been advocated, combined either with circumferential staged anterior and posterolateral fusion, or single stage combined posterolateral and posterior interbody fusion [51, 53–57]. In a retrospective study, Helenius et al. compared patients treated using posterolateral fusion, anterior fusion, or circumferential fusion without instrumentation for high grade isthmic spondylolisthesis. They concluded that uninstrumented circumferential fusion had improved correction of kyphosis, ODI, and SRS scores [58]. Partial, rather than complete reduction of the sagittal deformity when combined with wide decompression and stable fusion technique through combined anterior/posterior approaches or single posterior approach with interbody fusion, appears to provide stable, safe results with decreased rates of postoperative nerve root compression and cauda equina [57].

Direct comparison of reduction vs. fusion in situ with long-term follow-up yielded no difference in functional tests or clinical findings, with reduction of pain in both groups. However, reduction of slip, while resulting in improved slip percentage and sagittal alignment, was associated with longer operative time, higher blood loss, and higher complication rates including reoperation.

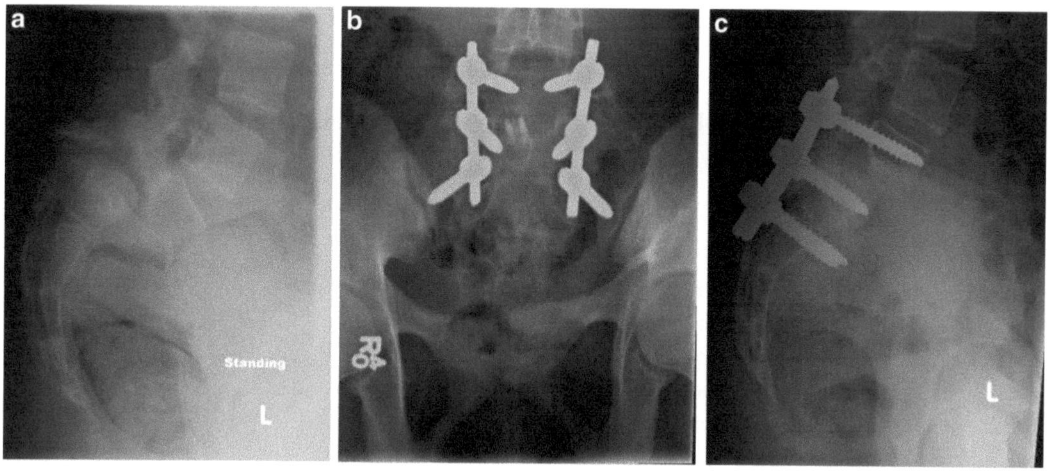

Fig. 24.3 (**a**) Preoperative lateral of high grade S1–S2 spondylolistheis. (**b**, **c**) Postoperative AP and lateral after reduction with posterolateral fusion L5–S2

These results, taken together, indicate that reduction should be predicated on specific goals such as improving neurologic signs and symptoms, clinical appearance, or possibly saving fusion levels in moderate slips [59] (Fig. 24.3).

Spondyloptosis

Grade V slip or 100 % displacement of the vertebral column relative to the inferior adjacent level (commonly L5–S1) is known as spondyloptosis. This, the greatest severity of sagittal deformity, carries unique challenges with surgical management. Like other high grade slips, fusion both in situ or with differing degrees of reduction have been utilized and been successful overall with regard to clinical outcomes, reduction of pain, and improvement of previous neurologic impingement [51, 56, 57, 60]. Posterior in situ fusion with posterior and interbody fibular graft was first described by Bohlman in 1982, and showed solid arthrodesis for both patients after 2-year follow-up [61]. A similar procedure has been described from an anterior transperitoneal approach, wherein all four patients achieved stable fusion at long-term follow-up with no worsening of neurologic deficit [62].

Additionally, complete vertebrectomy of the displaced level with reduction and fusion of the two adjacent levels has also been described as a viable, if not rare and technically challenging alternative. First performed by Gaines and Nichols in 1985, the first stage of the procedure consists of a vertebral body resection of L5 along with the L4–5 and L5–S1 discs. The second stage procedure consists of removal of the loose posterior element, the articular processes, and pedicles of L5 and reduction of L4 onto the sacrum which are subsequently fused. Long-term follow-up performed in 1994 and again in 2005 showed high incidence of neurologic deficit postoperatively (75 %), most commonly foot drop, the majority of which recovered. Despite these findings, the majority of patients reported extremely high satisfaction with improvement in pain, function, gait, and overall appearance [45, 63, 64]. A modified variant described by Kalra et al. resected only the lower half of L5 anteriorly, leaving the L5 pedicles in place for reduction screws and maintaining overall spinal column height. Performed in a single patient, outcomes at 2-year follow-up showed complete reduction of slip, resolution of neurologic deficit, and significant improvement in ODI score [65]. Current trends, however, have moved towards posterior-only approach with combined posterior and interbody in situ fusion.

Summary

Patients with low grade spondylolysis or spondylolisthesis rarely require surgery, as a majority respond to activity modification, NSAIDs, or physical therapy. For symptomatic patients who do not respond to conservative measures, surgical management is an option. This may be accomplished with direct pars interarticularis repair by compression screw, wiring technique, sublaminar-hook-screw construct, or modifications thereof. Additionally, posterolateral fusion with or without instrumentation offers similar subjective, clinical, and functional long-term outcomes to direct repair with a tradeoff of longer surgical time with greater exposure needed. Overall, both procedures offer good and excellent outcomes, even with radiographic findings of pseudarthrosis. For patients with high grade slip, in situ fusion or reduction and fusion are both valid options and depend upon surgeon experience and underlying patient function and neurologic status. For patients undergoing reduction, wide decompression and instrumentation with either circumferential or interbody fusion provide stable long-term results. Interbody fusion techniques show greater long-term fusion rates, achieve greater reduction, and appear to have higher functional outcome compared to posterior-only fusion. Reduction carries increased risk of neurologic injury, but the majority of these including cauda equina resolve. Long-term follow-up comparing in situ fusion to reduction with fusion of high grade spondylolisthesis has shown improved ODI and SRS scores with fusion in situ. Grade V spondylolisthesis presents several unique challenges for surgical repair and may be fused in situ from an anterior or posterior approach, with partial reduction, or Gaines procedure. Current trends have moved towards posterior-only approach with combined posterior and interbody fusion.

References

1. Wiltse LL, Newman PH, Macnab I. Classification of spondylolysis and spondylolisthesis. Clin Orthop Relat Res. 1976;117:23–9.
2. Meyerding HW. Spondylolisthesis. Surg Gynecol Obstet. 1932;54:371–7.
3. Kimura M. Seikei Geka. 1968;19(4):285–96. Japanese.
4. Buck JE. Direct repair of the defect in spondylolisthesis. Preliminary report. J Bone Joint Surg Br. 1970; 52:432–7.
5. Buck JE. Abstract: further thoughts on direct repair of the defect in spondylolysis. J Bone Joint Surg Br. 1979;61:123.
6. Pederson AK, Hagen R. Spondylolysis and spondylolisthesis. Treatment by internal fixation and bone-grafting of the defect. J Bone Joint Surg Am. 1988;70(1):15–24.
7. Hambly MF, Wiltse LL. A modification of the Scott wiring technique. Spine (Phila Pa 1976). 1994; 19(3):354–6.
8. Johnson GV, Thompson AG. The Scott wiring technique for direct repair of lumbar spondylolysis. J Bone Joint Surg Br. 1992;74(3):426–30.
9. Nicol RO, Scott JH. Lytic spondylolysis. Repair by wiring. Spine (Phila Pa 1976). 1986;11(10):1027–30.
10. Giudici F, Minoia L, Archetti M, Corriero AS, Zagra A. Long-term results of the direct repair of spondylolisthesis. Eur Spine J. 2011;20 Suppl 1:S115–20. doi:10.1007/s00586-011-1759-9.
11. Askar Z, Wardlaw D, Koti M. Scott wiring for direct repair of lumbar spondylolysis. Spine (Phila Pa 1976). 2003;28(4):354–7.
12. Songer MN, Rovin R. Repair of the pars interarticularis defect with a cable-screw construct. A preliminary report. Spine (Phila Pa 1976). 1998;23(2):263–9.
13. Schlenzka D, Remes V, Helenius I, Lamberg T, Tervahartiala P, Yrjönen T, Tallroth K, Osterman K, Seitsalo S, Poussa M. Direct repair for treatment of symptomatic spondylolysis and low-grade isthmic spondylolisthesis in young patients: no benefit in comparison to segmental fusion after a mean follow-up of 14.8 years. Eur Spine J. 2006;15(10):1437–47. Epub 2006 Feb 7.
14. Gillet P, Petit M. Direct repair of spondylolysis without spondylolisthesis, using a rod-screw construct and bone grafting of the pars defect. Spine (Phila Pa 1976). 1999;24(12):1252–6.
15. Kakiuchi M. Repair of the defect in spondylolysis. Durable fixation with pedicle screws and laminar hooks. J Bone Joint Surg Am. 1997;79(6):818–25.
16. Tokuhashi Y, Matsuzaki H. Repair of defects in spondylolysis by segmental pedicular screw hook fixation. A preliminary report. Spine (Phila Pa 1976). 1996; 21(17):2041–5.
17. Winter M, Jani L. Results of screw osteosynthesis in spondylolysis and low-grade spondylolisthesis. Arch Orthop Trauma Surg. 1989;108(2):96–9.
18. Karatas AF, Dede O, Atanda AA, Holmes L Jr, Rogers K, Gabos P, Shah SA. Comparison of direct pars repair techniques of spondylolysis in pediatric and adolescent patients: pars compression screw versus pedicle screw-rod-hook. J Spinal Disord Tech. 2012.
19. Shin MH, Ryu KS, Rathi NK, Park CK. Direct pars repair surgery using two different surgical methods:

pedicle screw with universal hook system and direct pars screw fixation in symptomatic lumbar spondylosis patients. J Korean Neurosurg Soc. 2012;51(1):14–9. doi:10.3340/jkns.2012.51.1.14. Epub 2012 Jan 31.
20. Noggle JC, Sciubba DM, Samdani AF, Anderson DG, Betz RR, Asghar J. Minimally invasive direct repair of lumbar spondylolysis with a pedicle screw and hook construct. Neurosurg Focus. 2008;25(2):E15. doi:10.3171/FOC/2008/25/8/E15.
21. Menga EN, Kebaish KM, Jain A, Carrino JA, Sponseller PD. Clinical results and functional outcomes after direct intralaminar screw repair of spondylolysis. Spine (Phila Pa 1976). 2014;39(1):104–10.
22. Girardo M, Bettini N, Dema E, Cervellati S. Uninstrumented posterolateral spinal arthrodesis: is it the gold standard technique for I degrees and II degrees grade spondylolisthesis in adolescence? Eur Spine J. 2009;18 Suppl 1:126–32. doi:10.1007/s00586-009-0983-z. Epub 2009 May 5.
23. Stanton RP, Meehan P, Lovell WW. Surgical fusion in childhood spondylolisthesis. J Pediatr Orthop. 1985;5(4):411–5.
24. Burkus JK, Lonstein JE, Winter RB, et al. Long-term evaluation of adolescents treated operatively for spondylolisthesis. A comparison of in situ arthrodesis only with in situ arthrodesis and reduction followed by immobilization in a cast. J Bone Joint Surg Am. 1992;74:693–704.
25. Velikas EP, Blackburne JS. Surgical treatment of spondylolisthesis in children and adolescents. J Bone Joint Surg Br. 1981;63-B(1):67–70.
26. Schlenzka D, Seitsalo S, Poussa M, Osterman K. Operative treatment of symptomatic lumbar spondylolysis and mild isthmic spondylolisthesis in young patients: direct repair of the defect or segmental spinal fusion? Eur Spine J. 1993;2(2):104–12.
27. Helenius I, Lamberg T, Osterman K, Schlenzka D, Yrjönen T, Tervahartiala P, Seitsalo S, Poussa M, Remes V. Scoliosis research society outcome instrument in evaluation of long-term surgical results in spondylolysis and low-grade isthmic spondylolisthesis in young patients. Spine (Phila Pa 1976). 2005;30(3):336–41.
28. Müslüman AM, Yılmaz A, Cansever T, Cavuşoğlu H, Colak I, Genç HA, Aydın Y. Posterior lumbar interbody fusion versus posterolateral fusion with instrumentation in the treatment of low-grade isthmic spondylolisthesis: midterm clinical outcomes. J Neurosurg Spine. 2011;14(4):488–96. doi:10.3171/2010.11.SPINE10281. Epub 2011 Feb 11.
29. Frennered AK, Danielson BI, Nachemson AL, Nordwall AB. Midterm follow-up of young patients fused in situ for spondylolisthesis. Spine (Phila Pa 1976). 1991;16(4):409–16.
30. Fu KM, Smith JS, Polly Jr DW, Perra JH, Sansur CA, Berven SH, Broadstone PA, Choma TJ, Goytan MJ, Noordeen HH, Knapp Jr DR, Hart RA, Donaldson 3rd WF, Boachie-Adjei O, Shaffrey CI. Morbidity and mortality in the surgical treatment of six hundred five pediatric patients with isthmic or dysplastic spondylolisthesis. Spine (Phila Pa 1976). 2011;36(4):308–12. doi:10.1097/BRS.0b013e3181cf3a1d.
31. Gill GG, Manning JG, White HL. Surgical treatment of spondylolisthesis without spine fusion; excision of the loose lamina with decompression of the nerve roots. J Bone Joint Surg Am. 1955;37-A(3):493–520.
32. Amuso SJ, Neff RS, Coulson DB, Laing PG. The surgical treatment of spondylolisthesis by posterior element resection. J Bone Joint Surg Am. 1970;52(3):529–36.
33. Osterman K, Lindholm TS, Laurent LE. Late results of removal of the loose posterior element (Gill's operation) in the treatment of lytic lumbar spondylolisthesis. Clin Orthop Relat Res. 1976;117:121–8.
34. Farrokhi MR, Rahmanian A, Masoudi MS. Posterolateral versus posterior interbody fusion in isthmic spondylolisthesis. J Neurotrauma. 2012;29(8):1567–73. doi:10.1089/neu.2011.2167. Epub 2012 Apr 2.
35. Grzegorzewski A, Kumar SJ. In situ posterolateral spine arthrodesis for grades III, IV, and V spondylolisthesis in children and adolescents. J Pediatr Orthop. 2000;20(4):506–11.
36. Newton PO, Johnston 2nd CE. Analysis and treatment of poor outcomes following in situ arthrodesis in adolescent spondylolisthesis. J Pediatr Orthop. 1997;17(6):754–61.
37. Lenke LG, Bridwell KH, Bullis D, Betz RR, Baldus C, Schoenecker PL. Results of in situ fusion for isthmic spondylolisthesis. J Spinal Disord. 1992;5(4):433–42.
38. Molinari RW, Bridwell KH, Lenke LG, Ungacta FF, Riew KD. Complications in the surgical treatment of pediatric high-grade, isthmic dysplastic spondylolisthesis. A comparison of three surgical approaches. Spine (Phila Pa 1976). 1999;24(16):1701–11.
39. Helenius I, Remes V, Poussa M. Uninstrumented in situ fusion for high-grade childhood and adolescent isthmic spondylolisthesis: long-term outcome. Surgical technique J Bone Joint Surg Am. 2008;90(Suppl 2 Pt 1):145–52. doi:10.2106/JBJS.G.01186.
40. Remes V, Lamberg T, Tervahartiala P, Helenius I, Schlenzka D, Yrjönen T, Osterman K, Seitsalo S, Poussa M. Long-term outcome after posterolateral, anterior, and circumferential fusion for high-grade isthmicspondylolisthesis in children and adolescents: magnetic resonance imaging findings after average of 17-year follow-up. Spine (Phila Pa 1976). 2006;31(21):2491–9.
41. Petraco DM, Spivak JM, Cappadona JG, Kummer FJ, Neuwirth MG. An anatomic evaluation of L5 nerve stretch in spondylolisthesis reduction. Spine. 1996;21:1133–8.
42. DeWald RL, Faut MM, Taddonio RF, Neuwirth MG. Severe lumbosacral spondylolisthesis in adolescents and children. Reduction and staged circumferential fusion. J Bone Joint Surg Am. 1981;63(4):619–26.
43. Smith JA, Deviren V, Berven S, Kleinstueck F, Bradford DS. Clinical outcome of trans-sacral interbody fusion after partial reduction for high-grade l5–s1 spondylolisthesis. Spine (Phila Pa 1976). 2001;26(20):2227–34.
44. Sasso RC, Shively KD, Reilly TM. Transvertebral transsacral strut grafting for high-grade isthmic

spondylolisthesis L5–S1 with fibular allograft. J Spinal Disord Tech. 2008;21(5):328–33. doi:10.1097/BSD.0b013e318149e7ea.
45. Lehmer SM, Steffee AD, Gaines Jr RW. Treatment of L5–S1 spondyloptosis by staged L5 resection with reduction and fusion of L4 onto S1 (Gaines procedure). Spine (Phila Pa 1976). 1994;19(17):1916–25.
46. Schoenecker PL, Cole HO, Herring JA, Capelli AM, Bradford DS. Cauda equina syndrome after in situ arthrodesis for severe spondylolisthesis at the lumbosacral junction. J Bone Joint Surg Am. 1990;72(3): 369–77.
47. Bozarth GR, Fogel GR, Toohey JS, Neidre A. Repair of pars interarticularis defect with a modified cable-screw construct. J Surg Orthop Adv. 2007;16(2): 79–83.
48. Maurice HD, Morley TR. Cauda equine lesions following fusion in situ and decompressive laminectomy for severe spondylolisthesis. Four case reports. Spine. 1989;1:214–6.
49. Smith MD, Bohlman HH. Spondylolisthesis treated by a single-stage operation combining decompression with in situ posterolateral and anterior fusion. An analysis of eleven patients who had long-term follow-up. J Bone Joint Surg Am. 1990;72(3):415–21.
50. Bradford DS, Boachie-Adjei O. Treatment of severe spondylolisthesis by anterior and posterior reduction and stabilization. A long-term follow-up study. J Bone Joint Surg Am. 1990;72(7):1060–6.
51. Boos N, Marchesi D, Zuber K, Aebi M. Treatment of severe spondylolisthesis by reduction and pedicular fixation. A 4-6-year follow-up study. Spine (Phila Pa 1976). 1993;18(12):1655–61.
52. Burkus JK, Lonstein JE, Winter RB, Denis F. Long-term evaluation of adolescents treated operatively for spondylolisthesis. A comparison of in situ arthrodesis only with in situ arthrodesis and reduction followed by immobilization in a cast. J Bone Joint Surg Am. 1992;74(5):693–704.
53. Schwend RM, Waters PM, Hey LA, Hall JE, Emans JB. Treatment of severe spondylolisthesis in children by reduction and L4–S4 posterior segmental hyperextension fixation. J Pediatr Orthop. 1992;12(6):703–11.
54. Laursen M, Thomsen K, Eiskjaer SP, Hansen ES, Bünger CE. Functional outcome after partial reduction and 360 degree fusion in grade III–V spondylolisthesis in adolescent and adult patients. J Spinal Disord. 1999;12(4):300–6.
55. Roca J, Ubierna MT, Cáceres E, Iborra M. One-stage decompression and posterolateral and interbody fusion for severe spondylolisthesis. An analysis of 14 patients. Spine (Phila Pa 1976). 1999;24(7):709–14.
56. Lenke LG, Bridwell KH. Evaluation and surgical treatment of high-grade isthmic dysplastic spondylolisthesis. Instr Course Lect. 2003;52:525–32.
57. Poussa M, Schlenzka D, Seitsalo S, Ylikoski M, Hurri H, Osterman K. Surgical treatment of severe isthmic spondylolisthesis in adolescents. Reduction or fusion in situ. Spine (Phila Pa 1976). 1993;18(7):894–901.
58. Helenius I, Lamberg T, Osterman K, Schlenzka D, Yrjönen T, Tervahartiala P, Seitsalo S, Poussa M, Remes V. Posterolateral, anterior, or circumferential fusion in situ for high-grade spondylolisthesis in young patients: a long-term evaluation using the Scoliosis Research Society questionnaire. Spine (Phila Pa 1976). 2006;31(2):190–6.
59. Hanson DS, Bridwell KH, Rhee JM, Lenke LG. Dowel fibular strut grafts for high-grade dysplastic isthmic spondylolisthesis. Spine (Phila Pa 1976). 2002;27(18):1982–8.
60. Lakshmanan P, Ahuja S, Lewis M, Howes J, Davies PR. Transsacral screw fixation for high-grade spondylolisthesis. Spine J. 2009;9(12):1024–9. doi:10.1016/j.spinee.2009.08.456. Epub 2009 Oct 12.
61. Bohlman HH, Cook SS. One-stage decompression and posterolateral and interbody fusion for lumbosacral spondyloptosis through a posterior approach. Report of two cases. J Bone Joint Surg Am. 1982; 64(3):415–8.
62. Jones AA, McAfee PC, Robinson RA, Zinreich SJ, Wang H. Failed arthrodesis of the spine for severe spondylolisthesis. Salvage by interbody arthrodesis. J Bone Joint Surg Am. 1988;70(1):25–30.
63. Gaines RW, Nichols WK. Treatment of spondyloptosis by two stage L5 vertebrectomy and reduction of L4 onto S1. Spine (Phila Pa 1976). 1985;10(7):680–6.
64. Gaines RW. L5 vertebrectomy for the surgical treatment of spondyloptosis: thirty cases in 25 years. Spine (Phila Pa 1976). 2005;30(6 Suppl):S66–70.
65. Kalra K, Kohli S, Dhar S. A modified Gaines procedure for spondyloptosis. J Bone Joint Surg Br. 2010;92(11): 1589–91. doi:10.1302/0301-620X.92B11.24382.

25 Complications Associated with Surgical Treatment of Adult Spondylolisthesis

Khalid Abbed and William E. Neway III

The surgical management of adult spondylolisthesis is challenging. Currently, there is no consensus on the best treatment option. This is likely secondary to the fact that numerous surgical procedures produce equivocal results. Despite the lack of a "gold standard" procedure, outcome studies have shown that by adhering to basic surgical tenants, surgeons can achieve a successful clinical result: maintenance or restoration of sagittal balance and obtaining a solid fusion.

The most recent published complication rate for the surgical management of spondylolisthesis is 9.2 % [1]. This was determined from a large retrospective review of 10,242 adult patients with degenerative or isthmic spondylolisthesis. Patients with degenerative spondylolisthesis had a significantly higher complication rate (8.5 %) compared with isthmic spondylolisthesis (6.6 %; $p=0.002$), as well as those with high-grade spondylolisthesis and advanced age (>65 years).

K. Abbed, M.D.
Department of Neurosurgery, Yale School of Medicine, Yale Spine Institute, 333 Cedar St. TMP 426, New Haven, CT 06510, USA
e-mail: Khalid.Abbed@yale.edu

W.E. Neway III, D.O. (✉)
Department of Orthopaedic Surgery, Spine Service, University of Alabama at Birmingham, 1720 2nd Ave South, FOT 901, Birmingham, AL 35294, USA
e-mail: wneway@uabmc.edu

Complications may occur despite both the surgeon and the patient making every attempt at prevention. It is important to acknowledge that adverse events happen even in the best environments.

The most common complications encountered in the surgical management of adult spondylolisthesis include pseudoarthrosis, neurologic injury, dural tears, slip progression, instrumentation failure, vascular events, and infection (Table 25.1).

When counseling a patient for the surgical correction of spondylolisthesis, it is important to identify those patients who are at an increased risk for a complication. This preoperative risk assessment is beneficial to both the surgeon and the patient as part of the informed consent. Factors which have been shown to have a higher complication rate include patients with a high-grade spondylolisthesis, diagnosis of degenerative spondylolisthesis, and patient age >65 years old [2]. There is no difference in complication rate among surgical approaches, including revision procedures.

Pseudoarthrosis

Pseudoarthrosis is defined as the failure to achieve a rigid osseous union between two bony segments one year after the index surgery. It is the most common complication following surgery for lumbar spinal fusion and occurs more frequently when done for spondylolisthesis than

A.L. Wollowick and V. Sarwahi (eds.), *Spondylolisthesis: Diagnosis, Non-Surgical Management, and Surgical Techniques*, DOI 10.1007/978-1-4899-7575-1_25,

Table 25.1 Complications of spondylolithesis

1. Neurologic
Nerve root injury
Compression
Traction
Dural tear
Autonomic dysfunction
Retrograde ejaculation
Cauda equina syndrome
Chronic pain
Peripheral neuropathy secondary to compression
2. Pseudoarthrosis
Severe grade spondylolithesis
3. Slip progression
Preoperative slip
Slip angle
4. Instrumentation failure
Bone-implant failure
Biologic failure
5. Vascular
Direct
Vessel injury
Indirect
PE/DVT
Ischemic optic neuropathy
6. Infection

lumbar disc degeneration [3]. The rate of pseudoarthrosis is higher in patients with a higher-grade spondylolisthesis and in adults [1]. The significance of a pseudoarthrosis varies between patients. While achieving a successful fusion does not always correlate with resolution of the patient's symptoms, there is a high statistical correlation between pseudoarthrosis and poor clinical outcome [4]. Historically, the rates for pseudoarthrosis of the lumbar spine are up to 56 % [5]. However, there have been no recent studies demonstrating pseudoarthrosis rates with the use of newer implant and bone grafting technology. In addition, this may not be truly representative of the actual pseudoarthrosis rate given that a certain percentage is asymptomatic and therefore underreported. Hence an asymptomatic pseudoarthrosis does not necessarily require treatment. On the other hand, persistent motion and instability would be surgical indications for a nonunion.

Factors contributing to the development of a pseudoarthrosis include excessive motion at the fusion site, poor surgical technique (insufficient decorticated host bone surface area and graft material), metabolic abnormalities (osteoporosis, Vit D deficiency, excessive alcohol use, malabsorption syndromes), smoking, trauma, and infection. The role that these risk factors play in leading to a nonunion is unclear and its etiology may likely be multifactorial [6].

By knowing some of the risk factors for a pseudoarthrosis, tactics aimed at decreasing the incidence include immobilization of the spondylotic segment, meticulous fusion bed preparation, optimal bone grafting, addressing nutritional status and smoking cessation.

Diagnosis of a pseudoarthrosis is complex and remains a difficult condition to assess. The presence of a nonunion is determined by combining the clinical symptoms and radiographic evidence, after ruling out other possible etiologies of the pain [7]. Symptoms suggestive of a pseudoarthrosis include back pain, signs or symptoms of neurologic irritation, progressive deformity, gait disturbance, and hamstring tightness. Symptoms beyond 1 year in duration are especially worrisome, as a solid fusion should be achieved in that time frame [8]. Evaluation of a patient with persistent symptoms should always start with a through history and physical examination. Plain radiographs (AP, lateral, flexion, and extension) of the lumbar spine should always be obtained prior to advanced imaging. While diagnosing a nonunion on plain radiographs can be difficult due to overlapping bony structures, they provide very valuable information. The absence of a fusion mass, gaps in the fusion mass, persistent motion on flexion and extension films, lucency around the implants, or implant failure are key radiographic findings suggestive of a pseudoarthrosis. Thin-cut CT scan may provide benefit when assessing interbody fusion mass and diagnosing a "locked pseudoarthrosis" [9]. They are less helpful in settings where plain radiographs show a large fusion mass or a pseudoarthrosis is evident. The risks of radiation exposure make the routine use of CT scans not possible despite superior results compared to other imaging sources. No single imaging modality should be used to confer the diagnosis of a pseudoarthrosis. Other signs that a pseudoarthrosis may be present include lucency around pedicle screws, broken implants, and slip progression.

Treatment of a pseudoarthrosis requires the surgeon to address the underlying pathology. If there is any broken hardware present, it should be removed and those levels re-instrumented, typically upsizing the pedicle screw by 1 mm. Intra-operative assessment of the fusion mass and localizing the pseudoarthrosis is required. Once localized, this area is meticulously prepped for bone grafting. Removal of soft tissue, adequate decortication to bleeding bone and packing the site with ample iliac crest bone graft. The use of bone morphogenic protein (BMP) can also be considered in this setting. It may improve local biology and improve the likelihood for successful bony healing. If anterior support was not used in the index procedure, the addition of an interbody in the lumbar region is indicated [3]. In the case of an uninstrumented pseudoarthrosis, the addition of pedicle screw and/or interbody should be considered. Lastly, the use of implanted or external bone stimulators to promote healing can be used, although their effectiveness is unclear in the literature. The successful treatment of a pseudoarthrosis depends on correction of the host factors and optimizing surgical technique.

Neurologic

Neurologic complications that may be encountered with surgery for spondylolisthesis include nerve root injury, cauda equina syndrome, autonomic dysfunction, dural tears, and chronic pain. Prior to surgery it is imperative to document a through neurological evaluation, noting any deficits. In addition, an upright lateral radiograph is required to assess the degree of spondylolisthesis. Advanced imaging of the spine, consisting of an MRI or CT myelogram, is useful to assess any compression on the spinal cord and exiting nerve roots.

Nerve root injury may result from compression, traction, or direct trauma mechanism. Compression on the exiting nerve roots can occur either at the intraforaminal or extraforaminal location. Soft tissue impingement caused by soft disc protrusions or fibrocartilaginous debris from attempted healing of a pars defect may cause compression [10]. Other sources of compression include post-operative epidural hematoma formation, which usually presents in a delayed fashion. In order to adequately assess these sources of potential compression, it is important to evaluate the exiting nerve root from the lateral recess and out the foramen. Complete exposure is particularly important when spondylolisthesis reduction is planned, as reduction into a narrowed foramen could exacerbate neural compression. Reduction maneuvers can lead to neurologic deficits via manipulation and/or nerve root traction. A cadaveric study showed a nonlinear relationship between nerve strain and reduction. In this model, 71 % of the strain experienced by the L5 nerve root occurred during the last 50 % of the reduction [11]. In support of this, recent studies have shown a decrease in neurologic complications using "partial reduction" techniques.

Traction injury has been described while placing the patient in the prone position on the Jackson table. It is theorized that the slip acutely worsens when the muscles are relaxed; the spine displaces dorsally causing traction on the nerve roots [10].

Direct trauma from manipulation of the dural sac may injure the lumbar or sacral nerve roots producing a multidermatomal deficit. Additionally, direct trauma may result during instrumentation of the vertebrae or decompression of the nerve.

Cauda equina syndrome has been known to occur in both the intra-operative and post-operative settings. During reduction of a slip, it is possible to displace the posterior cephalad portion of the disc into the canal. This situation can be minimized with careful evaluation of a preoperative sagittal MRI and inspection of the disc space both during and after reduction. Even without reduction, there have been reported cases of cauda equina syndrome, which can only be explained by a vascular phenomenon, hyperextension during positioning, or transient displacement during exposure.

A post-operative cause of cauda equina syndrome may result from an epidural hematoma producing compression on the thecal sac. Accumulation of the hematoma occurs over hours or days after surgery and can present with a delayed-onset neurologic deficit.

The key to cauda equina syndrome is prompt diagnosis and treatment as the outcome is time dependent. Obtaining an MRI or CT myelogram in an expedient manner and surgical decompression, if necessary, is paramount. If a large amount of reduction was obtained during the index surgery, adjusting the instrumentation to decrease the reduction is warranted.

Anterior approach to the lumbar spine can lead to autonomic nerve dysfunction that presents as retrograde ejaculation. In order to decrease the incidence of this rare complication, it is important to perform a careful dissection and avoid the use of electrocautery in the soft tissue overlying the sacral promontory area [10].

Chronic pain is a devastating complication that has significant effects on both the surgeon and patient. While fusions for discogenic disease have a less predictable outcome than for lytic spondylolisthesis, other sources of pain should be ruled out. Other causes of unexplained pain include spinal (pseudoarthrosis, nerve root compression, flat back syndrome, discogenic pain, adjacent segment disease) and non-spinal (complex regional pain syndrome, infection, endometriosis) etiologies and may require a multi-disciplinary approach [3].

Neurologic injury to the extremities can occur as a result of localized pressure on peripheral nerves. Care must be taken to inspect the trunk, extremities, head and bony prominences once the patient has been positioned. Placing the operating table in slight reverse Trendelenburg is important to prevent potential ocular complications. It is incumbent on the surgeon to ensure these regions are well padded to avoid such complications.

Slip Progression

Progression of spondylolisthesis has been shown to occur postoperatively. The two most important risk factors for progression are the magnitude of preoperative slip and slip angle. Slip angle is defined as the angle subtended by a line from the inferior endplate of the L5 vertebral body and the superior endplate of the sacrum. Other factors that play a role in slip progression include surgical technique and degenerative disk disease. Performing a Gill laminectomy, complete removal of the posterior elements at the slipped level, should never be done with an in situ fusion. This procedure requires posterior stabilization at a minimum. Progression of spondylolisthesis is most likely to occur 2 years from the index procedure [1]. Despite our ability to recognize these risk factors, predicting which slips will progress remains elusive. Slip progression may even occur in the face of an apparent solid fusion and it is usually later determined that the progression occurred through a nonunion [12].

Patients in whom the slip has progressed may present with worsening low back pain and sciatica. In those patients with intractable pain, disabling deformity, or neurologic symptoms, reoperation is warranted.

Instrumentation Failure

The role of instrumentation in the surgical management of spondylolisthesis is to assist with the reduction of spondylotic slips, maintain and stabilize the reduced vertebrae, and ultimately improve fusion rates. In order to decrease the risk of hardware failure, adherence to the basic principles of fusion surgery is paramount. While spinal implants are rapidly evolving, their purpose remains the same, which is to serve as an adjunct to spinal fusion surgery. They create a "temporary" fusion environment through immobilization, which optimizes the conditions for osteosynthesis. Instrument failure is defined as screw bending, breakage, pullout, dislodgement, or disassembly.

Instrumentation failure may occur for intrinsic or extrinsic reasons. Intrinsic instrumentation failure happens at the bone-implant interface as a result of excessive forces placed on the construct. This can occur during reduction of a severe slip, introducing non-physiologic lordosis or a lack of sufficient support creating a stress riser. This is particularly important for posterior column only constructs lacking an interbody. These constructs lacking anterior column support have been shown to have a relatively high failure rate [13]. They may experience larger flexion moments leading to instrument failure and eventually pseudoarthrosis, loss of reduction, or slip progression [6]. Additionally, proper surgical technique during assembly and locking of the implants is important to prevent dislodgement or disassembly. Attention must be paid to prevent cross-threading the locking screw caps, ensuring final tightening of screw caps with torque limiter and proper counter-torque technique, adequate rod length such that it protrudes from the tulip heads, both cranial and caudal.

A study on pedicle screw survivorship found that the incidence of instrumentation failure was the same in patients who had a solid fusion as in those with a pseudoarthrosis [14]. The reason for this finding was postulated that three-column instrumentation was performed with one-column (posterolateral) fusion. Thus, they also found that pedicle screw breakage in the absence of a pseudoarthrosis was not associated with poor outcomes. Lastly, they showed that implant failure was more likely in patients who had a major (Grade 3 or 4) reduction performed.

Extrinsic instrumentation failure is a secondary phenomenon that occurs as a result of biologic failure. A delayed union or nonunion may eventually lead to this type of "fatigue" failure of implants [10].

When addressing a patient with instrumentation failure it is important to identify the underlying cause prior to considering any revision procedures. The patients' symptoms should correlate with this specific etiology because instrumentation failure can occur in the post-operative period independently of a successful outcome (Figs. 25.1 and 25.2).

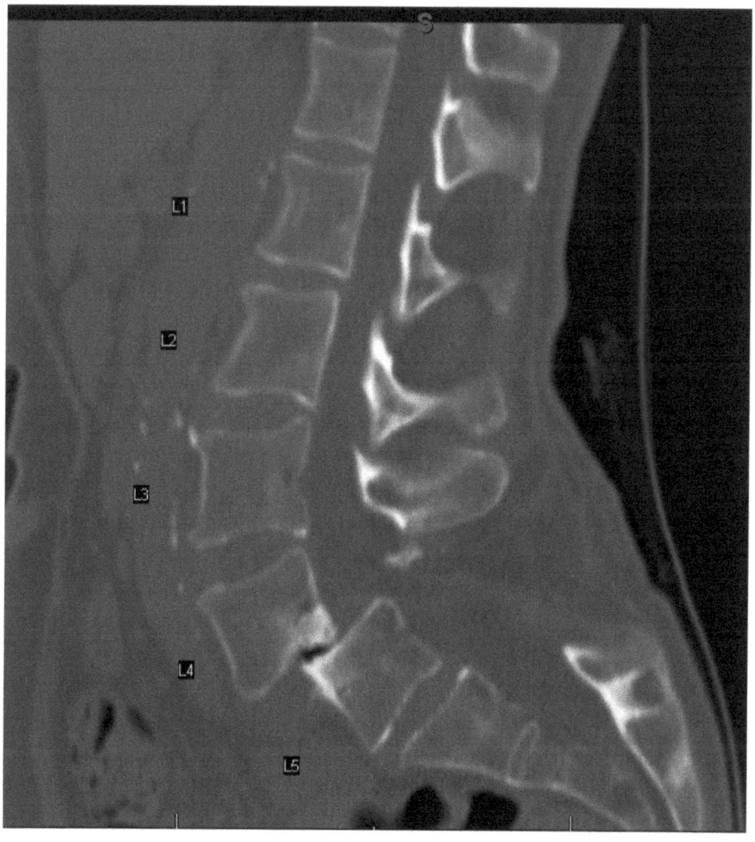

Fig. 25.1 Sixty-nine-year-old female with L4–5 spondylolisthesis and severe bilateral foraminal stenosis. She has complaints of bilateral lower extremity paresthesia and 4/5 weakness on exam

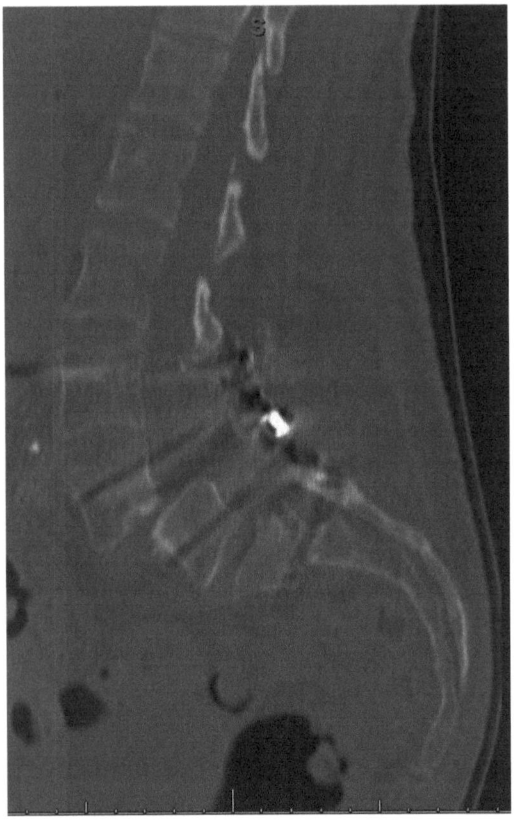

Fig. 25.2 Patient underwent L3–S1 decompression and posterior instrumented fusion with a successful outcome. Despite this, postoperatively the patient developed an acute grade II spondylolisthesis at S1–S2

Vascular

Vascular complications encountered during surgery for adult spondylolisthesis include pulmonary embolism, deep venous thrombosis, ischemic optic neuropathy, and direct vessel injury.

The prevalence of deep venous thrombosis formation is not well documented in the spine literature. Studies have shown mechanical prophylaxis decreases the rate of deep venous thrombosis formation from 10–15 % to 0.3–2 %. Risk factors for deep venous thrombosis formation to be aware of are prone positioning which compresses the femoral vessels, manipulation of great vessels during anterior approach, increased operative time, and prolonged post-operative recumbency which necessitates early ambulation with physical therapy [3].

Ischemic optic neuropathy is a rare but devastating complication of spine surgery that manifests as vision loss, which may or may not resolve over time. It is more common in spine surgery and estimated to occur approximately 0.2 % of the time. There are no patient demographics to help identify those at risk. It is common practice to introduce a slight amount of reverse Trendelenburg positioning for prone patients as this thought to decrease intraocular pressure [15].

Direct vessel injury may occur during spinal surgery can lead to excessive bleeding. Anterior approaches have a much higher incidence, especially at the L4–5 level as a result of the iliac bifurcation. When injury happens, it must be repaired immediately. Other sources of vessel injury may be from late erosion due to protruding implants. Postoperatively patients must be watched for abdominal and leg symptoms that could signify a vascular insufficiency.

Infection

Post-operative wound infections carry a significant morbidity and as a result surgeons need to maintain a high index of suspicion. Infections after instrumented spinal fusions have an incidence of 4–20 %. The most commonly involved organisms include coagulase-negative *Staphylococcus*, *S. aureus*, methicillin-resistant *S. aureus*, *Enterobacter*, *Pseudomonas*, and *Escherichia coli*. Patient risk factors to be identified preoperatively include advanced age, diabetes, obesity, smoking, and alcohol abuse [16, 17]. Infections can develop days to months postoperatively and typically present with various constitutional symptoms, persistent fever, pain, drainage from the wound, and erythema around the wound. Infections may be located either superficial or deep to the thoracolumbar fascia. Regardless, aggressive irrigation and debridement must be undertaken in the operating room, obtaining intra-operative cultures. Obtaining an infectious disease consult for appropriate antibiotic therapy is indicated. Patients with instrumented fusions it may be necessary to leave the instrumentation in place until the fusion occurs. It may be necessary to place the patient on suppressive, long-term antibiotic therapy while the fusion occurs with eventual removal of instrumentation to eradicate the infection.

Summary

The preceding chapter describes the most common complications encountered during the management and surgical treatment of adult spondylolisthesis. While it is comprehensive, it is by no means all-inclusive. Complications occur despite the surgeons' best efforts, as such, it is imperative to have a solid understanding of their evaluation and management. Early and aggressive intervention should be undertaken if a complication is suspected, including patient counseling, to ensure a successful outcome.

References

1. Boxall D, Bradford DS, Winter RB, Moe JH. Management of severe spondylolisthesis in children and adolescents. J Bone Joint Surg Am. 1979;61(4):479–95.
2. Sansur CA, Reames DL, Smith JS, Hamilton DK, Berven SH, et al. Morbidity and mortality in the surgical treatment of 10,242 patients with spondylolisthesis. J Neurosurg Spine. 2010;13:589–93.
3. Ogilvie JW. Complications in spondylolisthesis surgery. Spine. 2005;30(6S):S97–101.
4. Lenke LG, Bridwell KH, Bullis D, et al. Results of in situ fusion for isthmic spondylolisthesis. J Spinal Disord. 1992;5:433–42.
5. Rothman RH, Booth R. Failures of spinal fusion. Orthop Clin North Am. 1975;6(1):299–304.
6. Bradford DS, Boachie-Adjci O. Treatment of severe spondylolisthesis by anterior and posterior reduction and stabilization: a long-term follow-up study. J Bone Joint Surg Am. 1999;72(7):1060–6.
7. Lee C, Dorcil J, Radomisli TE. Nonunion of the spine: a review. Clin Orthop. 2004;419:71–5.
8. Raizman NM, O'Brien JR, Poehling-Monaghan KL, Yu WD. Pseudoarthrosis of the spine. J Am Acad Orthop Surg. 2009;17:494–503.
9. Shelby MD, Clark SR, Hall DJ, Freeman BJ. Radiographic assessment of spinal fusion. J Am Acad Orthop Surg. 2012;20:694–703.
10. Zeni A, Lubicky JP. Complications of sponylolysis/spondylolisthesis surgery. In: DeWald RL, Bridwell KH, editors. The textbook of spinal surgery. 3rd ed. Philadelphia: Lippincott Williams & Wilkins; 2011. p. 701–7.
11. Transfeldt FR, Dendrinos GK, Bradford DS. Paresis of proximal lumbar roots after reduction of L5–S1 spondylolisthesis. Spine. 1989;14(8):884–7.
12. Seitsalo S, Osterman K, Hyvarinen H, et al. Progression of spondylolisthesis in children and adolescents: a long-term follow-up of 272 patients. Spine (Phila Pa 1976). 1991;16(4):417–21.
13. Bridwell KH. Load sharing principles: the role and use of anterior structural support in adult deformity. Instr Course Lect. 1996;45:109–15.
14. McAfee PC, Weiland DJ, Carlow JJ. Survivorship analysis of pedicle spinal instrumentation. Spine. 1991;16(8 suppl):S422–7.
15. Pierce V, Kendrick P. Ischemic optic neuropathy after spine surgery. AANA J. 2010;78(2):141–5.
16. DeWald RL, Faut MM, Taddonio RF, et al. Severe lumbosacral spondylolisthesis in adolescents and children: reduction and staged circumferential fusion. J Bone Joint Surg Am. 1981;63(4):619–26.
17. Sailhan F, Gollogly S, Roussouly R, et al. Treatment of severe spondylolisthesis in adolescence with reduction and fusion of high-grade spondylolisthesis without decompression of the neural elements: a retrospective review of 44 patients. Spine. 2006;31(2):161–9.

Complications Associated with Surgical Treatment of Pediatric Spondylolisthesis

26

Dana Olszewski and Daniel J. Sucato

Introduction

Pediatric postsurgical populations are unique in their propensity to heal. They are also generally healthy patients with rare comorbidities when compared with their adult counterparts [1]. Unfortunately, there is no guarantee that the postoperative course of pediatric patients will remain entirely free of complications and they are sometimes afflicted with the same troubling consequences as adult patients. The definition of a complication is a "secondary condition that develops in the course of a primary disease or condition and arises either as a result of it or from independent causes" [2]. Obviously the easiest way to prevent operative complications is not to proceed down the surgical route at all. It is with this thought in mind that all surgical interventions should be approached in order to highlight the possible undesired outcomes and avoid unnecessary surgery.

D. Olszewski, M.D., M.P.H.
Department of Pediatric Orthopaedics,
Texas Scottish Rite Hospital, 2222 Welborn Street,
Dallas, TX 75219, USA
e-mail: dana.olszewski@tsrh.org

D.J. Sucato, M.D., M.S. (✉)
Department of Orthopaedic Surgery,
University of Texas at Southwestern Medical Center,
Texas Scottish Rite Hospital, 2222 Welborn Street,
Dallas, TX 75230, USA
e-mail: dan.sucato@tsrh.org

Children and adolescents diagnosed with spondylolisthesis, while usually healthy, oftentimes have significant preoperative deformity that requires aggressive surgical interventions. High-grade spondylolisthesis, for example, necessitates a reduction as part of the management and this carries a greater likelihood of surgical complications [3]. There are varying reports, from 10 to 47 %, of overall complication rates for spondylolisthesis surgery [3, 4]. Spondylolisthesis is distinguished from other spinal operations by the many options deemed appropriate for optimal surgical management and the specific negative sequelae that may follow.

In order to fully evaluate this patient population and their potential complications, we should remember several key questions. What are the complications that we most commonly see and how do they occur? Is there a specific patient or procedure that seems to have a higher rate of a particular complication? And perhaps the most important question, what can we do to prevent the complication from occurring?

General

There are some complications associated with surgery that occur in postoperative patients, irrespective of their type of surgery. After spinal surgery, infection can present with erythema, wound

A.L. Wollowick and V. Sarwahi (eds.), *Spondylolisthesis: Diagnosis, Non-Surgical Management, and Surgical Techniques*, DOI 10.1007/978-1-4899-7575-1_26,

dehiscence, increased drainage, pain, or a pseudoarthrosis. A septic and more emergent patient will present with constitutional symptoms such as a fever or chills, confusion, or lethargy.

The latest data from the Scoliosis Research Society (SRS) morbidity and mortality database define a 1.6 % infection incidence following spondylolisthesis surgery. This is equal to the average infection rate for all spine procedures but lower than the 2.1 % reported following scoliosis surgery [5]. Patients undergoing lumbar spine arthrodesis were found to have a 2.6 % rate of surgical site infection per Koutsoumbelis et al. There were four reported predictors of infection including increased intraoperative time and blood loss, incidental durotomy, and more than ten people being present in the operating room [6]. In general, the reported infection rate varies in the literature from 0 to 12 % [3, 7, 8]. Fu et al. reported a 1.2 % superficial infection and 0.8 % deep infection rate when looking at 605 patients [3].

The isolated pathogen in an acute surgical site infection is most commonly found to be Staphylococcus aureus, with methicillin resistant species increasing in prevalence [6, 9]. However, others have reported less commonly reported organisms in the setting of delayed infections. Vialle et al. reported on 40 patients status post surgery for high-grade spondylolisthesis in which five late infections (12 %) were identified. Of these five, cultures showed Escherichia coli to be the culprit in three cases, Staphylococcus aureus in one, and no bacteria was identified in the remaining patient. The high infection rate was thought to be secondary to the extensive dissection required for the double plate technique. Due to the high infection rate, double plating technique was not recommended.

In general most patients are given Ancef as a prophylactic antibiotic. A newer concept in infection prophylaxis is local administration of antibiotic powder to the wound and/or bone graft as an adjunct at the time of wound closure [10]. In a large series by Sweet et al. there was a 2.6 % infection rate for patients who were given cephalexin exclusively, however, this decreased to 0.2 % when 2 g of Vancomycin powder was added to patient's spinal wounds intraoperatively. This decrease was statistically significant ($p<0.0001$) [11]. Due to the decreased infection rate and lack of complications associated with vancomycin powder administration, we have adopted this as a standard practice for our patients.

In order to evaluate the extent of a postsurgical infection, advanced imaging may be helpful. Radiographs fail to show pertinent detail unless there is a latent infection, while Bone scan is limited by inability to differentiate between inflammation/postsurgical changes and infection. Gadolinium enhanced magnetic resonance imaging (MRI) is considered by many to be the gold standard for infection diagnosis [9]. MRI should be evaluated by a musculoskeletal radiologist to distinguish infection from normal postsurgical changes; rim enhancement being a specific finding confirming an infectious process. However presence of implants can degrade the quality of images due to artifacts. Computed tomography (CT) scan may be helpful in assessing the bony architecture and implant placement, but radiation is a concern.

In addition to imaging, laboratory work should be obtained including white blood cell count, erythrocyte sedimentation rate, C-reactive protein, and blood cultures. The first three are oftentimes repeated throughout the treatment course to ensure a downward trend in the values as supportive evidence that the treatment is working.

The management of spinal infections includes irrigation and debridement as well as intravenous antibiotics. Cultures are taken intraoperatively and antibiotic regimens are decided on the bacterial sensitivity. Infectious disease service is preferably involved in the management. If the cultures are negative, antibiotics are dosed according to the most common hospital wide postsurgical pathogens. Recommendations for duration of treatment vary based on the pathogen with most reports suggesting 6 weeks of antibiotics and increasing this to 8 weeks if MRSA is discovered [9].

Implant removal can be carried out for infections presenting late, especially when the fusion appears solid. Vialle et al. reported on removal of the instrumentation occurred in four of the five infected patients for delayed infections. None of their patients had a loss of correction.

Table 26.1 Postsurgical spondylolisthesis complications

Study	Method	GI	Neuro	Infection	Implant	Pseudoarthrosis
Vaille et al. [8]	Dual plating	2/40 (8 %)	12/40 (30 %)	5/40 (12 %)	9/40 (23 %)	0
Molinari et al. [7] (Group 1)	Posterior, no decompression	2/11 (18 %) (SMA)	0	0	NR	5/11 (45 %)
(Group 2)	Posterior, decompression	NR	2/7 (29 %)	0	2/7 (29 %)	2/7 (29 %)
(Group 3)	Circumferential, reduction	NR	2/19 (11 %)	1/19 (5 %)	2/19 (11 %)	0
Fu et al. [3]	All	NR	31/605 (5 %)	12/605 (2 %)	2/605 (0.3 %)	NR
Hu et al. [19]	Posterior, decompression	NR	4/16 (25 %)	NR	4/16 (25 %)	1/16 (6 %)

NR not reported

Experience with delayed infections in adolescent idiopathic scoliosis clearly defines the role of implant removal as an important part of successful treatment [12–14]. Acute infection is more challenging since complete fusion has not been achieved and rigid fixation with implants is necessary. Generally treatment consists of multiple irrigation and debridements until the wound is clean and final closure over drains followed by long-term antibiotics (6–10 weeks). The use of Wound VAC can help with wound closure in patients requiring multiple procedures. Recently, exchange of implants with titanium implants in patients with concern of lack of fusion or possible loss of correction has been reported. Experimental evidence indicates that titanium forms a thinner biofilm and has lower infection rate and may be more effective when attempting to clear infection [15].

As with any surgery, bleeding is a possibility and the amount varies significantly depending on several factors including, but not limited to the host, time spent in surgery, and the blood pressure maintained. One study looking at adult patients averaged a greater than 700 cc blood loss with 41 % of patients requiring a transfusion [16]. Pediatric patients, in contrast, have greater physiologic reserves when accommodating for blood loss. When hypotensive anesthesia is performed decreased blood flow can lead to other. There are rare reports of femoral head avascular necrosis occurring as a result of intraoperative hypotension [17]. All five hips in the three patients reported required total hip replacements for symptomatic relief.

No discussion of postsurgical complications is complete without postoperative urinary and gastrointestinal problems [18]. Vialle et al. reported on three out of 40 patients in their series, who had a small bowel obstruction presumed to be secondary to adhesions from transperitoneal approach [8]. Two patients required abdominal surgery for symptomatic resolution. In a small series examined by Molinari et al. 18 % of patients had superior mesenteric artery syndrome postoperatively due to casting. Another 8 % of patients in a different surgical subgroup, in their series, were found to have urinary retention for greater than 10 days. This resolved spontaneously within 2 weeks without the need for further intervention. Incidentally, these two patients had undergone a reduction of their listhesis. Overall, these concerns should always be discussed during informed surgical consent but are infrequent.

General reoperation rates vary and are typically reported in the literature according to the specific complication such as pseudarthrosis or instrumentation prominence. Cahill et al. grouped patients together and reported a reoperation rate of 37 %. Table 26.1 depicts the varying complication rates found in the literature by category.

A more sobering statistic is the mortality rate for all spine surgeries. Per the SRS database, there is a rate of 1.3 per 1,000 children who subsequently die after their operations [20]. This is an all encompassing number for spine surgeries and is not specific to spondylolisthesis procedures. When investigating operations for fixed sagittal deformities from the same database, there were three deaths (0.5 %) [21].

Pseudoarthrosis

Advancements in osteobiologics have improved fusion rates but pseudoarthrosis is still often times reported as the most common postoperative complication [4]. Rates vary from 0 to 45 % and are dependent on radiographic factors, patient factors, and surgical approaches [3, 7, 19, 22]. Molinari et al. reported that 16 % of their patients required repeat interventions for failure of fusion. The most common risk factors for pseudoarthrosis is a high-grade spondylolisthesis especially with significant kyphosis and when treated with a posterior fusion and instrumentation alone [23, 24] (Fig. 26.1). In order to evaluate for pseudoarthrosis, we look at three things: first is increased, second, is a defect in the fusion mass on XR or loss of reduction, and third is loss of fixation-implant breakage. If a robust fusion has occurred, radiographs may be sufficient for determining a diagnosis. Specifically, flexion and extension views will show instability at the vertebral segments in question and orthogonal views may assist in showing a gap in the bone formation in presence of nonunion. If in doubt, a CT scan may be helpful in assessing the fusion mass, particularly if utilizing metal subtraction techniques. Once the location of the pseudoarthrosis has been identified, an attempt should be made at determining the cause. If there is difficulty definitively diagnosing a pseudoarthrosis, the gold standard for identification is direct visualization in the operating room.

There are numerous reasons for the failure of fusion. The host may present a poor biologic platform for healing. Inadequate fixation may have been obtained or an infection may be present.

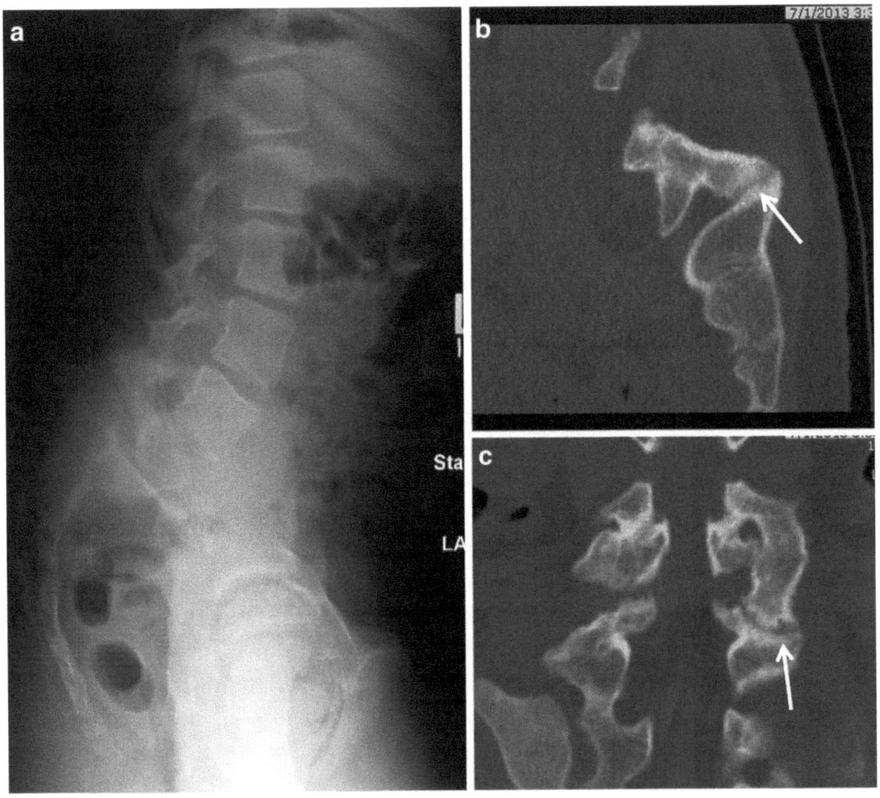

Fig. 26.1 Pseudoarthrosis of a high-grade spondylolisthesis. (**a**) The lateral radiograph of a patient 1 year following an in situ posterior spinal fusion through a Wiltse approach with continued pain. (**b**) The sagittal CT images demonstrating the pseudoarthrosis site (*arrow*). (**c**) Pseudoarthrosis depicted in coronal CT image (*arrow*)

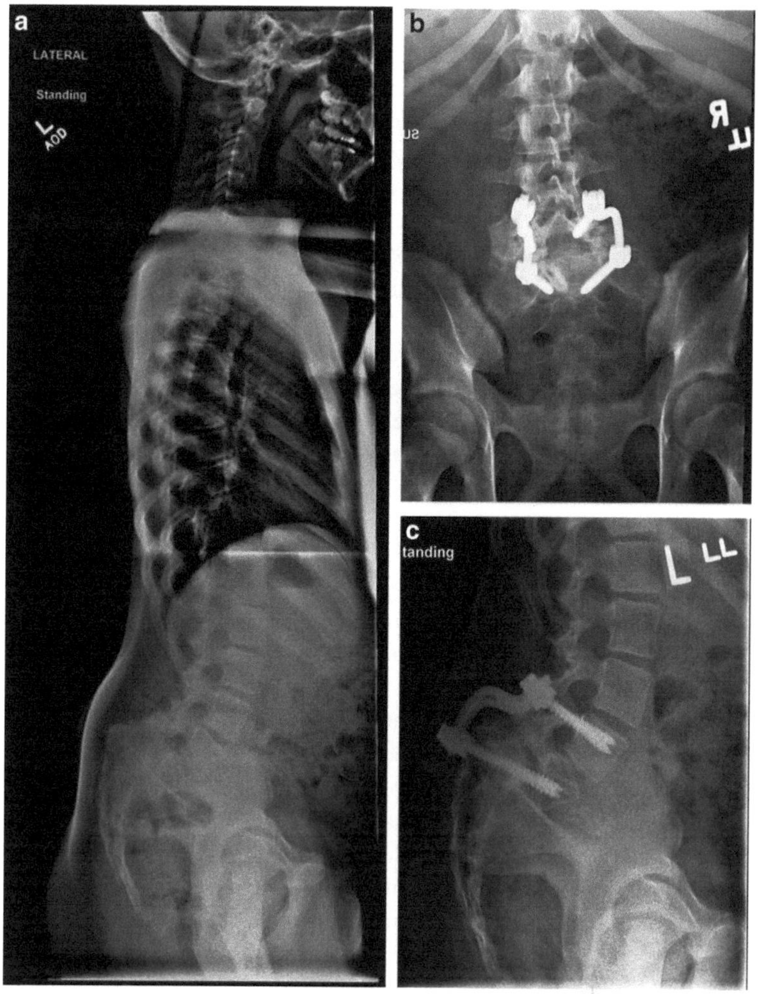

Fig. 26.2 (**a**) The lateral X-ray of the patient in Fig. 26.1 demonstrating overall excellent alignment. (**b**) The AP view (Ferguson view) and the (**c**) spot lateral of the patient after undergoing posterior instrumentation with pedicle screws at L4 and S1 and a Bohlman dowel graft from the sacrum to L5. The alignment has been maintained or slightly improved and a circumferential fusion has been done

Particular to the pediatric population, dysplastic L4 or L5 transverse processes create less potential surface area for fusion. Molinari et al. reported seven patients with a pseudoarthrosis after surgery for high-grade spondylolisthesis, all of whom had L5 transverse processes measuring less than 2 cm and averaging 1.6 cm. When compared with the group who had a solid fusion, the size difference in the transverse processes was determined to be statistically significant ($p=0.004$). In general, a thorough history and physical exam will aid in determining the underlying reason for pseudoarthrosis. Infection or nutrition labs may also assist in directing the surgeon to a specific diagnosis.

The treatment of a symptomatic pseudoarthrosis typically involves further surgical intervention. The explicit plan is detailed according to the diagnosis. For example, in the setting of an infection, irrigation and debridement is required prior to reattempting a fusion. The basic principle is to improve the rigidity of the construct and provide as much assistance to the biologic environment as is technically feasible. For those patients not infected, revision surgery is challenging but must include three basic principles: First, obtain adequate alignment to improve the degree of kyphosis present; second, obtain a circumferential fusion including anterior fusion through a formal anterior approach or via a transforaminal lumbar interbody fusion (TLIF) or posterolateral interbody fusion (PLIF); and finally, obtain stable, rigid fixation (Fig. 26.2).

Use of biologics to improve fusion and decrease pseudoarthrosis has its own complications. Rodgers et al. reported a case report where bone morphogenetic protein-2 (rhBMP2) was packed into an interbody cage at L4–5 level [25]. The patient developed a nonunion, which required revision surgery. It was during this second surgery that the left iliac vein was injured. The patient had an intraoperative cardiac arrest. The inflammatory reaction seen with the use of rhBMP-2 was believed to have caused the scarring and fibrosis surrounding the vessel making it more fragile during dissection. The patient subsequently healed without reported long-term affects.

Neurologic

Complications in this category vary from catastrophic neurologic compromise to resolving paresthesias from intraoperative positioning. According to the SRS database, neurologic deficits occur in 1.3 % of postoperative spondylolisthesis patients which is higher than that for all spine procedures, (1.1 %) but lower than that for scoliosis surgery (1.4 %) [5, 26]. The incidence of neurologic deficit is, in part, dependent on the procedure performed and should be a consideration when evaluating and determining treatment for these patients [27]. These numbers vary depending on the sampled patients and are found to be increased in patients with neuromuscular disorders [28]. Cahill et al. reported on 43 patients of which 5 (12 %) sustained a neurologic deficit. Four of the five patients had deficit at their final follow-up.

When specifically analyzing high-grade spondylolisthesis, there is an even higher rate of neurologic deficit identified in 15–30 % of patients [7, 19, 29]. Recovery most often occurs, with one study demonstrating 10 of 12 patients with complete recovery 18 months postoperatively [8]. Two had incomplete deficit of L5 with three out of five muscle strength in extensor hallucis longus.

Patients with high-grade spondylolisthesis who require a reduction have a complication rate that is nearly two times those who do not require a reduction [3]. While the burden of disease is an important underlying factor, the positioning of the patient on the table is the first time point when an iatrogenic complication may occur. All bony prominences should be appropriately padded. The table pads should be evaluated on a regular basis for cracking or thinning. Patients are typically positioned prone with their lower extremities in maximum extension to allow for ease with the reduction (Fig. 26.3). This extension may place an increased pressure at the site of the anterior superior iliac spines and, by anatomical association, the lateral femoral cutaneous nerve. While resulting postoperative paresthesias are usually transient, parents and patients should be warned about this risk.

There are many theoretical reasons for the increased risk that occurs with a reduction of one vertebral body on another. Sailhan et al. separated the theories into four possibilities [30]. The first is direct pressure of the spinal cord that occurs during decompression and the second is direct pressure on the nerve roots. After or during the reduction tension on the extradural nerves is another factor, while an extruded disc that with extension of the vertebral column, leads to volume reduction of the spinal canal is also a potential factor. Fu et al. reported that 10 % of patients who underwent a reduction ultimately suffered a neurologic deficit in contrast to only 2 % of patients who did not undergo a reduction [3].

Delayed neurologic deficits can also occur. Cahill et al. reported 33 % (4/12) of patients with a neurologic complication occurring several days after surgery during mobilization when early extension of the hips and knees may result in nerve stretch. Sailhan suggested a postoperative protocol to decrease possibility of nerve stretch by flexing hips and knees using pillows in the immediate postoperative period and then gradually extending the hips under careful physical examination [30]. Over the ensuing days, patient's lower extremities should be placed in more extension unless radicular pain or weakness occurred.

One unique deficit that is specific (but not exclusive) to spondylolisthesis surgery is an L5 nerve root stretch presenting as a foot drop or ankle dorsiflexion weakness with a rate between 5 and 35 % Although not completely understood, two different mechanisms may be in play, the first

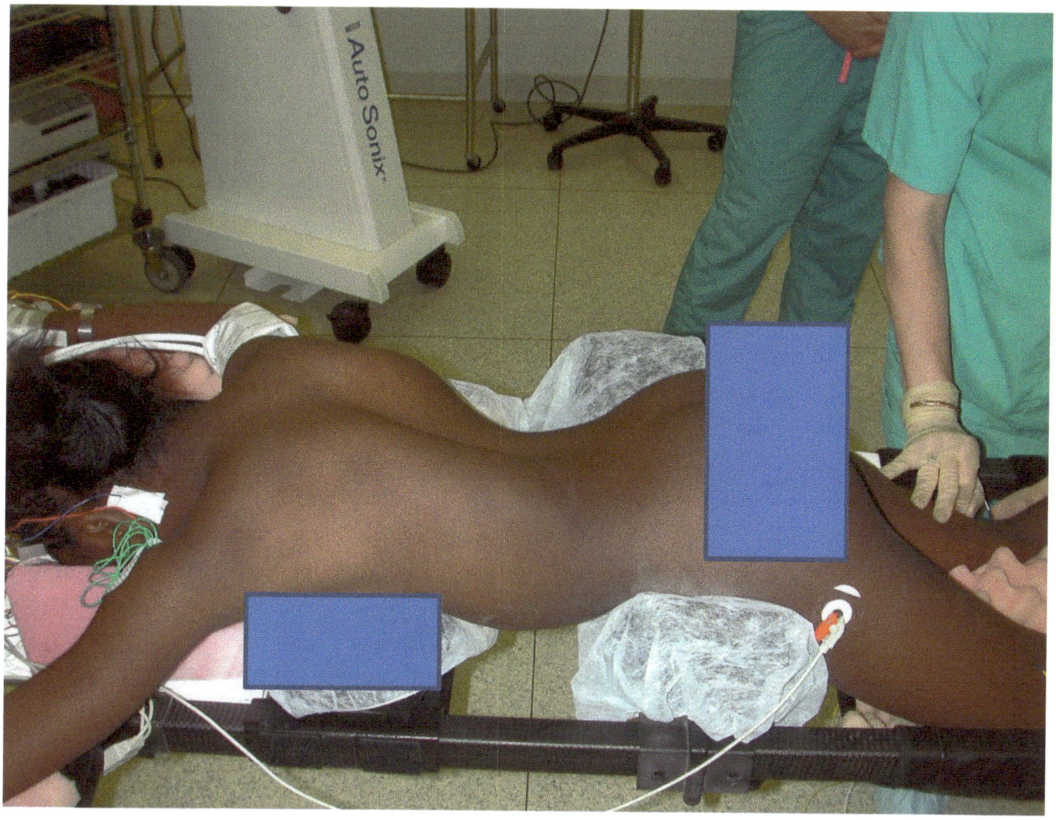

Fig. 26.3 Positioning on the OSI table for a posterior spinal approach for a spondylolisthesis. The anterior pads are placed on the anterior superior iliac spine distally to allow for the abdomen to be free and the hips to be extended while the proximal pads are placed distal enough to allow room in the axilla

is the inability to visualize the L5 nerve roots which are often deep and difficult to identify. Chen et al. reported on three out of 118 patients who had L5 nerve root injury [16]. Two were due to poor visualization. They concluded that complete exposure and hemostasis were critical factors in avoiding this complication. The second mechanism is excessive tension on the nerve root which may be due to either inadequate decompression and/or excessive reduction of the L5 vertebral body [31] (Fig. 26.4). Shufflebarger et al. reported on 25 patients undergoing surgery for spondylolisthesis at an average age of 13.5 years. Eleven of the 25 patients were found to have postoperative motor deficits, ten of whom had an L5 stretch injury [18]. All of these were found to have completely resolved within 3 months.

In addition to intraoperative and postoperative positioning, avoiding deficits of the L5 nerve root is dependent on a good decompression of the L5 nerve root at the time of surgery. Following removal of the posterior elements, the L5 nerve roots need to be identified and traced out laterally past the sacral ala to free up the roots and allow for reduction without tension (Fig. 26.5). The nerve roots should be visualized at all times especially during direct placement of the L5 pedicle screws and during the reduction maneuver.

Cauda equina syndrome was first described in association with lumbosacral spondylolisthesis in 1961. In 1990, Schoenecker et al. compiled a series of 12 patients who developed cauda equina syndrome following an in situ posterior arthrodesis [32]. Preoperatively all of these patients had either a Grade III or IV spondylolisthesis and 8 of the 12 patients had subtle abnormal preoperative physical exam findings such as decreased knee reflexes. Five of the 12 cases had

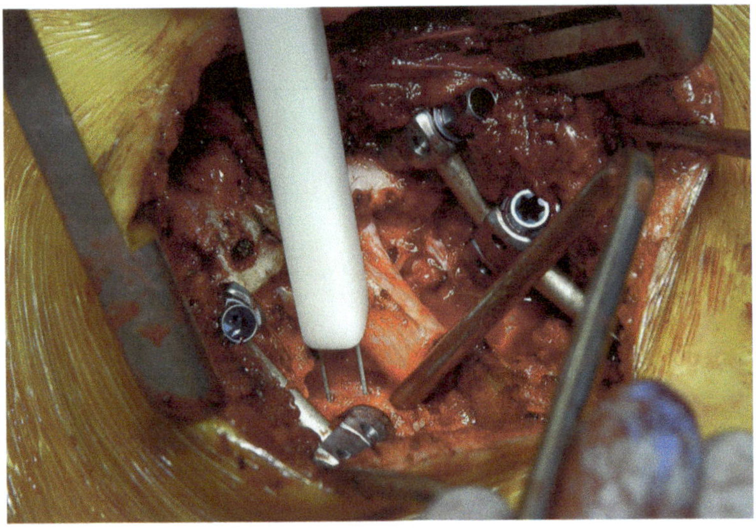

Fig. 26.4 Direct nerve stimulation of the L5 nerve root at the completion of the reduction of L5. The voltage necessary to elicit a response was similar to the baseline stimulation so it was thought that there would be a low likelihood for a neurologic deficit. The patient awoke without any deficits

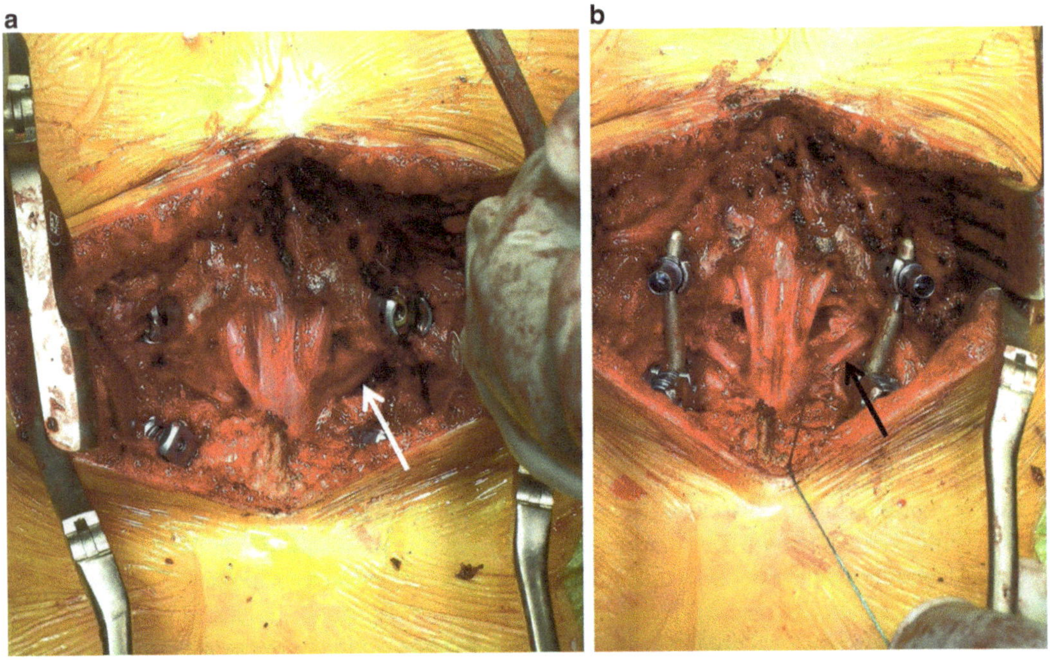

Fig. 26.5 Dissection of the L5 nerve roots. (**a**) The L4 and S1 screws are placed, and a PLIF approach allows for removal of the disc at L5–S1. The L5 nerve roots can be seen travelling out laterally past the sacral ala. (**b**) The same picture after the L5 screws have been placed under direction visualization to ensure the L5 nerve root is seen while the screws are placed. The reduction has been performed and the tension on the L5 nerve has been assessed throughout this reduction maneuver

complete resolution of their symptoms. The authors concluded that if there was the possibility of preoperative sacral compromise as demonstrated by some subtle neurologic findings, decompression of the nerve roots and sacral dome osteotomy should be considered rather than pure in situ fusion. This remains a rare occurrence and most reports, even with isolated in situ fusion, have not reported any cases of cauda equina syndrome.

Instrumentation

A misplaced screw may result in pain or a neurologic deficit and require further surgical intervention. Gundanna et al. reported on 186 patients, five patients had a new onset radiculopathy postoperatively [33]. Further imaging identified 8 malaligned screws. After removal or revision of all malaligned screws, the radicular pain completely resolved in all cases. Care should be taken during the placement of screws. Flouroscopy may be used as needed.

Other causes of implant problems include screw breakage or pullout. Poor host bone quality may lead to an increased risk of the screws backing out. A pseudoarthrosis due to infectious or biologic reasons may also be the cause of breakage or pullout.

Migration of cage may occur during compression to restore lordosis or may be due to inadequate fixation or inappropriate cage size (Fig. 26.6). Cages should be rigid enough to withstand the axial forces induced during normal motion in a patient but porous enough to allow for ingrowth. In a study by Chen et al. 4 out of 118 patients (3.3 %) had either subsidence or migration of a cage postoperatively [16]. All four of the patients required further surgery to achieve adequate fusion mass. The two cages that migrated were both found to be in a retropulsed position.

Molinari et al. provided a review of spondylolisthesis complications based on three different patient groups, separated according to their mode of fixation [7]. Group one consisted of patients who underwent in situ posterior fusion from L4 to the sacrum without undergoing decompression or instrumentation. Group two patients had a posterior fusion but hardware was now utilized for fixation. The third group of patients had a posterior decompression, reduction, instrumentation, and circumferential fusion. Patients who had a reduction experienced the greatest rates of instrumentation breakage or pullout. Two of the 19 patients in Group 3 subsequently had failure of their hardware. One patient experienced pullout of undersized screws and the second had failure of fixation distally resulting in a partial loss of reduction. The latter patient did not require further surgical intervention. Instrumentation is not beneficial when there is a failure to achieve adequate fixation. Hu et al. suggested obtaining tricortical S1 fixation or supplemental fixation in the S2 vertebral body may aid in eliminating this instrumentation problem [19]. McCord et al. reported that fixation into the ilium was the most stable construct when compared with nine other methods of fixation [34].

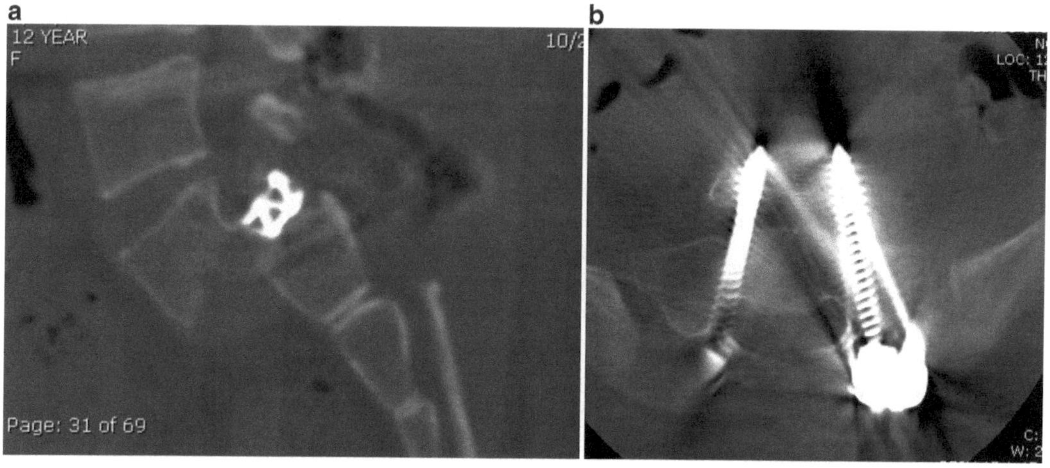

Fig. 26.6 Implant challenges for high-grade spondylolisthesis. (**a**) The anterior cage has migrated postoperatively resulting in some mild motor deficits. The patient returned to the operating room for removal of the cage. (**b**) Right L5–S1 screw is travelling medial

Approach Specific

There are several complications that are specific to the various surgical approaches that can be undertaken. With the anterior approach, there is the risk of retrograde ejaculation, dysuria, dyspareunia, and insufficient reduction and fixation [30, 35]. While it has been noted as a risk in adult male patients undergoing a transperitoneal approach, retrograde ejaculation seems to be more of a theoretical risk in the pediatric patient population. Frymoyer reported on a survey of surgeons from around the world and found a 0.42 % rate in patients who underwent an anterior lumbar interbody fusion [36]. Vaille et al. reported that, of the 15 male patients who underwent an anterior approach, there were no accounts of retrograde ejaculation [8]. Sailhan et al. reported that there was an increased risk of a loss of reduction postoperatively when a combined anterior and posterior approach was completed [30]. This was thought to be in part due to the greater risk of destabilization that occurs with disc removal between L5 and S1. This loss of reduction is typically identified within the first few months, prior to fusion occurring.

As was mentioned previously, a pure posterior approach can lead to an increase in the rate of pseudoarthrosis. An increase in the slip progression has also been seen when the posterior elements are removed [37].

Special Situations

Preoperative traction is written about more as a historical note now rather than a current reality. In the past, it was used as an adjunctive therapy to create a more favorable environment for closed reduction prior to posterior arthrodesis. Bradford reported two of six patients with resultant L5 radiculopathy after undergoing preoperative traction [38]. The improvements in instrumentation have made this an obsolete path for most surgeons.

Dural tears producing CSF leak are most frequently seen in lumbosacral spinal surgery [39]. Per the SRS M&M database, this is the most common complication of fixed sagittal plane deformity surgery at a rate of 5.9 % [21]. Dural tears have varying rates of occurrence and also seem to be dependent on the method of instrumentation. Chen et al. reported a 3.4 % rate of dural tears after performing posterior lumbar interbody fusions and found a direct correlation between the size of the cage and the rate of dural tears [16]. Most cases occurred during preparation for or insertion of the cage. Dural tears even superficial tears, that are noted during surgery but do not result in a cerebrospinal fluid leak, should be repaired. This is due to the risk of rupture postoperatively of the residual intact membranes during a valsalva maneuver. Dural tears should be taken seriously as leakage of cerebrospinal fluid may result in a pseudomeningocele or a meningocutaneous fistula, either of which may result in an infection or neurologic compromise.

Postoperative symptoms may include nausea, vomiting, a headache, dizziness, or clear wound drainage. The patient should initially be placed on bed rest. The duration of bed rest has not been standardized. Caffeine may assist in relieving headaches. Nonoperative management of dural tears may be attempted with the assistance of a drain. However, the management of these tears optimally consists of a primary repair. Adequate visualization is a necessity. The literature has not shown one particular suture type or method of closure to be superior. Fat grafts, fibrin glue, collagen matrix, a venous blood patch, and hydrogels have also all been attempted in order to create a water tight seal. While primary repair remains as the gold standard, there is a 5–10 % failure rate [39]. Therefore a combination of measures may be helpful in achieving complete resolution of this problem. The adjunct to primary repair is currently an evolving area and surgeon preference is an important factor.

Conclusion

Pediatric spondylolisthesis, due to the intricacies of both pathology and treatment, is an orthopedic problem that requires supervision by a physician trained in this area of subspecialization.

With proper precautions and knowledge of the deformity and anatomy, surgical management of spondylolisthesis can be a safe intervention. Education regarding the most common complications, how to avoid them, and what to warn patients and families about, is crucial.

References

1. Kalanithi PS, Patil CG, Boakye M. National complication rates and disposition after posterior lumbar fusion for acquired spondylolisthesis. Spine (Phila Pa 1976). 2009;34:1963–9.
2. Websters dictionary.
3. Fu K, Smith J, Polly D, Perra J, Sansur C, Berven S, et al. Morbidity and mortality in the surgical treatment of six hundred five pediatric patients with isthmic or dysplastic spondylolisthesis. Spine (Phila Pa 1976). 2011;36:308–12.
4. Cahill PJ, Samdani A, Smith J, Finlayson C, Marvil SC, Tantorski ME, Hammerberg K, Asghar J, Betz RR, Sturm PF. Complication rates in pediatric spondylolisthesis surgery: a dual center 16 year retrospective review. Scientific presentation at SRS, 23–26 September 2009.
5. Coe. SRS morbidity and mortality report. 2003.
6. Koutsoumbelis S, Hughes AP, Girardi FP, Cammisa FP, Finerty EA, Nguyen JT, Gausden E, Sama AA. Risk factors for postoperative infection following posterior lumbar instrumented arthrodesis. J Bone Joint Surg Am. 2011;93:1627–33.
7. Molinari R, Bridwell K, Lenke L, Ungacta F, Riew D. Complications in the surgical treatment of pediatric high-grade, isthmic dysplastic spondylolisthesis. Spine (Phila Pa 1976). 1999;24:1701–11.
8. Vialle R, Charosky S, Padovani JP, Rigault P, Glorion C. Surgical treatment of high grade lumbosacral spondylolisthesis in childhood, adolescent and young adult by the "double-plate" technique: a past experience. Eur Spine J. 2006;15:1210–8.
9. Hegde V, Meredith DS, Kepler CK, Huang RC. Management of postoperative spinal infections. World J Orthop. 2012;18:182–9.
10. American Academy of Orthopaedics. Recommendations for the use of intravenous antibiotic prophylaxis in primary total joint arthroplasty. Information Statement 1027. June 2004. www.aaos.org.
11. Sweet FA, Roh M, Sliva C. Intrawound application of vancomycin for prophylaxis in instrumented thoracolumbar fusions. Spine (Phila Pa 1976). 2011;36:2084–8.
12. Richards BS, Emara KM. Delayed infections after posterior TSRH spinal instrumentation for idiopathic scoliosis: revisited. Spine (Phila Pa 1976). 2001;26: 1990–6.
13. Hedequist D, Haugen A, Hresko T, et al. Failure of attempted implant retention in spinal deformity delayed surgical site infections. Spine (Phila PA 1976). 2009;34:60–4.
14. Kim HJ, Cunningham ME, Boachie-Adjei O. Revision spine surgery to manage pediatric deformity. J Am Acad Orthop Surg. 2010;18:739–48.
15. Glotzbecker MP, Riedel MD, Vitale MG, et al. What's the evidence? Systematic literature review of risk factors and preventive strategies for surgical site infection following pediatric spine surgery. J Pediatr Orthop. 2013;33:479–87.
16. Chen L, Tang T, Yang H. Complications associated with posterior lumbar interbody fusion using Bagby and Kuslich method for treatment of spondylolisthesis. Chin Med J. 2003;116(1):99–103.
17. Orpen N, Walker G, Fairlie N, Coghill S, Birch N. Avascular necrosis of the femoral head after surgery for lumbar spinal stenosis. Spine (Phila Pa 1976). 2003;28(18):E364–7.
18. Shufflebarger H, Geck M. High grade isthmicdysplastic spondylolisthesis: monosegmental surgical treatment. Spine (Phila Pa 1976). 2005;30:S42–9.
19. Hu SS, Bradford DS, Transfeldt EE, Cohen M. Reduction of high grade spondylolisthesis using Edwards instrumentation. Spine (Phila Pa 1976). 1996;21:367–71.
20. Smith JS, Saulle D, Chen C, Lenke L, Polly D, Kasliwal M, et al. Rates and causes of mortality associated with spine surgery based on 108,419 procedures. Spine (Phila Pa 1976). 2012;37:1975–82.
21. Smith JS, Sansur CA, Donaldson 3rd WF, Perra JH, Mudiyam R, Choma TJ, Zeller RD, et al. Short-term morbidity and mortality associated with correction of thoracolumbar fixed sagittal plane deformity: a report from the Scoliosis Research Society Morbidity and Mortality Committee. Spine (Phila Pa 1976). 2011;36: 958–64.
22. Burkus JK, Lonstein JE, Winter RB, Denis F. Long-term evaluation of adolescents treated operatively for spondylolisthesis. A comparison of in situ arthrodesis only with in situ arthrodesis and reduction followed by immobilization in a cast. J Bone Joint Surg. 1992;74:693–704.
23. Muschik M, Zippel H, Perka C. Surgical management of severe spondylolisthesis in children and adolescents. Anterior fusion in situ versus anterior spondylodesis with posterior transpedicular instrumentation and reduction. Spine (Phila Pa 1976). 1997;22(17): 2036–42. discussion 43.
24. Newton PO, Johnston 2nd CE. Analysis and treatment of poor outcomes following in situ arthrodesis in adolescent spondylolisthesis. J Pediatr Orthop. 1997; 17(6):754–61.
25. Rodgers SD, Marascalchi BJ, Grobelny BT, Smith ML, Samadani U. Revision surgery after interbody fusion with rhBMP-2: a cautionary tale for spine surgeons. J Neurosurg Spine. 2013;18(6):582–7.
26. Hamilton DK, Smith JS, Sansur CA, Glassman SD, Ames CP, Berven SH, Polly Jr DW, Perra JH, Knapp DR, Boachie-Adjei O, McCarthy RE, Shaffrey CI. Scoliosis Research Society Morbidity and Mortality Committee. Rates of new neurological deficit associated with spine surgery based on 108,419 procedures: a report of the scoliosis research society

morbidity and mortality committee. Spine (Phila Pa 1976). 2011;36:1218–28.

27. Smith J, Deviren V, Berven S, Kleinstueck F, Bradford D. Clinical outcome of trans-sacral interbody fusion after partial reduction for high-grade L5–S1 spondylolisthesis. Spine (Phila Pa 1976). 2001;26:2227–34.
28. Reames DL, Smith JS, Fu KM, Polly Jr DW, Ames CP, Berven SH, Perra JH, Glassman SD, McCarthy RE, Knapp Jr RD, Heary R, Shaffrey CI, Scoliosis Research Society Morbidity and Mortality Committee. Complications in the surgical treatment of 19,360 cases of pediatric scoliosis: a review of the Scoliosis Research Society Morbidity and Mortality database. Spine (Phila Pa 1976). 2011;36:1484–91.
29. Maurice HD, Morley TR. Cauda equina lesions following fusion in situ and decompressive laminectomy for severe spondylolisthesis: four case reports. Spine (Phila Pa 1976). 1989;14:214–6.
30. Sailhan F, Gollogly S, Roussouly P. The radiographic results and neurologic complications of instrumented reduction and fusion of high-grade spondylolisthesis without decompression of the neural elements: a retrospective review of 44 patients. Spine (Phila Pa 1976). 2006;31:161–9.
31. Petraco DM, Spivak JM, Cappadona JG, et al. An anatomic evaluation of L5 nerve stretch in spondylolisthesis reduction. Spine (Phila Pa 1976). 1996;21: 1133–8.
32. Schoenecker PL, Cole HO, Herring JA, Capelli AM, Bradford DS. Cauda equine syndrome after in situ arthrodesis for severe spondylolisthesis at the lumbosacral junction. J Bone Joint Surg. 1990;72(3):369–77.
33. Gundanna M, Eskenazi M, Bendo J, Spivak J, Moskovich R. Somatosensory evoked potential monitoring of lumbar pedicle screw placement for in situ posterior spinal fusion. Spine J. 2003;3(5):370–6.
34. McCord DH, Cunningham BW, Shono Y, Meyers JJ, McAfee PC. Biomechanical analysis of lumbosacral fixation. Spine (Phila Pa 1976). 1992;17:235–43.
35. Laursen M, Thomsen K, Eiskjaer SP, Hansen ES, Bunger CE. Functional outcome after partial reduction and 360 degree fusion in grade III–V spondylolisthesis in adolescent and adult patients. J Spinal Disord. 1999;12(4):300–6.
36. Frymoyer JW, Wiesel SW. The adult and pediatric spine. Philadelphia: Lippincott Williams and Wilkins Review; 2004. p. 415.
37. Seitsalo S, Osterman K, Hyvarinen H, Schlenzka D, Poussa M. Severe spondylolisthesis in children and adolescents. A long-term review of fusion in situ. J Bone Joint Surg. 1990;72(2):259–65.
38. Bradford DS. Closed reduction of spondylolisthesis: an experience in 22 patients. Spine (Phila Pa 1976). 1988;13:580–7.
39. Espiritu M, Rhyne A, Darden B. Dural tears in spinal surgery. J Am Acad Orthop Surg. 2010;18:537–45.

27 Intraoperative Neuro-Monitoring During Spondylolisthesis Surgery

Jahangir K. Asghar and Harry L. Shufflebarger

Electrophysiologic monitoring during spinal deformity is the standard of care in 2013.

With over 30 years employment in scoliosis surgery, there is no doubt that intraoperative neuro-monitoring (IONM) is the standard of care in the surgical management of spinal deformities and a similar statement can be made for most other aspects of spinal pathology [1, 2]. It is the authors' opinion that the development and maturation of the science and technology behind IONM has been fundamental in the evolution of modern spinal deformity surgery. Many of the currently utilized techniques for deformity releases and correction are only safe in the presence of reliable spinal cord monitoring. A number of studies have found that IONM is a highly sensitive and specific tool to recognize electrophysiologic changes at the level of the spinal cord [3–6].

Monitoring is not, however, without issues. Thuet et al. in 2010 authored a paper reviewing 3,400+ consecutively monitored pediatric patients; seven patients had changes in neurologic status that were not detected by multimodality protocols. 6 of the 7, including the only permanent deficit, were nerve root in origin. They argued that presently used nerve root monitoring methods are not sufficiently sensitive to detect all potential surgical risks. The inherently passive nature of spontaneous EMG monitoring may prevent assessment of changes in nerve root function because of indirect or insidious onset of stretch or compression [7, 8].

The literature describing the objective surgical outcomes for high-grade spondylolisthesis corroborates this finding with a seemingly high rate of transient and permanent neuropraxia. The incidence of transient neuropraxia may be as high as 25 % and permanent deficit may be up to 10 % based on surgical technique, severity, and approach [7]. This chapter will review several of the commonly used modalities for IONM and, also, present the authors' technique for using the multiple IONM modalities including triggered EMG of the nerve root to identify potential nerve root lesions secondary to compression and/or stretch during reduction and stabilization of spondylolisthesis.

Monitoring Modalities

Stagnara Wake-Up Test

Prior to the development and reliability of IONM, the only method to assess motor function during surgery was the Stagnara wake-up test, which

J.K. Asghar, M.D. • H.L. Shufflebarger, M.D. (✉)
Department of Orthopaedic Surgery,
Miami Children's Hospital, 3100 SW 62nd Ave,
Miami, FL 33155, USA
e-mail: jasghar01@gmail.com; hthook@aol.com

A.L. Wollowick and V. Sarwahi (eds.), *Spondylolisthesis: Diagnosis, Non-Surgical Management, and Surgical Techniques*, DOI 10.1007/978-1-4899-7575-1_27,

involved awakening patients intraoperative and demonstrated the ability to move the lower extremities. Although the gold standard, this technique has significant risks. It increases operative time, as it requires the cessation of all anesthetics until the patient has sufficient cognition to follow commands. Furthermore, the test lacks the obvious benefit of continuous assessment of neural function, and its use is limited in certain patients, such as those with cognitive or hearing deficits. It is difficult to grade weakness or identify sensory deficits. Finally, if the test is positive and the patient has sustained a deficit in extremity function, it is possible that a substantial period of time has elapsed between the injury, its detection, and the ultimate intervention. Despite its limitations and the advent of more sophisticated electrophysiologic testing, it remains a critical component of the intraoperative algorithm for electrophysiologic monitoring changes [6].

Somatosensory Evoked Potentials

Somatosensory evoked potentials (SSEPs) provide monitoring of the dorsal column-medial lemniscus pathway. These tracts mediate tactile discrimination, vibration sensation, form recognition, and conscious proprioception. Receptors generate information that correspond to these sensory modalities and relay signals to neuronal bodies located in dorsal root ganglia (DRG) at all spinal levels. SSEPs do not involve the spinothalamic (pain and temperature) pathway [4].

The axons from DRG project to the spinal cord give rise to the fasciculi gracilis and cuneatus, which carry the sensory information. These tracts ascend via the dorsal columns in the spinal cord. Following a decussation that occurs at the medullary level, it ascends to the thalamus and relays sensory information to the primary somatosensory cortex [9, 10].

In the upper extremities, the median nerve and ulnar nerve are frequently selected for monitoring. The posterior tibial nerve and peroneal nerve are typically used in the lower extremities stimulation of mixed sensory and motor fibers caudal to the region of the spinal cord at risk. Electrical stimulation in the extremities produces major positive and negative deflections as signals ascend via the somatosensory pathway. A negative potential measured at the scalp corresponds to the upper extremities at 20 ms (N20), and a positive potential measured at the scalp corresponds to the lower extremities at 37 ms (P37) [11].

A peripheral response recorded at the level of the brachial plexus (for the upper extremities) or the popliteal fossa (for the lower extremities) can be performed to ascertain adequacy of stimulation. These peripheral responses can also help to detect peripheral limb ischemia or nerve compression [8, 12, 13].

It is important to note that in the case of SSEPs, these earlier peaks tend to be less sensitive to anesthesia, and may therefore frequently be used to differentiate SSEP monitoring changes resulting from anesthetic effects from those relating to the surgical manipulation [14].

Alarm criteria of 50 % reduction in amplitude and/or 10 % increase in latency are usual guidelines for notifying the surgeon of a potential deficit, and corrective intervention should be considered if these changes correspond to a particular surgical manipulation. Factors that potentially affect the SSEP amplitude include halogenated agents, nitrous oxide, hypothermia, hypotension, and electrical interference. A common factor affecting SSEP latency readings is temperature [15]. Any SSEP changes with amplitude reduction of more than 50 % should also be considered relevant if they are temporally associated with a specific surgical intervention, such as during placement of spinal instrumentation or during correction of a spinal deformity [13, 16].

Nuwer et al. evaluated the clinical efficacy of intraoperative SSEP monitoring performed during scoliosis surgery in a large multicenter survey of 51,263 spinal surgeries. They reported an overall sensitivity of 92 % and specificity of 98.9 % in the ability of SSEPs to detect new postoperative neurological deficits [17]. Although SSEP signals are good indicators of spinal cord function, less information is provided regarding nerve root function. It is important to note, SSEPs are a composite of summated neural signals that enter the spinal cord through multiple segments. In addition, due to central amplification, it is possible for SSEPs to remain completely normal in the face of a nerve root injury [18–20].

Motor Evoked Potentials

As motor evoked potentials (MEPs) monitor function of the corticospinal tract, changes in MEPs are more sensitive in the detection of potential postoperative motor deficits. The corticospinal tract and dorsal columns lie in different vascular and anatomical territories, with the dorsal columns receiving the majority of perfusion via the posterior spinal arteries, and the lateral corticospinal tracts, the anterior corticospinal tracts, and the anterior horn cells receive the majority of their blood supply via the anterior spinal artery. Hence, it is possible to have significant spinal cord deficits that SSEPs alone would fail to demonstrate any alarm criteria. These caused by either direct mechanical trauma or vascular compromise of the corticospinal tracts [5, 21–23].

During scoliosis surgery, for example, small radiculomedullary arteries passing between the osseous rings of adjacent vertebrae may be stretched or compressed during correctional maneuvers, resulting in subsequent ischemia or infarction. If such an injury affects only the anterolateral funiculus, then postoperative motor deficits may occur without corresponding changes in SSEPs [24, 25].

During spine surgery, MEPs are stimulated trans-cranially (TcMEP). Trans-cranial stimulation can be performed either electrically or magnetically, with signal recording possible at the level of the muscle (compound muscle action potential), nerve (neurogenic MEP), or spinal cord (direct corticospinal wave [D-wave] recording).

Stimulation can also be performed in the spinal cord directly, with recording electrodes either in the nerve or the muscles. Although this technique offers the advantage of being less sensitive to anesthetic agents, responses obtained via direct spinal cord stimulation are less likely to represent motor function, but rather anti-dromic sensory responses [26, 27].

Common factors that may alter MEP wave form morphological characteristics include anesthetic fade, body temperature, blood pressure, surgical positioning, and technical pitfalls, among others. Although MEPs have become the gold standard for neuro-monitoring of the motor tracts, there are some disadvantages to MEP monitoring. The major drawback of MEP monitoring is the inability to perform continuous monitoring, requiring that MEPs be obtained intermittently during the surgery. Another inherent limitation of monitoring MEP signals is that they may be more technically challenging to obtain. If preoperative motor deficits exist at the time of surgery, the ability to obtain MEPs in the lower extremities is significantly lower [28, 29].

Anesthetic inhalants decrease the possible pool of motoneurons available for recruiting. Since the propagation of a peripheral motor response is effected, inhaled agents interfere with reliable MEP acquisition. Currently, total IV anesthesia (TIVA) is used, in which compounds such as nitrous oxide, volatile agents, and muscle relaxants are excluded, and short-acting agents such as fentanyl and propofol are relied upon to achieve anesthetic control. The use of TIVA offers clear benefits in obtaining MEPs over inhaled anesthetics. Even in cases in which TIVA is used, higher levels of propofol may cause suppression of motoneurons, a factor that should always be considered when interpreting MEP loss or amplitude reduction in this setting. There are several contraindications to MEP monitoring (i.e., Active Seizure disorder, VP shunt). They must always be weighed against the benefits provided by the technique. Although the technique is generally safe, tongue laceration (the most common complication) can occur due to forced contraction of facial muscles. Therefore, a bite block is mandatory [30–32].

Despite the potential anesthetic issues and contraindications, in the hands of an experienced anesthesia and neurophysiologic team, Kelleher et al. showed TcMEP had a 100 % sensitivity with 96 % specificity in cervico-thoracic spinal surgery [33].

Spontaneous EMG

Spontaneous EMG activity is used to monitor the corresponding nerve roots responsible for muscle innervation. This spontaneous motor activity can be measured with recording electrodes placed in the muscles of interest and based on the structures at risk. Although no stimulation is performed for this technique, surgical manipulation such as pulling, stretching, or compression of nerves produces neurotonic discharges resulting in activity in the corresponding innervated muscle(s). Specific muscles are normally paired with single nerve roots, yet in reality some redundancy in innervation occurs, and muscle selection should be made to maximize coverage based on the spinal level the surgeon will be working on. Spontaneous EMG tends to be quite sensitive to irritation of the nerve root due to retraction, irrigation, and manipulation during surgery. Relevant sEMG activity that is noted by neurophysiologists includes spikes, bursts, or trains [34].

During surgery, sEMG trains are of clinical significance, and the surgeon is typically notified if these occur. Trains are continuous, repetitive EMG firing caused by continuous force applied to the nerve root. Trains of higher frequency and/or amplitude tend to represent significant nerve fiber recruitment caused by excessive force on the nerve and are likely to indicate a high probability of nerve injury if a relevant manipulation is sustained. Spontaneous EMG spikes and bursts, on the other hand, often can inform the surgeon of proximity to the nerve root [35].

Not uncommonly, the electrodes will pick up interference from various sources that may be mistaken for spiking or training EMG activity. Sources of artifact responses picked up in the EMG window are cautery devices, electrocardiography leads, and high-speed drills. Anesthetic requirements for sEMG mandate that no paralytic agents are used, and that train-of-4 testing should indicate that at least 3 out of 4, if not 4 out of 4 twitches, be present for sEMG to be of value. It is also important to note that the underlying clinical condition of patients with various neurological disorders may interfere with the ability to acquire EMG signals. Muscular dystrophy is a classic example of neurological conditions that interfere with the acquisition of EMG signals [13, 36].

Triggered EMG

Triggered EMG is a method of active stimulation of the nerve root that was originally used to determine whether screws have breached the medial or inferior pedicle wall. When a pedicle screw is accurately placed, the surrounding bone acts as an insulator to electrical conduction, and a higher amount of electrical current is thus required to stimulate the surrounding nerve root. When a medial pedicle wall breach occurs, the stimulation threshold is significantly reduced [37, 38].

A monopolar electrode is used to directly stimulate the top of the pedicle screw at increasing current intensities. Needle electrodes in the appropriate muscle groups will measure CMAP time locked to the stimulation. To ensure that the stimulus current is delivered correctly, direct nerve root stimulation using <2 mA can be attempted to ensure a CMAP response in the appropriate distal muscle group [38].

A threshold response between 10 and 20 mA gives a reasonable probability that no breach of the medial wall has occurred, whereas thresholds >15 mA indicate a 98 % likelihood of accurate screw positioning on postoperative CT scan. Thresholds above 20 mA assure a strong probability that there is no breach of the medial pedicle wall. For thoracic pedicle screw placement, stimulation thresholds <6 mA suggest a medial pedicle breach. During pedicle screw stimulation, false-negative responses can occur as a result of various factors, including the use of muscle relaxants, current spread, or preexisting nerve damage [37, 39]. Lastly, advances in materials (Cobalt Chrome, HA coated screws) used in instrumentation may or may not be compatible with current monitoring techniques.

Multimodality Monitoring

In cervical and thoracic procedures, the spinal cord (and to a lesser degree, the nerve roots) are of greater importance when deciding which modalities to use [40, 41]. Conversely, in lumbar or sacral procedures the nerve roots are at greater risk of injury, and thus modalities that specifically taking advantage of the individual strengths of its various submodalities, and is thus able to provide a more global and accurate assessment of the dorsal and ventral function of the spinal cord [42]. When EMG is added, the overall function of the nervous system can be monitored, from the level of cortex to the spinal cord, nerve roots, and finally peripheral nerves and muscle. The combined use of SSEPs, MEPs, and both spontaneous and triggered EMG provide the necessary tools required to optimally monitor the functional integrity of the spinal cord during a broad spectrum of routine and complex spinal surgeries, while maximizing the diagnostic efficacy of monitoring in detecting neurological injury. The near real-time information relayed on the integrity of these systems provided by IOM provides an added layer of security for the surgical team during procedures in which neurological injury is a looming possibility [33, 43–46].

Lumbosacral Spine Surgery and Spondylolisthesis Reduction

In lumbosacral spinal procedures, the focus on preservation of neurological function shifts to the nerve root level, as only the thecal sac and nerve roots are encountered below the level of the conus medullaris. In this situation, SSEPs in combination with sEMG are the modalities of choice for optimal neurophysiological monitoring. In a 2004 study, Gunnarsson et al. analyzed the sensitivity and specificity of detecting new postoperative motor deficits using multimodality monitoring during thoracolumbar procedures. They reported that sEMG has a sensitivity of 100 % with a specificity of 23.7 %. On the other hand, SSEPs provided a sensitivity of 28.6 % with a specificity of 94.7 % [47]. Used concurrently, sEMG and SSEP monitoring are complimentary in preventing nerve root injury during lumbar spine surgery.

This is somewhat problematic in the reduction of spondylolisthesis, which occurs after nerve root decompression and creates an active stretch. As described earlier, the passive mechanism to assess a defect by sEMG spikes and burst or corresponding changes in SSEP and MEP may not be sufficient. Hence, the lumbosacral spine surgery model may not be sufficient for electrical monitoring in the reduction of spondylolisthesis. During surgery for release of a tethered spinal cord, multimodality monitoring—including SSEPs, sEMG, and tEMG—is routinely used to protect functional neural structures. The prognostic value of these modalities for tethered cord surgery is similar to the prognostic value for other lumbosacral procedures with regard to the high specificity (nearing 100 %) and relatively low sensitivity associated with SSEPs, complemented by a sensitivity of 100 % offered by sEMG/tEMG. sEMG will help warn the surgeon of inadvertent manipulation of the nerve roots, whereas tEMG aids the surgeon in localizing relevant neural structures [48]. A key maneuver during tethered cord surgery is stimulation of various structures in the surgical field performed in conjunction with tEMG monitoring to determine if they contain any functional neural elements. A technique described by Husain et al. involved comparing the motor threshold obtained with spinal cord stimulation before and after cord untethering. The expected response after untethering is a lower motor threshold, which can be explained in part by improved local cellular metabolism. However, if a higher threshold is observed following untethering, there is a significant likelihood of worsened postoperative motor function [49, 50].

Spondylolisthesis Reduction

Despite utilizing multimodal techniques of SSEP, MEP, sEMG in the surgical management for the reduction of high-grade spondylolisthesis, there still exists a high rate of L5 nerve root injury that is unrecognized in the intraoperative setting. Essentially, unless there is a spike or burst of sEMG there is no mechanism to determine if nerve root has been placed on excessive stretch. Given that 70 % of the L5 nerve root strain is seen in the second half of the reduction, some have advocated a partial reduction or 50 % reduction of L5 on S1. There, however, still remains a risk of unrecognized L5 root injury secondary to stretch, since there is no active monitoring of the root during reduction [51, 52].

A novel technique developed by the senior author, to attempt to address these concerns, utilizes a tEMG and direct nerve root stimulation to assess health of the nerve root. Using direct nerve root stimulation, a baseline threshold of the L5 nerve root is obtained after the laminectomy and prior to the reduction (Table 27.1) [52]. The direct nerve root stimulation is performed at the axilla of the nerve root prior to entering the foramen (Fig. 27.1). Direct nerve root stimulation is performed and the triggering threshold of the L5 nerve root is documented. The L5 nerve root stimulation is performed at strategic operative times (i.e., Laminectomy, Pre-reduction, and Post-reduction). Injured nerve roots will have higher triggering thresholds, with literature reports ranging from 6 to >10 mA for a chronically compressed root, as compared with 2 mA for a normal nerve root. If post-reduction, the triggered threshold increases by greater than a factor of 2, it is assumed that excess stretch has occurred and the reduction needs to be lessened [7]. The senior author's published neurologic outcome when using this technique ($n = 112$) to monitor reduction of high-grade spondylolisthesis shows no permanent neurologic injury and a substantially lower rate of transient neuropraxia (2.6 %, $n = 3$) when compared to that of the literature [52].

Conclusions

IONM is extremely valuable in the prevention of neurological injury during spine procedures. It is important to understand the spectrum of modalities available for neuro-monitoring—including SSEPs, MEPs, sEMG, and tEMG—and their limitations. With spondylolisthesis, utilizing all modalities including tEMG and direct nerve root stimulation helps maximize the diagnostic value of IOM during spinal procedures and mitigating the risk for neurologic injury.

Table 27.1 Expected threshold results in high-grade spondylolisthesis

Direct nerve root stimulation-L5	Threshold (mA)
Normal root threshold	1
First stimulation medial to pedicle	5–13
Lateral exposure and decompression of L5 root	3–8
Discectomy, sacral dome osteotomy	3–8
Reduction and inter-body graft placement	3–8
After compression	2–7

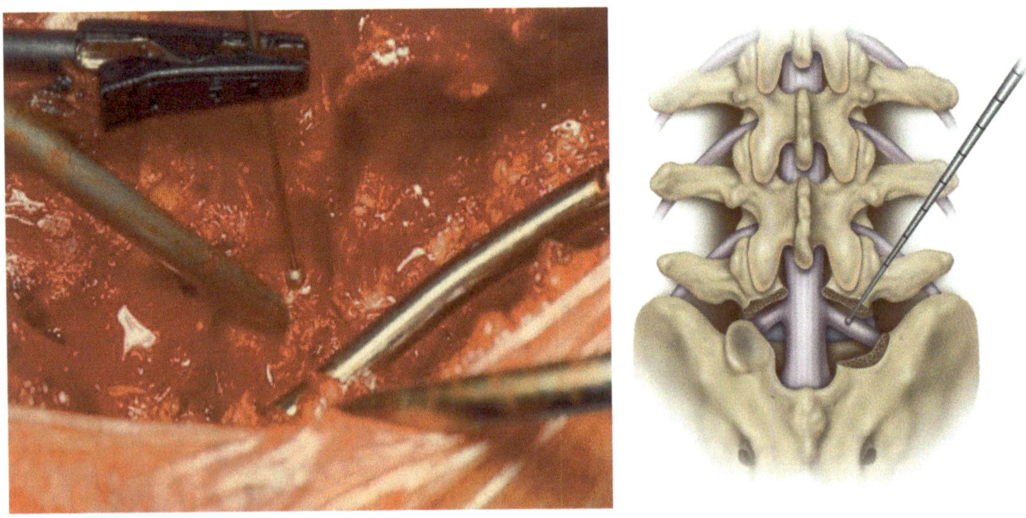

Fig. 27.1 After completion of L5 nerve root decompression, a stimulation probe directly stimulates nerve root to establish triggering threshold

References

1. Nash Jr CL, Lorig RA, Schatzinger LA, Brown RH. Spinal cord monitoring during operative treatment of the spine. Clin` Orthop Relat Res. 1977;126:100–5.
2. Vauzelle C, Stagnara P, Jouvinroux P. Functional monitoring of spinal cord activity during spinal surgery. Clin Orthop Relat Res. 1973;93:173–8.
3. Bose B, Sestokas AK, Schwartz DM. Neurophysiological monitoring of spinal cord function during instrumented anterior cervical fusion. Spine J. 2004;4:202–7.
4. Burke D, Hicks R, Stephen J, Woodforth I, Crawford M. Assessment of corticospinal and somatosensory conduction simultaneously during scoliosis surgery. Electroencephalogr Clin Neurophysiol. 1992;85: 388–96.
5. Chen X, Sterio D, Ming X, Para DD, Butusova M, Tong T, et al. Success rate of motor evoked potentials for intraoperative neurophysiologic monitoring: effects of age, lesion location, and preoperative neurologic deficits. J Clin Neurophysiol. 2007;24:281–5.
6. Gonzalez AA, Jeyanandarajan D, Hansen C, Zada G, Hsieh PC. Intraoperative neurophysiological monitoring during spine surgery: a review. Neurosurg Focus. 2009;27(4):E6.
7. Thuet ED, Winscher JC, Padberg AM, Bridwell KH, Lenke LG, Dobbs MB, Schootman M, Luhmann SJ. Validity and reliability of intraoperative monitoring in pediatric spinal deformity surgery: a 23-year experience of 3436 surgical cases. Spine (Phila Pa 1976). 2010;35(20):1880–6.
8. Tsai RY, Yang RS, Nuwer MR, Kanim LE, Delamarter RB, Dawson EG. Intraoperative dermatomal evoked potential monitoring fails to predict outcome from lumbar decompression surgery. Spine. 1997;22:1970–5.
9. Macdonald DB. Intraoperative motor evoked potential monitoring: overview and update. J Clin Monit Comput. 2006;20:347–77.
10. Merton PA, Morton HB. Stimulation of the cerebral cortex in the intact human subject. Nature. 1980; 285:227.
11. Keith RW, Stambough JL, Awender SH. Somatosensory cortical evoked potentials: a review of 100 cases of intraoperative spinal surgery monitoring. J Spinal Disord. 1990;3:220–6.
12. Chiappa K, Hill R. Short latency somatosensory evoked potentials methodology. In: Chiappa K, editor. Evoked potentials in clinical medicine. Philadelphia, PA: Lippincott-Raven; 1997.
13. Tsai TM, Tsai CL, Lin TS, Lin CC, Jou IM. Value of dermatomal somatosensory evoked potentials in detecting acute nerveroot injury: an experimental study with special emphasis on stimulus intensity. Spine. 2005;30:E540–6.
14. Sala F. Improving spinal cord monitoring: a neurosurgeon's view. Clin Neurophysiol. 2009;120:649–50.
15. Pechstein U, Nadstawek J, Zentner J, Schramm J. Isoflurane plus nitrous oxide versus propofol for recording of motor evoked potentials after high frequency repetitive electrical stimulation. Electroencephalogr Clin Neurophysiol. 1998;108:175–81.
16. Calancie B, Molano MR. Alarm criteria for motor-evoked potentials: what's wrong with the "presence-or-absence" approach? Spine. 2008;33:406–14.
17. Nuwer MR, Dawson EG, Carlson LG, Kanim LE, Sherman JE. Somatosensory evoked potential spinal cord monitoring reduces neurologic deficits after scoliosis surgery: results of a large multicenter survey. Electroencephalogr Clin Neurophysiol. 1995;96:6–11.
18. Holland NR. Intraoperative electromyography during thoracolumbar spinal surgery. Spine. 1998;23: 1915–22.
19. Jones SC, Fernau R, Woeltjen BL. Use of somatosensory evoked potentials to detect peripheral ischemia and potential injury resulting from positioning of the surgical patient: case reports and discussion. Spine J. 2004;4:360–2.
20. Jones SJ, Buonamassa S, Crockard HA. Two cases of quadriparesis following anterior cervical discectomy, with normal perioperative somatosensory evoked potentials. J Neurol Neurosurg Psychiatry. 2003;74:273–6.
21. Aglio LS, Romero R, Desai S, Ramirez M, Gonzalez AA, Gugino LD. The use of transcranial magnetic stimulation for monitoring descending spinal cord motor function. Clin Electroencephalogr. 2002;33:30–41.
22. Ben-David B, Haller G, Taylor P. Anterior spinal fusion complicated by paraplegia. A case report of a false negative somatosensory-evoked potential. Spine. 1987;12:536–9.
23. Ben-David B, Taylor PD, Haller GS. Posterior spinal fusion complicated by posterior column injury. A case report of a false-negative wake-up test. Spine. 1987;12:540–3.
24. Deletis V, Sala F. Intraoperative neurophysiological monitoring of the spinal cord during spinal cord and spine surgery: a review focus on the corticospinal tracts. Clin Neurophysiol. 2008;119:248–64.
25. Minahan RE, Sepkuty JP, Lesser RP, Sponseller PD, Kostuik JP. Anterior spinal cord injury with preserved neurogenic'motor' evoked potentials. Clin Neurophysiol. 2001;112:1442–50.
26. Langeloo DD, Lelivelt A, Louis Journee H, Slappendel R, deKleuver M. Transcranial electrical motor-evoked potential monitoring during surgery for spinal deformity: a study of 145 patients. Spine. 2003;28:1043–50.
27. Morota N, Deletis V, Constantini S, Kofler M, Cohen H, Epstein FJ. The role of motor evoked potentials during surgery for intramedullary spinal cord tumors. Neurosurgery. 1997;41:1327–36.
28. Hsu B, Cree AK, Lagopoulos J, Cummine JL. Transcranial motor-evoked potentials combined with response recording through compound muscle action potential as the sole modality of spinal cord monitoring in spinal deformity surgery. Spine. 2008;33:1100–6.
29. Quinones-Hinojosa A, Lyon R, Zada G, Lamborn KR, Gupta N, Parsa AT, et al. Changes in transcranial motor evoked potentials during intramedullary spinal cord tumor resection correlate with postoperative motor function. Neurosurgery. 2005;56:982–93.

30. Kalkman CJ, Drummond JC, Kennelly NA, Patel PM, Partridge BL. Intraoperative monitoring of tibialis anterior muscle motor evoked responses to transcranial electrical stimulation during partial neuromuscular blockade. Anesth Analg. 1992;75:584–9.
31. Kawaguchi M, Hayashi H, Yamamoto Y, Furuya H. Recent advances in the monitoring of myogenic motor-evoked potentials: development of post-tetanic motor-evoked potentials. J Anesth. 2008;22:489–92.
32. Pajewski TN, Arlet V, Phillips LH. Current approach on spinal cord monitoring: the point of view of the neurologist, the anesthesiologist and the spine surgeon. Eur Spine J. 2007;16(2 Suppl):S115–29.
33. Kelleher MO, Tan G, Sarjeant R, Fehlings MG. Predictive value of intraoperative neurophysiological monitoring during cervical spine surgery: a prospective analysis of 1055 consecutive patients. J Neurosurg Spine. 2008;8:215–21.
34. Owen JH, Padberg AM, Spahr-Holland L, Bridwell KH, Keppler L, Steffee AD. Clinical correlation between degenerative spine disease and dermatomal somatosensory-evoked potentials in humans. Spine. 1991;16(6 Suppl):S201–5.
35. Kothbauer KF, Deletis V, Epstein FJ. Motor-evoked potential monitoring for intramedullary spinal cord tumor surgery: correlation of clinical and neurophysiological data in a series of 100 consecutive procedures. Neurosurg Focus. 1998;4(5):e1.
36. Jimenez JC, Sani S, Braverman B, Deutsch H, Ratliff JK. Palsies of the fifth cervical nerve root after cervical decompression: prevention using continuous intraoperative electromyography monitoring. J Neurosurg Spine. 2005;3:92–7.
37. Calancie B, Madsen P, Lebwohl N. Stimulus-evoked EMG monitoring during transpedicular lumbosacral spine instrumentation. Initial clinical results. Spine. 1994;19:2780–6.
38. Shi YB, Binette M, Martin WH, Pearson JM, Hart RA. Electrical stimulation for intraoperative evaluation of thoracic pedicle screw placement. Spine. 2003;28:595–601.
39. Raynor BL, Lenke LG, Kim Y, Hanson DS, Wilson-Holde TJ, Bridwell KH, et al. Can triggered electromyograph thresholds predict safe thoracic pedicle screw placement? Spine. 2002;27:2030–5.
40. Fan D, Schwartz DM, Vaccaro AR, Hilibrand AS, Albert TJ. Intraoperative neurophysiologic detection of iatrogenic C5 nerve root injury during laminectomy for cervical compression myelopathy. Spine. 2002;27:2499–502.
41. Hilibrand AS, Schwartz DM, Sethuraman V, Vaccaro AR, Albert TJ. Comparison of transcranial electric motor and somatosensory evoked potential monitoring during cervical spine surgery. J Bone Joint Surg Am. 2004;86-A:1248–53.
42. MacDonald DB, Al Zayed Z, Khoudeir I, Stigsby B. Monitoring scoliosis surgery with combined multiple pulse transcranial electric motor and cortical somatosensory-evoked potentials from the lower and upper extremities. Spine. 2003;28:194–203.
43. Bindal RK, Ghosh S. Intraoperative electromyography monitoring in minimally invasive transforaminal lumbar interbody fusion. J Neurosurg Spine. 2007;6:126–32.
44. Khan MH, Smith PN, Balzer JR, Crammond D, Welch WC, Gerszten P, et al. Intraoperative somatosensory evoked potential monitoring during cervical spine corpectomy surgery: experience with 508 cases. Spine. 2006;31:E105–13.
45. Quraishi NA, Lewis SJ, Kelleher MO, Sarjeant R, Rampersaud YR, Fehlings MG. Intraoperative multimodality monitoring in adult spinal deformity: analysis of a prospective series of one hundred two cases with independent evaluation. Spine (Phila Pa 1976). 2009;34:1504–12.
46. Shufflebarger HL, Geck MJ. High-grade isthmic dysplastic spondylolisthesis: monosegmental surgical treatment. Spine (Phila Pa 1976). 2005;30(6 Suppl):S42–8.
47. Gunnarsson T, Krassioukov AV, Sarjeant R, Fehlings MG. Real-time continuous intraoperative electromyographic and somatosensory evoked potential recordings in spinal surgery: correlation of clinical and electrophysiologic findings in a prospective, consecutive series of 213 cases. Spine. 2004;29:677–84.
48. Paradiso G, Lee GY, Sarjeant R, Hoang L, Massicotte EM, Fehlings MG. Multimodality intraoperative neurophysiologic monitoring findings during surgery for adult tethered cord syndrome: analysis of a series of 44 patients with long-term follow-up. Spine (Phila Pa 1976). 2006;31:2095–102.
49. Husain AM, Shah D. Prognostic value of neurophysiologic intraoperative monitoring in tethered cord syndrome surgery. J Clin Neurophysiol. 2009;26:244–7.
50. Khealani B, Husain AM. Neurophysiologic intraoperative monitoring during surgery for tethered cord syndrome. J Clin Neurophysiol. 2009;26:76–81.
51. Petraco DM, Spivak JM, Cappadona JG, Kummer FJ, Neuwirth MG. An anatomic evaluation of L5 nerve stretch in spondylolisthesis reduction. Spine (Phila Pa 1976). 1996;21(10):1133–8. discussion 1139.
52. Sutter M, Eggspuehler A, Muller A, Dvorak J. Multimodal intraoperative monitoring: an overview and proposal of methodology based on 1,017 cases. Eur Spine J. 2007;16 Suppl 2:S153–61.

Value Considerations in the Surgical Management of Spondylolisthesis

28

Melissa Esparza and Sigurd H. Berven

Introduction

Value-based health care has become an important priority in the health care system in the USA. Value includes a consideration of both quality and cost—the value of a health care intervention is assessed by whether it provides an incremental benefit in outcome to justify an incremental increase in cost. Value considerations are particularly relevant to the management of spine-related conditions as the use of health care resources for the diagnosis and treatment of these conditions is increasing more rapidly than other areas of health care expenditures without a clear improvement of the health of the treated population. High and rising health care expenditures without a corresponding improvement in the health status of the population is an important challenge to sustainability in our health economy. The purpose of this chapter is to describe the role of value considerations in spine-related conditions and to provide a summary of the evidence on value-based care in the management of spondylolisthesis.

M. Esparza, B.A. • S.H. Berven, M.D. (✉)
Department of Orthopaedic Surgery,
UC San Francisco, 500 Parnassus Ave,
San Francisco, CA 94143, USA
e-mail: melissa.esparza@gmail.com;
bervens@orthosurg.ucsf.edu

Spinal disorders account for a significant proportion of the health care budget in the USA [1–3], contributing an estimated annual direct medical cost of $193.9 billion and an additional $14.0 billion in indirect costs through lost wages in the years 2002–2004 [2]. Martin et al. reported a 65 % increase in health care expenditures for patients with self-reported back and neck problems between 1997 and 2005 with no evidence of a corresponding improvement in self-assessed health status [3].

In addition to high spending, there is also a high degree of variability in the management of common spinal disorders, including spondylolisthesis. Variability is an important factor in value considerations as it affects both quality of care and cost of care. Variability in care pathways is a clear indication of the absence of an evidence-based approach among practitioners. Variability in costs indicates potential for decreasing costs in areas of high spending. Weinstein et al. found a 20-fold variation in the rates of lumbar spinal fusion between geographic regions of the USA between 1992 and 2003 [4]. Highly variable rates of spinal fusion have also been found between hospitals within the same geographic area and between surgeons within the same hospital [5, 6].

The combination of high spending, high variability, and an inconsistent demonstration of benefit in terms of patients' self-assessed health status raises important questions regarding the value of common interventions in spine surgery and the

A.L. Wollowick and V. Sarwahi (eds.), *Spondylolisthesis: Diagnosis, Non-Surgical Management, and Surgical Techniques*, DOI 10.1007/978-1-4899-7575-1_28,

appropriate rate of spinal surgery [7]. Value-enhancing procedures improve health-related quality of life and reduce cost over time by leading to improved long-term outcomes, a reduction in the need for further medical management, and lower rates of revision surgeries. Two recent systematic reviews of cost-utility analyses in spine care demonstrated the value added by numerous operative interventions in spine care as well as identified some interventions with less favorable cost-effectiveness [8, 9]. Establishing the value of operative and nonoperative interventions in spine care is an important priority in our current health care economy. An evidence-based approach to care is key in the effort to reduce variability and maximize value in health care [10].

An Evidence-Based Approach to the Management of Spondylolisthesis

Spondylolisthesis is a common spinal disorder that significantly impacts patients' health-related quality of life. Spondylolisthesis encompasses a spectrum of etiologies sharing the common pathology of forward displacement of one vertebra on the subjacent vertebra. Various classification systems have classified spondylolisthesis based on morphology, etiology, and severity [11–14]. This chapter will focus on two of the most common types of spondylolisthesis among adults, degenerative spondylolisthesis and isthmic spondylolisthesis.

The management of spondylolisthesis is characterized by significant variability in both operative and nonoperative treatment. Developing an evidence-based approach to care for spondylolisthesis involves addressing questions of the role of operative and nonoperative care as well as determining the surgical strategies that are most effective. Within the realm of surgery, questions include the role of decompression with or without fusion, the role of instrumentation in spinal fusion, and the role of circumferential arthrodesis compared with posterolateral arthrodesis. The first part of this chapter will review the literature to provide an evidence-based approach for addressing these questions and controversies. An evidence-based approach to care will provide a guide for reducing variability and improving quality of care in the management of spondylolisthesis.

The assessment of value is an important component in establishing an evidence-based approach to the management of spondylolisthesis. Defining the place of surgery for spondylolisthesis in a value-based healthcare economy includes an analysis of whether surgical care is cost-effective compared with alternative treatments and compared with other health care interventions that may compete for limited health care resources. The second part of this chapter will describe methods for value assessment in health care and review the literature for cost-effectiveness and cost-utility analyses of management approaches to spondylolisthesis.

Evidence for the Role of Operative versus Nonoperative Care: Degenerative Spondylolisthesis

Degenerative spondylolisthesis is characterized by the forward slippage of one vertebra on the subadjacent vertebra with the preservation of an intact neural arch [15]. Degeneration of the intervertebral disc and the facet joints permits displacement of the vertebrae with characteristic forward slippage and instability [16]. The natural history of the condition is not completely characterized, and often follows a stable course with slow progression over time, with significant variability between patients [17]. Surgical indications include progressive neural dysfunction related to neural compression. Surgery may also be indicated for patients with the persistence of leg pain, back pain, or neural symptoms despite nonoperative care [18]. Surgery is a discretionary procedure in such cases, and patients may choose to continue with nonoperative care or pursue operative treatment. In making an informed choice about their care, it is important for patients to have access to information on the outcomes of alternative interventions [19].

The Spine Patient Outcomes Research Trial (SPORT) [20] is an important study in assessing the outcomes and cost-effectiveness of different management approaches for three common spinal pathologies—intervertebral disc herniation, spinal stenosis, and degenerative spondylolisthesis. The study is a multicenter, prospective design including patients from 13 institutions in 11 states who were randomized to operative or nonoperative treatment, and a separate cohort of patients who were observed after choosing their care. Primary outcome measures included patient-reported health-related quality of life as measured by the SF-36 Health Status Questionnaire and the oswestry disability index (ODI). Secondary outcomes included preference-based measures of health status to estimate quality-adjusted life years (QALYs) and measures of resource utilization and cost. The SPORT was a pivotal trial in evaluating operative versus nonoperative treatment of three common spinal pathologies, and data from this trial has been used in many subsequent publications.

Using a subset of data from the SPORT, Weinstein et al. reported outcomes of surgical versus nonsurgical treatment for degenerative spondylolisthesis at 2-year follow-up [21] and 4-year follow-up [22]. Prior studies comparing operative and nonoperative care were limited by the inclusion of patients with mixed spinal pathologies, the lack of randomization, and the absence of standardized outcome instruments to assess results of care [23, 24].

The cohort studied by Weinstein et al. included patients diagnosed with degenerative spondylolisthesis who had at least 12 weeks of symptomatic neurogenic claudication or radicular pain with neural symptoms and were candidates for surgical care. Treatment options included lumbar laminectomy with or without fusion or nonoperative treatment, which did not follow a standardized protocol and could include education, physical therapy, injections, and pain medications. Surgeons chose between surgical strategies including laminectomy alone, noninstrumented posterolateral fusion, instrumented posterolateral fusion, and circumferential fusion. The primary outcome measures were patient self-assessments of health-related quality of life, including the SF-36 physical function and bodily pain domains and the ODI.

No significant difference was found in the outcomes of the operative group compared with the nonoperative group in the intent to treat analysis. However, there was a high rate of cross-over in the randomized cohort, with only 66 % of patients assigned to surgery undergoing operative care, and 54 % of patients assigned to nonoperative care undergoing surgery at 4-year follow-up. The as-treated analysis with careful control for confounding variables provides a more accurate assessment of the outcomes of care. An analysis of the randomized and observational cohorts combined demonstrated significant differences in favor of surgery for all the primary and secondary outcomes. The effect size favoring surgery was clinically significant with a difference of 15.3 points for bodily pain, 18.9 points for physical function, and 14.3 points for ODI.

Weinstein et al. provide the highest quality analysis of operative versus nonoperative care for degenerative spondylolisthesis; however, the study also has significant limitations. The high cross-over rate between study groups compromises the validity of the intent to treat analysis. Despite controlling for potential confounders in the as-treated analysis, the surgically treated group demonstrated a higher degree of disease severity with measurably more body pain, functional limitations, and disability at baseline than the patients treated nonoperatively. Another limitation of conclusions drawn from the as-treated analysis is that the demonstrated benefit of surgery may be related to patient preference for surgical intervention. Further studies that control for patient preference or include a placebo-controlled group may be useful in isolating the effect of surgery on clinical outcomes. Nonoperative management was consistent with the standard of care based on published guidelines, however lacked a standardized protocol of care. Further research on more clearly defined nonoperative protocols may be useful in demonstrating the value of specific nonoperative treatment modalities.

Evidence for the Role of Operative versus Nonoperative Care: Isthmic Spondylolisthesis

Isthmic spondylolisthesis is defined by the forward slippage of one vertebrae on the subadjacent vertebrae secondary to a defect in the pars interarticularis, which can arise from a stress fracture, an acute fracture, or elongation of the pars interarticularis [25]. In a long-term prospective study of the natural history of isthmic spondylolisthesis, Fredrickson et al. described a low rate of slip progression and clinical outcomes comparable to the general population of patients with isthmic spondylolisthesis at 45-year follow-up [26, 27]. Indications for surgery in adults with isthmic spondylolisthesis include high-grade slips, neural dysfunction, and the persistence of lower back pain or radicular pain after appropriate nonoperative care [28].

Several studies have compared conservative and operative treatment in the management of adult isthmic spondylolisthesis. Moller and Hedlund randomized 111 patients to posterolateral arthrodesis or an exercise program for the treatment of isthmic spondylolisthesis [29]. They found that patients treated with surgical arthrodesis had significantly improved functional outcomes and reduced pain compared with the nonoperatively treated patients. Limitations of the study include that nonoperative treatment was limited to a single exercise program, and outcomes were measured with a Visual Analogue Scale that does not provide a standardized measure of health-related quality of life that can be compared across studies.

L'Heureux et al. investigated the outcomes of surgical arthrodesis for the management of isthmic spondylolisthesis in a cohort of 31 adult patients [30]. Patients completed SF-36 questionnaires preoperatively and at 2-year follow-up and were asked additional satisfaction questions at follow-up. Patients demonstrated significant functional improvement and decreased pain rates at 2 years compared with preoperative scores. This study was useful in demonstrating that surgical arthrodesis is an appropriate management approach for patients with isthmic spondylolisthesis; however, it has significant limitations. The cohort consisted of only 31 patients and did not include a control group of patients treated nonoperatively that would allow for a comparison of nonoperative and operative treatment approaches. A range of operative techniques were used including circumferential arthrodesis and posterior only fusion, and both instrumented and noninstrumented fusions.

Overall, the literature supports operative management of adult isthmic spondylolisthesis for patients who have continued pain and functional disability after appropriate nonoperative management. Further investigation is necessary to guide specific surgical techniques for isthmic spondylolisthesis.

Evidence for Specific Surgical Strategies in the Management of Spondylolisthesis

The operative management of spondylolisthesis is variable and the effectiveness of different surgical techniques may be different based on etiology of the spondylolisthesis, severity of slippage, and patient factors. Current questions and controversies in the operative management of spondylolisthesis include the role for decompression, fusion, instrumentation, and circumferential fusion. Decision making in the use of these surgical strategies may be guided by an evidence-based approach to care.

Decompression and Fusion

Operative management of degenerative spondylolisthesis may consist of decompression alone or decompression with spinal fusion. Decompressive laminectomy alone has been shown to result in satisfactory outcomes. A meta-analysis by Mardjetko et al. identified eleven papers published between 1970 and 1993 that reported outcomes for 216 patients undergoing decompression without fusion for degenerative spondylolisthesis [31]. Sixty nine percent of patients had a satisfactory outcome and 31 % had unsatisfactory outcomes. Martin et al. performed a systematic review of the literature and identified eight studies between

1966 and 2005 comparing decompression alone to decompression and fusion [32]. The authors concluded that a satisfactory clinical outcome was more likely with fusion than with decompression alone, with a relative risk of 1.4, and a 95 % confidence interval (CI) of 1.04–1.89.

The highest quality evidence from the Martin et al review was a study by Herkowitz and Kurz of 50 consecutive patients with symptomatic degenerative spondylolisthesis randomized to decompression alone or to decompression with noninstrumented fusion [33]. Outcomes were rated as excellent, good, fair, and poor, based upon clinical improvement, patient activity tolerance, and medication usage. Compared to patients undergoing decompression alone, patients who underwent decompression and fusion had significantly less back and lower limb pain and were more likely to have outcomes rated as good or excellent. The degree of forward slippage increased in 24 of the 25 patients without fusion, and in only 7 of the 25 patients with fusion. Pseudarthrosis was present in 36 % of patients in the arthrodesis group, but 23 of the 25 arthrodesis patients had a complete union on at least one side. There were several limitations to this study. The outcomes measured represented surgeons' assessment of results and did not include any patient-reported outcomes on health-related quality of life. Decompressive technique in this study involved a midline decompression including the interspinous ligament and one half of the cephalad and caudad laminae of the involved vertebrae, together with medial caudad and cephalad facetectomy. More recent papers have included the study of minimally invasive surgery techniques that involve limited foraminotomies and spare midline spinal anatomy [34–36]. In an economic analysis of decompression with or without fusion, Kim et al. report on outcomes in the literature demonstrating that less-invasive decompressive techniques have good efficacy in certain subsets of patients with degenerative spondylolisthesis, although note that many of these studies also include patients with spinal stenosis without spondylolisthesis [36].

The management of isthmic spondylolisthesis may include decompression with fusion or fusion alone. Agabegi and Fischgrund performed a review of the literature in 2010 to describe current treatment strategies for isthmic spondylolisthesis [28]. The authors cite studies demonstrating lower rates of fusion for patients undergoing decompression and fusion compared with fusion alone for low-grade spondylolisthesis, but another study reporting only 57 % of adult patients with complete pain relief after undergoing fusion without decompression. Based on the literature, they recommend fusion with decompression for adult patients with radicular symptoms or neurologic deficits and evidence of compression of the neural elements.

Instrumentation

The systematic review by Martin et al. identified six studies comparing instrumented fusion to noninstrumented fusion [32]. The authors found no statistically significant difference in the relative risk of achieving a satisfactory clinical outcome for instrumented spinal fusion compared with the noninstrumented group, reporting a relative risk of 1.19 and a 95 % CI that spans one (0.92–1.54). However this study was limited by the inclusion of patients with as little as 1 year follow-up, cohorts as small as five patients per treatment group, and the inclusion of observational study designs. All of the effect sizes were larger in the randomized studies than in the observational studies. The highest quality study from this systematic review that assesses the effect of a solid fusion on long-term outcomes is the paper by Kornblum et al. [37].

Kornblum et al. performed a secondary analysis of patients randomized to noninstrumented posterolateral arthrodesis in two previous prospective, randomized clinical trials [37]. The 58 patients identified had a mean follow-up of 7.7 years (range 5–14 years). Outcomes measured included rating of excellent, good, fair, and poor based on pain relief and activity level. Pseudarthrosis, assessed by plain films at 2–4 year follow-up, developed in 25 of the 47 patients treated with a noninstrumented fusion. Compared to patients with a solid fusion, patients with incomplete union reported significantly worse pain and physical function and were observed to have significantly more segmental dynamic instability. This paper demonstrates improved outcomes for patients with solid fusion compared to those with an incomplete union at a minimum follow-up of 5 years; however, it does not assess the direct effect of instrumentation on fusion rates or clinical outcomes.

Agabegi and Fischgrund note that instrumented posterolateral fusion is the most common surgical technique for adult isthmic spondylolisthesis [28]. However they cite conflicting evidence in the literature for the role of instrumentation in low-grade spondylolisthesis, with four randomized trials showing no added benefit from instrumentation, and other studies demonstrating higher fusion rates and improved outcomes. For high-grade isthmic spondylolisthesis, the authors recommend instrumentation for posterolateral fusion from L4 to S1, and iliac screw fixation for severe slips or unstable cases. The role of instrumentation in adults with isthmic spondylolisthesis has a greater effect size than instrumentation in pediatric populations.

Circumferential Fusion

Definitive evidence for the role of circumferential arthrodesis in the management of both degenerative and isthmic spondylolisthesis is lacking. Videbaek et al. demonstrated significant improvement of clinical outcomes and fusion rates in patients with severe chronic low back pain undergoing circumferential fusion compared with posterolateral only fusion at 5- to 9-year follow-up [38]. In contrast, a study by Fritzell et al demonstrated no statistically significant difference in clinical outcomes between patients treated with circumferential arthrodesis compared with posterolateral fusion but a significantly higher rate of complications in the circumferential fusion group [39]. It must be noted that the cohorts in both the Videbaek et al. and Fritzell et al. consisted of patients with chronic low back pain with diagnoses that could include isthmic spondylolisthesis, degenerative spondylolisthesis, or other degenerative conditions of the spine. Agabegi and Fischgrund reviewed several additional studies of the role of circumferential fusion and concluded that anterior column support in addition to posterolateral fusion may be considered for patients with risk factors for pseudarthrosis and possibly for patients with large or hypermobile discs with low-grade isthmic spondylolisthesis. They advocate for circumferential fusion for high-grade isthmic spondylolisthesis in order to provide greater stability and increase fusion rates [28].

Evidence guiding the optimal strategies for surgical management of degenerative and isthmic spondylolisthesis remains limited. The literature demonstrates improved outcomes of decompression and fusion compared to traditional laminectomy alone for degenerative spondylolisthesis, but more study is necessary to evaluate the role of less-invasive decompression techniques without arthrodesis. For adult isthmic spondylolisthesis, the addition of decompression to spinal fusion is indicated for adult patients with radicular symptoms or neurologic deficits. The literature supports the use of instrumentation to increase fusion rates and demonstrates that patients with solid fusions have improved clinical outcomes. Further investigation is needed to determine the role of circumferential fusion in specific populations of patients with spondylolisthesis. The balance between fusion rates and possible complications and the need for revision surgery will also require further study. Finally, the role of biologics and innovative surgical techniques will have an impact on guidelines for specific surgical strategies.

Value Considerations in the Management of Spondylolisthesis

Value Assessment in Health Care Interventions

Assessing value in health care involves an analysis of the incremental benefits, measured by clinical outcomes, of one intervention compared to another relative to the incremental cost between those interventions. Determinants of clinical outcomes include change in the health-related quality of life, as well as complications and reoperation rates. Costs may be reported as direct costs, charges, or reimbursements. Indirect costs, including productivity costs, transportation, and the cost of caretakers, may also be included in cost calculations.

Cost-utility analysis is a specific type of cost-effectiveness analysis in which the benefit added by an intervention is quantified by a utility score. A utility score is a societal preference of a health state, measured on a scale of zero (death) to one (perfect health). Utility scores may be obtained via conversion of health-related quality of life scores from patient surveys, including general health status measures such as the SF-36 Health Status Questionnaire or disease-specific instruments such as the Scoliosis Research Society-22 (SRS-22) questionnaire and the ODI. Measurement of a utility score over time yields a QALY, which is calculated by multiplying the utility score by the number of years that score is maintained. The QALY measurement incorporates both quality and duration of the treatment effect, and is a standardized outcome measure that can be compared across fields and assigned value by society [40].

The value of an intervention may be expressed in terms of the incremental cost of the intervention necessary to achieve a gain of one QALY. The threshold for what a society may be willing to spend to improve quality of life through health care interventions affects the extent to which the intervention is determined to be cost-effective. In the USA, a threshold of $50,000 per QALY gained has been used to define an intervention as cost-effective, however there is not an established willingness-to-pay standard and a threshold of $100,000/QALY gained is also commonly used as the limit to define a cost-effective intervention [8, 41]. The relative value of one intervention over another may be expressed as an incremental cost-effectiveness ratio (ICER) or incremental cost-utility ratio (ICUR), calculated as the ratio between the difference in costs and the difference in benefits of two interventions.

In reviewing the evidence for the cost-effectiveness of various treatment options for spondylolisthesis, there are several important factors to consider, including research methodology, duration of follow-up, and methods for calculation of costs and benefits. As in all areas of research, the research methodology affects the quality of evidence. A prospective randomized controlled trial comparing the incremental cost-effectiveness between alternative interventions is the gold standard for determining the relative value of a health care intervention; however, other study designs offer valuable alternatives to evaluate cost-effectiveness when a randomized controlled trial is not feasible [42]. Economic modeling techniques and decision analysis models are useful tools in the economic assessment of alternative treatment options. These models may use previously published data to make assumptions about alternative outcomes of an intervention in order to predict long-term cost-effectiveness, thus the results of these studies are highly dependent on the underlying assumptions made. Sensitivity analysis may be used to determine the relative effect of various assumptions made in the study [43, 44].

Duration of follow-up is an important consideration when making value assessments of alternative treatment options. The value of an intervention may change over time based on the durability of the treatment effect. An intervention may have an initially higher cost compared to alternative treatments, but if its outcomes result in a reduction in the need for additional medical or surgical treatments including revision surgeries, then its initial costs may be significantly discounted over time. The relative value of treatment options in the management of spondylolisthesis may be different at 1 year after treatment compared to 10 years after treatment, and the true value of an intervention is best measured with long-term follow-up.

The value assessment of a technology is dependent on the manner by which costs and benefits are calculated. Costs may be reported from the perspective of the patient, hospital, third party payers, or society. Examples of direct costs include physician fees, medical devices, medications, and laboratory tests [43]. Charges include the cost of an intervention plus additional resources consumed during its utilization, and reflect what the patient is billed [45]. Reimbursements to the hospital may also be reported. Cost analyses that include indirect costs such as productivity costs, transportation, and the cost of caretakers, are more reflective of costs from a societal perspective. The benefits of an intervention are best measured by patient self-assessments of health status. Reporting the value of an intervention in terms of cost per QALY gained provides the best measure for value assessment as it allows for standardized comparisons of interventions.

Lastly, the application of results in guiding clinical practice should be limited to the populations in which they are studied. The majority of cost-effectiveness studies identified in the following literature review apply to degenerative spondylolisthesis; however, there is less evidence evaluating the cost-effectiveness of different management approaches for isthmic spondylolisthesis. Further study is necessary to clarify the value of alternative treatment strategies in different types of spondylolisthesis.

Evidence for the Cost-Effectiveness of Surgery for Spondylolisthesis

An evidence-based approach to care requires an assessment of the incremental value of alternative treatments. Value considerations in the management of spondylolisthesis include the relative value of operative compared to nonoperative care and the cost-effectiveness of specific surgical strategies, including decompression with or without fusion, the use of instrumentation in spinal fusions, and circumferential compared to posterolateral arthrodesis.

Value of Operative Versus Nonoperative Care

Tosteson et al. compared the value of operative and nonoperative care for patients from the SPORT cohort with spinal stenosis and degenerative spondylolisthesis, and found that operative management of degenerative spondylolisthesis significantly improved outcomes compared with nonoperative care, with a QALY gain of .23 (CI, 0.19–0.27) at 2-year follow-up [46]. The cost per QALY gained was $115,600 (CI $90,800–144,900) for degenerative spondylolisthesis compared to $77,600 (CI $49,600–120,000) for spinal stenosis alone. The authors attributed this difference to differences in the cost of the initial surgery, as fusion surgery was more common in the degenerative spondylolisthesis group than for patients in the stenosis group who more commonly underwent decompressive laminectomy alone.

Re-evaluation of outcomes at 4-year follow-up demonstrated an improvement in QALYs gained to .34 (CI 0.30–0.47) for patients undergoing surgery compared to nonoperative care for degenerative spondylolisthesis [47]. There was also an improvement in the value of operative management of spondylolisthesis, with a decrease in the cost per QALY gained to $64,300 (CI $32,864–83,117). This difference was accounted for by ongoing costs of the nonoperative treatment group in the 3rd and 4th years of the study predominantly because of productivity losses compared to the operatively treated group. These findings highlight how durability of treatment outcomes may discount the initial cost of an intervention and result in improved value over time. If these results continue to be maintained at longer-term follow-up, then the cost-effectiveness of surgical care will continue to improve with time compared to nonoperative treatment.

The cost-effectiveness analyses by Tosteson et al. have significant limitations. The studies used an as-treated analysis that demonstrated significant baseline differences between operative and nonoperative patients. Nonoperative care was not standardized, thus the cost-effectiveness of specific nonoperative treatment modalities could not be assessed. Costs were determined from patient self-reporting of resource utilization, time off from work, and caregiver time. A comprehensive database measuring actual expenditures on outpatient care and that assigns value to time off of work and activity limitations would more accurately characterize the relative costs of nonoperative care compared to surgery.

Value of Decompression with Fusion Versus Decompression Alone

The studies by Herkowitz et al., Martin et al., and others have guided current practice in making decompression with fusion the treatment of choice in the surgical management of degenerative spondylolisthesis [33, 32]. However, there have been few studies addressing the relative cost-effectiveness of fusion versus decompression alone. The analysis by Tosteson et al. includes data on the cost per QALY of decompression alone ($17,000, CI cost saving to $234,460) and fusion surgery ($66,300, CI $34,863–84,416), however the authors caution against drawing conclusions from this data given the low number of patients undergoing decompression alone ($n=23$ versus 356 undergoing fusion) [47]. Kuntz et al. performed a cost-utility analysis using a Markov model to assess the cost-effectiveness of types of surgical interventions for degenerative spondylolisthesis [48]. The analysis compared laminectomy alone to laminectomy with fusion either with or without instrumentation, and found laminectomy with noninstrumented fusion to have a cost/QALY gained of $56,500. The authors note that this value compares favorably with other well-accepted surgical interventions and is highly sensitive to assumptions made in the model including cost calculations, complication and reoperation rates, the level to which patients value changes in quality of life, and the true effectiveness of the surgeries to alleviate symptoms.

Another cost-utility analysis by Kim et al. used a Markov model comparing decompression with fusion to a minimally invasive midline-sparing decompression technique for stable Grade I degenerative spondylolisthesis. The base-case analysis found an incremental cost-utility ratio of $185,878 per QALY gained for decompression plus instrumented fusion compared with decompression alone. The authors conclude that while most of the literature supports more successful outcomes for fusion compared to traditional laminectomy alone, a midline facet-preserving decompression has comparable outcomes and is more cost-effective than decompression with instrumented fusion in a subset of patients with leg-dominant pain and a stable Grade I degenerative spondylolisthesis [36].

Value of Instrumented Versus Noninstrumented Fusion

The literature demonstrates that higher rates of fusion are achieved with spinal instrumentation compared with noninstrumented fusion in degenerative spondylolisthesis. The systematic review by Martin et al found that patients undergoing instrumented fusion achieved higher rates of solid fusion compared to patients undergoing noninstrumented fusion, with a relative risk of successful fusion of 1.37, and a 95 % CI of 1.07–1.75 [32]. Kornblum et al. demonstrate that solid arthrodesis is associated with less segmental instability and better outcomes than pseudarthrosis [37]. However, conclusions about the cost-effectiveness of instrumented fusions compared to noninstrumented fusions have been variable.

Kuntz et al. evaluated the cost-effectiveness of instrumentation in fusions for degenerative spondylolisthesis and found instrumented fusion to have an ICER of $3,112,800 per QALY compared to noninstrumented fusions [48]. As with other economic modeling studies, results were dependent on assumptions made in the base-case analysis. Sensitivity analysis showed the ICER to decrease to $82,400 per QALY if the proportion of patients whose symptoms were relieved after instrumented fusion was 90 % instead of 80 % compared to noninstrumented fusion. A major limitation of cost-effectiveness studies has been the poor sensitivity of outcomes measures to different techniques, high variability in surgical outcomes, and limited follow-up on small numbers of patients.

Tosteson et al. found a slightly more favorable economic value for instrumented fusion (cost/QALY $118,100; CI $91,200–153,100) compared to noninstrumented fusion (cost/QALY 119,900; CI $72,200–192,000) at 2 years [46], with a further improvement in value for instrumented fusion (cost/QALY $64,900; CI $33,708–88,574) versus noninstrumented fusion (cost/QALY $71,200, CI $28,515–99,673) at 4-year follow-up [47]. However, the differences in cost and QALYs were not statistically significant and they note that their analysis was not powered to detect differences in surgical strategies. The authors point out that the findings by Kornblum et al showing better long-term outcomes for patients with a solid fusion compared to patients with pseudarthrosis suggest that the higher fusion rates associated with instrumentation may lead to improved outcomes and thus better value over time.

Value of Circumferential versus Posterolateral Fusion

Another controversy in the value of different surgical techniques for spondylolisthesis is the use of circumferential fusion compared to posterolateral fusion. The Tosteson et al analysis was not powered to detect differences in these two approaches, but does present data on results between posterolateral and circumferential fusion at 2 and 4-year follow-up. At 2 years, circumferential arthrodesis had the most favorable cost-effective ratio of the different fusion types, with a cost per QALY of $107,000 (CI $65,100–166,700) [46]. While the absolute cost/QALY of circumferential fusion decreased to $66,900 (CI $26,855–111,555) at 4 years, its relative cost/QALY compared to posterolateral fusion ($64,100, CI $30,972–93,819) was less favorable [47].

Soegaard et al performed a cost-utility analysis of circumferential fusion compared to posterolateral fusion in the management of patients with severe chronic low back pain from degenerative conditions of the spine including degenerative and isthmic spondylolisthesis [49]. At 2-year follow-up, patients randomized to undergo circumferential fusion demonstrated higher fusion rates and lower rates of revision surgeries. By 8-year follow-up, patients who underwent circumferential fusion also had a significant improvement in physical and psychosocial disability scores compared to patients who had posterolateral fusion. The ICUR between the two groups favored the circumferential approach, with an incremental savings of $49,306/QALY compared to posterolateral fusions. Despite a higher initial cost for the index procedure, circumferential fusion was dominant over posterolateral fusion in that it was both significantly more effective and less costly over time. A significant limitation of this study is that clinical outcomes were drawn from the study by Videbaek et al [38] that included both patients with isthmic spondylolisthesis, degenerative spondylolisthesis and other degenerative conditions. Further research is needed to determine the cost-effectiveness of circumferential versus posterolateral fusion in the treatment of specific spinal pathologies.

Conclusion

Value-based health care is an increasingly important priority in our health care economy. Minimizing variability of care between practitioners is an important priority for healthcare value and quality. An evidence-based approach to care is fundamental to reducing variability and optimizing value in health care. This chapter provided a review of the literature on value considerations in the management of spondylolisthesis.

Establishing the value of different treatment options for spondylolisthesis is useful as it allows for a comparison with alternative medical interventions that may compete for the health care dollar. The value of spinal surgery is in the range of other health care interventions that society pays for routinely [50]. Current evidence on value of surgery for spondylolisthesis demonstrates costs and outcomes that are comparable with other spinal and orthopedic conditions. The durability of clinical outcomes of surgery for spondylolisthesis has resulted in an improved cost-effectiveness with longer-term follow-up [22]. If this improvement in clinical outcomes is maintained, the value of surgery for spondylolisthesis will continue to improve over time.

Accurate information on the incremental value of different surgical strategies is useful in guiding an evidence-based approach to surgical planning and techniques. The literature demonstrates that decompression with fusion compared with traditional laminectomy alone to have improved outcomes and a value that compares favorably with other well-accepted surgical interventions. The incremental cost of instrumented fusion compared with noninstrumented fusion is high; however, the high cost of spinal instrumentation may be discounted over time given the evidence showing higher fusion rates with instrumented fusion and improved outcomes associated with solid fusions. Circumferential fusion has been shown to be dominant over posterolateral fusion in the surgical management of patients with various spinal pathologies but the specific role of circumferential fusion for spondylolisthesis has not been clearly established.

Further study is necessary to establish the relative value of surgical care for spondylolisthesis and the value of specific surgical strategies, including minimally invasive surgical techniques, the use of biologics for spinal fusions, and other emerging technologies and innovations in surgical technique. More investigation may clarify the value of various surgical techniques in specific populations of patients with spondylolisthesis. From the perspective of the patient and society, the true value of a health care intervention is measured over a lifetime. Investigation of value considerations in spine care should continue to be measured over time in order to evaluate the cost-effectiveness of alternative treatment options at long-term follow-up. In guiding recommendations for the management of spondylolisthesis, an evidence-based approach to care is fundamental to the goal of reducing variability, improving outcomes, and maximizing value over time.

Disclosure Presentation of this work was made possible by R25MD006832 from the National Institute on Minority Health and Health Disparities. The views expressed do not necessarily reflect the official policies of the DHHS.

References

1. Luo X, Pietrobon R, Sun SX, Liu GG, Hey L. Estimates and patterns of direct health care expenditures among individuals with back pain in the United States. Spine. 2004;29(1):79–86. doi:10.1097/01.BRS.0000105527.13866.0F.
2. United States Bone and Joint Initiative. The burden of musculoskeletal diseases in the United States. 2nd ed. Rosemont, IL: American Academy of Orthopaedic Surgeons; 2011.
3. Martin BI, Deyo RA, Mirza SK, et al. Expenditures and health status among adults with back and neck problems. JAMA. 2008;299(6):656–64.
4. Weinstein JN, Lurie JD, Olson PR, Bronner KK, Fisher ES. United States' trends and regional variations in lumbar spine surgery: 1992–2003. Spine. 2006;31(23):2707–14.
5. Abraham DJ, Herkowitz HN, Katz JN. Indications for thoracic and lumbar spine fusion and trends in use. Orthop Clin North Am. 1998;29(4):803.
6. Deyo RA, Mirza SK. Trends and variations in the use of spine surgery. Clin Orthop. 2006;443:139–46.
7. Deyo RA, Mirza SK. The case for restraint in spinal surgery: does quality management have a role to play? Eur Spine J. 2009;18 Suppl 3:331–7.
8. Kepler CK, Wilkinson SM, Radcliff KE, et al. Cost-utility analysis in spine care: a systematic review. Spine J. 2012;12(8):676–90.
9. Indrakanti SS, Weber MH, Takemoto SK, Hu SS, Polly D, Berven SH. Value-based care in the management of spinal disorders: a systematic review of cost-utility analysis. Clin Orthop. 2012;470(4):1106–23.
10. Berven SH, Herkowitz HN. Evidence-based medicine for the spine: degenerative spondylolisthesis. Semin Spine Surg. 2009;21(4):238–45.
11. Wiltse LL, Newman PH, Macnab I. Classification of spondylolisis and spondylolisthesis. Clin Orthop. 1976;117:23–9.
12. Marchetti PG, Bartolozzi P. Spondylolisthesis: classification of spondylolisthesis as a guideline for treatment. In: deWald R, Bridwell K, editors. The textbook of spinal surgery. 2nd ed. Philadelphia, PA: Lippincott Williams & Wilkins; 1997. p. 1211–54.
13. Meyerding H. Spondylolisthesis. Surg Gynecol Obstet. 1932;54:371–7.
14. Taillard WF. Etiology of spondylolisthesis. Clin Orthop. 1976;117:30–9.
15. Macnab I. Spondylolisthesis with an intact neural arch; the so-called pseudo-spondylolisthesis. J Bone Joint Surg Br. 1950;32-B(3):325–33.
16. Newman PH. Degenerative spondylolisthesis. Orthop Clin North Am. 1975;6(1):197–8.
17. Matsunaga S, Sakou T, Morizono Y, Masuda A, Demirtas AM. Natural history of degenerative spondylolisthesis. Pathogenesis and natural course of the slippage. Spine. 1990;15(11):1204–10.
18. Majid K, Fischgrund JS. Degenerative lumbar spondylolisthesis: trends in management. J Am Acad Orthop Surg. 2008;16(4):208–15.
19. Weinstein JN, Clay K, Morgan TS. Informed patient choice: patient-centered valuing of surgical risks and benefits. Heal Aff. 2007;26(3):726–30.
20. Birkmeyer NJO, Weinstein JN, Tosteson ANA, et al. Design of the Spine Patient Outcomes Research Trial (SPORT). Spine. 2002;27(12):1361–72.
21. Weinstein JN, Lurie JD, Tosteson TD, et al. Surgical versus nonsurgical treatment for lumbar degenerative spondylolisthesis. N Engl J Med. 2007;356(22):2257–70.
22. Weinstein JN, Lurie JD, Tosteson TD, et al. Surgical compared with nonoperative treatment for lumbar degenerative spondylolisthesis. Four-year results in the Spine Patient Outcomes Research Trial (SPORT) randomized and observational cohorts. J Bone Joint Surg Am. 2009;91(6):1295–304.
23. Atlas SJ, Keller RB, Robson D, Deyo RA, Singer DE. Surgical and nonsurgical management of lumbar spinal stenosis: four-year outcomes from the maine lumbar spine study. Spine. 2000;25(5):556–62.
24. Malmivaara A, Slätis P, Heliövaara M, et al. Surgical or nonoperative treatment for lumbar spinal stenosis? A randomized controlled trial. Spine. 2007;32(1):1–8.
25. Hu SS, Tribus CB, Diab M, Ghanayem AJ. Spondylolisthesis and spondylolysis. Instr Course Lect. 2008;57:431–45.

26. Fredrickson BE, Baker D, McHolick WJ, Yuan HA, Lubicky JP. The natural history of spondylolysis and spondylolisthesis. J Bone Joint Surg Am. 1984;66(5): 699–707.
27. Beutler WJ, Fredrickson BE, Murtland A, Sweeney CA, Grant WD, Baker D. The natural history of spondylolysis and spondylolisthesis: 45-year follow-up evaluation. Spine. 2003;28(10):1027–35. discussion 1035.
28. Agabegi SS, Fischgrund JS. Contemporary management of isthmic spondylolisthesis: pediatric and adult. Spine J. 2010;10(6):530–43.
29. Möller H, Hedlund R. Surgery versus conservative management in adult isthmic spondylolisthesis–a prospective randomized study: part 1. Spine. 2000; 25(13):1711–5.
30. L'Heureux Jr EA, Perra JH, Pinto MR, Smith MD, Denis F, Lonstein JE. Functional outcome analysis including preoperative and postoperative SF-36 for surgically treated adult isthmic spondylolisthesis. Spine. 2003;28(12):1269–74.
31. Mardjetko SM, Connolly PJ, Shott S. Degenerative lumbar spondylolisthesis. A meta-analysis of literature 1970–1993. Spine. 1994;19(20 Suppl):2256S–65S.
32. Martin CR, Gruszczynski AT, Braunsfurth HA, Fallatah SM, O'Neil J, Wai EK. The surgical management of degenerative lumbar spondylolisthesis: a systematic review. Spine. 2007;32(16):1791–8.
33. Herkowitz HN, Kurz LT. Degenerative lumbar spondylolisthesis with spinal stenosis. A prospective study comparing decompression with decompression and intertransverse process arthrodesis. J Bone Joint Surg Am. 1991;73(6):802–8.
34. Sasai K, Umeda M, Maruyama T, Wakabayashi E, Iida H. Microsurgical bilateral decompression via a unilateral approach for lumbar spinal canal stenosis including degenerative spondylolisthesis. J Neurosurg Spine. 2008;9(6):554–9.
35. Ikuta K, Tono O, Oga M. Clinical outcome of microendoscopic posterior decompression for spinal stenosis associated with degenerative spondylolisthesis–minimum 2-year outcome of 37 patients. Minim Invasive Neurosurg. 2008;51(5):267–71.
36. Kim S, Mortaz Hedjri S, Coyte PC, Rampersaud YR. Cost-utility of lumbar decompression with or without fusion for patients with symptomatic degenerative lumbar spondylolisthesis. Spine J. 2012;12(1):44–54.
37. Kornblum MB, Fischgrund JS, Herkowitz HN, Abraham DA, Berkower DL, Ditkoff JS. Degenerative lumbar spondylolisthesis with spinal stenosis: a prospective long-term study comparing fusion and pseudarthrosis. Spine. 2004;29(7):726–33. discussion 733–734.
38. Videbaek TS, Christensen FB, Soegaard R, et al. Circumferential fusion improves outcome in comparison with instrumented posterolateral fusion: long-term results of a randomized clinical trial. Spine. 2006;31(25):2875–80.
39. Fritzell P, Hägg O, Jonsson D, Nordwall A. Cost-effectiveness of lumbar fusion and nonsurgical treatment for chronic low back pain in the Swedish Lumbar Spine Study: a multicenter, randomized, controlled trial from the Swedish Lumbar Spine Study Group. Spine. 2004;29(4):421–34. discussion Z3.
40. Rihn JA, Berven S, Allen T, et al. Defining value in spine care. Am J Med Qual. 2009;24(6 Suppl):4S–14.
41. Wong DA. Commentary: implications and limitations of cost-utility analysis. Spine J. 2012;12(8):691–2.
42. Bozic KJ, Pierce RG, Herndon JH. Health care technology assessment. Basic principles and clinical applications. J Bone Joint Surg Am. 2004;86-A(6): 1305–14.
43. Meltzer MI. Introduction to health economics for physicians. Lancet. 2001;358(9286):993–8.
44. Tarride J-E, Blackhouse G, Bischof M, et al. Approaches for economic evaluations of health care technologies. J Am Coll Radiol. 2009;6(5):307–16.
45. Kamerlink JR, Quirno M, Auerbach JD, et al. Hospital cost analysis of adolescent idiopathic scoliosis correction surgery in 125 consecutive cases. J Bone Joint Surg Am. 2010;92(5):1097–104.
46. Tosteson ANA, Lurie JD, Tosteson TD, et al. Surgical treatment of spinal stenosis with and without degenerative spondylolisthesis: cost-effectiveness after 2 years. Ann Intern Med. 2008;149(12):845–53.
47. Tosteson ANA, Tosteson TD, Lurie JD, et al. Comparative effectiveness evidence from the Spine Patient Outcomes Research Trial: surgical versus non-operative care for spinal stenosis, degenerative spondylolisthesis, and intervertebral disc herniation. Spine. 2011;36(24):2061–8.
48. Kuntz KM, Snider RK, Weinstein JN, Pope MH, Katz JN. Cost-effectiveness of fusion with and without instrumentation for patients with degenerative spondylolisthesis and spinal stenosis. Spine. 2000;25(9): 1132–9.
49. Soegaard R, Bünger CE, Christiansen T, Høy K, Eiskjaer SP, Christensen FB. Circumferential fusion is dominant over posterolateral fusion in a long-term perspective: cost-utility evaluation of a randomized controlled trial in severe, chronic low back pain. Spine. 2007;32(22):2405–14.
50. Katz JN, Losina E. Cost-effectiveness of spine surgery: the jury is out. Ann Intern Med. 2008;149(12): 901–3.

Index

A.L. Wollowick and V. Sarwahi (eds.), *Spondylolisthesis: Diagnosis, Non-Surgical Management, and Surgical Techniques*, DOI 10.1007/978-1-4899-7575-1,

L

M

P